BIOCHEMISTRY RESEARCH TRENDS

PRINCIPLES OF FREE RADICAL BIOMEDICINE

VOLUME III

BIOCHEMISTRY RESEARCH TRENDS

Additional books in this series can be found on Nova's website
under the Series tab.

Additional E-books in this series can be found on Nova's website
under the E-books tab.

BIOCHEMISTRY RESEARCH TRENDS

PRINCIPLES OF FREE RADICAL BIOMEDICINE

VOLUME III

KOSTAS PANTOPOULOS
AND
HYMAN M. SCHIPPER
EDITORS

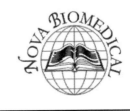

Nova Science Publishers, Inc.
New York

Copyright ©2012 by Nova Science Publishers, Inc.

All rights reserved. No part of this book may be reproduced, stored in a retrieval system or transmitted in any form or by any means: electronic, electrostatic, magnetic, tape, mechanical photocopying, recording or otherwise without the written permission of the Publisher.

For permission to use material from this book please contact us:
Telephone 631-231-7269; Fax 631-231-8175
Web Site: http://www.novapublishers.com

NOTICE TO THE READER

The Publisher has taken reasonable care in the preparation of this book, but makes no expressed or implied warranty of any kind and assumes no responsibility for any errors or omissions. No liability is assumed for incidental or consequential damages in connection with or arising out of information contained in this book. The Publisher shall not be liable for any special, consequential, or exemplary damages resulting, in whole or in part, from the readers' use of, or reliance upon, this material. Any parts of this book based on government reports are so indicated and copyright is claimed for those parts to the extent applicable to compilations of such works.

Independent verification should be sought for any data, advice or recommendations contained in this book. In addition, no responsibility is assumed by the publisher for any injury and/or damage to persons or property arising from any methods, products, instructions, ideas or otherwise contained in this publication.

This publication is designed to provide accurate and authoritative information with regard to the subject matter covered herein. It is sold with the clear understanding that the Publisher is not engaged in rendering legal or any other professional services. If legal or any other expert assistance is required, the services of a competent person should be sought. FROM A DECLARATION OF PARTICIPANTS JOINTLY ADOPTED BY A COMMITTEE OF THE AMERICAN BAR ASSOCIATION AND A COMMITTEE OF PUBLISHERS.

Additional color graphics may be available in the e-book version of this book.

Library of Congress Cataloging-in-Publication Data

ISSN: 2159-9343

ISBN 978-1-61324-184-4

Published by Nova Science Publishers, Inc.†New York

Contents

Preface		**vii**
Chapter 1	Pulmonary Diseases *Nurlan Dauletbaev and Larry C. Lands*	**1**
Chapter 2	Disorders of Iron Homeostasis *Giada Sebastiani and Kostas Pantopoulos*	**29**
Chapter 3	Wilson Disease *Maryam Moini and Michael L. Schilsky*	**49**
Chapter 4	Oxidative Stress in Liver Diseases *Giada Sebastiani*	**65**
Chapter 5	Reactive Oxygen Species in Renal Glomerular Diseases *Andrey V. Cybulsky*	**107**
Chapter 6	Carcinogenesis *Undurti N. Das*	**123**
Chapter 7	Cancer Chemotherapy *Zuanel Diaz and Wilson Miller*	**143**
Chapter 8	Oxidative Stress in Arterial Hypertension and Atherosclerosis *Ernesto L. Schiffrin and Rhian M. Touyz*	**169**
Chapter 9	Diabetes Mellitus *Peter Rösen*	**201**
Chapter 10	Redox Neurology *Hyman M. Schipper*	**229**
Chapter 11	Redox Ophthalmology *Alex F. Thompson and Leonard A. Levin*	**263**
Chapter 12	Skin Diseases: Role of Reactive Oxygen and Nitrogen *Mohammad Athar, Arianna L. Kim, Levy Kopelovich, Craig A. Elmets and David R. Bickers*	**285**

Chapter 13	Oxidative Stress in Male Reproduction	**305**
	Rakesh K. Sharma, Aaron Thompson,	
	Shiva Kothari and Ashok Agarwal	
Chapter 14	Oxidative Stress in Female Reproduction	**329**
	Sajal Gupta, Sarah Brickner, Rathna Shenoy BS,	
	Chin Kun Baw and Ashok Agarwal	
Chapter 15	Oxidative Stress in Exercise and Training	**351**
	Stelios Kokkoris, Theodoros Vassilakopoulos	
	and Sabah N. A. Hussain	
Chapter 16	Reactive Metabolites and Oxygen Species in Toxicology	**367**
	Jennifer J. Schlezinger and Koren K. Mann	
Index		**385**

Preface

Recent years have witnessed an avalanche of new knowledge implicating free radicals in virtually every aspect of biology and medicine. It is now axiomatic that the regulated accumulation of reactive oxygen species (ROS) contributes to organismal health and well-being and that ROS serve as signaling molecules involved in cell growth, differentiation, gene regulation, replicative senescence and apoptosis. This book is an interdisciplinary text broken up into three consecutive volumes on the biochemistry and cellular/molecular biology of free radicals, transition metals, oxidants and antioxidants, and the role of oxidative stress in human health and disease. The sixteen chapters comprising Volume III address the perceived roles of reactive species and oxidative stress in a wide range of human medical conditions.

Chapter 1 - The respiratory tract is unique because of its continuous exposure to ROS and reactive nitrogen species (RNS), and presence of high concentrations of extracellular antioxidants. Depending on circumstances, ROS/RNS can be necessary or harmful. This Chapter reviews the sources of ROS/RNS in the respiratory tract under normal and pathological conditions, contemporary diagnostic techniques used to measure ROS/RNS in pulmonary diseases, and current knowledge concerning the possible role(s) of ROS/RNS in the pathophysiology of these diseases.

Chapter 2 - In healthy individuals, the rate of dietary iron absorption and the levels of body iron are tightly controlled. Misregulation of iron homeostasis can lead to pathological conditions, ranging from anemias caused by iron deficiency or defective iron trafficking, to iron overload (hemochromatosis). Pathophysiological and clinical aspects of iron-related disorders and the role of oxidative stress are discussed.

Chapter 3 - Copper is an essential trace element and plays an integral role in cellular and trace metal metabolism. However, at high intracellular concentrations, copper is toxic. This Chapter focuses on the pathogenesis of Wilson disease, an inherited disorder of copper metabolism, and the resultant copper-induced free radical injury in the liver, nervous system and other organs of affected patients.

Chapter 4 - This Chapter provides an overview of the epidemiology of liver diseases and outlines mechanisms for ROS-mediated liver fibrogenesis. Emphasis is given on the role of oxidative stress in chronic viral hepatitis (C or B), alcoholic liver disease, non-alcoholic fatty liver disease, hepatocellular carcinoma and acetaminophen toxicity.

Chapter 5 - The clinical manifestations of immune glomerular diseases range from isolated albuminuria or hematuria, to nephrotic syndrome, nephritic syndrome and/or rapidly progressive glomerulonephritis. This Chapter reviews the role of ROS as mediators of renal glomerular damage.

Chapters 6-7 - Free radicals have direct effects on cell growth, developmentand survival, and play a significant role in cancer. ROS have both beneficial and harmful actions. They are needed for signal-transduction pathways and cell survival; however, excessive amounts of ROS may start lethal chain reactions and lead to cell death. Chapter 6 deals with the effects of free radicals in tumor cell biology and carcinogenesis. Chapter 7 is focused on pro- or anti-oxidant therapies that have been proposed for cancer treatment and prevention, based on the dichotomous property of ROS in determining cell fate. In addition, it describes our current appreciation of approaches aimed at modulation of oxidative stress in cancer and their essential mechanisms.

Chapter 8 - This Chapter highlights the role of oxidative stress an important cause of vascular injury in hypertension and a contributor to the development and progression of atherosclerosis. ROS/RNS are produced under physiological conditions in a highly regulated fashion at low concentrations and function as signaling molecules that control endothelial and vascular smooth muscle cell function. In pathological situations increased ROS production leads to endothelial dysfunction, enhanced contractility and growth of vascular smooth muscle cells, lipid peroxidation, inflammation and increased deposition of extracellular matrix proteins. These processes contribute to vascular injury, triggering atherosclerosis and the development of hypertension.

Chapter 9 - Diabetes mellitus is one of the fastest growing health problems in the world. There is emerging evidence that ROS contribute to destruction of pancreatic β-cells in both type I and type II diabetes and that they additionally play an important role in the complex network of interactions leading to insulin resistance. As discussed herein, this realization may offer unique therapeutic options to treat diabetes and its complications.

Chapters 10-12 - The objectives of Chapter 10 are to facilitate an appreciation of biological features which render the nervous system uniquely prone to free radical injury, describe major etiopathogenetic mechanisms mediating oxidative neural damage, and discuss select diseases which illustrate key principles of 'redox neurology'. Chapter 11 focuses on 'redox ophthalmology' and the role of ROS in the pathogenesis of age-related macular degeneration (AMD), diabetic retinopathy, glaucoma and corneal diseases. Chapter 12 outlines principles of 'redox dermatology', and includes discussions of the roles of ROS in the pathogenesis of vitiligo, allergic skin reactions, varicose ulcers and drug-induced photosensitization.

Chapters 13-14 - ROS have also been implicated in the etiopathogenesis of various medical conditions affecting male and female reproduction. Chapter 13 highlights the physiological and pathological effects of ROS on the male reproductive system, enumerates their importance in the field of assisted reproductive technology, and proposes possible ways of mitigating oxidative stress in order to achieve positive results in infertile couples with male factor infertility. Chapter 14 deals with the effects of oxidative stress on female reproduction, gametes, embryos, and their environments, including follicular fluid, hydrosalpingeal fluid, and peritoneal fluid. The state of these microenvironments influences pregnancy outcomes by directly affecting oocyte quality, sperm-oocyte interaction, implantation, and early embryo development.

Chapter 15 - This Chapter elaborates on the role of ROS in exercise physiology. Acute physical exercise induces production of ROS in skeletal muscle via different mechanisms. ROS formation during vigorous physical exertion can result in oxidative stress and modulate contractile function. Furthermore, involvement of ROS in the regulation of gene expression via redox-sensitive transcription pathways represents an important regulatory mechanism involved in the process of training adaptation.

Chapter 16 - Toxicology is defined as the study of adverse effects of chemicals or xenobiotics. This final Chapter provides an understanding on the contribution of ROS to toxicological mechanisms and describes ROS-dependent detoxification pathways.

In: Principles of Free Radical Biomedicine, Volume III
Editors: K. Pantopoulos and H. M. Schipper

ISBN 978-1-61324-184-4
©2012 Nova SciencePublishers, Inc.

Chapter 1

Pulmonary Diseases

Nurlan Dauletbaev[1] and Larry C. Lands[1, 2]

[1]Research Institute of McGill University Health Centre, Montreal, Canada
[2]Montreal Children's Hospital, 2300 Tupper Street, Montreal, Quebec
H3H 1P3, Canada

1. Introduction

The respiratory tract comprises the upper and lower airways and lungs. Its function is to warm, clean, and humidify inhaled air, and to carry out the exchange of oxygen and carbon dioxide between the air and the blood circulating through the lungs. The respiratory tract is unique because of its continuous exposure to reactive oxygen species (ROS) and reactive nitrogen species (RNS), and presence of high concentrations of extracellular antioxidants. *ROS/RNS in the respiratory tract originate from both within (endogenous ROS/RNS) and outside (exogenous ROS/RNS) of our body.* Depending on circumstances, ROS/RNS can be necessary or harmful. There are several lines of antioxidant defense in the respiratory tract whose function is to prevent ROS/RNS from causing harm to host cells. When ROS/RNS exceed the neutralizing capacity of the antioxidant defense system, pathological overexposure ensues. Overexposure to ROS/RNS triggers or aggravates pulmonary diseases. This Chapter will review the sources of ROS/RNS in the respiratory tract under normal and pathological conditions, current diagnostic techniques used to study the role of ROS/RNS in pulmonary diseases, and possible pathophysiology of ROS/RNS in these diseases.

1.1. Endogenous and Exogenous Sources of ROS/RNS in the Respiratory Tract

Both non-immune and immune cells in the respiratory tract are capable of producing ROS/RNS [1, 2]. ROS are reactive metabolites of oxygen (Vol. I, Chapter 2). The most prominent sources of ROS are the mitochondrial respiratory chain [3], NADPH oxidases [1,

2, 4], and lipooxygenases [5, 6]. Other sources are intracellular enzymes (xanthine oxidase, cyclooxygenases, etc) capable of generating ROS [7, 8]. RNS include nitrogen oxide (•NO), which is synthesized by the enzyme •NO synthase [9], and reactive metabolites of •NO (Vol. I, Chapter 3).

The ROS/RNS levels are low in healthy respiratory tract. Unstimulated respiratory epithelial cells and pulmonary macrophages, the most abundant cells in healthy respiratory tract, produce only negligible amounts of ROS/RNS. Under these conditions, other ROS/RNS-generating cells (e.g neutrophils, eosinophils, lymphocytes etc) are present in low quantities and are dormant. *ROS/RNS levels increase dramatically during immune responses to pathogens.* Pulmonary macrophages generate ROS/RNS within their specialized compartments or in the extracellular space (Figure 1).

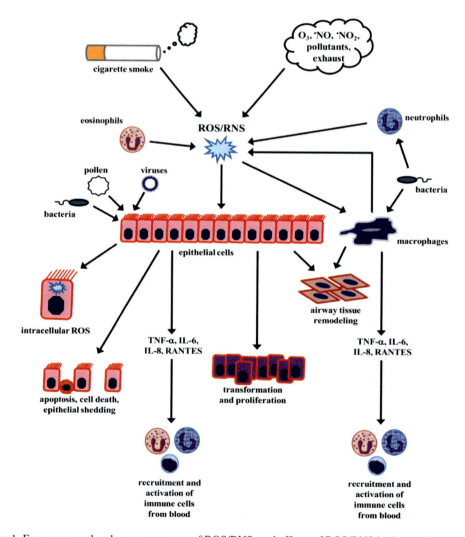

Figure 1. Exogenous and endogenous sources of ROS/RNS, and effects of ROS/RNS in the respiratory tract.

Further, other professional immune cells (i.e. neutrophils and eosinophils) are recruited from blood and activated, and produce enormous amounts of ROS/RNS (Figure 1). ROS are also generated intracellularly by respiratory epithelium when it is exposed to pollen NADPH oxidases or viruses (Figure 1). The main purpose of ROS/RNS generation by immune and non-immune cells is elimination of pathogens. Therefore, generation of ROS/RNS is essential for homeostasis within the respiratory tract. As ROS/RNS can also be harmful to respiratory cells, there are intrinsic mechanisms to prevent excessive injury. These mechanisms include abundant intra- and extracellular antioxidant defense systems and elimination of ROS/RNS-generating cells by apoptosis.

ROS/RNS that originate from outside of our body are brought into the respiratory tract with inhaled air. Examples of these ROS/RNS include ozone (O_3), •NO, nitric dioxide (•NO_2), and other gaseous substances in the ambient air (Figure 1). Other important sources are particulate air pollutants and diesel exhaust particles, which either contain or are capable of generating ROS/RNS (Figure 1). *A very prominent source of ROS/RNS is cigarette smoke.* Cigarette smoke contains gaseous ROS/RNS and oxidizing particular matter (tar), which penetrates through cigarette filters [10] (Figure 1). The gaseous ROS/RNS include hydrogen peroxide (H_2O_2), •NO, and •NO_2; tar contains the quinone-hydroquinone-semiquinone system that generates superoxide anion ($O_2^{\bullet-}$) [10, 11]. *A further source of ROS is bacteria*, such as *Pseudomonas aeruginosa* that producesphenazine pigments (e.g. pyocyanin [12]) (Figure 1). Phenazine pigments react with molecular oxygen to produce $O_2^{\bullet-}$ and H_2O_2. It is thought that *Pseudomonas aeruginosa* uses phenazine pigments as "redox-active" antibiotics to suppress growth of other bacteria [13, 14]. These pigments are highly toxic to bacteria, other than Pseudomonas, and to respiratory cells. *Under pathological conditions, the amount of ROS/RNS within the respiratory tract exceeds the neutralizing capacity of the antioxidant defense systems. Then, overabundant ROS/RNS alter normal cell functioning and cause various deleterious effects.* Often, the harmful effects of ROS/RNS are not limited to the respiratory tract, and extend to other organs and systems.

1.2. Sampling Techniques to Document Overabundance of ROS/RNS in the Respiratory Tract

Sampling techniques differ in their ability to gather volatile substances, fluids, and cells from the respiratory tract. Some techniques sample volatile substances only; others provide mixtures of fluids and cells, or exclusively collect cells. There are non-invasive, minimally invasive, and invasive sampling techniques. Techniques that are less invasive represent a minimal burden on the patient and elicit fewer complications. Sampling techniques can be used to analyze directly ROS/RNS and/or evidence of cell injury (i.e. products of protein/lipid/DNA oxidation), or to collect cells to evaluate their ROS/RNS generating activity. Current sampling techniques gather information from different compartments of the respiratory tract, which is divided into two parts, upper and lower (Figure 2). The upper respiratory tract includes nose, nasal cavities, sinuses, throat, and larynx. The lower respiratory tract comprises trachea, proximal bronchi, distal bronchi and bronchioles, and alveoli. The lower respiratory tract can be further divided into proximal (i.e. larger bronchi) and distal portion (i.e. distal bronchi and alveoli). The majority of techniques used to study ROS/RNS in pulmonary diseases predominantly sample the airway lumen and the surface of the respiratory mucosa.

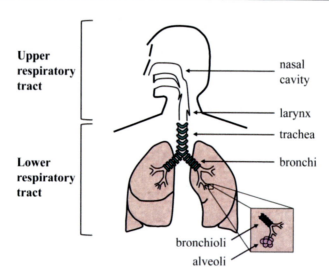

Figure 2. Schematic representation of the human respiratory tract.

These techniques, which include nasal lavage, analyses of exhaled air and exhaled breath condensate, induced sputum, bronchial wash samples, and broncho-alveolar lavage (Table 1 and Figure 2), will be highlighted in this Chapter. The deleterious effects of overabundant ROS/RNS often extend beyond the respiratory tract. To document the extra-respiratory effects of ROS/RNS, other tissues and cells (e.g. blood plasma or serum, erythrocytes, skeletal muscles, etc) can be sampled.

1.3. Nasal Lavage

Nasal lavage collects secretions and cells from the nasal cavity. *Nasal lavage is a popular technique to study oxidative stress and inflammation in the nasal cavity.* It is minimally invasive and represents only a slight discomfort for a patient. Nasal lavage is conducted by instillation of a small volume of pre-warmed sterile isotonic saline into individual's nostrils. The collected lavage is separated into supernatant and cells. Most often, oxidative stress is documented in the supernatants as the presence of oxidized proteins or lipids. Further, decreased concentrations of antioxidants can also indicate the presence of oxidative stress.

1.4. Analyses of Exhaled Air and Exhaled Breath Condensate

Exhaled air contains gases other than O_2 and CO_2, (e.g. •NO, CO), water vapor, volatile substances (e.g. H_2O_2), and small quantities of non-volatile substances (e.g. products of lipid oxidation, polypeptides) (Figure 3). Exhaled gases (e.g. •NO or CO) can be analyzed directly in exhaled air, as specialized and highly sensitive equipment exists to monitor these substances. Exhaled •NO is representative of the lower respiratory tract; further, a modified procedure exists to sample nasal •NO. *The analyses of exhaled •NO and CO are non-invasive and do not cause any discomfort for patients.* Other substances, both volatile (e.g. H_2O_2) and non-volatile (e.g. products of lipid oxidation), cannot be analyzed directly in the exhaled air. These substances can be detected when the exhaled air vapor is cooled down in a specialized device and forms a condensate called *exhaledbreath condensate* (Figure 3).

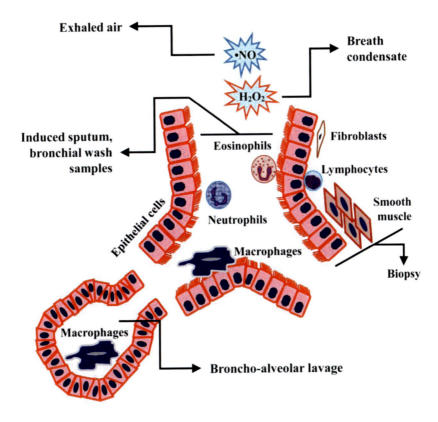

Figure 3. Sampling techniques to study ROS/RNS in the respiratory tract.

The analysis of breath condensate usually requires a collection of exhaled air vapor from multiple breathing cycles. The vast majority of the volume of exhaled breath condensate is water; H_2O_2 and other substances are present in minute, yet detectable, quantities. It is believed that H_2O_2 obtained with exhaled breath condensate originates from the proximal portion of the lower respiratory tract. Various cells (respiratory epithelial cells, macrophages, neutrophils, eosinophils, lymphocytes) produce H_2O_2. H_2O_2 is either generated directly in the extracellular space [15-18] or escapes cells through aquaporin channels [19]. *Exhaled breath condensate is a non-invasive procedure with minimal discomfort for subjects.*

Table 1. Major techniques used to study oxidative/nitrosative processes in the airway lumen

Technique	What it samples	Degree of invasiveness; patient discomfort; complications	Comments
Nasal lavage	Lumen of nasal cavity, surface of the nasal mucosa	Minimally invasive; minimal discomfort; minimal complications	Unsophisticated technique, routinely applied to study oxidative/nitrosative processes in the upper respiratory tract
Exhaled air	Gases present in the proximal portion of the lower respiratory tract *	Non-invasive; no discomfort; no complications	Requires specialized, expensive equipment capable of on-line detection of gases
Exhaled breath condensate	Non-gaseous, volatile and non-volatile substances from the proximal portion of the lower respiratory tract [#]	Non-invasive; minimal discomfort; no complications	Requires specialized, moderately expensive equipment
Induced sputum	Tracheobronchial secretions and cells from the proximal portion of the lower respiratory tract [§¶]	Relatively non-invasive; mild discomfort; minor complications	Requires specialized, moderately expensive equipment
Bronchial wash samples and broncho-alveolar lavage (BAL)	Tracheobronchial secretions and cells from the proximal portion (bronchial wash samples) or the distal portion (BAL) of the lower respiratory tract	Invasive; substantial discomfort; heightened risk of complications	The required specialized equipment is routinely available in most respiratory centers

Footnote: * modification of this technique exists to sample air from the nasal cavity; [#] modification of this technique exists to sample substances from the distal portion of the lower respiratory tract; [§] samples need to be purified from contaminating saliva; [¶] modification of this technique exists to study low-molecular weight thiols, such as glutathione

1.5. Induced Sputum and Bronchial Wash Samples

The healthy respiratory tract produces small quantities of tracheobronchial secretions. These secretions are a complex mixture of mucins and other secreted proteins, ions, antioxidants, antimicrobial peptides, proteins from blood plasma, and some immune cells. Their function is to trap and neutralize bacteria and particles that are continuously brought into the respiratory tract with inhaled air.

In the diseased respiratory tract, the amount of tracheobronchial secretions is elevated and their composition changes. The secretions may become so abundant that patients can voluntarily expectorate them. Voluntarily expectorated tracheobronchial secretions are called *spontaneous sputum*. Not all patients with pulmonary diseases and extremely few healthy individuals can voluntarily expectorate sputum. Until the early 1990s, bronchoscopic procedures (described in more detail below) were required to obtain tracheobrochial secretions from the individuals who could not voluntarily expectorate sputum.

It was also known that an inhalation of hypertonic saline (3-5% NaCl) promotes expectoration. In 1992, a group of Canadian pulmonologists pioneered the use of hypertonic saline to obtain tracheobronchial secretions from healthy individuals and patients with mild bronchial asthma to study inflammatory processes in the respiratory tract [20]. The tracheobronchial secretions expectorated during and immediately after inhalation of hypertonic saline are called *induced sputum* (Figure 3).

Since 1992, induced sputum has been widely used to document ROS/RNS, antioxidants, and inflammation in the proximal portion of the lower respiratory tract in patients with pulmonary diseases. Since induced sputum is a mixture of airway secretions and cells, these have to be separated prior to analyses. The separation often involves pre-treatment with reducing agents, such as dithiothreitol, to break disulfide bonds which interlock mucinmultimers. The use of dithiothreitol should be avoided when protein or low-molecular weight disulfides are to be studied [21].

Highly purulent secretions, such as in patients with cystic fibrosis, contain high amount of DNA released from decaying cells. DNA is charged and interferes with sputum solubilization. The use of recombinant DNAses is effective to solubilize such induced sputum samples [22]. Induced sputum is a relatively non-invasive procedure with mild discomfort for subjects. In some subjects, especially in young children, induced sputum is not always successful. In such cases, tracheobronchial secretions can still be obtained through a traditional, invasive procedure called bronchoscopy. During bronchoscopy, a flexible tube (bronchoscope) is inserted into the respiratory tract through the subject's nose or mouth after mild sedation. The bronchoscope is equipped with a camera. Tracheobronchial secretions are aspirated through the bronchoscope.

Sometimes, the amount of secretions is low; in these cases, a small amount of sterile isotonic saline is instilled into the airways and immediately aspirated through the bronchoscope. The secretions obtained during this procedure are called *bronchial wash samples* (Figure 3). Bronchoscopic collection of bronchial wash samples is an invasive procedure with substantial discomfort and potential complications for subjects. Bronchial wash samples represent slightly diluted secretions from the proximal portion of the lower respiratory tract.

1.6. Broncho-Alveolar Lavage

Broncho-alveolar lavage (BAL) is the classic diagnostic technique in respiratory medicine employed for several decades to obtain secretions from the distal portion of the lower respiratory tract (Figure 3). It is performed using a bronchoscope. The bronchoscope is inserted in the respiratory tract and advanced until the diameter of the bronchus will not allow any further insertion ("wedge position").

A small aliquot of sterile saline is instilled through the bronchoscope into the respiratory tract and immediately aspirated. Normally, the first aliquot contains mostly fluids and cells retrieved from the terminal bronchi. When subsequent aliquots of sterile saline are instilled and aspirated, fluids and cells from the alveoli are retrieved. BAL is an invasive procedure with a substantial discomfort and potential side effects for subjects. It provides fluids and cells from the distal portion of the lower respiratory tract.

2. Pulmonary Diseases and Conditions with Exposure to Overabundant ROS/RNS

It is likely that many acute respiratory infections (e.g. upper respiratory tract infections, pneumonia) are associated with exposure of the respiratory cells to overabundant ROS/RNS. *These ROS/RNS are generated by the host as part of the immune response to pathogens.* Further, pathogens can exacerbate the exposure to ROS/RNS by depleting intracellular antioxidant defenses.

Upper respiratory tract infections exemplify this. The vast majority of these infections are caused by viruses; among them, rhinoviruses are the most frequently encountered viral species [23-25]. Rhinoviruses have been demonstrated experimentally to stimulate intracellular production of superoxide anion through activation of xanthine oxidase [26] (Figure 1). This is accompanied by the depletion of intracellular gluthathione, a key low-molecular weight antioxidant [26] (see Vol. II, Chapter 1). Other viruses implicated in the upper respiratory tract infections (e.g. influenza or respiratory syncytial viruses) have also been shown to promote production of ROS and/or deplete intracellular antioxidants [27-29] (Figure 1). The presence of overabundant ROS/RNS in the respiratory tract during these infections has been documented.

For example, concentrations of H_2O_2 in exhaled breath condensate transiently increase during acute upper respiratory tract infections and fall back following resolution [30]. Lower respiratory tract infections (i.e. pneumonia) have also been associated with elevated levels of H_2O_2 in breath condensate [31]. Acute respiratory tract infections normally resolve within a few days, either spontaneously or after pharmacological interventions. Therefore, the exposure to ROS/RNS is of transient nature. It is possible, though, that limiting the deleterious effects of ROS/RNS during these infections may facilitate recovery.

In contrast to acute respiratory tract infections, many chronic respiratory diseases are associated with protracted overexposure to ROS/RNS. In addition, certain acute respiratory conditions are accompanied by a massive overexposure to ROS/RNS. These major pulmonary diseases and conditions will be highlighted in this Chapter, with emphasis on asthma, chronic obstructive pulmonary disease, and cystic fibrosis.

2.1. Allergic Rhinitis

Allergic rhinitis is a symptomatic disorder of the nose induced after allergen exposure by an immunoglobulin E (IgE)-mediated inflammation [32, 33]. It is typically characterized by runny nose, sneezing, nasal congestion, and itchy nose and/or eyes. Allergic rhinitis is caused by airborne indoor or outdoor allergens. Depending on the symptoms' frequency, it is divided into intermittent and persistent forms [33]. Allergic rhinitis is associated with overexposure to ROS/RNS of endogenous and exogenous origins. Endogenous ROS/RNS in allergic rhinitis originate from respiratory epithelial cells and immune cells, such as eosinophils. Respiratory epithelium expresses specialized enzymes that generate ROS/RNS upon inflammatory stimulation [1, 9]. Further, there are elevated numbers of eosinophils in nasal mucosa and secretions [34-36]. Activated eosinophils generate superoxide anion and H_2O_2 (Figure 1); their enzyme, eosinophil peroxidase, uses H_2O_2 as a substrate to produce hypobromous acid[37, 38], which is highly toxic to mucosal cells. Allergic rhinitis can be worsened by exogenous ROS/RNS derived from allergens, airborne pollutants, cigarette smoke, and respiratory viruses; these are discussed in a greater detail below ("Bronchial asthma"). Exposure to ROS/RNS stimulates or aggravates inflammatory responses from nasal mucosa. Further, remodeling processes in the respiratory tract are activated by chronic overexposure to ROS/RNS, although the magnitude of these processes seems to be less prominent than in asthma [39].

2.2. Bronchial Asthma

Asthma is currently defined as a chronic inflammatory disorder of the airways in which many cells and cellular elements play a role. The chronic inflammation is associated with airway hyperresponsiveness that leads to recurrent episodes of wheezing, breathlessness, chest tightness, and coughing, particularly at night or in the early morning. These episodes are usually associated with widespread, but variable, airflow obstruction within the lung that is often reversible either spontaneously or with treatment [40]. It is believed that ROS/RNS are a prominent contributing factor in the pathogenesis of asthma. As with allergic rhinitis, ROS/RNS in asthma originate from both endogenous and exogenous sources. Allergens and airborne pollutants are principal exogenous sources. Pollen contains NADPH oxidases [41, 42], which generate superoxide anion and cause oxidative injury to cells in the respiratory tract mucosa [43] (Figure 1). Further, ROS/RNS are inhaled with ambient air (ozone, •NO, •NO$_2$, diesel exhaust, particulate matter) and promote oxidative/nitrosative injury in the lung [9, 44-47] (Figure 1). Another prominent source of exogenous ROS/RNS is cigarette smoke [10, 11] (Figure 1). Both active and secondhand smoking are known to aggravate asthma [48-50]. Excessive ROS/RNS also originate from viral infections [26-29, 51] (Figure 1), which are widely recognized as a risk factor for asthma exacerbations [52]. Endogenous ROS/RNS are produced as part of chronic inflammatory processes in the respiratory tract of patients with asthma. Immune cells, respiratory epithelium, airway smooth muscles are capable of generating ROS/RNS [1, 2, 6, 9, 17] (Figure 1). For instance, allergic inflammation in asthma is associated with increased numbers of eosinophils and, occasionally, neutrophils in the lumen of the respiratory tract. Along with pulmonary macrophages, both these cell types generate excessive amounts of ROS/RNS (Figure 1). These ROS/RNS include highly toxic species, such as hypobromous acid, hypochlorous acid, hydroxyl radicals, peroxynitrite, etc. which are believed to damage the respiratory epithelium. Compared to healthy individuals, patients with asthma often exhibit lower concentrations of antioxidants in the respiratory tract [53, 54]. The relative deficiency of antioxidants is likely to further aggravate the deleterious effects of ROS/RNS in asthmatic airways. The presence of overabundant ROS/RNS in the respiratory tract of patients with asthma is well documented. Thus, concentrations of H_2O_2 in exhaled breath condensate are higher in asthmatics compared to healthy individuals [55-59]. H_2O_2 concentrations are also elevated in BAL samples of patients with asthma [54]. Further, concentrations of •NO in exhaled air and other RNS in respiratory tract secretions are greatly increased in asthma [60-62]. *While physiological elevation of •NO can be beneficial for asthma because of its anti-obstructive and anti-viral effects, supraphysiological increases of this molecule can lead to nitrosative stress.* Besides ROS/RNS, samples from the respiratory tract of patients with asthma demonstrate the endproducts of oxidative/nitrosative injury [63-65]. There are several ways how chronic or acute exposure to overabundant ROS/RNS in asthma can aggravate clinical disease. First, ROS/RNS can trigger inflammatory responses in the respiratory tract cells (Figure 1). The molecular mechanisms for ROS/RNS-induced inflammatory responses involve activation of transcription factors and MAP kinases, and inactivation of anti-inflammatory phosphatases (Vol. II, Chapter 21). Further, ROS/RNS can potentiate the existing immune and inflammatory responses in the allergic respiratory tract. The allergic immune response in asthma is orchestrated by $CD4^+$ T helper type 2 (Th2) lymphocytes [66], and ROS have been shown to promote differentiation of naïve $CD4^+$ T cells into Th2 cells [67]. The inflammatory responses can be potentiated through endogenous, mitochondria-derived, ROS [68] or environmental ROS [69, 70]. Next, ROS/RNS can trigger or potentiate apoptosis and cell death in the respiratory epithelium [71], or interfere with epithelial repair processes [72]. These processes lead to epithelial cell desquamation in the respiratory tract and disturbance of its integrity. Consequently, allergens, environmental and microbial factors can reach the normally inaccessible immune (e.g. lymphocytes) and structural cells (fibroblasts and airway smooth muscle cells) underneath the respiratory epithelium [73]. Exposed to challenges, these cells respond by proliferation, maturation, and secretion of inflammatory cytokines, which leads to amplification of inflammation in the respiratory tract and airway remodeling (Figure 1). Airway remodeling is linked to airway hyperresponsiveness [74], which is a characteristic feature of asthma. To summarize, exogenous and endogenous ROS/RNS can contribute to development and clinical course of bronchial asthma. *The multiple effects of ROS/RNS in asthma include inflammation, alteration of adaptive immune response, and airway remodeling.*

2.3. Chronic Obstructive Pulmonary Disease (COPD)

COPD is currently defined as a preventable and treatable disease with some significant extrapulmonary effects that may contribute to the severity in individual patients. Its pulmonary component is characterized by airflow limitation that is not fully reversible. The airflow limitation is usually progressive and associated with an abnormal inflammatory response of the lung to noxious particles or gases. Cigarette smoking is the major risk factor for COPD [75]. However, nonsmokers can also develop COPD [75-78], albeit with a lower incidence. Further risk factors for both smokers and nonsmokers include occupational dusts and chemicals, biomass fuel smoke, airborne pollutants, and previous chronic pulmonary diseases (tuberculosis, asthma) [75, 78].

Similar to asthma, COPD is characterized by airway obstruction. However, unlike in asthma, bronchial obstruction is, most commonly, not fully reversible in COPD. Further, pathological processes in COPD involve the distal portion of the respiratory tract, whereas obstruction in the proximal portion is more associated with asthma. Interestingly, many pathological mechanisms seen in asthma are also present in COPD; however, the clinical features of these two diseases are often very different. It is possible that these differences are due to the fact that COPD, most frequently, is initiated and sustained by a frequent exposure to exuberant amounts of exogenous ROS/RNS. These exogenous ROS/RNS are present in high amounts in cigarette smoke [10, 11] (Figure 1). Acute inhalation of cigarette smoke results in significantly elevated levels of ROS/RNS in the respiratory tract [79-81]; these ROS/RNS exert a wide spectrum of deleterious effects. Many possible ROS/RNS-driven mechanisms of COPD are currently debated.

First, ROS/RNS are clearly pro-inflammatory in COPD. They stimulate the respiratory tract cells, such as epithelial cells and macrophages, to produce various cytokines and chemokines (TNFα, IL-1β, IL-6, IL-8 etc), growth factors (G-CSF, GM-CSF etc), proteolytic enzymes (matrix metalloproteinases, MMPs), adhesion molecules (ICAM-1) and mucins (Figure 1). Chemokines and growth factors recruit from blood and activate neutrophils and lymphocytes, whose activity further propagates inflammation in the respiratory tract (Figure 1). MMPs and neutrophil elastase cause tissue destruction. The inflammation in advanced COPD is not restricted to the respiratory tract (local inflammation), but spreads to many organs and systems (systemic inflammation). Stimulated cells in the respiratory tract also generate ROS/RNS. These endogenous ROS/RNS are likely to be responsible for elevated levels of many markers of oxidative/nitrosative stress detected in the respiratory tract after smoking cessation [82-84]. Unlike in asthma, the main blood-derived immune cell in the lumen of the respiratory tract of COPD patients is the neutrophil. Activated neutrophils produce many types of ROS, including highly toxic hypochlorous acid, which is a product of a chemical reaction between H_2O_2 and chlorine, catalyzed by myeloperoxidase, a neutrophil enzyme. The physiological role of hypochlorous acidis bacterial killing. However, in COPD, this compound can contribute to the damage to the respiratory epithelial monolayer. As discussed above with regard to bronchial asthma, the integrity of the respiratory epithelial monolayer is essential in preventing allergens, particles, and viruses from reaching cells beneath the monolayer (lymphocytes, dendritic cells, airway smooth muscle cells, fibroblasts). ROS/RNS in cigarette smoke also interfere with epithelial repair. Inadequate repair processes combined with increased cell apoptosis stimulated by ROS/RNS are believed to engender destruction of the alveolar structure (Figure 1).

Further, discordant damage and repair result in remodeling of small airways in COPD [85, 86]. One of the possible mechanisms for increased cell apoptosis observed in the respiratory tract of patients with COPD may be associated with ceramide, the apoptosis-inducing sphingolipid constituent of the plasma membrane. Experimental models suggest that augmentation of ceramide causes increased cell apoptosis and tissue damage [87] similar to those seen in human COPD. Clinical data indicate increased expression of ceramide-synthesizing enzymes in the lungs of COPD patients [88]. In cell culture models, the expression of these enzymes is up-regulated by ROS/RNS, including those derived from cigarette smoke [89, 90]. Ceramide levels are inversely correlated with the levels of intracellular glutathione [91]. An increased consumption of intracellular glutathione by ROS/RNS in COPD may potentiate ceramide-induced apoptosis.

While inflammation and cell death are constantly present in the respiratory tract of COPD patients, they are further aggravated by air pollution, viral and bacterial infections. Air pollutants and viruses have been demonstrated to cause oxidative stress in the respiratory epithelium. In turn, oxidative stress potentiates inflammatory responses to viral and bacterial pathogens in the respiratory epithelium [92].

In addition, overexposure to oxidants impairs innate anti-bacterial and anti-viral immunity in the respiratory tract [93], which hinders pathogen clearance and sustains pathogen-induced inflammatory responses. Deleterious effects of ROS/RNS are often detected beyond the respiratory tract. Thus, protein carbonyls, the markers of protein oxidation, are found in increased quantities in skeletal muscles of patients with COPD [94, 95]. Increased protein oxidation in skeletal muscles may be further aggravated by physical exercise in these patients, and can explain the myopathy often observed in COPD [96-98]. The oxidative stress in skeletal muscles is likely caused by local overproduction of ROS [99], which is a consequence of systemic inflammation. ROS/RNS may be especially harmful in individuals with inhered or acquired imbalances in antioxidant defense systems. Possible predisposing factors for these imbalances have been discussed in recent reviews [100-102]. In particular, polymorphism of superoxide dismutase 3 (SOD3) gene, an extracellular antioxidant enzyme (Vol. II, Chapter 5), has attracted attention as a risk factor for COPD and impaired lung function / bronchial hyperresponsiveness in the general population [102-105].

In summary, overexposure to ROS/RNS, which most commonly originate from cigarette smoke, initiate and sustain pathological processes which lead to COPD. *The multiple effects of ROS/RNS in COPD include local and systemic inflammation, oxidative/nitrosative stress, apoptosis and cell death, and airway remodeling.*

2.4. α_1-Antitrypsin Deficiency

Above, inherent impairment of antioxidant defenses was discussed as a risk factor for COPD. Another inherent risk factor for COPD is deficiency of α_1-antitrypsin (AAT) whose function is to inhibit neutrophil elastase. Most commonly, this deficiency is caused by mutations in the AAT gene, SERPINA 1 [106, 107]. Some mutations lead to significantly lower systemic concentrations of AAT; others result in a decreased functional activity [107]. Individuals, who smoke and have the AAT deficiency develop emphysema far quicker than individuals with functional AAT. The ATT deficiency can be further aggravated by oxidation of the protein by ROS. As discussed in Vol. II, Chapter 21, AAT contains a sulfur-based methionine residue within its active centre that binds neutrophil elastase. The enzyme's active center can be transiently inactivated by oxidation of methionine. Oxidation of the enzyme hinders its binding to neutrophil elastase; uninhibited neutrophil elastase is pro-inflammatory and contributes to tissue damage. This ROS-induced inactivation of ATT is transient; therefore, the importance of this inactivation is not clear in patients with COPD who have normal levels of AAT. However, oxidation of ATT in individuals with AAT deficiency is likely to be more pertinent to clinical disease.

2.5. Cystic Fibrosis

Cystic fibrosis (CF) is the most common recessively inherited genetic condition affecting Caucasian populations. The most important clinical manifestation in CF is progressive lung disease, which is associated with recurrent lower respiratory tract illnesses, respiratory failure, and death [108]. The disease is caused by mutations in the gene encoding for CF transmembrane conductance regulator (CFTR). In respiratory epithelium, CFTR is an ion channel whose primary function is secretion of chloride and bicarbonate ions [109]. CFTR also participates in excretion of glutathione [110-114]. The normal respiratory tract, especially its distal portion, contain high concentrations of glutathione [115]. Extracellular glutathione originates from cells in the respiratory tract (epithelial cells, macrophages, dendritic cells, lymphocytes etc) [116]. The relationship between respiratory tract glutathione and CF is complex. The distal portion of the respiratory tract of patients with CF, sampled by BAL, often exhibits low levels of glutathione [117]. Alternatively, the otherwise normal levels of GSH are decreased during lung infection [118], probably consumed by oxidatively-stressed cells in the respiratory tract [118]. Impaired glutathione secretion by the respiratory epithelium [110-114], lack of essential constituents due to malnutrition [119], or increased consumption of glutathione during lung infection [118] are likely to cause these low levels of glutathione. The proximal portion of the CF respiratory tract, represented by induced sputum, often shows normal or even elevated concentrations of extracellular glutathione [120]. The discrepancy between BAL and sputum can be explained by the presence of high numbers of apoptotic neutrophils in the latter [121]. Apoptotic neutrophils are known to excrete glutathione [122] and can also excrete catalase, an antioxidant enzyme (Vol. II, Chapter 7) found at high levels in CF sputum [123]. High concentrations of glutathione [120], catalase [123], and mucins [124] in sputum explain low levels of H_2O_2 in exhaled breath condensate samples from patients with CF [125]. Exhaled H_2O_2 originates in the proximal portion of the lower respiratory tract [126], which is also the site harboring sputum. Therefore, antioxidants in CF sputum can neutralize H_2O_2 before it vaporizes. The lack of elevated H_2O_2 in exhaled air should not be interpreted as the evidence of absent oxidative/nitrosative stress in the CF respiratory tract. Rather, it is likely to be an indication that *oxidative/nitrosative stress in CF is distinct from that seen in asthma and COPD*. The studies on concentrations of exhaled •NO in patients with CF support the disparity between CF and other chronic pulmonary inflammatory diseases. Unlike in asthma, most studies reported decreased or normal concentrations of •NO in the CF respiratory tract [127-134]. This may be due to impaired activity of •NO synthase [135-138], increased concentrations of arginases in CF sputum [139] that consume L-arginine (the amino acid precursor for •NO synthesis) [139], and/or diversion of •NO into other RNS [133, 140-142]. Although concentrations of exhaled •NO are often decreased in patients with CF, there is an ample evidence of nitrosative stress in the CF respiratory tract [133, 140, 141]. Furthermore, the CF respiratory tract is unique because it contains high numbers of neutrophils early on in life, and these cells have been shown to produce vigorously oxidants when stimulated with bacterial products [143-146]. The presence of oxidative stress in the CF respiratory tract is highlighted by studies revealing abundant protein and lipid oxidation products in CF airway secretions or exhaled air [118, 147-154]. *Pseudomonas aeruginosa*, the pathogen specific for the CF respiratory tract, produces a pigment called pyocyanin [12], which causes oxidative stress in CF respiratory epithelium and provokes an inflammatory response [155-161]. In response to *Pseudomonas aeruginosa* infection, glutathione levels in the non-CF respiratory tract are quickly up-regulated [162]. By contrast, the CF respiratory tract cannot up-regulate glutathione levels as vigorously [162] which aggravates the oxidative insult conferred by Pseudomonas infection. Beside glutathione, patients with CF are frequently deficient in fat-soluble antioxidants, such as vitamin E [163, 164]. The vast majority of patients with CF have pancreatic insufficiency [165]. The deficiency of pancreatic enzymes causes fat malabsorption and, subsequently, inadequate absorbance of vitamin E and other fat-soluble antioxidants (see Vol. II, Chapter 3). To summarize, overexposure to ROS/RNS is likely pertinent to CF lung disease, yet it is distinct from asthma and COPD. *The sources of ROS/RNS include neutrophils and bacterial products, both overabundant in the CF respiratory tracts. The overexposure to ROS/RNS is aggravated by relative deficiency of antioxidants due to CF mutation or malnutrition.*

2.6. Lung Cancer

Lung cancer refers to rapid and uncontrolled growth of lung cells, often associated with invasion into neighboring tissues or spread into other organs (metastasis). Lung cancer is the leading cause of cancer-related death [166]. There are different types of lung cancer; however, current or former smoking and secondhand smoking have been singled out as the major risk factor for many types of lung cancer [166]. Among the smokers, those with airway obstruction are at heightened risk for developing lung cancer [167]; consequently, lung cancer is frequently associated with COPD [168]. However, not every smoker or COPD patient develops lung cancer, which implicates individual susceptibility to cancer development. The current view of carcinogenesis is that it is a multifactorial process involving genetic and epigenetic modulations of expression of tumor suppressors/oncogenes, activation of growth factor receptors and transcription factors, and local immune responses (see Chapters 6 and 7 in this Volume). Cigarette smoke contains multiple carcinogens, many of which are or give rise to ROS/RNS [11]. The radical and non-radical carcinogens promote genetic mutations through carcinogen binding to DNA [11, 169]. Oxidative DNA damage, such as formation of 8-oxoguanine, are elevated in smokers [170], and an inherently inadequate capacity to repair oxidative DNA damage is associated with lung cancer [171]. Formation of 8-oxoguanine can occur within the coding sequence of the gene or within the gene promoters [172]. The latter alters the transcription factor binding which is essential for initiating gene expression. Oxidative damage to genes can occur in an epigenetic manner. Thus, cytosine oxidation at CpG islands in the gene promoter regions results in attenuated expression of corresponding proteins [173, 174]. When the targeted proteins are tumor suppressors, the influence of oncogenes is magnified. Smoking has also been shown to increase expression of epidermal growth factor receptor (EGFR) in respiratory epithelial cells [175, 176]. EGFR plays a key role in the development of non-small cell lung cancer [177], the most frequent form of lung cancer. Further, EGFR genetic abnormalities are frequently associated with lung cancer in non-smokers [178]. Cigarette smoke activates "pro-survival" transcription factors, such as NF-κB and STAT-3. Persistent activation of these transcription factors have been linked to lung cancer [179, 180].

Smoking also suppresses innate and acquired immunity [93, 181, 182], which can diminish the body's ability to purge mutated cells. Risk factors for non-smokers include exposure to inhaled environmental (radon gas, pollutants) and occupational (asbestos) hazards; oxidative/nitrosative cell damage appears to be a significant component mediating their hazardous effects [183-185]. In summary, cigarette smoking and associated chronic inflammation and obstruction in the respiratory tract are major risk factors for development of lung cancer. Other factors include genetic predisposition and exposure to hazardous environmental and occupational inhalants.

2.7. Other Pulmonary Diseases and Conditions Associated With Overexposure to ROS/RNS

Interstitial lung diseases include several clinical entities caused by occupational (e.g. asbestosis), infectious (e.g. atypical pneumonias), and idiopathic (e.g. pulmonary fibrosis, sarcoidosis) factors. In contrast to obstructive lung diseases (asthma, COPD, most of CF), pathological processes largely involve the lung parenchyma outside of the alveoli. The understanding of the role of ROS/RNS in interstitial lung diseases is far from complete. However, clinical evidence indicates the presence of elevated levels of H_2O_2 and lipid peroxidation products in exhaled breath condensate samples of these patients [186-189]. This is likely to be a result of increased generation of ROS by the respiratory cells [188]. The role of exhaled •NO is even less clear, because elevated •NO levels may indicate enhanced antibacterial defenses.

Acute respiratory distress syndrome (ARDS) is a severe form of lung injury and a syndrome of acute pulmonary inflammation [190]. The causes for ARDS include direct (acid aspiration of gastric contents, pneumonia) and indirect (sepsis, severe trauma) lung injury [191]. The mechanisms responsible for this syndrome have not been fully elucidated, but oxidative and nitrosative stress is a relevant pathophysiological feature. The lung injury is neutrophil-dependent [191], and activated neutrophils are a major source of pathological ROS/RNS production in the respiratory tract [192, 193]. Other sources include ischemia/reperfusion and oxygen therapy [194]. The deleterious effects of ROS/RNS are associated with excessive inflammation and increased cell death [194, 195].

3. Therapeutic Measures

With the recognition of diverse pathophysiological roles of ROS/RNS in pulmonary diseases, several preventive and pharmacological interventions are being currently explored.

The most important preventive measure for many pulmonary diseases is cessation of active smoking [196, 197]. Further, secondhand smoking is a recognized risk factor for developing inflammatory lung diseases and allergies, especially in children [198]. Therefore, minimizing exposure to cigarette smoke at home or in public is another valid preventative measure. Further important preventative measure is *daily consumption of a diet rich in antioxidants, especially in early lifewhile the immune system is undergoing development* [199]. Direct supplementation of antioxidants has also been tried, albeit with mixed successes. Thus, N-acetylcysteine, an antioxidant drug and precursor to glutathione (see Vol. II, Chapters 11, and Chapter 10 in this Volume), appears to modulate favorably the oxidant/antioxidant balance by decreasing H_2O_2 levels in the respiratory tract [200, 201] and augmenting extra- and intracellular glutathione [202, 203]. However, inflammation and clinical outcomes in respiratory tract conditions are mostly uninfluenced by N-acetylcysteine administration [203-208]. Other antioxidant supplements have also shown ambiguous efficacy in clinical studies. Therefore, current interest has shifted to diet-derived antioxidants and anti-inflammatory agents (nutriceuticals) such as curcumin, and to stimulation of the master up-regulator of protein antioxidants, Nrf2 (Vol. II, Chapters 13 and 21).

Conclusions

The normal respiratory tract is constantly exposed to ROS/RNS and this exposure may be greatly enhanced under diverse pathological conditions, including asthma, COPD, CF, and lung cancer. In the latter, augmented oxidative/nitrosative stress may contribute to disease etiopathogenesis by mediating inflammatory reactions, apoptosis or uncontrolled cell growth. The advent of safe and effective medications and nutriceuticals to combat these untoward processes and restore redox homeostasis would greatly assist in the management of the pulmonary conditions discussed in this Chapter.

References

[1] Fischer H. Mechanisms and function of DUOX in epithelia of the lung. *Antioxid. Redox. Signal,* 2009;11:2453-65.

[2] van der Vliet A. NADPH oxidases in lung biology and pathology: host defense enzymes, and more. *Free Radic. Biol. Med.* 2008;44:938-55.

[3] Murphy MP. How mitochondria produce reactive oxygen species. *Biochem J.* 2009;417:1-13.

[4] Lambeth JD, Kawahara T, Diebold B. Regulation of Nox and Duox enzymatic activity and expression. *Free Radic. Biol. Med.* 2007;43:319-31.

[5] Bochkov VN, Oskolkova OV, Birukov KG, Levonen AL, Binder CJ, Stockl J. Generation and biological activities of oxidized phospholipids. *Antioxid. Redox. Signal,* 2010;12:1009-59.

[6] Bove PF, van der Vliet A. Nitric oxide and reactive nitrogen species in airway epithelial signaling and inflammation. *Free Radic. Biol. Med.* 2006;41:515-27.

[7] Droge W. Free radicals in the physiological control of cell function. *Physiol. Rev.* 2002;82:47-95.

[8] Novo E, Parola M. Redox mechanisms in hepatic chronic wound healing and fibrogenesis. *Fibrogenesis Tissue Repair* 2008;1:5.

[9] Reynaert NL, Ckless K, Wouters EF, van der Vliet A, Janssen-Heininger YM. Nitric oxide and redox signaling in allergic airway inflammation. *Antioxid. Redox. Signal.* 2005;7:129-43.

[10] Pryor WA, Stone K. Oxidants in cigarette smoke. Radicals, hydrogen peroxide, peroxynitrate, and peroxynitrite. *Ann. N Y Acad. Sci.* 1993;686:12-27.

[11] Pryor WA. Cigarette smoke radicals and the role of free radicals in chemical carcinogenicity. *Environ. Health Perspect.* 1997;105 Suppl 4:875-82.

[12] Lau GW, Hassett DJ, Ran H, Kong F. The role of pyocyanin in Pseudomonas aeruginosa infection. *Trends Mol. Med.* 2004;10:599-606.

[13] Dietrich LE, Teal TK, Price-Whelan A, Newman DK. Redox-active antibiotics control gene expression and community behavior in divergent bacteria. *Science,* 2008;321:1203-6.

[14] Price-Whelan A, Dietrich LE, Newman DK. Rethinking 'secondary' metabolism: physiological roles for phenazine antibiotics. *Nat. Chem. Biol.* 2006;2:71-8.

[15] Segal AW. How neutrophils kill microbes. *Annu. Rev. Immunol.* 2005;23:197-223.

[16] Reth M. Hydrogen peroxide as second messenger in lymphocyte activation. *Nat. Immunol.* 2002;3:1129-34.

[17] Kariyawasam HH, Robinson DS. The eosinophil: the cell and its weapons, the cytokines, its locations. *Semin. Respir. Crit. Care Med.* 2006;27:117-27.

[18] Forman HJ, Torres M. Reactive oxygen species and cell signaling: respiratory burst in macrophage signaling. *Am. J. Respir. Crit. Care Med.* 2002;166:S4-S8.

[19] Bienert GP, Moller AL, Kristiansen KA et al. Specific aquaporins facilitate the diffusion of hydrogen peroxide across membranes. *J. Biol. Chem.* 2007;282:1183-92.

[20] Pin I, Gibson PG, Kolendowicz R et al. Use of induced sputum cell counts to investigate airway inflammation in asthma. *Thorax,* 1992;47:25-9.

[21] Dauletbaev N, Rickmann J, Viel K, Buhl R, Wagner TO, Bargon J. Glutathione in induced sputum of healthy individuals and patients with asthma. *Thorax,* 2001;56:13-8.

[22] Smountas AA, Lands LC, Mohammed SR, Grey V. Induced sputum in cystic fibrosis: within-week reproducibility of inflammatory markers. *Clin. Biochem.* 2004;37:1031-6.

[23] Gwaltney JM, Jr., Hendley JO, Simon G, Jordan WS, Jr. Rhinovirus infections in an industrial population. I. The occurrence of illness. *N. Engl. J. Med.* 1966;275:1261-8.

[24] Arden KE, McErlean P, Nissen MD, Sloots TP, Mackay IM. Frequent detection of human rhinoviruses, paramyxoviruses, coronaviruses, and bocavirus during acute respiratory tract infections. *J. Med. Virol.* 2006;78:1232-40.

[25] Monto AS. Epidemiology of viral respiratory infections. *Am. J. Med.* 2002;112 Suppl 6A:4S-12S.

[26] Papi A, Contoli M, Gasparini P et al. Role of xanthine oxidase activation and reduced glutathione depletion in rhinovirus induction of inflammation in respiratory epithelial cells. *J. Biol. Chem.* 2008;283:28595-606.

[27] Buffinton GD, Christen S, Peterhans E, Stocker R. Oxidative stress in lungs of mice infected with influenza A virus. *Free Radic. Res. Commun.* 1992;16:99-110.

[28] Hennet T, Peterhans E, Stocker R. Alterations in antioxidant defences in lung and liver of mice infected with influenza A virus. *J. Gen. Virol.* 1992;73 (Pt 1):39-46.

[29] Hosakote YM, Liu T, Castro SM, Garofalo RP, Casola A. Respiratory syncytial virus induces oxidative stress by modulating antioxidant enzymes. *Am. J. Respir. Cell Mol. Biol.* 2009;41:348-57.

[30] Jobsis RQ, Schellekens SL, Fakkel-Kroesbergen A, Raatgeep RH, de Jongste JC. Hydrogen peroxide in breath condensate during a common cold. *Mediators Inflamm.* 2001;10:351-4.

[31] Majewska E, Kasielski M, Luczynski R, Bartosz G, Bialasiewicz P, Nowak D. Elevated exhalation of hydrogen peroxide and thiobarbituric acid reactive substances in patients with community acquired pneumonia. *Respir. Med.* 2004;98:669-76.

[32] Bousquet J, Van CP, Khaltaev N. Allergic rhinitis and its impact on asthma. *J. Allergy Clin. Immunol.* 2001;108:S147-S334.

[33] Bousquet J, Khaltaev N, Cruz AA et al. Allergic Rhinitis and its Impact on Asthma (ARIA) 2008 update (in collaboration with the World Health Organization, GA(2)LEN and AllerGen). *Allergy* 2008;63 Suppl 86:8-160.

[34] Ahlstrom-Emanuelsson CA, Greiff L, Andersson M, Persson CG, Erjefalt JS. Eosinophil degranulation status in allergic rhinitis: observations before and during seasonal allergen exposure. *Eur. Respir. J.* 2004;24:750-7.

[35] Ciprandi G, Vizzaccaro A, Cirillo I, Tosca M, Massolo A, Passalacqua G. Nasal eosinophils display the best correlation with symptoms, pulmonary function and inflammation in allergic rhinitis. *Int. Arch. Allergy Immunol.* 2005;136:266-72.

[36] Watanabe K, Misu T, Inoue S, Edamatsu H. Cytolysis of eosinophils in nasal secretions. *Ann. Otol. Rhinol. Laryngol.* 2003;112:169-73.

[37] Aldridge RE, Chan T, van Dalen CJ et al. Eosinophil peroxidase produces hypobromous acid in the airways of stable asthmatics. *Free Radic. Biol. Med.* 2002;33:847-56.

[38] Weiss SJ, Test ST, Eckmann CM, Roos D, Regiani S. Brominating oxidants generated by human eosinophils. *Science* 1986;234:200-3.

[39] Bousquet J, Jacot W, Vignola AM, Bachert C, Van CP. Allergic rhinitis: a disease remodeling the upper airways? *J. Allergy Clin. Immunol.* 2004;113:43-9.

[40] GINA - the Global Initiative for Asthma. www.ginasthma.com. 2009.

[41] Dharajiya NG, Bacsi A, Boldogh I, Sur S. Pollen NAD(P)H oxidases and their contribution to allergic inflammation. *Immunol. Allergy Clin. North Am.* 2007;27:45-63.

[42] Wang XL, Takai T, Kamijo S, Gunawan H, Ogawa H, Okumura K. NADPH oxidase activity in allergenic pollen grains of different plant species. *Biochem. Biophys. Res. Commun.* 2009;387:430-4.

[43] Boldogh I, Bacsi A, Choudhury BK et al. ROS generated by pollen NADPH oxidase provide a signal that augments antigen-induced allergic airway inflammation. *J. Clin. Invest.* 2005;115:2169-79.

[44] Li N, Hao M, Phalen RF, Hinds WC, Nel AE. Particulate air pollutants and asthma. A paradigm for the role of oxidative stress in PM-induced adverse health effects. *Clin. Immunol.* 2003;109:250-65.

[45] Pandya RJ, Solomon G, Kinner A, Balmes JR. Diesel exhaust and asthma: hypotheses and molecular mechanisms of action. *Environ. Health Perspect.* 2002;110 Suppl 1:103-12.

[46] Gershwin LJ. Effects of air pollutants on development of allergic immune responses in the respiratory tract. *Clin. Dev. Immunol.* 2003;10:119-26.

[47] Peden DB, Setzer RW, Jr., Devlin RB. Ozone exposure has both a priming effect on allergen-induced responses and an intrinsic inflammatory action in the nasal airways of perennially allergic asthmatics. *Am. J. Respir. Crit. Care Med.* 1995;151:1336-45.

[48] Pietinalho A, Pelkonen A, Rytila P. Linkage between smoking and asthma. *Allergy,* 2009;64:1722-7.

[49] Vozoris N, Lougheed MD. Second-hand smoke exposure in Canada: prevalence, risk factors, and association with respiratory and cardiovascular diseases. *Can. Respir. J.* 2008;15:263-9.

[50] ten Brinke A. Risk factors associated with irreversible airflow limitation in asthma. *Curr. Opin. Allergy Clin. Immunol.* 2008;8:63-9.

[51] de Gouw HW, Grunberg K, Schot R, Kroes AC, Dick EC, Sterk PJ. Relationship between exhaled nitric oxide and airway hyperresponsiveness following experimental rhinovirus infection in asthmatic subjects. *Eur. Respir. J.* 1998;11:126-32.

[52] Jackson DJ, Johnston SL. The role of viruses in acute exacerbations of asthma. *J. Allergy Clin. Immunol.* 2010;125:1178-87.

[53] Kelly FJ, Mudway I, Blomberg A, Frew A, Sandstrom T. Altered lung antioxidant status in patients with mild asthma. *Lancet*, 1999;354:482-3.

[54] Fitzpatrick AM, Teague WG, Holguin F, Yeh M, Brown LA. Airway glutathione homeostasis is altered in children with severe asthma: evidence for oxidant stress. *J. Allergy Clin. Immunol.* 2009;123:146-52.

[55] Antczak A, Nowak D, Shariati B, Krol M, Piasecka G, Kurmanowska Z. Increased hydrogen peroxide and thiobarbituric acid-reactive products in expired breath condensate of asthmatic patients. *Eur. Respir. J.* 1997;10:1235-41.

[56] Dohlman AW, Black HR, Royall JA. Expired breath hydrogen peroxide is a marker of acute airway inflammation in pediatric patients with asthma. *Am. Rev. Respir. Dis.* 1993;148:955-60.

[57] Emelyanov A, Fedoseev G, Abulimity A et al. Elevated concentrations of exhaled hydrogen peroxide in asthmatic patients. *Chest,* 2001;120:1136-9.

[58] Jobsis Q, Raatgeep HC, Hermans PW, de Jongste JC. Hydrogen peroxide in exhaled air is increased in stable asthmatic children. *Eur. Respir. J.* 1997;10:519-21.

[59] Loukides S, Bouros D, Papatheodorou G, Panagou P, Siafakas NM. The relationships among hydrogen peroxide in expired breath condensate, airway inflammation, and asthma severity. *Chest,* 2002;121:338-46.

[60] Fitzpatrick AM, Brown LA, Holguin F, Teague WG. Levels of nitric oxide oxidation products are increased in the epithelial lining fluid of children with persistent asthma. *J. Allergy Clin. Immunol.* 2009;124:990-6.

[61] Perez-de-Llano LA, Carballada F, Castro AO et al. Exhaled nitric oxide predicts control in patients with difficult-to-treat asthma. *Eur. Respir. J.* 2010;35:1221-7.

[62] van Veen IH, ten BA, Sterk PJ et al. Exhaled nitric oxide predicts lung function decline in difficult-to-treat asthma. *Eur. Respir. J.* 2008;32:344-9.

[63] Baraldi E, Giordano G, Pasquale MF et al. 3-Nitrotyrosine, a marker of nitrosative stress, is increased in breath condensate of allergic asthmatic children. *Allergy,* 2006;61:90-6.

[64] Montuschi P, Corradi M, Ciabattoni G, Nightingale J, Kharitonov SA, Barnes PJ. Increased 8-isoprostane, a marker of oxidative stress, in exhaled condensate of asthma patients. *Am. J. Respir. Crit. Care Med.* 1999;160:216-20.

[65] Hasan RA, Thomas J, Davidson B, Barnes J, Reddy R. 8-Isoprostane in the exhaled breath condensate of children hospitalized for status asthmaticus. *Pediatr. Crit. Care Med.* 2010.

[66] Paul WE, Zhu J. How are T(H)2-type immune responses initiated and amplified? *Nat. Rev. Immunol.* 2010;10:225-35.

[67] King MR, Ismail AS, Davis LS, Karp DR. Oxidative stress promotes polarization of human T cell differentiation toward a T helper 2 phenotype. *J. Immunol.* 2006;176:2765-72.

[68] Aguilera-Aguirre L, Bacsi A, Saavedra-Molina A, Kurosky A, Sur S, Boldogh I. Mitochondrial dysfunction increases allergic airway inflammation. *J. Immunol.* 2009;183:5379-87.

[69] Stenfors N, Bosson J, Helleday R et al. Ozone exposure enhances mast-cell inflammation in asthmatic airways despite inhaled corticosteroid therapy. *Inhal. Toxicol.* 2010;22:133-9.

[70] Vagaggini B, Bartoli ML, Cianchetti S et al. Increase in markers of airway inflammation after ozone exposure can be observed also in stable treated asthmatics with minimal functional response to ozone. *Respir. Res.* 2010;11:5.

[71] Bucchieri F, Puddicombe SM, Lordan JL et al. Asthmatic bronchial epithelium is more susceptible to oxidant-induced apoptosis. *Am. J. Respir. Cell Mol. Biol.* 2002;27:179-85.

[72] Persinger RL, Blay WM, Heintz NH, Hemenway DR, Janssen-Heininger YM. Nitrogen dioxide induces death in lung epithelial cells in a density-dependent manner. *Am. J. RespirCell Mol. Biol.* 2001;24:583-90.

[73] Holgate ST. The airway epithelium is central to the pathogenesis of asthma. *Allergol. Int.* 2008;57:1-10.

[74] Siddiqui S, Martin JG. Structural aspects of airway remodeling in asthma. *Curr, AllergyAsthma Rep.* 2008;8:540-7.

[75] GOLD - the Global Initiative for Chronic Obstructive Lung Disease. www.goldcopd.com. 2009.

[76] Menezes AM, Perez-Padilla R, Jardim JR et al. Chronic obstructive pulmonary disease in five Latin American cities (the PLATINO study): a prevalence study. *Lancet,* 2005;366:1875-81.

[77] Brito-Mutunayagam R, Appleton SL, Wilson DH, Ruffin RE, Adams RJ. GOLD stage 0 is associated with excess FEV1 decline in a representative population sample. *Chest,* 2010.

[78] Salvi SS, Barnes PJ. Chronic obstructive pulmonary disease in non-smokers. *Lancet,* 2009;374:733-43.

[79] Guatura SB, Martinez JA, Santos Bueno PC, Santos ML. Increased exhalation of hydrogen peroxide in healthy subjects following cigarette consumption. *Sao Paulo Med. J.* 2000;118:93-8.

[80] Chambers DC, Tunnicliffe WS, Ayres JG. Acute inhalation of cigarette smoke increases lower respiratory tract nitric oxide concentrations. *Thorax,*1998;53:677-9.

[81] Balint B, Donnelly LE, Hanazawa T, Kharitonov SA, Barnes PJ. Increased nitric oxide metabolites in exhaled breath condensate after exposure to tobacco smoke. *Thorax,* 2001;56:456-61.

[82] Dekhuijzen PN, Aben KK, Dekker I et al. Increased exhalation of hydrogen peroxide in patients with stable and unstable chronic obstructive pulmonary disease. *Am. J. Respir. Crit. Care Med.* 1996;154:813-6.

[83] Louhelainen N, Rytila P, Haahtela T, Kinnula VL, Djukanovic R. Persistence of oxidant and protease burden in the airways after smoking cessation. *BMC Pulm. Med.* 2009;9:25.

[84] Nowak D, Kasielski M, Antczak A, Pietras T, Bialasiewicz P. Increased content of thiobarbituric acid-reactive substances and hydrogen peroxide in the expired breath condensate of patients with stable chronic obstructive pulmonary disease: no significant effect of cigarette smoking. *Respir. Med.* 1999;93:389-96.

[85] Hogg JC, McDonough JE, Gosselink JV, Hayashi S. What drives the peripheral lung-remodeling process in chronic obstructive pulmonary disease? *Proc. Am. Thorac. Soc.* 2009;6:668-72.

[86] Puchelle E, Zahm JM, Tournier JM, Coraux C. Airway epithelial repair, regeneration, and remodeling after injury in chronic obstructive pulmonary disease. *Proc. Am. Thorac. Soc.* 2006;3:726-33.

[87] Petrache I, Natarajan V, Zhen L et al. Ceramide upregulation causes pulmonary cell apoptosis and emphysema-like disease in mice. *Nat. Med.* 2005;11:491-8.

[88] Filosto S, Castillo S, Danielson A et al. Neutral Sphingomyelinase 2: A Novel Target in Cigarette Smoke-induced Apoptosis and Lung Injury. Am J Respir *Cell Mol. Biol.* 2010.

[89] Castillo SS, Levy M, Thaikoottathil JV, Goldkorn T. Reactive nitrogen and oxygen species activate different sphingomyelinases to induce apoptosis in airway epithelial cells. *Exp. Cell Res.* 2007;313:2680-6.

[90] Levy M, Khan E, Careaga M, Goldkorn T. Neutral sphingomyelinase 2 is activated by cigarette smoke to augment ceramide-induced apoptosis in lung cell death. *Am. J. Physiol. Lung Cell Mol. Physiol.* 2009;297:L125-L133.

[91] Lavrentiadou SN, Chan C, Kawcak T et al. Ceramide-mediated apoptosis in lung epithelial cells is regulated by glutathione. *Am. J. Respir. Cell Mol. Biol.* 2001;25:676-84.

[92] Schneider D, Ganesan S, Comstock AT et al. Increased Cytokine Response of Rhinovirus-infected Airway Epithelial Cells in Chronic Obstructive Pulmonary Disease. *Am. J. Respir. Crit. Care Med.* 2010.

[93] Herr C, Beisswenger C, Hess C et al. Suppression of pulmonary innate host defence in smokers. *Thorax,* 2009;64:144-9.

[94] Marin-Corral J, Minguella J, Ramirez-Sarmiento AL, Hussain SN, Gea J, Barreiro E. Oxidised proteins and superoxide anion production in the diaphragm of severe COPD patients. *Eur. Respir. J.* 2009;33:1309-19.

[95] Barreiro E, Gea J, Matar G, Hussain SN. Expression and carbonylation of creatine kinase in the quadriceps femoris muscles of patients with chronic obstructive pulmonary disease. *Am. J. Respir. Cell Mol. Biol.* 2005;33:636-42.

[96] Couillard A, Koechlin C, Cristol JP, Varray A, Prefaut C. Evidence of local exercise-induced systemic oxidative stress in chronic obstructive pulmonary disease patients. *Eur. Respir. J.* 2002;20:1123-9.

[97] Couillard A, Maltais F, Saey D et al. Exercise-induced quadriceps oxidative stress and peripheral muscle dysfunction in patients with chronic obstructive pulmonary disease. *Am. J. Respir. Crit. Care Med.* 2003;167:1664-9.

[98] van Helvoort HA, Heijdra YF, de Boer RC, Swinkels A, Thijs HM, Dekhuijzen PN. Six-minute walking-induced systemic inflammation and oxidative stress in muscle-wasted COPD patients. *Chest,* 2007;131:439-45.

[99] Heunks LM, Vina J, van Herwaarden CL, Folgering HT, Gimeno A, Dekhuijzen PN. Xanthine oxidase is involved in exercise-induced oxidative stress in chronic obstructive pulmonary disease. *Am. J. Physiol.* 1999;277:R1697-R1704.

[100] Bentley AR, Emrani P, Cassano PA. Genetic variation and gene expression in antioxidant related enzymes and risk of COPD: a systematic review. *Thorax,* 2008;63:956-61.

[101] Kinnula VL. Focus on antioxidant enzymes and antioxidant strategies in smoking related airway diseases. *Thorax,* 2005;60:693-700.

[102] Oberley-Deegan RE, Regan EA, Kinnula VL, Crapo JD. Extracellular superoxide dismutase and risk of COPD. *COPD* 2009;6:307-12.

[103] Dahl M, Bowler RP, Juul K, Crapo JD, Levy S, Nordestgaard BG. Superoxide dismutase 3 polymorphism associated with reduced lung function in two large populations. *Am. J. Respir. Crit. Care Med.* 2008;178:906-12.

[104] Siedlinski M, van Diemen CC, Postma DS, Vonk JM, Boezen HM. Superoxide dismutases, lung function and bronchial responsiveness in a general population. *Eur. Respir. J.* 2009;33:986-92.

[105] Ganguly K, Depner M, Fattman C et al. Superoxide dismutase 3, extracellular (SOD3) variants and lung function. *Physiol. Genomics.* 2009;37:260-7.

[106] Senn O, Russi EW, Imboden M, Probst-Hensch NM. alpha1-Antitrypsin deficiency and lung disease: risk modification by occupational and environmental inhalants. *Eur. Respir.J.* 2005;26:909-17.

[107] Stoller JK, Aboussouan LS. Alpha1-antitrypsin deficiency. Lancet 2005;365:2225-36.

[108] Lands LC, Stanojevic S. Oral non-steroidal anti-inflammatory drug therapy for cystic fibrosis. *Cochrane Database Syst. Rev.* 2007;CD001505.

[109] Riordan JR. CFTR function and prospects for therapy. *Annu. Rev. Biochem.* 2008;77:701-26.

[110] l'Hoste S, Chargui A, Belfodil R et al. CFTR mediates apoptotic volume decrease and cell death by controlling glutathione efflux and ROS production in cultured mice proximal tubules. *Am. J. Physiol. Renal. Physiol.* 2010;298:F435-F453.

[111] Kariya C, Leitner H, Min E, van HC, van HA, Day BJ. A role for CFTR in the elevation of glutathione levels in the lung by oral glutathione administration. *Am. J. Physiol. LungCell Mol. Physiol.* 2007;292:L1590-L1597.

[112] Kogan I, Ramjeesingh M, Li C et al. CFTR directly mediates nucleotide-regulated glutathione flux. *EMBO J.* 2003;22:1981-9.

[113] Gao L, Kim KJ, Yankaskas JR, Forman HJ. Abnormal glutathione transport in cystic fibrosis airway epithelia. *Am. J. Physiol.* 1999;277:L113-L118.

[114] Linsdell P, Hanrahan JW. Glutathione permeability of CFTR. *Am. J. Physiol.* 1998;275:C323-C326.

[115] Cantin AM, North SL, Hubbard RC, Crystal RG. Normal alveolar epithelial lining fluid contains high levels of glutathione. *J. Appl. Physiol.* 1987;63:152-7.

[116] Cantin AM, Begin R. Glutathione and inflammatory disorders of the lung. *Lung,* 1991;169:123-38.

[117] Roum JH, Buhl R, McElvaney NG, Borok Z, Crystal RG. Systemic deficiency of glutathione in cystic fibrosis. *J. Appl. Physiol.* 1993;75:2419-24.

[118] Hull J, Vervaart P, Grimwood K, Phelan P. Pulmonary oxidative stress response in young children with cystic fibrosis. *Thorax* 1997;52:557-60.

[119] Lands LC, Grey V, Smountas AA, Kramer VG, McKenna D. Lymphocyte glutathione levels in children with cystic fibrosis. *Chest* 1999;116:201-5.

[120] Dauletbaev N, Viel K, Buhl R, Wagner TO, Bargon J. Glutathione and glutathione peroxidase in sputum samples of adult patients with cystic fibrosis. *J. Cyst. Fibros,* 2004;3:119-24.

[121] Watt AP, Courtney J, Moore J, Ennis M, Elborn JS. Neutrophil cell death, activation and bacterial infection in cystic fibrosis. *Thorax,* 2005;60:659-64.

[122] van den Dobbelsteen DJ, Nobel CS, Schlegel J, Cotgreave IA, Orrenius S, Slater AF. Rapid and specific efflux of reduced glutathione during apoptosis induced by anti-Fas/APO-1 antibody. *J. Biol. Chem.* 1996;271:15420-7.

[123] Worlitzsch D, Herberth G, Ulrich M, Doring G. Catalase, myeloperoxidase and hydrogen peroxide in cystic fibrosis. *Eur. Respir. J.* 1998;11:377-83.

[124] Cantin AM, White TB, Cross CE, Forman HJ, Sokol RJ, Borowitz D. Antioxidants in cystic fibrosis. Conclusions from the CF antioxidant workshop, Bethesda, Maryland, November 11-12, 2003. *Free Radic. Biol. Med.* 2007;42:15-31.

[125] Ho LP, Faccenda J, Innes JA, Greening AP. Expired hydrogen peroxide in breath condensate of cystic fibrosis patients. *Eur. Respir. J.* 1999;13:103-6.

[126] Moller W, Heimbeck I, Weber N et al. Fractionated exhaled breath condensate collection shows high hydrogen peroxide release in the airways. *J. Aerosol. Med. Pulm. Drug. Deliv* 2010;23:129-35.

[127] Grasemann H, Michler E, Wallot M, Ratjen F. Decreased concentration of exhaled nitric oxide (NO) in patients with cystic fibrosis. *Pediatr. Pulmonol.* 1997;24:173-7.

[128] Ho LP, Innes JA, Greening AP. Exhaled nitric oxide is not elevated in the inflammatory airways diseases of cystic fibrosis and bronchiectasis. *Eur. Respir. J.* 1998;12:1290-4.

[129] Elphick HE, Demoncheaux EA, Ritson S, Higenbottam TW, Everard ML. Exhaled nitric oxide is reduced in infants with cystic fibrosis. *Thorax,* 2001;56:151-2.

[130] Franklin PJ, Hall GL, Moeller A, Horak F, Jr., Brennan S, Stick SM. Exhaled nitric oxide is not reduced in infants with cystic fibrosis. *Eur. Respir. J.* 2006;27:350-3.

[131] Keen C, Gustafsson P, Lindblad A, Wennergren G, Olin AC. Low levels of exhaled nitric oxide are associated with impaired lung function in cystic fibrosis. *Pediatr. Pulmonol.* 2010;45:241-8.

[132] Hofer M, Mueller L, Rechsteiner T, Benden C, Boehler A. Extended nitric oxide measurements in exhaled air of cystic fibrosis and healthy adults. *Lung* 2009;187:307-13.

[133] Ho LP, Innes JA, Greening AP. Nitrite levels in breath condensate of patients with cystic fibrosis is elevated in contrast to exhaled nitric oxide. *Thorax,* 1998;53:680-4.

[134] Thomas SR, Kharitonov SA, Scott SF, Hodson ME, Barnes PJ. Nasal and exhaled nitric oxide is reduced in adult patients with cystic fibrosis and does not correlate with cystic fibrosis genotype. *Chest* 2000;117:1085-9.

[135] Steagall WK, Elmer HL, Brady KG, Kelley TJ. Cystic fibrosis transmembrane conductance regulator-dependent regulation of epithelial inducible nitric oxide synthase expression. *Am. J. Respir. Cell Mol. Biol.* 2000;22:45-50.

[136] Liang G, Stephenson AH, Lonigro AJ, Sprague RS. Erythrocytes of humans with cystic fibrosis fail to stimulate nitric oxide synthesis in isolated rabbit lungs. *Am. J. Physiol. Heart Circ. Physiol.* 2005;288:H1580-H1585.

[137] Grasemann H, Knauer N, Buscher R, Hubner K, Drazen JM, Ratjen F. Airway nitric oxide levels in cystic fibrosis patients are related to a polymorphism in the neuronal nitric oxide synthase gene. *Am. J. Respir. Crit. Care Med.* 2000;162:2172-6.

[138] Meng QH, Springall DR, Bishop AE et al. Lack of inducible nitric oxide synthase in bronchial epithelium: a possible mechanism of susceptibility to infection in cystic fibrosis. *J. Pathol.* 1998;184:323-31.

[139] Grasemann H, Schwiertz R, Matthiesen S, Racke K, Ratjen F. Increased arginase activity in cystic fibrosis airways. *Am. J. Respir. Crit. Care Med.* 2005;172:1523-8.

[140] Balint B, Kharitonov SA, Hanazawa T et al. Increased nitrotyrosine in exhaled breath condensate in cystic fibrosis. *Eur. Respir. J.* 2001;17:1201-7.

[141] Formanek W, Inci D, Lauener RP, Wildhaber JH, Frey U, Hall GL. Elevated nitrite in breath condensates of children with respiratory disease. *Eur. Respir. J.* 2002;19:487-91.

[142] Morrissey BM, Schilling K, Weil JV, Silkoff PE, Rodman DM. Nitric oxide and protein nitration in the cystic fibrosis airway. *Arch. Biochem. Biophys.* 2002;406:33-9.

[143] Kolpen M, Hansen CR, Bjarnsholt T et al. Polymorphonuclear leucocytes consume oxygen in sputum from chronic Pseudomonas aeruginosa pneumonia in cystic fibrosis. *Thorax*, 2010;65:57-62.

[144] McKeon DJ, Cadwallader KA, Idris S et al. Cystic fibrosis neutrophils have normal intrinsic reactive oxygen species generation. *Eur. Respir. J.* 2010;35:1264-72.

[145] Hughes JE, Stewart J, Barclay GR, Govan JR. Priming of neutrophil respiratory burst activity by lipopolysaccharide from Burkholderia cepacia. *Infect. Immun.* 1997;65:4281-7.

[146] Kronborg G, Fomsgaard A, Jensen ET, Kharazmi A, Hoiby N. Induction of oxidative burst response in human neutrophils by immune complexes made in vitro of lipopolysaccharide and hyperimmune serum from chronically infected patients. *APMIS* 1993;101:887-94.

[147] Paredi P, Kharitonov SA, Leak D et al. Exhaled ethane is elevated in cystic fibrosis and correlates with carbon monoxide levels and airway obstruction. *Am. J. Respir. Crit. Care Med.* 2000;161:1247-51.

[148] Starosta V, Rietschel E, Paul K, Baumann U, Griese M. Oxidative changes of bronchoalveolar proteins in cystic fibrosis. *Chest*, 2006;129:431-7.

[149] Ciabattoni G, Davi G, Collura M et al. In vivo lipid peroxidation and platelet activation in cystic fibrosis. *Am. J. Respir. Crit. Care Med.* 2000;162:1195-201.

[150] Benabdeslam H, Abidi H, Garcia I, Bellon G, Gilly R, Revol A. Lipid peroxidation and antioxidant defenses in cystic fibrosis patients. *Clin. Chem. Lab. Med.* 1999;37:511-6.

[151] Collins CE, Quaggiotto P, Wood L, O'Loughlin EV, Henry RL, Garg ML. Elevated plasma levels of F2 alpha isoprostane in cystic fibrosis. *Lipids*, 1999;34:551-6.

[152] Dominguez C, Gartner S, Linan S, Cobos N, Moreno A. Enhanced oxidative damage in cystic fibrosis patients. *Biofactors* 1998;8:149-53.

[153] Brown RK, Wyatt H, Price JF, Kelly FJ. Pulmonary dysfunction in cystic fibrosis is associated with oxidative stress. *Eur. Respir. J.* 1996;9:334-9.

[154] Portal BC, Richard MJ, Faure HS, Hadjian AJ, Favier AE. Altered antioxidant status and increased lipid peroxidation in children with cystic fibrosis. *Am. J. Clin. Nutr.* 1995;61:843-7.

[155] Schwarzer C, Fischer H, Kim EJ et al. Oxidative stress caused by pyocyanin impairs CFTR Cl(-) transport in human bronchial epithelial cells. *Free. Radic. Biol. Med.* 2008;45:1653-62.

[156] Rada B, Lekstrom K, Damian S, Dupuy C, Leto TL. The Pseudomonas toxin pyocyanin inhibits the dual oxidase-based antimicrobial system as it imposes oxidative stress on airway epithelial cells. *J. Immunol.* 2008;181:4883-93.

[157] Schwarzer C, Fu Z, Fischer H, Machen TE. Redox-independent activation of NF-kappaB by Pseudomonas aeruginosa pyocyanin in a cystic fibrosis airway epithelial cell line. *J. Biol. Chem.* 2008;283:27144-53.

[158] O'Malley YQ, Reszka KJ, Spitz DR, Denning GM, Britigan BE. Pseudomonas aeruginosa pyocyanin directly oxidizes glutathione and decreases its levels in airway epithelial cells. *Am. J. Physiol. Lung Cell Mol. Physiol.* 2004;287:L94-103.

[159] Denning GM, Wollenweber LA, Railsback MA, Cox CD, Stoll LL, Britigan BE. Pseudomonas pyocyanin increases interleukin-8 expression by human airway epithelial cells. *Infect. Immun.* 1998;66:5777-84.

[160] Britigan BE, Rasmussen GT, Cox CD. Augmentation of oxidant injury to human pulmonary epithelial cells by the Pseudomonas aeruginosa siderophore pyochelin. *Infect. Immun.* 1997;65:1071-6.

[161] Britigan BE, Roeder TL, Rasmussen GT, Shasby DM, McCormick ML, Cox CD. Interaction of the Pseudomonas aeruginosa secretory products pyocyanin and pyochelin generates hydroxyl radical and causes synergistic damage to endothelial cells. Implications for Pseudomonas-associated tissue injury. *J. Clin. Invest.* 1992;90:2187-96.

[162] Day BJ, van Heeckeren AM, Min E, Velsor LW. Role for cystic fibrosis transmembrane conductance regulator protein in a glutathione response to bronchopulmonary pseudomonas infection. *Infect Immun.* 2004;72:2045-51.

[163] Lagrange-Puget M, Durieu I, Ecochard R et al. Longitudinal study of oxidative status in 312 cystic fibrosis patients in stable state and during bronchial exacerbation. *Pediatr. Pulmonol.* 2004;38:43-9.

[164] Sokol RJ, Reardon MC, Accurso FJ et al. Fat-soluble vitamins in infants identified by cystic fibrosis newborn screening. *Pediatr. Pulmonol. Suppl.* 1991;7:52-5.

[165] Lands LC. Nutrition in pediatric lung disease. *Paediatr. Respir. Rev.* 2007;8:305-11.

[166] Alberg AJ, Samet JM. Epidemiology of lung cancer. *Chest,* 2003;123:21S-49S.

[167] Tockman MS, Anthonisen NR, Wright EC, Donithan MG. Airways obstruction and the risk for lung cancer. *Ann. Intern. Med.* 1987;106:512-8.

[168] Wasswa-Kintu S, Gan WQ, Man SF, Pare PD, Sin DD. Relationship between reduced forced expiratory volume in one second and the risk of lung cancer: a systematic review and meta-analysis. *Thorax,* 2005;60:570-5.

[169] Sato M, Shames DS, Gazdar AF, Minna JD. A translational view of the molecular pathogenesis of lung cancer. *J. Thorac Oncol.* 2007;2:327-43.

[170] Asami S, Hirano T, Yamaguchi R, Tomioka Y, Itoh H, Kasai H. Increase of a type of oxidative DNA damage, 8-hydroxyguanine, and its repair activity in human leukocytes by cigarette smoking. *Cancer Res.* 1996;56:2546-9.

[171] Kohno T, Kunitoh H, Toyama K et al. Association of the OGG1-Ser326Cys polymorphism with lung adenocarcinoma risk. *Cancer Sci.* 2006;97:724-8.

[172] Evans MD, Cooke MS. Factors contributing to the outcome of oxidative damage to nucleic acids. *Bioessays,* 2004;26:533-42.

[173] Weitzman SA, Turk PW, Milkowski DH, Kozlowski K. Free radical adducts induce alterations in DNA cytosine methylation. *Proc. Natl. Acad. Sci. U S A* 1994;91:1261-4.

[174] Cerda S, Weitzman SA. Influence of oxygen radical injury on DNA methylation. *Mutat. Res.* 1997;386:141-52.

[175] Barsky SH, Roth MD, Kleerup EC, Simmons M, Tashkin DP. Histopathologic and molecular alterations in bronchial epithelium in habitual smokers of marijuana, cocaine, and/or tobacco. *J. Natl. Cancer Inst.* 1998;90:1198-205.

[176] O'Donnell RA, Richter A, Ward J et al. Expression of ErbB receptors and mucins in the airways of long term current smokers. *Thorax*, 2004;59:1032-40.

[177] Yoshida T, Zhang G, Haura EB. Targeting epidermal growth factor receptor: Central signaling kinase in lung cancer. *Biochem. Pharmacol.* 2010.

[178] Burns TF, Rudin CM. Lung cancer in 'never-smokers': beyond EGFR mutations and EGFR-TK inhibitors. *Oncology* (Williston Park) 2010;24:48-9.

[179] Deng J, Fujimoto J, Ye XF et al. Knockout of the tumor suppressor gene Gprc5a in mice leads to NF-kappaB activation in airway epithelium and promotes lung inflammation and tumorigenesis. *Cancer Prev. Res.* (Phila Pa) 2010;3:424-37.

[180] Yu H, Pardoll D, Jove R. STATs in cancer inflammation and immunity: a leading role for STAT3. *Nat. Rev. Cancer,* 2009;9:798-809.

[181] Mehta H, Nazzal K, Sadikot RT. Cigarette smoking and innate immunity. *Inflamm. Res.* 2008;57:497-503.

[182] Stampfli MR, Anderson GP. How cigarette smoke skews immune responses to promote infection, lung disease and cancer. *Nat. Rev. Immunol.* 2009;9:377-84.

[183] Chow S, Campbell C, Sandrini A, Thomas PS, Johnson AR, Yates DH. Exhaled breath condensate biomarkers in asbestos-related lung disorders. *Respir. Med.* 2009;103:1091-7.

[184] Pelclova D, Fenclova Z, Kacer P, Kuzma M, Navratil T, Lebedova J. Increased 8-isoprostane, a marker of oxidative stress in exhaled breath condensate in subjects with asbestos exposure. *Ind. Health,* 2008;46:484-9.

[185] Sperati A, Abeni DD, Tagesson C, Forastiere F, Miceli M, Axelson O. Exposure to indoor background radiation and urinary concentrations of 8-hydroxydeoxyguanosine, a marker of oxidative DNA damage. *Environ. Health Perspect.* 1999;107:213-5.

[186] Psathakis K, Mermigkis D, Papatheodorou G et al. Exhaled markers of oxidative stress in idiopathic pulmonary fibrosis. *Eur. J. Clin. Invest.* 2006;36:362-7.

[187] Psathakis K, Papatheodorou G, Plataki M et al. 8-Isoprostane, a marker of oxidative stress, is increased in the expired breath condensate of patients with pulmonary sarcoidosis. *Chest* 2004;125:1005-11.

[188] Piotrowski WJ, Kurmanowska Z, Antczak A, Marczak J, Ciebiada M, Gorski P. Exhaled 8-isoprostane in sarcoidosis: relation to superoxide anion production by bronchoalveolar lavage cells. *Inflamm. Res.* 2010.

[189] Kwiatkowska S, Szkudlarek U, Luczynska M, Nowak D, Zieba M. Elevated exhalation of hydrogen peroxide and circulating IL-18 in patients with pulmonary tuberculosis. *Respir. Med.* 2007;101:574-80.

[190] Bernard GR, Artigas A, Brigham KL et al. The American-European Consensus Conference on ARDS. Definitions, mechanisms, relevant outcomes, and clinical trial coordination. *Am. J. Respir. Crit. Care Med.* 1994;149:818-24.

[191] Ware LB, Matthay MA. The acute respiratory distress syndrome. *N. Engl. J. Med.* 2000;342:1334-49.

[192] Sznajder JI, Fraiman A, Hall JB et al. Increased hydrogen peroxide in the expired breath of patients with acute hypoxemic respiratory failure. *Chest,* 1989;96:606-12.

[193] Baldwin SR, Simon RH, Grum CM, Ketai LH, Boxer LA, Devall LJ. Oxidant activity in expired breath of patients with adult respiratory distress syndrome. *Lancet* 1986;1:11-4.

[194] Chabot F, Mitchell JA, Gutteridge JM, Evans TW. Reactive oxygen species in acute lung injury. *Eur. Respir. J.* 1998;11:745-57.

[195] Tasaka S, Amaya F, Hashimoto S, Ishizaka A. Roles of oxidants and redox signaling in the pathogenesis of acute respiratory distress syndrome. *Antioxid. Redox. Signal,* 2008;10:739-53.

[196] Tashkin DP, Murray RP. Smoking cessation in chronic obstructive pulmonary disease. *Respir. Med.* 2009;103:963-74.

[197] Thomson NC, Chaudhuri R. Asthma in smokers: challenges and opportunities. *Curr. Opin. Pulm. Med.* 2009;15:39-45.

[198] Metsios GS, Flouris AD, Koutedakis Y. Passive smoking, asthma and allergy in children. *Inflamm Allergy Drug Targets,* 2009;8:348-52.

[199] Kelly FJ. Vitamins and respiratory disease: antioxidant micronutrients in pulmonary health and disease. *Proc. Nutr. Soc.* 2005;64:510-26.

[200] De BF, Aceto A, Dragani B et al. Long-term oral n-acetylcysteine reduces exhaled hydrogen peroxide in stable COPD. *Pulm. Pharmacol. Ther.* 2005;18:41-7.

[201] Kasielski M, Nowak D. Long-term administration of N-acetylcysteine decreases hydrogen peroxide exhalation in subjects with chronic obstructive pulmonary disease. *Respir. Med.* 2001;95:448-56.

[202] Dauletbaev N, Fischer P, Aulbach B et al. A phase II study on safety and efficacy of high-dose N-acetylcysteine in patients with cystic fibrosis. *Eur. J. Med. Res.* 2009;14:352-8.

[203] Tirouvanziam R, Conrad CK, Bottiglieri T, Herzenberg LA, Moss RB, Herzenberg LA. High-dose oral N-acetylcysteine, a glutathione prodrug, modulates inflammation in cystic fibrosis. *Proc. Natl. Acad. Sci. U S A* 2006;103:4628-33.

[204] Decramer M, Rutten-van MM, Dekhuijzen PN et al. Effects of N-acetylcysteine on outcomes in chronic obstructive pulmonary disease (Bronchitis Randomized on NAC Cost-Utility Study, BRONCUS): a randomised placebo-controlled trial. *Lancet* 2005;365:1552-60.

[205] Dauletbaev N, Rickmann J, Viel K et al. Antioxidant properties of cystic fibrosis sputum. *Am. J. Physiol. Lung Cell Mol. Physiol.* 2005;288:L903-L909.

[206] Schermer T, Chavannes N, Dekhuijzen R et al. Fluticasone and N-acetylcysteine in primary care patients with COPD or chronic bronchitis. *Respir. Med.* 2009;103:542-51.

[207] Nash EF, Stephenson A, Ratjen F, Tullis E. Nebulized and oral thiol derivatives for pulmonary disease in cystic fibrosis. *Cochrane Database Syst. Rev.* 2009;CD007168.

[208] Black PN, Morgan-Day A, McMillan TE, Poole PJ, Young RP. Randomised, controlled trial of N-acetylcysteine for treatment of acute exacerbations of chronic obstructive pulmonary disease [ISRCTN21676344]. *BMC Pulm. Med.* 2004;4:13.

In: Principles of Free Radical Biomedicine, Volume III
Editors: K. Pantopoulos and H. M. Schipper

ISBN 978-1-61324-184-4
©2012 Nova SciencePublishers, Inc.

Chapter 2

Disorders of Iron Homeostasis

Giada Sebastiani[1,2,] and Kostas Pantopoulos[2]*
[1]Venetian Institute of Molecular Medicine (VIMM), Padova, Italy
[2]Lady Davis Institute for Medical Research, Sir Mortimer B. Davis Jewish General
Hospital, and Department of Medicine, McGill University, Montreal, Quebec, Canada

1. Introduction

In healthy individuals, the rate of dietary iron absorption and the levels of body iron are tightly controlled (see Vol. II, Chapter 19). *Misregulation of systemic iron homeostasis can lead to pathological conditions, ranging from anemias caused by iron deficiency or defective iron traffic, to iron overload (hemochromatosis)* [1].

Other iron-related disorders are characterized by local accumulation of the metal in mitochondria, as a result of gene mutations that affect directly or indirectly iron regulatory pathways.

Secondary iron overload develops as a complication of another disease. Thus, repeated blood transfusions, an inevitable treatment of various anemias characterized by ineffective erythropoiesis, promote transfusional siderosis, while chronic liver diseases are often associated with mild to moderate secondary iron overload.

Pathophysiological and clinical aspects of iron-related disorders are discussed below. Diseases involving iron overload in the central nervous system (CNS) are discussed separately in Chapter 10 of this Volume.

---

[*]E-mails: giagioseba@iol.it and kostas.pantopoulos@mcgill.ca

2. Anemias Caused by Iron Deficiency or Defective Iron Traffic

2.1. Iron deficiency

Dietary iron absorption serves to compensate for non-specific iron losses. Maintenance of body iron levels is essential to satisfy the high metabolic requirements of this metal for erythropoiesis. Inadequate iron absorption may result in gradual depletion of body iron stores and culminates in *iron deficiency anemia* (IDA) [2]. This condition occurs when iron becomes limiting for erythropoiesis and is caused by low availability or malabsorption of nutritional iron, or chronic blood losses related to confounding disorders. IDA is associated with complications such as disability, impaired thermoregulation, immune dysfunction and neurocognitive defects. Nutritional iron deficiency affects approximately 2 billion people worldwide, mostly in developing countries, and poses a serious health care challenge [3]. IDA is normally treated by iron supplementation therapy and can be prevented by fortification of foods with iron.

2.2. Defective Iron Traffic

Iron may become limiting for erythropoiesis even in the presence of adequate stores. This is a common side effect of prolonged inflammation, in response to infectious or autoimmune disorders or cancer. The hallmark of the *anemia of inflammation* or *anemia of chronic disease* (ACD) is the retention of iron within reticuloendothelial macrophages, accompanied by decreased dietary iron absorption that leads to hypoferremia [4]. The diversion of iron traffic from the circulation into storage sites is thought to be part of an iron withholding defense strategy of the host to deplete invading pathogens of an essential nutrient [5]. The pathogenesis of ACD is tightly associated with the induction of the iron regulatory hormone hepcidin via the IL-6/STAT3 signaling pathway [6-8], which inhibits the efflux of iron from macrophages and enterocytes via ferroportin. Inflammatory cytokines also trigger reduced proliferation of erythroid progenitor cells and altered expression of iron metabolism genes that contribute to hypoferremia. ACD is the most frequent anemia among hospitalized patients in industrial countries. Even though ACD is not lifethreatening *per se*, it can affect disease progression [9] and should be treated to improve the patient's quality of life. Treatment of the underlying primary disease provides a good therapeutic option. Targeted pharmacological correction of ACD can be achieved by administration of recombinant erythropoietin and, in acute cases, by blood transfusion. Iron supplementation therapy is controversial because it may promote bacteremia; however, it can be useful for ACD patients who also suffer from IDA. New powerful pharmacological tools for the treatment of ACD are expected to emerge from the development of small molecule inhibitors or blocking antibodies of the hepcidin pathway. Such drugs would be particularly valuable for the subset of ACD patients that respond poorly to erythropoietin. A rare congenital form of *iron refractory iron deficiency anemia* (IRIDA) is caused by mutations in the transmembrane serine protease matriptase (TMPRSS6) that leads to pathological increase in hepcidin levels and aberrant iron traffic [10]. Mice with targeted [11] or chemically-induced [12] disruption of the TMPRSS6 gene recapitulate this phenotype. Patients with IRIDA respond poorly to oral and parenteral iron therapy.

3. Hereditary Hemochromatosis

Hereditary hemochromatosis is characterized by chronic hyperabsorption of dietary iron, at a rate that may reach 8-10 mg/day [13, 14]. This results in *gradual saturation of circulating transferrin with iron (from physiological ~30% up to 100%), and the buildup of a pool of redox-active non-transferrin-bound iron (NTBI) in plasma. The toxic NTBI is eventually taken up by tissues, especially the liver and pancreas, and iron accumulates within parenchymal cells.*

Notably, macrophages and enterocytes fail to retain iron and exhibit an iron deprivation phenotype, especially at the early stages of the disease. The CNS is spared from iron overload. Excessive iron deposition in the liver parenchyma predisposes for fibrosis, cirrhosis and hepatocellular carcinoma [15-17], and may exacerbate other types of chronic liver disease [18, 19].

Iron overload is also associated with cardiomyopathy, diabetes mellitus, hypogonadism, arthritis and skin pigmentation [1]. Organ damage can be easily prevented by therapeutic phlebotomy, which reduces the iron burden. Early diagnosed and phlebotomized patients have a normal life span. Untreated patients develop clinical symptoms mostly after the fourth decade of life. Various forms of hereditary iron overload disorders are discussed below. Molecules and tissues (or cell types) implicated in disease pathogenesis are highlighted in Figure 1.

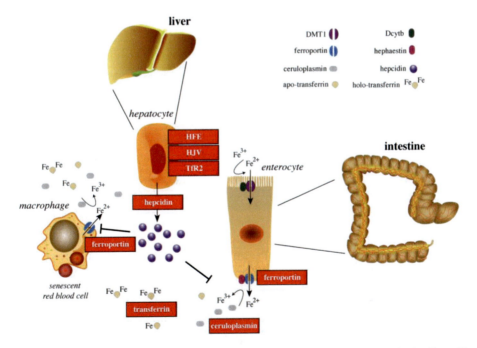

Figure 1. Misregulation of systemic iron homeostasis leads to hemochromatosis. Molecules implicated in the pathogenesis of hereditary iron overload are highlighted in red.

3.1. HFE Hemochromatosis

The most common form of hereditary iron overload (classified as hemochromatosis type 1), with autosomal recessive pattern of transmission and high prevalence in Caucasians of Northern European ancestry, is related to mutations in the hemochromatosis gene HFE [13, 14]. This was first discovered in 1996 by linkage disequilibrium and haplotype analysis from a large cohort of patients [20]. Earlier studies revealed that the hemochromatosis gene is located close to the major histocompatibility complex (MHC) locus on the short arm of chromosome 6 [21, 22]. Indeed, the HFE protein is an atypical MHC class I molecule, consisting of 3 extracellular subunits ($\alpha 1$, $\alpha 2$ and $\alpha 3$) a transmembrane domain and a cytoplasmic tail. As expected, HFE interacts with β_2-microglobulin and is expressed on the plasma membrane following processing in the endoplasmic reticulum (ER) and Golgi network. The groove between the $\alpha 1$ and $\alpha 2$ subunits of HFE is smaller to that of typical MHC class I proteins; this presumably renders it insufficient for peptide antigen presentation [23]. Nonetheless, an immunological capacity of HFE cannot be excluded [24, 25].

The majority of hemochromatosis patients express HFE with a C282Y substitution. This point mutation disrupts a disulphide bond that is essential for the association of HFE with β_2-microglobulin. Consequently, HFE C282Y is retained in the ER and fails to reach the plasma membrane [26, 27]. Eventually, the mutant protein undergoes degradation by the proteasome [28]. The frequency of the homozygous HFE C282Y genotype is approximately 1:200; however, its clinical penetrance is debatable [13-15, 29, 30]. Further disease-associated HFE mutations include H63D or S65C substitutions [31], often in compound heterozygosity with C282Y. Conceivably, apart from HFE mutations, the development of iron overload requires the contribution of additional, yet incompletely understood, environmental, genetic and/or epigenetic factors [32]. Importantly, the targeted disruption of HFE [33, 34] or β_2-microglobulin [35, 36] promotes iron overload in mice, to variable degrees among different strains [37-41]. Likewise, knock-in mice with orthologous HFE C282Y [42] and H63D [43] substitutions exhibit a similar hemochromatosis phenotype. Together with the previous genetic and clinical data, these animal studies highlight the significance of HFE in the control of body iron homeostasis.

Even though the function of HFE remains obscure, it is well established that this protein operates upstream of the hepcidin pathway and controls the expression of the iron-regulatory hormone in response to iron, possibly as part of a putative "iron sensing complex" [44] (see also Vol. II, Chapter 19). Thus, patients with HFE hemochromatosis express inappropriately low hepcidin levels [45, 46] and exhibit blunted hepcidin responses to iron challenge [47], despite high transferrin saturation and increased body iron stores. Similar results emerged from the analysis of HFE-/- mice [48-51].

3.2. Juvenile Hemochromatosis

Juvenile hemochromatosis (classified as hemochromatosis type 2) is a rare autosomal recessive disease of hereditary iron overload with early onset in the late teens and early twenties [52, 53]. Its trait is mostly found in pedigrees from Greece, Southern Italy and the Saguenay region of Quebec, Canada. The disease usually manifests with hypogonadism, cardiomyopathy and diabetes mellitus. The major locus of the juvenile hemochromatosis gene maps to the 1q chromosome [54, 55] (subtype 2A). Iron overload is caused by pathogenic mutations in the HFE2 gene encoding hemojuvelin (HJV) [56]. The most frequent is a HJV G320V substitution, but a wide spectrum of additional mutations is known [31]. Affected patients [56] and HJV-/- mice [57, 58] express extremely low levels of hepcidin, despite high iron indexes (transferrin saturation and body iron stores). These data are consistent with the function of HJV as a bone morphogenetic protein (BMP) co-receptor that is essential for efficient signaling to hepcidin [59] (Vol. II, Chapter 19). A relatively less frequent 1q-unlinked genotype of juvenile hemochromatosis has also been described [60, 61] (subtype 2B). Here, iron overload is caused by mutations in the hepcidin gene (called HAMP) on chromosome 19, leading to complete silencing of hepcidin expression [62]. The first two reported cases exhibited either a nonsense mutation leading to a premature termination codon (R56X), or a frameshift mutation yielding aberrant pro-hepcidin [62]. Disruption of the HAMP gene promotes a similar phenotype of severe tissue iron overload in mice [63, 64].

3.3. TfR2 Hemochromatosis

Another rare type of non-HFE hemochromatosis is caused by several pathogenic mutations in the transferrin receptor 2 (TfR2) gene at the chromosome 7q22 (classified as hemochromatosis type 3). Its clinical phenotype and transmission pattern are similar to that of classical HFE hemochromatosis [65, 66]. The first reported case was due to a nonsense mutation leading to a premature termination codon (Y250X) of TfR2 [67], but further mutations have been mapped [31]. TfR2-/- [68] or TfR2 knock-in mice with an orthologous Y250 substitution [69] develop iron overload and constitute models for hemochromatosis type 3. Humans [70] and mice [71] lacking functional TfR2 express inappropriately low levels of hepcidin, suggesting that TfR2 operates upstream of the hepcidin pathway, possibly as part of a putative iron sensing complex (Vol. II, Chapter 19).

3.4 Dysregulation of Hepcidin as a Common Denominator in Hereditary Hemochromatosis

Hereditary hemochromatosis comprises a genetically heterogenous group of diseases that vary in the clinical symptoms and the underlying causative mutations. *Iron overload is eventually caused by molecular defects in the hepcidin pathway that lead to inappropriately low hepcidin expression. Importantly, the impairment of this pathway quantitatively correlates with the degree of iron accumulation.* Thus, genetic disruption of the HAMP gene or severe hepcidin insufficiency due to mutations in HJV lead to early onset juvenile hemochromatosis, the most aggressive form of hereditary iron overload. On the other hand, relatively milder hepcidin insufficiency, due to mutations in HFE or TfR2, leads to late onset hemochromatosis of type 1 or 3, respectively. Considering that pathological overexpression of hepcidin promotes the development of ACD, the function of this iron regulatory hormone is analogous to that of a rheostat that controls systemic iron traffic and homeostasis (Figure 2).

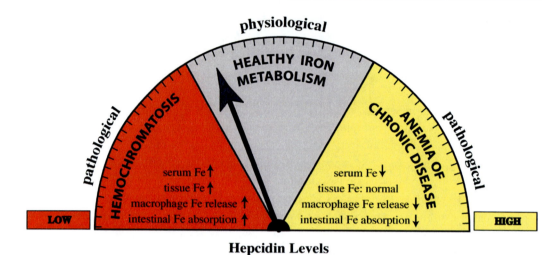

Figure 2. Hepcidin, a rheostat for systemic iron homeostasis. Physiological hepcidin levels indicate healthy iron metabolism. Pathologically low hepcidin levels are associated with mild to severe hemochromatosis; the degree of iron loading is indirectly proportional to hepcidin expression. Pathologically high hepcidin levels are associated with anemia of chronic disease (also known as anemia of inflammation).

3.5. Ferroportin Disease

Hepcidin regulates systemic iron homeostasis by binding to ferroportin and promoting its degradation, which in turn limits iron efflux from intestinal cells and macrophages. Because a failure to maintain hepcidin levels within a physiological window leads to iron related disorders, it is expected that mutations on its target ferroportin impairing iron export are incompatible with health. The "ferroportin disease" is a distinct condition of hereditary iron overload (also classified as hemochromatosis type 4) that is caused by mutations in the SLC40A1 gene on chromosome 2q32 encoding ferroportin [72] and appears to be associated with high hepcidin levels [73]. In contrast to other types of hemochromatosis, the ferroportin disease exhibits an autosomal dominant transmission pattern. It is more frequent than type 2 and 3 hemochromatosis. While the first reported cases were attributed to ferroportin N144H [74] or A77D [75] substitutions, several additional missense mutations and deletions were subsequently documented [31].

The ferroportin disease is heterogenous, with diverse phenotypes ranging from macrophage iron loading and low transferrin saturation (subtype 4A) to parenchymal iron loading and relatively high transferrin saturation analogous to classical hemochromatosis (subtype 4B). Patients with subtype 4A show reduced tolerance to phlebotomy and are prone to develop anemia in response to this treatment, despite persistently elevated serum ferritin levels. The phenotypic diversity of the ferroportin disease mirrors the effects of the underlying mutation on ferroportin function. Subtype 4A mutations impair ferroportin trafficking, resulting in macrophage iron loading. By contrast, subtype 4B mutations inhibit the binding of hepcidin to ferroportin, promoting parenchymal iron loading. The autosomal dominant inheritance can be explained by a dominant negative effect of mutations on the ferroportin dimer [76]. The *flatiron* mouse, carrying a H32R substitution in one allele of the SLC40A1 gene, recapitulates phenotypic hallmarks of subtype 4A ferroportin disease [77].

4. Hereditary Disorders of Systemic Iron Overload Unlinked to the Hepcidin Pathway

Other conditions of hereditary iron overload have been described that are not caused by defects in the hepcidin pathway. These include aceruloplasminemia and the extremely rare hypo- or atransferrinemia and heme oxygenase-1 deficiency.

4.1. Aceruloplasminemia

Loss-of-function mutations in the ceruloplasmin gene on chromosome 3q23-q24 lead to aceruloplasminemia [78]. The disease exhibits some phenotypic similarities with ferroportin disease of subtype 4A, consistent with the function of ceruloplasmin in iron efflux from macrophages and intestinal cells. These include iron overload in visceral organs (liver, pancreas and spleen), associated with low serum iron and mild microcytic anemia.

However, in contrast to ferroportin disease, aceruloplasminemia also leads to brain iron overload and neurological abnormalities [79] (for details see Chapter 10 in this Volume). This is atypical for all other forms of hemochromatosis, where excess of iron does not cross the blood-brain barrier.

Brain iron overload may result from inactivation of the astrocyte-specific glycophosphatidylinositol (GPI)-anchored ceruloplasmin isoform, which serves to stabilize ferroportin in these cells and thereby control iron efflux from the CNS [80, 81]. Clinical symptoms of aceruloplasminemia are also observed in ceruloplasmin knockout (Cp-/-) mice [82, 83].

4.2. Hypotransferrinemia or Atransferrinemia

This disease is caused by partial or complete functional inactivation of the plasma iron carrier transferrin, due to mutations in its gene on chromosome 3q21 [84, 85]. Clinical manifestations include microcytic anemia, increased dietary iron absorption and tissue iron overload.

Hypotransferrinemic (*hpx*) mice, which express inappropriately low levels of transferrin due to a spontaneous splicing defect, develop similar symptoms [86]. The deficiency in functional transferrin deprives erythroid cells of adequate iron and leads to ineffective erythropoiesis, which in turn stimulates excessive iron absorption and the buildup of NTBI in plasma. NTBI eventually accumulates in tissue parenchymal cells.

4.3. Heme Oxygenase-1 (HO-1) Deficiency

This fatal disease has been reported in a single case of a 6-year old Japanese male who presented with severe growth retardation, persistent hemolytic anemia, endothelial cell injury and massive inflammation, and succumbed soon thereafter [87]. Iron deposits in the liver and kidney were documented at biopsy and autopsy. HO-1 knockout mice survive to adulthood, but display severe pathological features including hepatic and renal iron overload [88, 89].

5. Hereditary Disorders of Mitochondrial Iron Overload

Other, rare, hereditary conditions are associated with local intracellular iron accumulation within mitochondria. Diseases of mitochondrial iron overload are caused by mutations in proteins involved in heme biosynthesis [90, 91] (such as ALAS2) or iron-sulfur cluster biogenesis [92] (such as frataxin, glutaredoxin 5, Abcb7 or ISCU). These pathways (described inVol. II, Chapter 19) consume the majority of internalized metabolic iron with key reactions taking place in mitochondria.

5.1. X-Linked Sideroblastic Anemia (XLSA)

Sporadic and familial forms of this disease are caused by mutations in ALAS2, the erythroid-specific isoform of delta-aminolevulinic acid synthase [91], which catalyzes the first step in heme biosynthesis (Vol. II, Chapter 19). Excess iron is deposited in ring-shaped granules within mitochondria, yielding iron-loaded erythroblasts (sideroblasts). A treatment with pyridoxine is efficient for most patients bearing mutations in ALAS2 that negatively affect the binding of its cofactor 5'-pyridoxal phosphate. By contrast, patients with mutations in other domains of ALAS2 do not respond to this drug. In severe cases of XLSA, systemic secondary iron overload may develop in response to blood transfusions (transfusional siderosis). In addition, primary iron overload may be triggered by ineffective erythropoiesis, combined with increased iron absorption. The zebrafish *sauternes* (sau) mutant recapitulates phenotypic hallmarks of XLSA [93].

5.2. Friedreich's Ataxia (FRDA)

This autosomal recessive neurodegenerative disorder is caused by diminished expression of frataxin, due to expansion of the GAA triplet repeat in its gene [94]. FRDA is associated with early onset gait and limb ataxia, muscle weakness and cardiomyopathy, which are linked to mitochondrial iron overload [95]; see also Chapter 10 in this Volume.

The disruption of frataxin suffices to promote mitochondrial iron overload in yeast [96], while frataxin knockout mice represent animal models of FRDA [97]. Conditional frataxin knockout mice respond to therapy with mitochondrial-specific chelators, which reduces mitochondrial iron burden [98].

5.3. X-Linked Sideroblastic Anemia with Ataxia (XLSA/A)

This rare form of XLSA is caused by missense mutations in the ATP-binding cassette of the mitochondrial transporter Abcb7 [99]. Apart from sideroblastic anemia, patients also develop early onset cerebellar ataxia. The disruption of mouse Abcb7 is embryonically lethal [100] and no animal models of XLSA/A are currently available (see also Chapter 10 in this Volume).

5.4. Deficiency in ISCU

Splicing defects resulting in low expression of the scaffold protein ISCU manifest as a hereditary myopathy with exercise intolerance and lactic acidosis [101, 102]. The insufficiency of ISCU associates with aberrant mitochondrial iron metabolism. Muscles of affected patients exhibit reduced levels of IRP1 (Vol. II, Chapter 19), possibly due to iron-dependent destabilization of accumulated apo-IRP1 [103, 104].

5.5. Deficiency in Glutaredoxin 5

A splicing defect resulting in reduced expression of the iron-sulfur cluster assembly co-factor glutaredoxin 5 (Grx5), has been linked to a sideroblastic-like form of microcytic anemia and blood transfusion-related systemic iron overload [105]. The complete disruption of Grx5 promotes severe anemia and early embryonic lethality in the *shiraz* zebrafish mutant [106]. In these animals, the lack of Grx5 allows accumulation of apo-IRP1 that represses ALAS2 mRNA and thereby inhibits heme biosynthesis.

6. Transfusional Siderosis and Iron Chelation Therapy

Patients suffering from hereditary or acquired anemias associated with ineffective erythropoiesis (such as thalassemias, sickle cell disease, XLSA, aplastic or hemolytic anemias, congenital dyserythropoietic anemias or myelodysplastic syndromes) require frequent blood transfusion therapy. *Transfused red cells add substantial amounts of iron to the recipient's organism (up to ~ 1 mg/ml of red cells), eventually leading to the development of transfusional siderosis, a form of secondary ironoverload* [107]. Ineffective erythropoiesis also triggers increased dietary iron absorption in the intestine via silencing of hepcidin expression. In thalassemias, hepcidin mRNA transcription is blocked by upregulation of growth differentiation factor 15 (GDF15), a member of the transforming growth factor β (TGFβ) superfamily [108] (see alsoVol. II, Chapter 19). *Iron from transfused red blood cells initially accumulates in reticuloendothelial macrophages of the recipient. At later stages, iron deposits are also formed within tissue parenchymal cells, where they are considered to be more toxic.* Excess of iron in myocardial fiber cells triggers cardiomyopathy and heart failure, a common complication of transfusional siderosis. Iron chelation therapy can mitigate rapidly progressive heart failure and arrhythmias [109].

Iron chelators can be bidentate, tridentate or hexadentate molecules that offer two, three or six atoms, respectively, for iron coordination in an octahedral orientation [110, 111]. *Clinically applied chelators diminish iron's redox reactivity by occupying its coordination site and sterically inhibiting its interaction with reactive oxygen species.* Hexadentate chelators tend to be more efficient in this regard than chelators with lower denticity because they form more stable complexes in a 1:1 stoichiometry [112]. The full occupation of iron's coordination sphere requires two or three molecules of tri- or bidentate chelators, respectively.

Desferrioxamine (DFO), a hexadentate chelator of the hydroxamate class, has been the most widely applied drug for the treatment of transfusional siderosis over the past 40 years [109, 110]. This natural siderophore is generated by *Streptomyces pilosus* and secreted to capture extracellular iron for metabolic purposes. While DFO is generally safe and exhibits high efficacy in clinical settings, its administration is cumbersome and requires prolonged parenteral infusions. The reduced oral bioavailability of DFO is related to its relatively high molecular mass (Mw 561) and hydrophilicity that prevent passive diffusion of the drug across cellular membranes. Cells take up circulating DFO by fluid phase endocytosis [113]. Following chelation of intracellular iron, the drug is excreted in the urine and stool.

A wide range of small molecules with iron chelating properties can reduce iron burden in cell culture and animal models. However, only few compounds have been approved for clinical use. Deferiprone (L1), an orally absorbed, lipophilic bidentate chelator, has been clinically applied as an alternative to DFO. However, L1 monotherapy has also been associated with agranulocytosis, neutropenia, liver dysfunction and other adverse effects, while a combined DFO/L1 regimen appears to be better tolerated [109]. Deferasirox, a more recently developed lipophilic tridentate oral chelator, appears to be efficacious and safe for the treatment of transfusional siderosis [109].

7. Iron Overload Secondary to Chronic Liver Diseases

Hereditary hemochromatosis and transfusional siderosis are associated with severe iron overload that can eventually lead to multiple organ failure, including liver damage. Interestingly, patients with non-hemochromatotic chronic liver diseases frequently exhibit minimal to modest accumulation of excess hepatic iron. *A downregulation of hepcidin expression in response to oxidative stress* [114, 115] *very likely contributes to this type of secondary iron overload, at least in chronic hepatitis C* [116] (see also Chapter 4 in this Volume). Deposition of excess iron may exacerbate liver injury and predispose to hepatic fibrosis [19, 117, 118].

Its negative impact has been documented in several conditions that are highly prevalent in the general population, such as chronic infection by hepatitis C (HCV) and B (HBV) viruses, alcoholic and non-alcoholic fatty liver diseases, insulin resistance-hepatic iron overload syndrome and porphyria cutanea tarda. The role of iron in the progression of chronic liver diseases is extensively discussed in Chapter 4 of this Volume.

8. Hereditary Hyperferritinemia-Cataract Syndrome (HHCS)

HHCS is not an iron-related disorder in a strict sense. This autosomal dominant condition is characterized by early onset cataract and a profound (up to 20-fold) increase in serum ferritin levels without iron overload or any other abnormalities in systemic or local iron homeostasis [119]. HHCS is etiologically linked to mutations in L-ferritin IRE (seeVol. II,

Chapter 19) that prevent the binding of IRPs and result in unrestricted L-ferritin mRNA translation [120].

Several HHCS-associated mutations in L-ferritin IRE, including deletions and point mutations, have been reported [119]. The biochemical phenotype of HHCS correlates well with the degree of inhibition of IRP-binding [121]. Nevertheless, individuals sharing the same mutation may present with variable clinical phenotypes, indicating an involvement of additional factors in disease progression [119].

Experiments in lymphoblastoid cell lines and in surgery-recovered lens from HHCS patients suggest that the overproduction of L-ferritin disrupts the H-/L- equilibrium in holo-ferritin [122]. The accumulation of L-homopolymers may trigger the development of cataract. The generation of animal models for HHCS is expected to shed more light on the pathogenetic mechanism.

9. Stepwise Decision Tree for the Diagnosis of Systemic Iron Overload

The management of iron overload states should be a sequential process that initiates with the clinical suspicion and diagnosis (Figure 3). Clinical manifestations include asthenia, fatigue, arthralgias, skin pigmentation, impotence, diabetes, osteopenia, hepatomegaly, and cardiac abnormalities including rhythm disturbances and heart failure. Early age at presentation may indicate juvenile hemochromatosis, with symptoms mostly related to heart, liver and endocrine glands. Elevated serum ferritin concentration (>200 µg/L in females and >300 µg/L in males) is a typical biochemical index of an iron overload state. However, before considering the possibility for hereditary hemochromatosis, it is essential to exclude other frequent unrelated causes of hyperferritinemia; for example metabolic syndrome (obesity or increased body mass index in conjunction with one or more among hypertension, non-insulin-dependent diabetes, hyperlipidemia and hyperuricemia), inflammatory or neoplastic conditions. Secondary iron overload due to transfusional siderosis or chronic liver disease (that is associated with mild to moderate hyperferritinemia), as well as the rare possibility of HHCS should also be excluded. The next step is to evaluate visceral iron excess by non-invasive techniques (magnetic resonance imaging) or by liver biopsy with Perls' iron staining. The absence of severe liver fibrosis can be predicted by clinical and biochemical variables (a combination of absence of hepatomegaly at clinical examination, normal aspartate aminotransferase and serum ferritin <1000 µg/L) [123]. In chronic hepatitis C, a cut-off of serum ferritin of 450 µg/L for males and of 350 µg/L for females may exclude significant hepatic iron overload (≥ grade II on a four grade scale) with high certainty [124]. Liver biopsy serves not only for the diagnosis and quantification of hepatic iron deposition, but also for staging liver disease through semiquantification of liver fibrosis and necroinflammatory activity. Over the past few years, systematic efforts to reduce the need for liver biopsy have culminated in the development of non-invasive diagnostic approaches for liver fibrosis in chronic liver diseases, by means of instrumental devices and/or serum biochemical markers [125]. Thus far, these new methods have found only limited applications in hemochromatosis patients [126] and future longitudinal, prospective studies are expected to establish their diagnostic potential in this context.

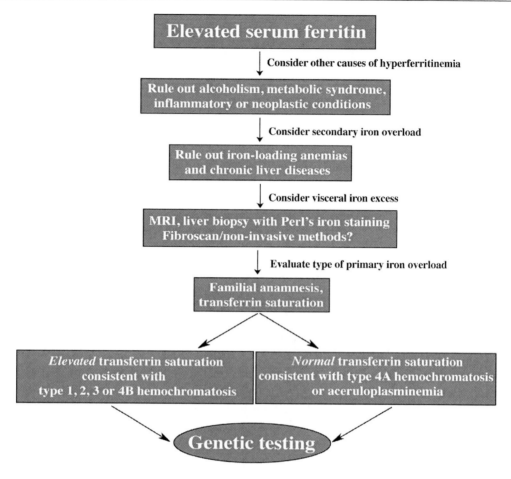

Figure 3. Stepwise decision tree for the clinical management of iron overload states.

If the suspicion for primary iron overload persists after exclusion of the aforementioned conditions, a careful familial anamnesis (account of medical history) and the determination of all serum iron indices are necessary. Familial anamnesis, especially related to first-degree relatives, may lead to the identification of further patients with late or early onset.

Elevated transferrin saturation in Caucasians (>60% in males and >50% in females) is consistent with HFE-hemochromatosis (type 1), which can be confirmed by genotyping (C282Y homozygosity or other less frequent mutations, such as C282Y/H63D compound heterozygosity).

If typical HFE-related genotypes are absent or the patient is not Caucasian or of Northern European ancestry, other types of non-HFE hemochromatosis should be considered. Juvenile hemochromatosis (subtypes 2A or 2B) is likely in younger patients (<30 years), and TfR2-related hemochromatosis (type 3) or ferroportin disease (subtype 4B) are possible in older patients. When normal or low transferrin saturation is found (<45%), plasma ceruloplasmin should be determined to examine the possibility for aceruloplasminemia, especially in patients with anemia and/or neurological symptoms.

If ceruloplasmin levels are normal, the most likely diagnosis is ferroportin disease (subtype 4A). Once the genotype of hemochromatosis has been established, family screening should be performed.

Conclusions

The regulation of systemic and cellular iron metabolism is critical for health and its disruption leads to disease. Here, we provided an overview of the clinical features, molecular pathogenesis and management of various iron-related disorders. The overwhelming majority of such clinically relevant conditions are linked to defects in the hepcidin pathway. The development of novel drugs to pharmacologically control this pathway poses a challenge for the management of iron-related disorders.

Acknowledgments

GS is funded by an unrestricted grant from Roche-Italia. KP is funded by the Canadian Institutes for Health Research (CIHR) and holds a *Chercheur National* career award from the *Fonds de la recherche en santé du Quebec* (FRSQ).

References

[1]   Andrews NC. Disorders of iron metabolism. *N. Engl. J. Med.* 1999;341:1986-95.
[2]   Clark SF. Iron deficiency anemia. *Nutr. Clin. Pract.* 2008;23:128-41.
[3]   Zimmermann MB, Hurrell RF. Nutritional iron deficiency. *Lancet,* 2007;370:511-20.
[4]   Weiss G, Goodnough LT. Anemia of chronic disease. *N. Engl. J. Med.* 2005;352:1011-23.
[5]   Weinberg ED. Iron availability and infection. *Biochim. Biophys. Acta,* 2009;1790:600-5.
[6]   Wrighting DM, Andrews NC. Interleukin-6 induces hepcidin expression through STAT3. *Blood,* 2006;108:3204-9.
[7]   Pietrangelo A, Dierssen U, Valli L, et al. STAT3 is required for IL-6-gp130-dependent activation of hepcidin in vivo. *Gastroenterology,* 2007;132:294-300.
[8]   Verga Falzacappa MV, Vujic Spasic M, Kessler R, Stolte J, Hentze MW, Muckenthaler MU. STAT3 mediates hepatic hepcidin expression and its inflammatory stimulation. *Blood,* 2007;109:353-8.
[9]   Spivak JL. The anaemia of cancer: death by a thousand cuts. *Nat. Rev. Cancer.* 2005;5:543-55.
[10] Finberg KE, Heeney MM, Campagna DR, et al. Mutations in TMPRSS6 cause iron-refractory iron deficiency anemia (IRIDA). *Nat. Genet.* 2008;40:569-71.
[11] Folgueras AR, Martin de Lara F, Pendas AM, et al. The membrane-bound serine protease matriptase-2 (Tmprss6) is an essential regulator of iron homeostasis. *Blood,* 2008;112:2539-45.
[12] Du X, She E, Gelbart T, et al. The Serine Protease TMPRSS6 Is Required to Sense Iron Deficiency. *Science,* 2008;320:1088-92.
[13] Pietrangelo A. Hereditary hemochromatosis - a new look at an old disease. *N. Engl. J. Med.* 2004;350:2383-97.

[14] Beutler E. Hemochromatosis: genetics and pathophysiology. *Annu. Rev. Med.* 2006;57:331-47.

[15] Adams PC, Barton JC. Haemochromatosis. *Lancet,* 2007;370:1855-60.

[16] Ramm GA, Ruddell RG. Hepatotoxicity of iron overload: mechanisms of iron-induced hepatic fibrogenesis. *Semin. Liver Dis.* 2005;25:433-49.

[17] Kowdley KV. Iron, hemochromatosis, and hepatocellular carcinoma. *Gastroenterology,* 2004;127:S79-86.

[18] Pietrangelo A. Iron-induced oxidant stress in alcoholic liver fibrogenesis. *Alcohol,* 2003;30:121-9.

[19] Sebastiani G, Walker AP. HFE gene in primary and secondary hepatic iron overload. *World J. Gastroenterol.* 2007;13:4673-89.

[20] Feder JN, Gnirke A, Thomas W, et al. A novel MHC class I-like gene is mutated in patients with hereditary haemochromatosis. *Nat. Genet.* 1996;13:399-408.

[21] Simon M, Bourel M, Fauchet R, Genetet B. Association of HLA-A3 and HLA-B14 antigens with idiopathic haemochromatosis. *Gut,* 1976;17:332-4.

[22] Jazwinska EC, Lee SC, Webb SI, Halliday JW, Powell LW. Localization of the hemochromatosis gene close to D6S105. *Am. J. Hum. Genet.* 1993;53:347-52.

[23] Lebrón JA, Bennet MJ, Vaughn DE, et al. Crystal structure of the hemochromatosis protein HFE and characterization of its interaction with transferrin receptor. *Cell.* 1998;93:111-23.

[24] Rohrlich PS, Fazilleau N, Ginhoux F, et al. Direct recognition by alphabeta cytolytic T cells of Hfe, a MHC class Ib molecule without antigen-presenting function. *Proc. Natl. Acad. Sci. USA,* 2005;102:12855-60.

[25] de Almeida SF, Carvalho IF, Cardoso CS, et al. HFE cross-talks with the MHC class I antigen presentation pathway. *Blood,* 2005;106:971-7.

[26] Feder JN, Tsuchihashi Z, Irrinki A, et al. The hemochromatosis founder mutation in HLA-H disrupts b_2-microglobulin interaction and cell surface expression. *J. Biol. Chem.* 1997;272:14025-8.

[27] Waheed A, Parkkila S, Zhou XY, et al. Hereditary hemochromatosis: Effects of C282Y and H63D mutations on association with b_2-microglobulin, intracellular processing, and cell surface expression of the HFE protein in COS-7 cells. *Proc. Natl. Acad. Sci. USA,* 1997;94:12384-9.

[28] de Almeida SF, Fleming JV, Azevedo JE, Carmo-Fonseca M, de Sousa M. Stimulation of an unfolded protein response impairs MHC class I expression. *J. Immunol.* 2007;178:3612-9.

[29] Allen KJ, Gurrin LC, Constantine CC, et al. Iron-overload-related disease in HFE hereditary hemochromatosis. *N. Engl. J. Med.* 2008;358:221-30.

[30] Waalen J, Beutler E. Iron-overload-related disease in HFE hereditary hemochromatosis. *N. Engl. J. Med.* 2008;358:2293-4; author reply 4-5.

[31] Lee PL, Beutler E. Regulation of hepcidin and iron-overload disease. *Annu. Rev. Pathol.* 2009;4:489-515.

[32] Beutler E. Iron storage disease: facts, fiction and progress. *Blood Cells Mol. Dis.* 2007;39:140-7.

[33] Zhou XY, Tomatsu S, Fleming RE, et al. HFE gene knockout produces mouse model of hereditary hemochromatosis. *Proc. Natl. Acad. Sci. USA,* 1998;95:2492-7.

[34] Bahram S, Gilfillan S, Kühn LC, et al. Experimental hemochromatosis due to MHC class I HFE deficiency: immune status and iron metabolism. *Proc. Natl. Acad. Sci. USA,* 1999;96:13312-7.

[35] de Sousa M, Reimao R, Lacerda R, Hugo P, Kaufmann SHE, Porto G. Iron overload in b$_2$-microglobulin-deficient mice. *Immunol. Lett.* 1994;39:105-11.

[36] Rothenberg BE, Voland JR. b$_2$ knockout mice develop parenchymal iron overload: a putative role for class I genes of the major histocompatibility complex in iron metabolism. *Proc. Natl. Acad. Sci. USA,* 1996;93:1529-34.

[37] Fleming RE, Holden CC, Tomatsu S, et al. Mouse strain differences determine severity of iron accumulation in Hfe knockout model of hereditary hemochromatosis. *Proc. Natl. Acad. Sci. USA,* 2001;98:2707-11.

[38] Levy JE, Montross LK, Andrews NC. Genes that modify the hemochromatosis phenotype in mice. *J. Clin. Invest.* 2000;105:1209-16.

[39] Sproule TJ, Jazwinska EC, Britton RS, et al. Naturally variant autosomal and sex-linked loci determine the severity of iron overload in beta 2-microglobulin-deficient mice. *Proc. Natl. Acad. Sci. USA,* 2001;98:5170-4.

[40] Bensaid M, Fruchon S, Mazeres C, Bahram S, Roth MP, Coppin H. Multigenic control of hepatic iron loading in a murine model of hemochromatosis. *Gastroenterology,* 2004;126:1400-8.

[41] Wang F, Paradkar PN, Custodio AO, et al. Genetic variation in Mon1a affects protein trafficking and modifies macrophage iron loading in mice. *Nat. Genet.* 2007;39:1025-32.

[42] Levy JE, Montross LK, Cohen DE, Fleming MD, Andrews NC. The C282Y mutation causing hereditary hemochromatosis does not produce a null allele. *Blood,* 1999;94:9-11.

[43] Tomatsu S, Orii KO, Fleming RE, et al. Contribution of the H63D mutation in HFE to murine hereditary hemochromatosis. *Proc. Natl. Acad. Sci. USA,* 2003;100:15788-93.

[44] Pantopoulos K. Function of the hemochromatosis protein HFE: Lessons from animal models. *World J. Gastroenterol.* 2008;14:6893-901.

[45] Bridle KR, Frazer DM, Wilkins SJ, et al. Disrupted hepcidin regulation in HFE-associated haemochromatosis and the liver as a regulator of body iron homoeostasis. *Lancet,* 2003;361:669-73.

[46] Gehrke SG, Kulaksiz H, Herrmann T, et al. Expression of hepcidin in hereditary hemochromatosis: evidence for a regulation in response to serum transferrin saturation and non-transferrin-bound iron. *Blood,* 2003;102:371-6.

[47] Piperno A, Girelli D, Nemeth E, et al. Blunted hepcidin response to oral iron challenge in HFE-related hemochromatosis. *Blood,* 2007;110:4096-100.

[48] Ahmad KA, Ahmann JR, Migas MC, et al. Decreased liver hepcidin expression in the hfe knockout mouse. *Blood Cells Mol. Dis.* 2002;29:361-6.

[49] Muckenthaler M, Roy CN, Custodio AO, et al. Regulatory defects in liver and intestine implicate abnormal hepcidin and Cybrd1 expression in mouse hemochromatosis. *Nat. Genet.* 2003;34:102-7.

[50] Constante M, Jiang W, Wang D, Raymond VA, Bilodeau M, Santos MM. Distinct requirements for Hfe in basal and induced hepcidin levels in iron overload and inflammation. *Am. J. Physiol. Gastrointest. Liver Physiol.* 2006;291:G229-37.

[51] Ludwiczek S, Theurl I, Bahram S, Schumann K, Weiss G. Regulatory networks for the control of body iron homeostasis and their dysregulation in HFE mediated hemochromatosis. *J. Cell Physiol.* 2005;204:489-99.

[52] Camaschella C, Roetto A, De Gobbi M. Juvenile hemochromatosis. *Semin. Hematol.* 2002;39:242-8.

[53] Pietrangelo A. Juvenile hemochromatosis. *J. Hepatol.* 2006;45:892-4.

[54] Roetto A, Totaro A, Cazzola M, et al. Juvenile hemochromatosis locus maps to chromosome 1q. *Am. J. Hum. Genet.* 1999;64:1388-93.

[55] Rivard SR, Lanzara C, Grimard D, et al. Juvenile hemochromatosis locus maps to chromosome 1q in a French Canadian population. *Eur. J. Hum. Genet.* 2003;11:585-9.

[56] Papanikolaou G, Samuels ME, Ludwig EH, et al. Mutations in HFE2 cause iron overload in chromosome 1q-linked juvenile hemochromatosis. *Nat. Genet.* 2004;36:77-82.

[57] Huang FW, Pinkus JL, Pinkus GS, Fleming MD, Andrews NC. A mouse model of juvenile hemochromatosis. *J. Clin. Invest.* 2005;115:2187-91.

[58] Niederkofler V, Salie R, Arber S. Hemojuvelin is essential for dietary iron sensing, and its mutation leads to severe iron overload. *J. Clin. Invest.* 2005;115:2180-6.

[59] Babitt JL, Huang FW, Wrighting DM, et al. Bone morphogenetic protein signaling by hemojuvelin regulates hepcidin expression. *Nat. Genet.* 2006;38:531-9.

[60] Papanikolaou G, Politou M, Roetto A, et al. Linkage to chromosome 1q in Greek families with juvenile hemochromatosis. *Blood Cells Mol. Dis.* 2001;27:744-9.

[61] Papanikolaou G, Papaioannou M, Politou M, et al. Genetic heterogeneity underlies juvenile hemochromatosis phenotype: analysis of three families of northern Greek origin. *Blood Cells Mol. Dis.* 2002;29:168-73.

[62] Roetto A, Papanikolaou G, Politou M, et al. Mutant antimicrobial peptide hepcidin is associated with severe juvenile hemochromatosis. *Nat. Genet.* 2003;33:21-2.

[63] Nicolas G, Bennoun M, Devaux I, et al. Lack of hepcidin gene expression and severe tissue iron overload in upstream stimulatory factor 2 (USF2) knockout mice. *Proc. Natl. Acad. Sci. USA,* 2001;98:8780-5.

[64] Lesbordes-Brion JC, Viatte L, Bennoun M, et al. Targeted disruption of the hepcidin 1 gene results in severe hemochromatosis. *Blood,* 2006;108:1402-5.

[65] Pietrangelo A. Non-HFE hemochromatosis. *Hepatology,* 2004;39:21-9.

[66] Wallace DF, Subramaniam VN. Non-HFE haemochromatosis. *World J. Gastroenterol.* 2007;13:4690-8.

[67] Camaschella C, Roetto A, Cali A, et al. The gene TFR2 is mutated in a new type of haemochromatosis mapping to 7q22. *Nat. Genet.* 2000;25:14-5.

[68] Wallace DF, Summerville L, Subramaniam VN. Targeted disruption of the hepatic transferrin receptor 2 gene in mice leads to iron overload. *Gastroenterology,* 2007;132:301-10.

[69] Fleming RE, Ahmann JR, Migas MC, et al. Targeted mutagenesis of the murine transferrin receptor-2 gene produces hemochromatosis. *Proc. Natl. Acad. Sci. USA,* 2002;99:10653-8.

[70] Nemeth E, Roetto A, Garozzo G, Ganz T, Camaschella C. Hepcidin is decreased in TFR2 hemochromatosis. *Blood,* 2005;105:1803-6.

[71] Kawabata H, Fleming RE, Gui D, et al. Expression of hepcidin is down-regulated in TfR2 mutant mice manifesting a phenotype of hereditary hemochromatosis. *Blood,* 2005;105:376-81.

[72] Pietrangelo A. The ferroportin disease. *Blood Cells Mol. Dis.* 2004;32:131-8.

[73] Papanikolaou G, Tzilianos M, Christakis JI, et al. Hepcidin in iron overload disorders. *Blood,* 2005;105:4103-5.

[74] Njajou OT, Vaessen N, Joosse M, et al. A mutation in SLC11A3 is associated with autosomal dominant hemochromatosis. *Nat. Genet.* 2001;28:213-4.

[75] Montosi G, Donovan A, Totaro A, et al. Autosomal-dominant hemochromatosis is associated with a mutation in the ferroportin (SLC11A3) gene. *J. Clin. Invest.* 2001;108:619-23.

[76] De Domenico I, Ward DM, Nemeth E, et al. The molecular basis of ferroportin-linked hemochromatosis. *Proc. Natl. Acad. Sci. USA,* 2005;102:8955-60.

[77] Zohn IE, De Domenico I, Pollock A, et al. The flatiron mutation in mouse ferroportin acts as a dominant negative to cause ferroportin disease. *Blood,* 2007;109:4174-80.

[78] Yoshida K, Furihata K, Takeda S, et al. A mutation in the ceruloplasmin gene is associated with systemic hemosiderosis in humans. *Nat. Genet.* 1995;9:267-72.

[79] Nittis T, Gitlin JD. The copper-iron connection: Hereditary aceruloplasminemia. *Semin. Hematol.* 2002;39:282-9.

[80] Jeong SY, David S. Glycosylphosphatidylinositol-anchored ceruloplasmin is required for iron efflux from cells in the central nervous system. *J. Biol. Chem.* 2003;278:27144-8.

[81] De Domenico I, Ward DM, di Patti MC, et al. Ferroxidase activity is required for the stability of cell surface ferroportin in cells expressing GPI-ceruloplasmin. *EMBO J.* 2007;26:2823-31.

[82] Harris ZL, Durley AP, Man TK, Gitlin JD. Targeted gene disruption reveals an essential role for ceruloplasmin in cellular iron efflux. *Proc. Natl. Acad. Sci. USA,* 1999;96:10812-7.

[83] Patel BN, Dunn RJ, Jeong SY, Zhu Q, Julien JP, David S. Ceruloplasmin regulates iron levels in the CNS and prevents free radical injury. *J. Neurosci.* 2002;22:6578-86.

[84] Hayashi A, Wada Y, Suzuki T, Shimizu A. Studies on familial hypotransferrinemia: unique clinical course and molecular pathology. *Am. J. Hum. Genet.* 1993;53:201-13.

[85] Beutler E, Gelbart T, Lee P, Trevino R, Fernandez MA, Fairbanks VF. Molecular characterization of a case of atransferrinemia. *Blood,* 2000;96:4071-4.

[86] Trenor CC, Campagna DR, Sellers VM, Andrews NC, Fleming MD. The molecular defect in hypotransferrinemic mice. *Blood,* 2000;96:1113-8.

[87] Yachie A, Niida Y, Wada T, et al. Oxidative stress causes enhanced endothelial cell injury in human heme oxygenase-1 deficiency. *J. Clin. Invest.* 1999;103:129-35.

[88] Poss KD, Tonegawa S. Heme oxygenase 1 is required for mammalian iron reutilization. *Proc. Natl. Acad. Sci. USA,* 1997;94:10919-24.

[89] Poss KD, Tonegawa S. Reduced stress defense in heme oxygenase 1-deficient cells. *Proc. Natl. Acad. Sci. USA,* 1997;94:10925-30.

[90] Ryter SW, Tyrrell RM. The heme synthesis and degradation pathways: role in oxidant sensitivity. Heme oxygenase has both pro- and antioxidant properties. *Free Radic. Biol. Med.* 2000;28:289-309.

[91] Ponka P. Tissue-specific regulation of iron metabolism and heme synthesis: distinct control mechanisms in erythroid cells. *Blood*, 1997;89:1-25.

[92] Lill R. Function and biogenesis of iron-sulphur proteins. *Nature*, 2009;460:831-8.

[93] Brownlie A, Donovan A, Pratt SJ, et al. Positional cloning of the zebrafish sauternes gene: a model for congenital sideroblastic anaemia. *Nat. Genet.* 1998;20:244-50.

[94] Campuzano V, Montermini L, Molto MD, et al. Friedreich's ataxia: autosomal recessive disease caused by an intronic GAA triplet repeat expansion. *Science*, 1996;271:1423-7.

[95] Pandolfo M. Friedreich's ataxia: clinical aspects and pathogenesis. *Semin. Neurol.* 1999;19:311-21.

[96] Babcock M, de Silva D, Oaks R, et al. Regulation of mitochondrial iron accumulation by Yfh1p, a putative homolog of frataxin. *Science,* 1997;276:1709-12.

[97] Puccio H, Simon D, Cossee M, et al. Mouse models for Friedreich ataxia exhibit cardiomyopathy, sensory nerve defect and Fe-S enzyme deficiency followed by intramitochondrial iron deposits. *Nat. Genet.* 2001;27:181-6.

[98] Whitnall M, Rahmanto YS, Sutak R, et al. The MCK mouse heart model of Friedreich's ataxia: Alterations in iron-regulated proteins and cardiac hypertrophy are limited by iron chelation. *Proc. Natl. Acad. Sci. U S A* 2008;105:9757-62.

[99] Allikmets R, Raskind WH, Hutchinson A, Schueck ND, Dean M, Koeller DM. Mutation of a putative mitochondrial iron transporter gene (ABC7) in X-linked sideroblastic anemia and ataxia (XLSA/A). *Hum. Mol. Genet.* 1999;8:743-9.

[100] Pondarre C, Antiochos BB, Campagna DR, et al. The mitochondrial ATP-binding cassette transporter Abcb7 is essential in mice and participates in cytosolic iron-sulfur cluster biogenesis. *Hum. Mol. Genet.* 2006;15:953-64.

[101] Mochel F, Knight MA, Tong WH, et al. Splice mutation in the iron-sulfur cluster scaffold protein ISCU causes myopathy with exercise intolerance. *Am. J. Hum. Genet.* 2008;82:652-60.

[102] Olsson A, Lind L, Thornell LE, Holmberg M. Myopathy with lactic acidosis is linked to chromosome 12q23.3-24.11 and caused by an intron mutation in the ISCU gene resulting in a splicing defect. *Hum. Mol. Genet.* 2008;17:1666-72.

[103] Clarke SL, Vasanthakumar A, Anderson SA, et al. Iron-responsive degradation of iron-regulatory protein 1 does not require the Fe-S cluster. *EMBO J.* 2006;25:544-53.

[104] Wang J, Fillebeen C, Chen G, Biederbick A, Lill R, Pantopoulos K. Iron-dependent degradation of apo-IRP1 by the ubiquitin-proteasome pathway. *Mol. Cell Biol.* 2007;27:2423-30.

[105] Camaschella C, Campanella A, De Falco L, et al. The human counterpart of zebrafish shiraz shows sideroblastic-like microcytic anemia and iron overload. *Blood* 2007;110:1353-8.

[106] Wingert RA, Galloway JL, Barut B, et al. Deficiency of glutaredoxin 5 reveals Fe-S clusters are required for vertebrate haem synthesis. *Nature* 2005;436:1035-9.

[107] Pippard MJ. Secondary iron overload. London: W. B. Saunders Company Ltd; 1994, 271-309.

[108] Tanno T, Bhanu NV, Oneal PA, et al. High levels of GDF15 in thalassemia suppress expression of the iron regulatory protein hepcidin. *Nat. Med.* 2007;13:1096-101.

[109] Cappellini MD, Pattoneri P. Oral iron chelators. *Annu. Rev. Med.* 2009;60:25-38.

[110] Tam TF, Leung-Toung R, Li W, Wang Y, Karimian K, Spino M. Iron chelator research: past, present, and future. *Curr. Med. Chem.* 2003;10:983-95.

[111] Kontoghiorghes GJ, Pattichis K, Neocleous K, Kolnagou A. The design and development of deferiprone (L1) and other iron chelators for clinical use: targeting methods and application prospects. *Curr. Med. Chem.* 2004;11:2161-83.

[112] Liu ZD, Hider RC. Design of clinically useful iron(III)-selective chelators. *Med. Res. Rev.* 2002;22:26-64.

[113] Doulias PT, Christoforidis S, Brunk UT, Galaris D. Endosomal and lysosomal effects of desferrioxamine: protection of HeLa cells from hydrogen peroxide-induced DNA damage and induction of cell-cycle arrest. *Free Radic. Biol. Med.* 2003;35:719-28.

[114] Nishina S, Hino K, Korenaga M, et al. Hepatitis C virus-induced reactive oxygen species raise hepatic iron level in mice by reducing hepcidin transcription. *Gastroenterology,* 2008;134:226-38.

[115] Miura K, Taura K, Kodama Y, Schnabl B, Brenner DA. Hepatitis C virus-induced oxidative stress suppresses hepcidin expression through increased histone deacetylase activity. *Hepatology* 2008;48:1420-9.

[116] Fujita N, Sugimoto R, Motonishi S, et al. Patients with chronic hepatitis C achieving a sustained virological response to peginterferon and ribavirin therapy recover from impaired hepcidin secretion. *J. Hepatol.* 2008;49:702-10.

[117] Adams P, Brissot P, Powell LW. EASL International Consensus Conference on Haemochromatosis. *J. Hepatol.* 2000;33:485-504.

[118] Alla V, Bonkovsky HL. Iron in nonhemochromatotic liver disorders. *Semin. Liver Dis.* 2005;25:461-72.

[119] Roetto A, Bosio S, Gramaglia E, Barilaro MR, Zecchina G, Camaschella C. Pathogenesis of hyperferritinemia cataract syndrome. *Blood Cells Mol. Dis.* 2002;29:532-5.

[120] Beaumont C, Leneuve P, Devaux I, et al. Mutation in the iron responsive element of the L ferritin mRNA in a family with dominant hyperferritinaemia and cataract. *Nat. Genet.* 1995;11:444-6.

[121] Allerson CR, Cazzola M, Rouault TA. Clinical severity and thermodynamic effects of iron-responsive element mutations in hereditary hyperferritinemia-cataract syndrome. *J. Biol. Chem.* 1999;274:26439-47.

[122] Levi S, Girelli D, Perrone F, et al. Analysis of ferritins in lymphoblastoid cell lines and in the lens of subjects with hereditary hyperferritinemia-cataract syndrome. *Blood,* 1998;91:4180-7.

[123] Guyader D, Jacquelinet C, Moirand R, et al. Noninvasive prediction of fibrosis in C282Y homozygous hemochromatosis. *Gastroenterology* 1998;115:929-36.

[124] Sebastiani G, Vario A, Ferrari A, Pistis R, Noventa F, Alberti A. Hepatic iron, liver steatosis and viral genotypes in patients with chronic hepatitis C. *J. Viral. Hepat.* 2006;13:199-205.

[125] Sebastiani G, Alberti A. Non invasive fibrosis biomarkers reduce but not substitute the need for liver biopsy. *World J. Gastroenterol.* 2006;12:3682-94.

[126] Adhoute X, Foucher J, Laharie D, et al. Diagnosis of liver fibrosis using FibroScan and other noninvasive methods in patients with hemochromatosis: a prospective study. *Gastroenterol. Clin. Biol.* 2008;32:180-7.

In: Principles of Free Radical Biomedicine, Volume III
Editors: K. Pantopoulos and H. M. Schipper

ISBN 978-1-61324-184-4
©2012 Nova SciencePublishers, Inc.

Chapter 3

Wilson Disease

*Maryam Moini[1] and Michael L. Schilsky[2, *]*

[1]Shiraz Organ Transplant Center, Division of Gastroenterology and Hepatology,
Department of Internal Medicine, Shiraz University of Medical Sciences, Shiraz, Iran
[2]Section of Transplantation and Immunologyg and Yale New Haven Transplantation
Center, Division of Digestive Diseases, Departments of Medicine and Surgery, Yale
University Medical Center, New Haven, Connecticut, U.S.A.

1. Introduction

Copper is an essential trace element and plays an integral role in cellular and trace metal metabolism. This metal is involved in several intracellular enzymatic activities including cellular respiration, neurotransmitter biosynthesis, connective tissue formation and free radical eradication. However, in high intracellular concentration copper may induce tissue injury. The liver plays a central role in copper metabolism and is a site for copper storage. The liver is also the target organ of injury in the inherited disorder of copper metabolism, Wilson disease, although many other organs may also be affected at different stages of the illness. This Chapter focuses on the pathogenesis of Wilson disease and the resultant copper-induced free radical injury in the liver, neurologic system and other organs of affected patients.

2. Cellular Copper Transport

Copper enters the cells through a membrane transporter protein named CTR1 (for details see Vol. II, Chapter 20 on copper metabolism). CTR1 is expressed in all human tissues, especially in liver [1]. The structure of this transporter reveals three transmembrane domains, an extracellular amino terminus and an intracellular carboxyl terminus [2]. An MXXXM

---

*Phone: 203-737-1592, Fax: 203-785-6645, E-mail: Michael.Schilsky@yale.edu

motif located in the second domain is essential for copper uptake, while the methionine rich motif in the first is important for copper uptake under copper-limiting conditions [3]. CTR1 acts functionally as a trimer with a region of low electron density in the center that creates a pore for copper ion transport [4]. Copper is taken up by CTR1 in the reduced form Cu^{1+} rather than Cu^{2+}. This change in copper oxidation state may be the result of metalloreductase function located on the cell plasma membrane [5]. In high copper conditions CTR1 is endocytosed into intracellular vesicles and degraded [6]. Copper transported into the cytosol by CTR1 is followed by its binding to metallochaperones that brings copper to a number of enzymes, compartments and other metal ion transporters. Atox1 is the metallochaperone known to be involved in copper transport to the membrane bound copper transporting P-type ATPases ATP7A and ATP7B [7]. ATP7A and ATP7B play a role in intracellular copper homeostasis by the transport of copper from the cytosol to other compartments using an energy dependent mechanism. ATP7B also functions in the incorporation of copper into copper dependent proteins by transporting copper to the trans- Golgi network (TGN) [8].

While ATP7A is expressed in many tissues, ATP7B is most highly expressed in hepatocytes, but is also present in kidney and placenta and to a lesser degree in brain, heart and lung [9]. This explains the importance of ATP7B to hepatocellular copper metabolism. In the cytosol, copper transporting ATPases receive copper from the metallochaperone, Atox1. Atox1 shuttles the copper from its surface to repeated cysteine- and methionine-rich metal binding domains (MBD) on the amino terminus of the ATPases. In basal conditions where copper is relatively low, ATP7A moves between the TGN and the plasma membrane. In conditions where copper concentration is elevated, ATP7A moves towards the basolateral membrane within vesicles to export cellular copper. ATP7B is located mainly in cells in the TGN under normal conditions. When cells are exposed to high concentrations of copper, ATP7B transports the copper molecules to vesicles that move toward the apical membrane (in the liver the apical membrane is the bile canalicular membrane) for excretion. ATP7B may also remain within vesicles near the apical membrane. These vesicles fuse with the canalicular membrane to release the copper into bile. ATP7B then recycles back to the TGN. This cycling is dependent on phosphorylation and dephosphorylation of ATP7B [9,10]. Another protein involved in the biliary excretion of copper, COMMD1, may directly interact with ATP7B. How COMMD1 functions in copper transport is still undefined. However, there is no evidence of any copper overload disorder uniquely related to impaired COMMD1 function in human beings, though copper overload in Bedlington terriers is due to mutated *COMMD1* [11,12].

3. Wilson Disease

Wilson disease is an autosomal recessive disorder, which affects one out of 30,000 births. It was first described by Kinnier Wilson as "Progressive Lenticular Degeneration" in 1912 [13]. The mutated gene is located on chromosome 13 and encodes the copper transporting ATPase ATP7B. Over 500 mutations involving the *ATP7B* gene are discovered and recorded [14]. The most common mutation of *ATP7B* is H1069Q in exon 14, which is seen in patients of European origin and the R778L mutation that is more commonly present in Asian patients [15]. However, most patients carry two different *ATP7B* mutations [16]. *ATP7B dysfunction or absence resulting from these mutations is responsible for the pathogenesis of Wilson disease. Impaired excretion of copper leads to its hepatocellular accumulation and consequent hepatic and/or neurologic injury that is the hallmark of this disease.* In addition, impaired ATP7B function reduces the incorporation of copper into ceruloplasmin peptide. Due to the decreased half-life of the apoceruloplasmin in the circulation there is a decrease in the steady state plasma levels of ceruloplasmin. This is a useful marker of Wilson disease and can be useful for clinical screening. *As the major route of copper excretion into bile is defective in Wilson disease, copper serum levels increase and copper accumulates in other tissues as well, leading to the extrahepatic manifestations of this disease.*

4. Cytopathic Effect of Copper Overload

The most accepted mechanism for copper-induced cellular injury is copper's role in the generation of reactive oxygen species (ROS). In the presence of reducing agents Cu^{++} is reduced to Cu^{+}. Cu^{+} is reoxidized to Cu^{++} in the presence of molecular oxygen and this can produce $O_2\bullet$ from molecular oxygen and $OH\bullet$ from H_2O_2 via the Fenton reaction [17, 18]. Hydroxyl radicals are very potent and can react with other molecules to induce oxidative damage. The free radicals are also capable of inducing DNA oxidation and breaks. Experimental studies have shown that after incubating isolated hepatocytes with copper, ROS production rapidly increases. In part, the resultant cellular toxicity by excess copper is due to mitochondrial ROS production rather than cytosolic ROS production due to redox cycling [19].

In vivo studies show that peroxidative damage to membrane lipids is one of the consequences of copper overload. ROS can interact with lipids to produce lipid radicals. Lipid peroxidation is induced by peroxy radical formation as a result of the reaction of lipid radicals with oxygen. Peroxy radicals can damage cellular membrane permeability. They are also able to attack DNA and other intracellular molecules, directly. Lipid peroxidation occurs in mitochondrial and lysosomal membranes of damaged hepatocytes. There is also evidence of reduction in the activity of cytochrome *c* oxidase and impairment of liver mitochondrial respiration as a result of copper overload [17].

Levels of antioxidants in liver cells influence copper's ability to cause liver injury. Administration of vitamin E (α-tocopherol) as an antioxidant lipid-soluble vitamin delays the presentation of acute liver injury in an animal model of Wilson disease; the Long-Evans Cinnamon (LES) rat [20]. Vitamin E derivatives may prevent lipid peroxidation in copper overloaded hepatocytes [21]. There are also some reports of symptom improvement after adding vitamin E to therapeutic regimens in patients with Wilson disease [22].

Intracellular antioxidant defense system may also play a role in the suppression of copper induced oxidative injury. Glutathione (GSH) is a tri-peptide reducing agent with a high concentration in the cytosol of hepatocytes that has potent antioxidant properties (Vol. II, Chapter 1). It also functions as an intracellular free radical scavenger. High intracellular GSH levels have been detected in hepatocytes of asymptomatic carriers of Wilson disease in a recent study [23]. Although these individuals have modestly increased hepatic copper concentration compared to control, they have no significant pathologic findings on their liver biopsies. The increased GSH level may represent a cellular response to overcome copper-induced oxidative injury. By contrast, decreased GSH was detected in hepatocytes of Wilson disease patients with mild to severe liver involvement. This may be due to GSH consumption in a pathway of defense against the severe oxidative stress in copper-laden hepatocytes or alternatively, a decreased capacity for its production [23]. Decreased cytosolic GSH in periportal hepatocytes after copper overload has been demonstrated, likely making these cells more vulnerable to oxidative injury caused by copper in animal models [24]. This may be very important in that the periportal region contains most of the liver's progenitorcells for hepatocytes and biliary cells, and injury to this region could inhibit hepatic regeneration [24]. *In acute liver failure due to Wilson disease, a secondary insult leading to a decrease in antioxidant capacity of hepatocytes may play a critical role in the sudden clinical decompensation* [25].

Copper is also capable of evoking apoptotic cellular injury in the setting of acute liver failure in Wilson disease. Acute copper exposure leads to activation of the CD95 system and induction of apoptosis [26]. Copper induced apoptosis may also develop through its effect on a so called anti-apoptotic protein, X-linked inhibitor of apoptosis (XIAP). Copper binds XIAP and induces conformational changes. These changes make XIAP unstable with a resultant decrease in its steady state level and impaired inhibition of activation of the caspase cascade, thereby lowering the threshold for apoptosis [27].

5. Free Radical-Dependent Liver Fibrogenesis

Fibrosis (Chapter 4 in this Volume) is the result of excessive accumulation of extracellular matrix (ECM) in the liver tissue produced by hepatic stellate cells (HSCs). ROS and lipid peroxidation byproducts resulting from oxidative insults to hepatocytes are able to activate the HSC to produce a marked amount of ECM. It is thought that free radicals can activate the HSCs in both direct and indirect ways. The direct way is through the effect of free radicals on *ECM* genes in HSC or attacking HSC membrane, which activates the cell after triggering an intracellular cascade. The indirect way is via the effect of inflammatory cytokines. The cytokines released by activated inflammatory cells during oxidative stress may activate HSC in a paracrine fashion. It is also supposed that there is a mitogenic role for free radicals in interaction with HSCs, but whether this is a direct effect of free radicals on these cells or mediated through cytokine activation is uncertain [18]. A summary of how copper toxicity affects the liver is shown in Figure 1.

6. Copper Toxicity in the Nervous System

Though copper accumulates throughout the brain, it is the accumulation of copper in the basal ganglia and injury to this region in particular that leads to the parkinsonian features of this disorder suggesting an increased susceptibility of the basal ganglia to oxidative injury (see also Chapter 10 in this Volume). This selective vulnerability of grey matter of brain for degenerative changes in Wilson disease may be due to the presence of protoplasmic glial cells in these areas. These cells have a particular susceptibility to copper-induced damage. These glial cells also contain metallothionein (MT), a metal binding protein (see next paragraph) that could participate in metal detoxification and storage. However accumulated MT-bound copper may become harmful when byproducts of the oxidative process attack the binding sites of the complex. This could also contribute to injury in these glial cells. Another potential role for copper induced cellular toxicity in the central nervous system is neurotransmitter dysregulation. There is evidence of interaction between copper and dopamine in substantia nigra neurons of animal models with neurodegeneration as a consequence of copper overload [28, 29].

7. Cellular Adaptive Responses to Copper Overload

When the cell is exposed to a high level of copper an intracellular stress response is evoked. This may include an increase in the generation of heat shock proteins and other changes common to cellular stress responses. Upon copper exposure hepatocytes were shown to be able to increase many fold the expression of genes responsible for heat shock protein synthesis [30]. Small heat shock proteins, called α-crystallins have selective binding sites for Cu^{++} and may play a role in intracellular copper sequestration, thereby decreasing the resultant oxidative damage [31]. However for metal induced injury, the induction of MT is uniquely important. MTs are cysteine-rich proteins that play a protective role in copper and several other heavy metal exposures. The synthesis of MT is induced after high copper exposure through the interaction of copper with metal response elements (MRE) of the *MT* gene and metal transcription factor (MTF)-1 [32, 33]. MTF1 contains a six-zinc finger DNA-binding domain, which binds to the MRE to induce the *MT* gene [34]. MT is thought to function in metal ion homeostasis for essential metalssuch as zinc and copper, as well as play an important role in the cellular detoxification of these metals and free radical scavenging [32]. The intracellular location of copper-bound Cu-MT may determine whether Cu-MT promotes or attenuates cellular injury by copper. The sequestration of copper in the form of Cu-MT by the lysosome is supposed to have a cytoprotective effect in animal models of copper overload [35]. By contrast, the presence of high amount of Cu-MT complexes in the nucleus may promote DNA injury and apoptosis and thus play a role in overall copper-induced cellular injury [36].

8. Pathology

The transition from copper overload in hepatocytes to cellular injury visible on histological examination of tissues differs between individuals. However, most individuals progress from the simple accumulation of copper to cellular injury with time. Early structural changes visible on light microscopy include steatosis, both microvesicular and macrovesicular. At this stage of the disease, electron microscopic evaluation of liver cells shows evidence of abnormal looking mitochondria with dilated cristae and increased number of dense bodies. In the mitochondria, the intercristal space between inner and outer membrane of cristae is widened. These changes disappear with progression of the disease or with treatment. Other histologic findings in liver biopsy specimens of patients with Wilson disease include focal necrosis, glycogenated nuclei in hepatocytes and apoptotic bodies. Routine histochemical staining for copper is not positive in early phases of the disease when copper is mainly cytosolic, but may be seen when copper has accumulated in lysosomes. This may also be observed on ultrastructural analysis as dense deposits in lysosomes. With disease progression there is inflammation and portal and bridging fibrosis that will eventually lead to cirrhosis. In some cases, findings of chronic active hepatitis or submassive necrosis with Mallory bodies may be evident [37].

9. Clinical Manifestations of Wilson Disease

There is a wide range of clinical presentations of Wilson disease in patients, however most commonly there are two major organ specific presentations. Patients may present with hepatic manifestations ranging from only biochemical abnormalities to liver failure. Others may present with neuropsychiatric manifestations, and these patients are typically a decade older than those with hepatic presentations. Some may present with a mixture of both hepatic and neuropsychiatric symptoms. In addition, a significant number of patients are asymptomatic and are diagnosed during family screening or routine checkups.

9.1. Hepatic Manifestations

The spectrum of liver manifestation of Wilson disease varies between asymptomatic patients with abnormal biochemical studies to acute liver failure or liver failure with decompensated cirrhosis. Children may have hepatomegaly or abnormal liver tests. In some asymptomatic individuals biochemical tests and histologic findings of hepatic steatosis are evident. Some patients report an episode of acute illness resembling viral hepatitis. Some affected individuals, mostly very young patients, have features in common with autoimmune hepatitis with positive serological markers and even inflammatory changes on biopsy that include plasma cell infiltrates. The presenting feature in some others is compatible with chronic hepatitis and/or signs and symptoms of liver cirrhosis. There are rare reports of hepatocellular carcinoma and cholangiocarcinoma occurring in patients with Wilson disease [11, 22, 38].

Acute liver failure may be the first presentation of Wilson disease in about 5% of patients. Patients with acute liver failure have concomitant Coombs-negative hemolytic anemia and more frequently have evidence of acute renal failure compared to patients with acute liver failure of other etiologies. These patients with very rare exception will not survive without liver transplantation.

9.2. Neuropsychiatric Manifestations

The first neuropsychiatric manifestations may comprise behavioral changes, deterioration in hand writing, and in children, changes in school performance. The hallmark of neurologic involvement in Wilson disease is parkinsonian features and a progressive movement disorder. Common neurologic disturbances include tremor, impaired fine motor skills, drooling, dysarthria, dystonia, spasticity, dysphagia with risk of aspiration and ataxia. Autonomic dysfunction can also occur, but this is typically in patients with other neurological findings [39]. Depression, anxiety and frank psychosis are among psychiatric presentations, and may occur concurrently with other neurological manifestations or even in patients with hepatic disease without clinically apparent neurological findings [11, 15, 22].

10. Further Pathological Features

10.1. Eye Involvement

The deposition of copper in Descemet's membrane of cornea produces a yellowish brown discoloration ring in the outer border of the cornea known as Kayser-Fleischer (K-F) ring. K-F rings are detected in about 50% of Wilson patients presenting with hepatic manifestations and they are almost invariably present in patients with neurologic involvement. Although K-F rings may sometimes be visible to the naked eye, slit lamp examination is necessary to confirm the presence or absence of K-F rings. The presence of K-F ring is regarded as one of the diagnostic criteria in Wilson disease. However, it is not 100% specific for this disease and may be rarely detected in other types of chronic liver disease, especially in those with longstanding cholestasis.

Sunflower cataracts are another common ophthalmologic finding in Wilson disease due to copper deposition in the lens. It does not lead to any visual impairment and its detection requires slit lamp examination. Both of these ophthalmologic findings will reverse gradually after appropriate treatment for Wilson disease is started. Their reappearance in a previously successfully treated patient is suggestive of noncompliance [11, 22].

10.2. Renal Involvement

Renal tubular dysfunction (Chapter 5 in this Volume) is a known complication of untreated Wilson disease. This may be the result of copper-induced chronic injury of the renal tubular system leading to the aminoaciduria, glucosuria, phosphaturia and uricosuria known as Fanconi syndrome. There is also evidence of hypercalciuria and increase incidence of nephrolithiasis in patients with Wilson disease [40]. However, acute kidney injury may be induced when there is a sudden release of high concentrations of copper into the circulation in patients presenting with acute liver failure. There is also report of acute kidney injury due to rhabdomyolysis (release of myoglobin from damaged skeletal muscle), a rare complication of Wilson disease [41].

10.3. Other Organs

Coomb's-negative hemolysis (both acute and chronic), pancreatitis, hypoparathyroidism, infertility, skeletal abnormalities (arthritis, osteoporosis) are among other extrahepatic manifestations of Wilson disease [22]. Cardiac involvement in patients with Wilson disease includes left ventricular (LV) parietal thickening, concentric LV remodeling, benign supraventricular tachycardias and extrasystolic beats [42]. Rarely is this clinically significant.

11. Screening for Wilson Disease

Screening for Wilson disease should be performed in patients presenting with suggestive signs and symptoms of liver or neuropsychiatric disease and in siblings of individuals diagnosed with the condition. Screening tests include clinical and biochemical studies. (1) Initially, liver tests and blood counts should be performed to determine whether there is acute or chronic liver injury. (2) Measurement of 24 hour urine copper excretion should be performed on all patients under consideration for Wilson disease. The level of urinary copper in most symptomatic Wilson patients is greater than 100 μg per day; however in some patients and in asymptomatic affected siblings it may be lower. Any subject with a 24 hour urine copper excretion over 40 μg per day should be evaluated further for Wilson disease. (3) Slit lamp examination for K-F rings should be performed in all suspected cases over the age of 5 years. K-F rings are present in almost all patients with neuropsychiatric presentations but in only ~ 50% of patients presenting with liver disease (4) Serum ceruloplasmin levels are less than 20 mg/dl in most patients with Wilson disease. However, serum ceruloplasmin assay as a single test should not be used to diagnose or exclude Wilson disease, as about 10-25% of patients have serum ceruloplasmin concentrations within the normal range and about 5% of heterozygous carriers also have low values [22]. (5) Liver biopsy should be performed in all patients under investigation for Wilson disease who do not exhibit K-F rings and whose serum ceruloplasmin levels are low (see below). (6) Molecular testing should be used for family screening if the proband has been identified (see below).

11.1. Diagnosis

Establishing a diagnosis of Wilson disease is based on a combination of clinical and laboratory findings; however molecular diagnosis is also possible. In a patient with unexplained liver or neurological disease and positive K-F ring whose ceruloplasmin level and 24-hr urine copper are abnormal, a diagnosis of Wilson disease is established and there is no need for further diagnostic evaluation. Further testing with liver biopsy may provide additional information with respect to the stage of the liver disease. If there is uncertainty about the diagnosis in patients without K-F rings, liver biopsy and hepatic copper measurement should be performed. Copper concentrations of more than 250 μg/g dry weight of liver are considered to be diagnostic for Wilson disease; however the threshold for the sensitivity of the diagnosis is improved if this level is lowered to 70 μg/g dry weight with some reduced specificity given the overlap with some heterozygotes. When the diagnosis remains indeterminate or when family screening is needed, molecular genetic testing may be useful. Currently there are over 500 different mutations of *ATP7B* described, and most patients are compound heterozygotes. In some populations, specific mutations may dominate and then selective testing for these mutations can precede a full gene search, although advances in DNA sequencing has made possible full *ATP7B* gene screening.

11.2. Family Screening

First degree relatives of patients with documented Wilson disease should undergo screening evaluation. This includes liver function tests, serum ceruloplasmin level, serum and 24 hour urine copper measurement and evaluation for K-F rings via slit lamp. There may be a need for further examination with liver biopsy for copper measurement and histological evaluation as well as molecular analysis for *ATP7B* mutations in debated cases. Molecular genetic analysis is useful as a screening tool in families in whom the mutated gene of the affected person (proband) is detected [11]. A more simplified process of screening for specific mutations compared to genome-wide surveys is possible for these individuals.

12. Management of Wilson Disease

The aim of treatment in Wilson disease is to prevent, stop or even reverse the copper-induced damage in affected tissues (Table 1). *The goal is to decrease cellular copper storage to sub-toxic levels where oxidative stress could be easily overcome.*

Table 1. Treatment of Wilson Disease

Copper Removal	Chelation Therapy: Dimercaptopropanol Penicillamine Trientine Ammonium Tetrathiomolybdate
Preventing Copper Absorption	Diet; restriction of copper containing food Zinc
Increasing Cellular Defense	Antioxidants; Vitamin E GSH Inducers; NAC (?) Metallothionein Stimulators; Zinc
Gene Therapy	Transfection of liver cells with *ATP7B* gene (Experimental)
Liver and Hepatocyte Cell Transplantation	Transplant with liver from unaffected or heterozygote donor Infuse hepatocytes from unaffected donor (Experimental)

12.1. Diet

Limiting dietary copper intake and its intestinal absorption is a reasonable way to decrease the rate of copper accumulation in tissues. Shellfish, nuts, chocolate, mushrooms, and organ meats are rich in copper and their ingestion should be avoided or minimized. It is also advisable to check the amount of copper in drinking water and to use a purifying system if the copper concentration is high [22].

12.2. Chelators

Chelation therapy is recommended as the initial therapy in symptomatic patients. The mechanism of action for these medications is to bind copper molecules in the circulation and facilitate their excretion by the kidney. The first chelating agent used for the treatment of Wilson disease was British anti-Lewisite BAL; dimercaptopropanol) which was administered by intramuscular injection. This agent was replaced by orally-available D-penicillamine. Apart from the chelating action of D-penicillamine, it may also induce tissue MT. D-penicillamine can interfere with collagen cross-linking and in addition possesses immunosuppressant properties.

The second oral chelating agent that was developed was trientine, initially for patients intolerant to D-penicillamine. Trientine has gained popularity due to its better safety profile. A third oral chelator still under investigation is ammonium tetrathiomolybdate (TM). TM functions by interfering with copper absorption in the gut if given with food, and in addition binds copper in the circulation in a complex with albumin. TM thus far has a reduced incidence of neurological deterioration following treatment initiation, though there are reported reversible hematological and liver test abnormalities associated with its use [22].

12.3. Zinc

Zinc is another oral agent introduced for the treatment of Wilson disease with different mechanisms of action. *Zinc interferes with copper uptake in gut indirectly. Zinc induces MT in enterocytes, and MT acts as an endogenous chelator with more affinity for copper than zinc.*

The copper bound to MT in enterocytes does not enter the circulation and is lost in stool during enterocyte shedding. Zinc also is capable of inducing MT in hepatocytes, thus playing a role in hepatocyte protection against copper-induced injury (See under Cellular adaptive responses to copper overload) [22].

12.4. Combination Therapy

Though not prospectively analyzed, the combination of a chelator and zinc may have an additive effect for treating Wilson disease since each modality has a different mechanism of action [43]. In a retrospective analysis, patients with decompensated cirrhosis improved with treatment with both zinc and trientine given temporally apart to avoid interaction [44]. Whether combination treatment is more effective than chelation therapy alone has not been established, but the theoretical value of a multimodal treatment regimen suggests its clinical utility. Further study will be needed to establish a proper duration of dual therapy because frequent dosages that require administration apart from food are inconvenient for most individuals.

12.5. Liver Transplantation

Liver transplantation is the treatment of choice for patients with Wilson disease who present with acute liver failure or suffer end-stage liver disease unresponsive to medical therapy. Although liver transplantation may be performed in patients with neurologic involvement, the less favorable outcome in terms of neurologic recovery in this group should be considered when contemplating this treatment modality [45].

12.6. Treatment of the Patient with Acute Liver Failure - MARS, Plasmapheresis, Hemodiafiltration

In addition to initiation of supportive care as in any form of acute liver failure, some special treatment modalities are of particular use in acute liver failure due to Wilson disease. The liver support systems providing albumin dialysis exchange as molecular adsorbent recirculating system (MARS), plasmapheresis or hemodiafiltration might be helpful as a bridge to the liver transplantation by virtue of their ability to reduce excess circulating copper concentrations and thus help to decrease the toxicity of copper in affected organs [45].

12.7. Adjunctive Care

Beside management aimed at reducing body copper storage in Wilson disease, some other treatment modalities may be also necessary or beneficial. In advanced chronic liver disease, there may be a need for treatment of portal hypertension and its complications. Nonselective β-blockers are administered to decrease portal pressure. Diuretics and/or large volume paracentesis for control of ascites (abdominal fluid accumulation) and lactulose or non-absorbable antibiotics for hepatic encephalopathy are used as well in the setting of these complications.

Patients with neuropsychiatric manifestations may benefit from symptomatic treatment of movement disorders, depression and other psychiatric problems. *Vitamin E concentrations are reportedly low in hepatocytes of patients with Wilson disease [46]. It therefore may be worthwhile to consider the supplementation of vitamin E as an adjunctive treatment, though there is limited evidence in support of its clinical efficacy* (See Cytopathic effect of copper overload).

N-acetylcysteine (NAC), an antidote for acute liver failure due to acetaminophen toxicity, (Vo. III, Chapter 4) may be beneficial in other forms of acute liver failure [47]. As the major hepatoprotective function of NAC is felt to be replenishment of GSH stores in hepatocytes, its use may be beneficial in acute liver failure due to Wilson disease. There are other proposed cytoprotective mechanisms for NAC, which may be of value in the setting of copper-induced injury. Induction of cytoprotective proteins with free radical-scavenging properties, enhanced metabolic activity of pyruvate dehydrogenase, stabilization of mitochondrial function, and influence on cytokine synthesis are among the mechanisms considered [48].

13. Experimental Treatment Modalities

Using animal models (see also Vol. II, Chapter 20) to achieve new treatment modalities for Wilson disease has resulted in some successes in two fields; hepatocyte transfusion and gene therapy. Isolated hepatocyte transplantation from an unaffected donor to an animal model of Wilson disease has yielded promising results [49]. However there are some limitations in applying these results to humans. The needs for life-long immunosuppression, problems in inducing a suitable stimulus for transplanted hepatocyte repopulation without injuring remaining liver cells, and finding a reliable source of human hepatocytes are among these limitations [45]. The basis of gene therapy is the transfection of hepatocytes with *ATP7B* gene using adenoviral and lentiviral vectors [50]. However, despite the early promising results in animal models, concerns about potential side effects and complications of gene therapy in general have delayed human trials. Particular concerns are questions about the safety of integration of the virus into the host genome and the risk of developing antibodies against viral or transfected proteins [45].

Conclusions

The pathobiology of injury in copper overload that occurs in Wilson disease highlights the mechanisms of free radical injury to liver cells and the role of the liver in copper metabolism. A better understanding of the molecular basis for Wilson disease has evolved since the recognition of the genetic defect being mutation of the copper transporting ATPase, ATP7B that is expressed mainly in liver. This defect causes reduced copper export from the liver and results in pathologic copper accumulation that causes injury to the liver and other tissues, mainly the central nervous system. *Injury to liver cells that can result in necrosis or apoptosis is perpetuated via free radical formation and reduced function of the antioxidant systems that normally confer protection to these cells. Important molecules involved in cytoprotection include MT and GSH, and possibly heat shock proteins. Treatment for Wilson disease involves medical therapy to remove copper or prevent its absorption. In addition, antioxidant therapy may be a useful adjunct to medical treatment.* For those with liver failure due to Wilson disease, hepatic replacement by liver transplantation is curative. Future potential therapies include gene replacement therapy with *ATP7B*, *ATP7B* repair and cell-based therapies such as hepatocyte transplantation. A better understanding of the cellular mechanisms responsible for copper-induced injury and cytoprotection may lead to other novel interventions for this disorder in the future.

References

[1] Zhou B, Gitschier J. hCTR1: a human gene for copper uptake identified by complementation in yeast. *Proc. Natl. Acad. Sci. U S A,* 1997;94:7481-6.

[2] Eisses JF, Kaplan JH. Molecular characterization of hCTR1, the human copper uptake protein. *J. Biol. Chem.* 2002;277:29162-71.

[3] Puig S, Lee J, Lau M, Thiele DJ. Biochemical and genetic analyses of yeast and human high affinity copper transporters suggest a conserved mechanism for copper uptake. *J. Biol. Chem.* 2002;277:26021-30.

[4] Aller SG, Unger VM. Projection structure of the human copper transporter CTR1 at 6-A resolution reveals a compact trimer with a novel channel-like architecture. *Proc. Natl. Acad. Sci. U S A,* 2006;103:3627-32.

[5] Hassett R, Kosman DJ. Evidence for Cu(II) reduction as a component of copper uptake by Saccharomyces cerevisiae. *J. Biol. Chem.* 1995;270:128-34.

[6] Petris MJ, Smith K, Lee J, Thiele DJ. Copper-stimulated endocytosis and degradation of the human copper transporter, hCtr1. *J. Biol. Chem.* 2003;278:9639-46.

[7] Wernimont AK, Huffman DL, Lamb AL, O'Halloran TV, Rosenzweig AC. Structural basis for copper transfer by the metallochaperone for the Menkes/Wilson disease proteins. *Nat. Struct. Biol.* 2000;7:766-71.

[8] Lutsenko S, Barnes NL, Bartee MY, Dmitriev OY. Function and regulation of human copper-transporting ATPases. *Physiol. Rev.* 2007;87:1011-46.

[9] La Fontaine S, Mercer JF. Trafficking of the copper-ATPases, ATP7A and ATP7B: role in copper homeostasis. *Arch. Biochem. Biophys.* 2007;463:149-67.

[10] Nyasae L, Bustos R, Braiterman L, Eipper B, Hubbard A. Dynamics of endogenous ATP7A (Menkes protein) in intestinal epithelial cells: copper-dependent redistribution between two intracellular sites. *Am. J. Physiol. Gastrointest. Liver Physiol.* 2007;292: G1181-94.

[11] Ala A, Walker AP, Ashkan K, Dooley JS, Schilsky ML. Wilson's disease. *Lancet,* 2007;369:397-408.

[12] Tao TY, Liu F, Klomp L, Wijmenga C, Gitlin JD. The copper toxicosis gene product Murr1 directly interacts with the Wilson disease protein. *J. Biol. Chem.* 2003;278:41593-6.

[13] Wilson SAK. Progressive lenticular degeneration: a familial nervous disease associated with cirrhosis of the liver. *Brain,* 1912;34:295-509.

[14] Wilson Disease Mutation Database, http://www.medicalgenetics.med.ualberta.ca/ wilson /index.php.

[15] Ferenci P. Regional distribution of mutations of the ATP7B gene in patients with Wilson disease: impact on genetic testing. *Hum. Genet.* 2006;120:151-9.

[16] Shah AB, Chernov I, Zhang HT, et al. Identification and analysis of mutations in the Wilson disease gene (ATP7B): population frequencies, genotype-phenotype correlation, and functional analyses. *Am. J. Hum. Genet.* 1997;61:317-28.

[17] Gaetke LM, Chow CK. Copper toxicity, oxidative stress, and antioxidant nutrients. *Toxicology,* 2003;189:147-63.

[18] Pietrangelo A. Metals, oxidative stress, and hepatic fibrogenesis. *Semin. Liver Dis.* 1996;16:13-30.

[19] Pourahmad J, O'Brien PJ. A comparison of hepatocyte cytotoxic mechanisms for Cu2+ and Cd2+. *Toxicology,* 2000;143:263-73.

[20] Yamazaki K, Ohyama H, Kurata K, Wakabayashi T. Effects of dietary vitamin E on clinical course and plasma glutamic oxaloacetic transaminase and glutamic pyruvic transaminase activities in hereditary hepatitis of LEC rats. *Lab. Anim. Sci.* 1993;43:61-7.

[21] Sokol RJ, McKim JM,Jr, Devereaux MW. Alpha-Tocopherol Ameliorates Oxidant Injury in Isolated Copper-Overloaded Rat Hepatocytes. *Pediatr. Res.* 1996;39:259-63.

[22] Roberts EA, Schilsky ML, American Association for Study of Liver Diseases (AASLD). Diagnosis and treatment of Wilson disease: an update. *Hepatology,* 2008;47:2089-111.

[23] Nagasaka H, Takayanagi M, Tsukahara H. Children's toxicology from bench to bed--Liver Injury (3): Oxidative stress and anti-oxidant systems in liver of patients with Wilson disease. *J. Toxicol. Sci.* 2009;34 Suppl 2:SP229-36.

[24] Roy DN, Mandal S, Sen G, Biswas T. Superoxide anion mediated mitochondrial dysfunction leads to hepatocyte apoptosis preferentially in the periportal region during copper toxicity in rats. *Chem. Biol. Interact.* 2009;182:136-47.

[25] Schilsky ML, Thiele DJ. Copper Metabolism and the Liver. In: *The Liver, Biology and Pathology.* 5th ed. John Wiley and Sons, 2009.

[26] Strand S, Hofmann WJ, Grambihler A, et al. Hepatic failure and liver cell damage in acute Wilson's disease involve CD95 (APO-1/Fas) mediated apoptosis. *Nat. Med.* 1998;4:588-93.

[27] Mufti AR, Burstein E, Duckett CS. XIAP: cell death regulation meets copper homeostasis. *Arch. Biochem. Biophys.* 2007;463:168-74.

[28] Paris I, Dagnino-Subiabre A, Marcelain K, et al. Copper neurotoxicity is dependent on dopamine-mediated copper uptake and one-electron reduction of aminochrome in a rat substantia nigra neuronal cell line. *J. Neurochem.* 2001;77:519-29.

[29] Hoogenraad T. U. Wilson Disease. In: Major Problems in Neurology. Philadelphia: W .B. Saunders Company, 1996.

[30] Song MO, Freedman JH. Expression of copper-responsive genes in HepG2 cells. *Mol. Cell Biochem.* 2005;279:141-7.

[31] Ahmad MF, Singh D, Taiyab A, Ramakrishna T, Raman B, Rao C. Selective Cu2+ binding, redox silencing, and cytoprotective effects of the small heat shock proteins alphaA- and alphaB-crystallin. *J. Mol. Biol.* 2008;382:812-24.

[32] Mattie MD, Freedman JH. Copper-inducible transcription: regulation by metal- and oxidative stress-responsive pathways. *Am. J. Physiol. Cell Physiol.* 2004;286:C293-301.

[33] Heuchel R, Radtke F, Georgiev O, Stark G, Aguet M, Schaffner W. The transcription factor MTF-1 is essential for basal and heavy metal-induced metallothionein gene expression. *EMBO J.* 1994;13:2870-5.

[34] Laity JH, Andrews GK. Understanding the mechanisms of zinc-sensing by metal-response element binding transcription factor-1 (MTF-1). *Arch. Biochem. Biophys.* 2007;463:201-10.

[35] Sternlieb I. Hepatic lysosomal copper-thionein. Experientia Suppl 1987;52:647-53.

[36] Deng DX, Ono S, Koropatnick J, Cherian MG. Metallothionein and apoptosis in the toxic milk mutant mouse. *Lab. Invest.* 1998;78:175-83.

[37] Scheinberg I.H. and Sternlieb I. Wilson Disease. In: *Major Problems in Internal Medicine*. Philadelphia: W. B. Saunders Company, 1984.

[38] Kosminkova EN, Generalova SI, Ponomarev AB. The development of diffuse cholangiocarcinoma in a female patient with long-term undiagnosed Wilson's disease. Ter Arkh 1995;67:85-7.

[39] Bhattacharya K, Velickovic M, Schilsky M, Kaufmann H. Autonomic cardiovascular reflexes in Wilson's disease. *Clin. Auton. Res.* 2002;12:190-2.

[40] Azizi E, Eshel G, Aladjem M. Hypercalciuria and nephrolithiasis as a presenting sign in Wilson disease. *Eur. J. Pediatr.* 1989;148:548-9.

[41] Propst A, Propst T, Feichtinger H, Judmaier G, Willeit J, Vogel W. Copper-induced acute rhabdomyolysis in Wilson's disease. *Gastroenterology*, 1995;108:885-7.

[42] Hlubocka Z, Marecek Z, Linhart A, et al. Cardiac involvement in Wilson disease. *J. Inherit. Metab. Dis.* 2002;25:269-77.

[43] Schilsky ML. Treatment of Wilson's disease: what are the relative roles of penicillamine, trientine, and zinc supplementation? *Curr. Gastroenterol. Rep.* 2001;3:54-9.

[44] Askari FK, Greenson J, Dick RD, Johnson VD, Brewer GJ. Treatment of Wilson's disease with zinc. XVIII. Initial treatment of the hepatic decompensation presentation with trientine and zinc. *J. Lab. Clin. Med.* 2003;142:385-90.

[45] Schilsky ML. Wilson disease: current status and the future. *Biochimie*, 2009;91:1278-81.

[46] Sokol RJ, Twedt D, McKim JM,Jr, et al. Oxidant injury to hepatic mitochondria in patients with Wilson's disease and Bedlington terriers with copper toxicosis. *Gastroenterology*, 1994;107:1788-98.

[47] Lee WM, Hynan LS, Rossaro L, et al. Intravenous N-acetylcysteine improves transplant-free survival in early stage non-acetaminophen acute liver failure. *Gastroenterology*, 2009;137:856,64, 864.e1.

[48] Koch A, Trautwein C. N-acetylcysteine on its way to a broader application in patients with acute liver failure. *Hepatology,* 2009;51:338-40.

[49] Malhi H, Joseph B, Schilsky ML, Gupta S. Development of cell therapy strategies to overcome copper toxicity in the LEC rat model of Wilson disease. *Regen Med.* 2008;3:165-73.

[50] Merle U, Encke J, Tuma S, Volkmann M, Naldini L, Stremmel W. Lentiviral gene transfer ameliorates disease progression in Long-Evans cinnamon rats: an animal model for Wilson disease. *Scand. J. Gastroenterol.* 2006;41:974-82.

In: Principles of Free Radical Biomedicine, Volume III
Editors: K. Pantopoulos and H. M. Schipper

ISBN 978-1-61324-184-4
©2012 Nova SciencePublishers, Inc.

Chapter 4

Oxidative Stress in Liver Diseases

Giada Sebastiani[*]
Venetian Institute of Molecular Medicine (VIMM), Padova, Italy
Lady Davis Institute for Medical Research, Jewish General Hospital, Montreal,
Quebec, Canada

1. Introduction

Free radicals are naturally generated in biological systems through a variety of processes. Polyunsaturated lipids are essential to the entire supporting system of cells, including cell membranes, endoplasmic reticulum (ER) and mitochondria. Peroxidation of lipids is a major effect of free radicals (Vol. I, Chapter 7).

Reactive oxygen and nitrogen species (ROS and RNS) are highly reactive molecules that are normally produced in small amounts during cellular metabolism, with beneficial effects including cytotoxicity against pathogens (Vol. I, Chapters 2 and 3).

Indeed, some enzymes involved in cellular metabolism are aimed to produce free radicals including ROS and RNS. However, free radicals may also damage normal tissue if the balance between prooxidants and antioxidants molecules is disrupted. When an imbalance favoring prooxidants occurs, a situation of oxidative stress is established. Oxidative stress has been proposed as a critical mechanism of damage in various diseases, including liver diseases.

---

[*]E-mail: giada.sebastiani@gmail.com

2. Epidemiology of Liver Diseases: The Dimension of the Problem

Liver diseases pose an important health concern worldwide. Overall, chronic liver diseases represent a major cause of morbidity and mortality. The major etiologies are chronic infection with hepatitis B (HBV) and C (HCV) viruses, and alcoholic and non-alcoholic fatty liver disease. Chronic hepatitis B and C are the leading causes of cirrhosis and of hepatocellular carcinoma (HCC) worldwide.

Approximately 400 million people are chronically infected with HBV and 25-40% of them die of cirrhosis and of its end-stage complications [1, 2]. HBV is the most important carcinogen after tobacco and the incidence of HCC is 300,000 cases per year. Epidemiological studies have demonstrated an approximately 100-fold increase in the relative risk of HCC among HBV carriers compared to non-carriers [3, 4]. Chronic hepatitis C is a major health concern with around 200 million individuals affected worldwide, with a greater prevalence in Western countries [5]. The acute infection with HCV frequently does not resolve and 80% of the infected individuals become chronic carriers and may then progress towards severe liver disease. Natural history studies indicate that approximately 10-20% of chronically infected hepatitis C patients will develop severe liver cirrhosis and 1-5% will develop HCC within two to three decades [6]. Once liver cirrhosis is established in HCV patients, HCC develops at a yearly rate of 5-7% [7].

Alcoholic liver disease (ALD) is one of the leading causes of end-stage chronic liver disease. Data from the World Health Organization (WHO) indicate that ALD is the third cause of death and disability in most developed countries, with an increasing morbidity also in developing countries [8]. It is well established that only a minority of heavy drinkers, estimated between 10% and 30%, will ever develop advanced ALD and that the risk increases with cumulative alcohol intake [9].

Non-alcoholic fatty liver disease (NAFLD) has become the most common cause of chronic liver disease and impaired liver function in industrialized countries, where 10-23% of the adult population is estimated to be affected [10, 11]. The high incidence of NAFLD in developed countries is related to the widespread presence of risk factors including metabolic disorders such as obesity, dyslipidemias, type 2 diabetes and insulin resistance, but also use of drugs, parenteral nutrition, and gastric bypass surgery [12, 13]. The disease has a spectrum ranging from fatty liver alone to non-alcoholic steatohepatitis (NASH) and progressive steatofibrosis. Many cases of cryptogenic cirrhosis may be end-stage forms of NASH [14]. Liver biopsy studies in obese subjects have shown that 30-40% of patients develop more than simple steatosis. In patients with NASH, 74% will have fibrosis and one third of the cases will have cirrhosis at the time of the first liver biopsy [15, 16].

In all forms of chronic liver diseases, once cirrhosis is established, there is no actual therapy to prevent the end-stage complications apart from follow-up and monitoring for complications including gastrointestinal bleeding, hepatorenal syndrome and HCC. The only definitive therapy for liver cirrhosis is liver transplantation; however this procedure is costly and access to donor transplants is limited. *Oxidative stress has been implicated in the pathogenesis of various forms of chronic liver diseases through both common mechanisms and etiology-specific mechanisms. Moreover, oxidative stress is the main causative agent for* two frequent conditions that lead to acute liver injury, intoxication with paracetamol and the ischemia-reperfusion injury related to liver transplantation and major hepatic surgery.

3. Progression of Liver Diseases: The Role of Oxidative Stress in Liver Fibrogenesis

Independently of etiology, chronic liver diseases are characterised by a common physiopathological pathway: the progressive accumulation of fibrosis in the liver that leads to structural and hemodynamic changes, culminating in cirrhosis and its end-stage liver complications.

Liver fibrosis and cirrhosis represent the consequence of a persistent wound healing response to chronic liver injury that can derive from various causes including hepatotropic viruses, autoimmune diseases, drug-related damage, and cholestatic and metabolic diseases. Cirrhosis, the most advanced stage of liver fibrosis, implies not only more scarring than simple fibrosis, but also a progressive distortion of the liver architecture associated with nodule formation, altered blood flow and increased risk of liver failure.

Fibrosis is a structural change in the liver that accompanies chronic injury; fibrogenesis refers to the production of extracellular matrix (ECM) [17]. The key step in the pathophysiology of liver fibrogenesis is the balance between ECM deposition and removal. The main protagonists in this balance are the hepatic stellate cells (HSCs) that, from a quiescent form, may transform into a myofibroblast-like phenotype [18, 19]. This phenotypic modification implies activation of signalling and cross-talk between different types of cells. Cross-talks between parenchymal and nonparenchymal cells represent the main event in liver fibrogenesis.

Cytokines and ROS are the most important factors in these cross-talks and ROS are mainly involved in necrosis and apoptosis of hepatocytes and HSC activation. HSC activation leads to accumulation of ECM whose main components are represented by collagens, hyaluronan, laminin, elastin, fibronectin, tenascin, undulin, entactin, fibulin, fibrillin, thrombospondin (1 and 2) and proteoglycans. Many factors and cytokines are involved in this dynamic process, including activating factors (tumor necrosis factor alpha, TNFα), chemotactic factors (monocyte chemotactic protein 1, MCP-1; platelet-derived growth factor, PDGF), proliferative factors (PDGF), fibrogenetic factors (transforming growth factor beta 1, TGFβ1; connective tissue growth factor, CTGF), contractility factors (endothelin 1, ET-1), enzymes involved in matrix degradation (metalloproteinases, MMPs, and their inhibitors) and other mediators of fibrogenesis (nitric oxide, NO). The main pathways in the activation of HSCs are summarised in Figures 1 and 2. The two main phases in the activation of HSCs are initiation and perpetuation [18, 20].

3.1. HSCs Initiation

The initiation phase includes rapid changes in gene expression and cell phenotype, and early changes in ECM composition [18]. It involves cross-talks between many cells through several cytokines (Figure 1).

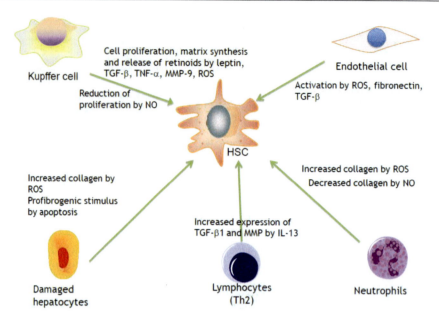

Figure 1. Cross-talks between parenchymal and nonparenchymal cells during hepatic stellate cell (HSC) initiation. TGFβ, transforming growth factor beta; TNFα, tumor necrosis factor alpha; MMP, metalloproteinase; ROS, reactive oxygen species; NO, nitric oxide; IL, interleukin; Th, T helper.

HSCs themselves activate through trans-differentiation, with production of cytoskeletal proteins like α-smooth muscle actin and glial fibrillary acidic protein. Kupffer cells induce HSC proliferation, matrix synthesis and release of retinoids by HSCs through cytokines, such as TGFβ and TNFα, and through MMPs, ROS and RNS. *ROS and RNS can regulate Kupffer cell activation and signalling to control the HSCs' fibrogenic response* [21]. *Kupffer cells also produce NO, which mitigates the effect of ROS by reducing HSC proliferation and contractility.* Damaged hepatocytes may also act in the initiation phase of HSC activation through production of ROS and apoptosis. Lymphocytes, especially Th2 CD4, favour fibrogenesis through production of inflammatory cytokines (interleukins, IL), such as IL-4, IL-6, IL-13, which increase collagen production and TGFβ1 and MMP expression by macrophages. Neutrophils actively contribute to initiate HSCs through production of ROS and, as counterbalance, through production of NO. Endothelial cells may also contribute to HSC initiation phase through production of fibronectin and production of TGFβ.

3.2. HSC Perpetuation

The perpetuation phase includes events that amplify the activated phenotype of HSCs [18]. HSCs are stimulated by both paracrine and autocrine stimuli and the low-density subendothelial matrix is progressively replaced by one rich in fibril-forming collagen. HSCs are sensitive to cytokines and ROS as a result of paracrine stimulation from injured hepatocytes, Kupffer cells and endothelial cells, in addition to rapid changes in ECM composition. Phenotypic responses of activated HSCs include many mechanisms underlying the perpetuation of the response initiated during the activation phase. These can be summarised as follows (Figure 2):

1) Proliferation. PDGF is the most potent mitogen for HSCs; its production is upregulated in the fibrotic liver and its inhibition attenuates experimental liver fibrogenesis. PDGF activates mitogen-activated protein kinase signaling [22]. Interestingly, nicotinamide adenine dinucleotide phosphate (NADPH) is expressed in HSCs and produces ROS, which in turn induce the production of PDGF; again, this molecule increases mitosis of HSCs [23]. This result strongly suggests that ROS play an important role in fibrogenesis by increasing PDGF throughout.

2) Contractility. It represents an important mechanism underlying increased portal resistance during liver injury. ET-1 is the key contractile stimulus. Two G-protein-coupled receptors (ET receptor types A and B) mediate the effects of ET-1 and are expressed on both quiescent and activated HSCs. NO produced by HSCs is the antagonist of ET-1 [24].

3) Fibrogenesis. TGFβ1 is the most potent fibrogenic factor for HSCs, which are also its most important source [25]. Disruption of TGFβ synthesis or signaling pathway prevents scar formation in experimental liver fibrosis [26]. TGFβ stimulates additionally the expression of CTGF, an important amplifier of the profibrogenic action of TGFβ1, and of ET-1. Fibrogenesis is also stimulated by leptin, a profibrogenic hormone of the liver. Leptin acts directly on liver fibrogenesis by promoting α1-collagen production in activated HSCs. Leptin increases the phagocytic activity and cytokine secretion by Kupffer cells and serves as a stimulus for endothelial cells to proliferate and release ROS [21, 27]. In contrast, adiponectin, an adipocyte-derived soluble matrix protein with anti-inflammatory properties markedly inhibits liver fibrogenesis.

4) Matrix degradation. HSCs express all the components for matrix degradation [18]. MMPs are calcium-dependent enzymes that specifically degrade collagens. MMP-1 is the main human protease that degrades type I collagen. Through up-regulation of tissue inhibitors of MMPs, TIMP-1 and TIMP-2, HSCs can inhibit the activity of interstitial collagenases, which additionally increase scar tissue.

5) HSC chemotaxis. HSCs increase in number in areas of liver injury, and this is likely due to both proliferation and migration. The main identified chemoattractants include PDGF, insulin-like growth factor 1 (IGF-1), ET-1 and MCP-1. MCP-1 is the main chemoattractant for monocytes [18].

6) Retinoid loss. Quiescent HSCs are characterized by accumulation of intracellular retinoid. Loss of intracellular retinoid is a notable feature of HSCs activation but the causal relationship between retinoid loss and HSCs activation remains unclear [20].

3.3. Destiny of Activated HSCs

During tissue recovery from acute liver injury, the number of activated HSCs decreases as tissue integrity is restored. This event may be due to two different destinies of activated HSCs in the course of fibrosis resolution: reversion of the activated phenotype or cell apoptosis. Reversion of HSCs is mediated by peroxisome proliferator-activated receptor γ (PPARγ) [20].

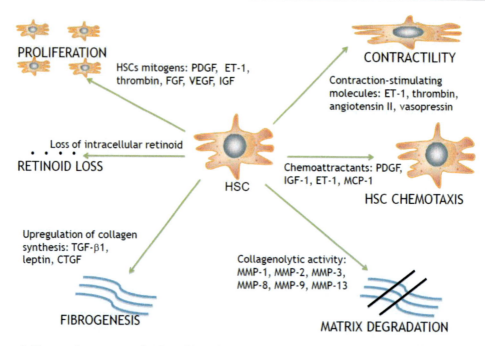

Figure 2. Phenotypic responses of activated hepatic stellate cell (HSC) during the perpetuation phase and involved mediators. PDGF, platelet derived growth factor; ET-1, endothelin 1; FGF, fibroblast growth factor; VEGF, vascular endothelial growth factor; IGF, insulin-like growth factor; TGFβ, transforming growth factor beta; MMP, metalloproteinase; CTGF, connective tissue growth factor; MCP, monocyte chemotactic protein.

PPARγ seems to play a pivotal role in regulation of HSCs activation since activated HSCs can be phenotypically reversed to quiescent cells by forced expression of PPARγ [28]. Apoptosis of HSCs is likely to be involved in the decreased number of HSCs during resolution of hepatic fibrosis. Some mediators have been found to have antiapoptotic activity and may be involved in the fibrogenetic process: IGF-1, TNFα, nuclear factor κB (NF-κB) and TIMP-1 [18].

4. Oxidative Stress and Chronic Hepatitis C

The natural course of chronic hepatitis C is characterised by progressive fibrosis in the inflamed liver with development of cirrhosis and hemodynamic changes, which may be followed by end-stage complications. The progression of fibrosis in chronic hepatitis C is highly variable. Several factors may favour progression, including alcohol, co-infection with other viruses, young age at the time of infection and male sex [6]. However, the pathogenesis of chronic hepatitis C is not yet completely understood. HCV is a positive-stranded RNA virus of the *Flaviviridae* family, with a genome size of ~9.6 kb [29]. The structural genes of HCV genome include core, E1 and E2; the nonstructural genes include NS2, NS3, NS5A and NS5B. This genome encodes a polyprotein, which is translated in a cap-independent way (Figure 3). Its translation requires an internal ribosomal entry site (IRES) that includes most of the 5'-untranslated region and the first nine codons of the polyprotein coding sequence.

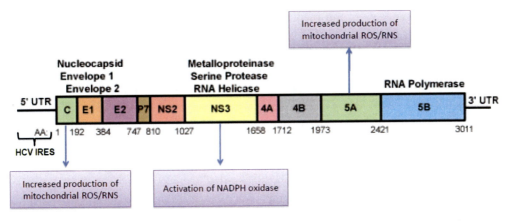

Figure 3. Genome organization of hepatitis C virus (HCV) with the role of HCV proteins in oxidative stress. IRES, internal ribosomal entry site; UTR, untranslated region; ROS, reactive oxygen species; RNS, reactive nitrogen species; NADPH, nicotinamide adenine dinucleotide phosphate. Modified from http://www.microbiologybytes.com/virology/HCV.html.

The HCV polyprotein is cleaved by cellular and viral proteases to generate mature viral gene products, including the core protein that forms the viral capsid and the non-structural proteins NS3, possessing protease and helicase activity, NS5A, and NS5B, the viral RNA polymerase.

Virions are assembled by the formation of the capsid by the core protein and the internalization of the genome, which then likely buds into the ER. The virions, which are enveloped by lipid membranes and viral proteins, are exported from the cell via the normal host secretory pathway [30].

4.1. Oxidative Stress and Pathogenesis of HCV-Induced Liver Injury

Despite continued studies, the molecular mechanism by which HCV induces pathogenic changes in the liver remains largely unclear. Oxidative stress has emerged as having a key role in the pathogenesis of HCV-induced damage to the liver. Indeed, *infection with HCV is characterized by increased levels of ROS and RNS and decreased antioxidant levels in patients*. Moreover, increased lipid peroxidation levels in liver, serum and peripheral mononuclear blood cells of HCV patients have been reported [31].

Other indicators of oxidative stress and oxidative DNA damage, like 4-hydroxynonenal (4-HNE) and 8-hydroxydeoxyguanosine, are increased during HCV infection. On the other hand, glutathione (GSH) content decreases both in blood and liver [32]. *Various mechanisms may be responsible for the severe increase in oxidative stress that is observed in HCV infection. These include: chronic inflammation, iron overload, activation of Kupffer cells, direct increase of ROS and RNS by HCV proteins, both structural and nonstructural (Table 1)* [31]. Necroinflammation is a common feature of chronic HCV infection and it can lead to oxidative stress through activation of phagocytic NADPH oxidase.

However, this mechanism is quite nonspecific, as necroinflammation is a common feature in several chronic liver diseases. The other mechanisms may be considered more specific for HCV chronic infection.

Table 1. Main events, cells and mediators implicated in HCV-induced oxidative stress.

Event/cell/mediator	Mechanism
Chronic inflammation	Activation of phagocytic NADPH oxidase.
Iron	Oxidative stress
Kupffer cells	Production of proinflammatory cytokines (TNFα, IL-1), and profibrogenic cytokines (TGFβ), with subsequent ROS increase, activation of HSCs and liver fibrosis.
HCV core proteins	Mitochondrial dysfunction, ER stress and immune cell-mediated oxidative bursts; Direct increase of oxidative stress, lipid peroxidation; decrease of intracellular GSH levels and mitochondrial NADPH content; production of mediators (cyclooxygenase-2, inducible nitric oxide synthase) which increase ROS and RNS.
Nonstructural proteins	Mitochondrial dysfunction, ER stress and immune cell-mediated oxidative bursts

Legend:HCV, hepatitis C virus;NADPH, nicotinamide adenine dinucleotide phosphate; TNFα, tumor necrosis factor alpha; IL-1, interleukin 1; TGFβ, transforming growth factor beta; ROS, reactive oxygen species; HSCs, hepatic stellate cells; ER, endoplasmic reticulum; GSH, glutathione; RNS, reactive nitrogen species.

4.2. Iron

It is well established that iron could induce oxidative stress through several oxidative reactions that may lead to production of ROS (Vol. I, Chapter 5 and Vol. II, Chapter 19). Differently from chronic HBV infection, a frequent elevation of serum iron indices during chronic infection with HCV has been reported in several studies [33-35]. Elevation of the serum ferritin concentration was found in 20 to 60% of patients with chronic hepatitis C; stainable hepatic iron deposits were detected in 3-38% but in most cases hepatic iron concentration was not significantly increased [35-37].Elevated serum ferritin levels in HCV infection may be mainly explained by several associated conditions, in the absence of iron overload, such as cytolytic necroinflammation, hepatic steatosis and diabetes mellitus, which are commonly associated with hepatitis C infection [35, 38, 39].

However, even in relatively low concentrations, iron has been suggested as a cofactor that may both promote the progression of liver disease and reduce the response to antiviral therapy [40, 41]. Mechanisms proposed include excess ROS formation, increased fibrogenesis through activation of HSCs and impairment of the host immune response [42]. Considering the central role of hepcidin in the control of systemic iron homeostasis (Vol. II, Chapter 19), it is reasonable to hypothesize that hepatic iron deposition during HCV infection may be related to effects of HCV on the hepcidin pathway. In clinical studies, hepcidin expression was found to be significantly lower in HCV- as compared to HBV-infected patients and HCV-negative controls.

Importantly, hepcidin expression was reversed upon HCV eradication with pegylated interferon plus ribavirin therapy, with a concomitant improvement of iron indices [43]. A mouse model expressing an HCV polyprotein transgene exhibits iron accumulation in the liver with decreased hepcidin mRNA and serum pro-hepcidin levels, resulting in increased expression of ferroportin (see Vol. II, Chapter 19) in the duodenum, spleen and liver [44]. *Nishina et al* [44] *proposed a model for HCV-induced iron overload where HCV, oxidative stress and iron act in a "ménage a trois"*: HCV promotes oxidative stress, down-regulating the C/EBPα (CCAAT/enhancer-binding protein α) transcription factor, which is essential for basal hepcidin transcription. Reduction of hepcidin expression leads to increased iron fluxes from the duodenum and macrophages and, eventually, hepatic iron deposition.

Further experiments in an HCV replicon cell culture model showed that HCV-induced oxidative stress suppresses hepcidin expression through increased histone deacetylase activity that reduces the binding of C/EBPα and STAT3 (signal transducer and activator of transcription 3) to the hepcidin promoter [45]. The role of mutations in the HFE gene responsible for hereditary hemochromatosis (Chapter 2 in this Volume) as a risk factor for iron overload in chronic hepatitis C has also been studied in different populations, with somewhat discordant results [35].

4.3. Kupffer Cells

Activation of Kupffer cells by ROS produced by the neighboring hepatocytes is a key event in enhancing oxidative stress during HCV infection [31]. These cells express many proinflammatory and profibrogenic cytokines and, when ROS levels increase, they release mediators in the ECM, including TNFα, IL-1, IL-6, IL-8 and TGFβ. The rising concentrations of ROS induce lipid peroxidation (Vol. I, Chapter 7), which eventually disrupts cellular membranes and can induce mitochondrial dysfunction.

4.4. HCV Core Protein

The main mechanisms through which HCV proteins contribute to oxidative stress include mitochondrial dysfunction, ER stress and immune cell-mediated oxidative bursts [46]. *The HCV core protein, localized in the outer mitochondrial membrane, seems particularly potent in producing mitochondrial abnormalities and oxidative stress* (Figure 4). It facilitates the uptake of calcium into the mitochondria and induces mitochondrial permeability transition. The accumulation of calcium leads to a stimulation of electron transport, which eventually increases ROS production [47].

NO synthase activity is also stimulated, with formation of NO and its derivates, and subsequent inflammation, DNA damage and apoptosis [48]. The depletion of GSH and the release of cytochrome c impair the function of mitochondria and further elevate ROS in hepatocytes [31].

During HCV replication, the HCV core protein also associates with the ER. HCV replicates in the ER membrane, leading to production of viral proteins. Due to overload of chaperones, the ER may fail to export synthesized proteins properly, leading to accumulation of misfolded proteins. These misfolded proteins generate an unfolded protein response (Vol. II, Chapter 18) that can eventually lead to ER dysfunction and cell death. The consequent loss of ER function may lead to stress and activation of inflammatory signaling pathways [46].

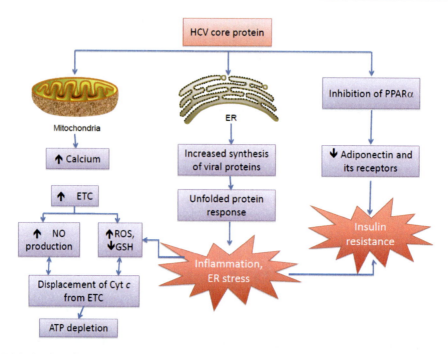

Figure 4. Mechanisms for hepatitis C virus (HCV) core protein-induced oxidative stress. PPARα, peroxisome proliferator-activated receptor alpha; ETC, electron transport chain; NO, nitric oxide; ER, endoplasmic reticulum; GSH, glutathione; ATP, adenosine triphosphate.

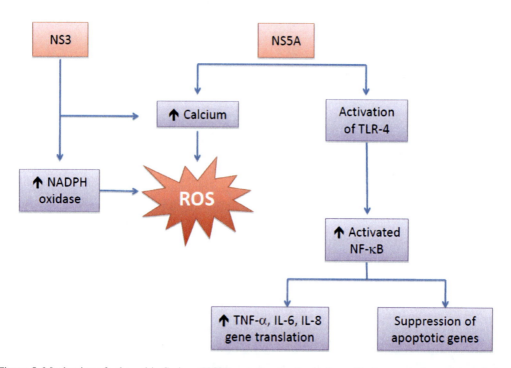

Figure 5. Mechanisms for hepatitis C virus (HCV) non-structural proteins oxidative stress through association with endoplasmic reticulum (ER). NADPH, nicotinamide adenine dinucleotide phosphate; ROS, reactive oxygen species; TLR-4, toll-like receptor 4; NF-κB, nuclear factor-κB; TNFα, tumor necrosis factor alpha; IL, interleukin.

The HCV core protein also inhibits PPARα and PPARγ expressed in macrophages, adipocytes and hepatocytes. PPARα induces gene transcription of enzymes involved in mitochondrial and peroxisomal oxidation, required for metabolism of triglycerides. The accumulation of hepatic triglycerides deriving from inhibition of PPARα by HCV core protein is associated with loss of adiponectin receptors in the liver and, together with reduction of circulating adiponectin, contributes to systemic insulin resistance, metabolic abnormalities and oxidative stress [49]. Adiponectin is a soluble matrix protein produced by adipocytes or adipose tissues found around kidney, heart and liver that has anti-inflammatory properties [50]. It enhances the insulin sensitivity of hepatocytes and therefore it plays an important role in fatty acid metabolism. Insulin may have a direct effect on the liver through its ability to produce ROS [51]. Furthermore, insulin may also be directly involved in causing ER stress along with the unfolding protein response and apoptosis.

4.5. Nonstructural HCV Proteins

Of the HCV non-structural proteins, NS3 and NS5A act as key mediators in the induction of oxidative stress and inflammation (Figure 5). Indeed, the association of NS5A with the ER has been suggested to stimulate mitochondrial production of ROS by releasing calcium from the ER [49].

Moreover, NS5A may activate NF-κB (Vol. II, Chapter 12) by binding to Toll-like receptor 4 (TLR-4) found on the plasma membranes of hepatocytes and B cells [52]. NS5A-induced mitochondrial production of ROS is thought to activate NF-κB, which in turn up-regulates genes involved in cytokine production, such as TNFα, IL-6 and IL-8 [49]. This response may play an important role in inflammation, immune response and HCC development [53]. NS3 has been shown to activate NADPH oxidase that generates ROS [54] and can thereby lead to a large number of pathological events in the liver. NS3-induced ER and oxidative stress may activate NF-κB and increase the risk of inflammation, insulin resistance and HCC [49]. *Nonstructural proteins may also modulate the host redox status by HCV. Indeed, host antioxidant defenses, mediated by GSH, catalase and heme oxygenase-1, are augmented suggesting adaptation to oxidative stress* [55].

5. Oxidative Stress and Chronic Hepatitis B

HBV is a partially double-stranded DNA virus, member of *Hepadnaviruses*, containing a genome of 3.2 kb, which encodes four genes named C, S, P and X. The C genes code for the core protein and the serum e antigen, the S gene encodes three related viral envelope proteins known as surface antigens (including the large, pre-S1+pre-S2+S, the middle, pre-S2+S and the small S), the P gene encodes the viral DNA polymerase, and the X gene a 16.5 kDa protein (Figure 6).

In chronic hepatitis B, HBV DNA can be integrated into the host genome [56]. HBx protein has been shown to activate cellular transcription factors via oxidative stress in cells [57, 58]. While most of the available evidence points to a predominantly cytoplasmic distribution [59, 60], HBxhas also been found associated to mitochondria, causing a decrease in the mitochondrial membrane potential and a subsequent elevation of ROS [58, 61]. HBx-induced oxidative stress leads to the activation of a series of transcription factors including STAT3 and NF-κB [58]. NF-κB was one of the first HBx-responsive elements identified [62]. HBx constitutively upregulates STAT3, that is normally activated by cytokines such as IL-6 [58, 63].

Activated STAT forms dimers or multimers that are then transported into the nucleus, where they bind to DNA and activate gene expression. Oxidative stress triggers STAT3 tyrosine phosphorylation and nuclear translocation, which correlates with high DNA binding activity [63, 64]. Similarly to HCV NS5A, Meyer and colleagues showed that also HBV surface antigen is localized to the ER and transactivates NF-κB [57]. Moreover, the HBV activates the unfolded protein response [65].

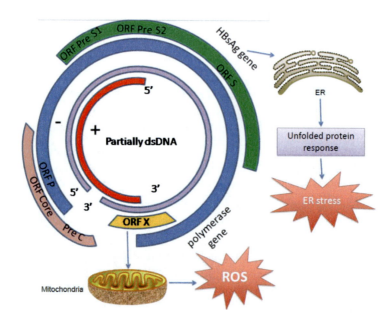

Figure 6. Genome organization of hepatitis B virus (HBV) with the role of individual proteins in oxidative stress. ORF, open reading frame; dsDNA, double stranded DNA; HBsAg, hepatitis B surface antigen; ER, endoplasmic reticulum.

6. Oxidative Stress and Alcoholic Liver Disease

Acute and chronic alcohol consumption increases the productions of ROS, lowers antioxidant levels and enhances oxidative stress in many tissues, especially in the liver. Indeed, the ability of alcohol to increase ROS, RNS and to induce peroxidation of lipids, DNA and proteins has been demonstrated in various biological systems and in humans [66].

Nowadays it is clear that alcohol-induced oxidative stress plays a key role in the pathogenesis of liver injury in ALD. Alcohol alters cell function either directly via its solvent action on cellular membranes and indirectly by its metabolism. Several pathways and enzymes are implicated in the mechanisms of alcohol-induced oxidative stress [55, 67] (Table 2).

Table 2. Pathways involved in alcohol-induced oxidative stress

Pathway	Mechanism
Redox state changes (changes in the NAD^+/NADH ratio)	Result of alcohol oxidation by alcohol and aldehyde dehydrogenase, which eventually triggers ROS formation
Production of the reactive product acetaldehyde	Acetaldehyde interacts with proteins and lipids leading to radical formation and cell damage
Damage to mitochondria	Decreased production of ATP
Alcohol direct membrane effects	Interaction of hydrophobic alcohol with phospholipids, proteins or enzymes
Alcohol-induced hypoxia	Mainly affecting the pericentral zone of the liver acinus where extra oxygen is required for alcohol metabolism
Effects on the immune system	Altered production of signaling molecules and cytokines
Increase in bacterial-derived endotoxin	Activation of Kupffer cells with subsequent production of ROS
Induction of CYP2E1	Production of ROS through alcohol metabolism
Increase in the levels of free iron	Iron-mediated production of ROS
Effects on antioxidants	Effect on antioxidant enzymes and chemicals, especially glutathione
Generation of alcohol-derived radicals	One electron oxidation of alcohol to 1-hydroxyethyl radical
Conversion of xanthine dehydrogenase to xanthine oxidase	Generation of ROS

Legend: NAD, nicotinamide adenine dinucleotide; ATP, adenosine triphosphate; CYP2E1, cytochrome P450 2E1; ROS, reactive oxygen species.

6.1. Molecular Mechanisms for Alcohol Metabolism

In the case of moderate and short-term alcohol consumption, the majority of alcohol is metabolized by alcohol dehydrogenase (ADH), which is located in the cytoplasm of hepatocytes. Through this enzyme, alcohol is oxidized to acetaldehyde via a reversible reaction and NAD^+ is reduced to NADH. Acetaldehyde is then oxidized to acetate via an irreversible reaction by aldehyde dehydrogenase (ALDH), which also requires the reduction of NAD^+ to NADH. The acetate is metabolized to acetylcoenzyme A and oxidized in the Krebs cycle (Figure 7) [68]. There are five classes (I-V) of ADH, but the hepatic form that is primarily used in humans is class I. Class I ADH isoenzymes consists of α, β, and γ subunits that are encoded by the genes ADH1A, ADH1B and ADH1C, respectively [69]. The enzyme is contained in the lining of the stomach and in the liver. It forms a dimer (i.e., consists of two polypeptides), with each dimer containing two zinc ions (Zn^{2+}). One of those ions is crucial for enzyme function: it is located at the catalytic site and holds the hydroxyl group of the alcohol in place. ADH activity varies between men and women, between young and old, and among different populations.

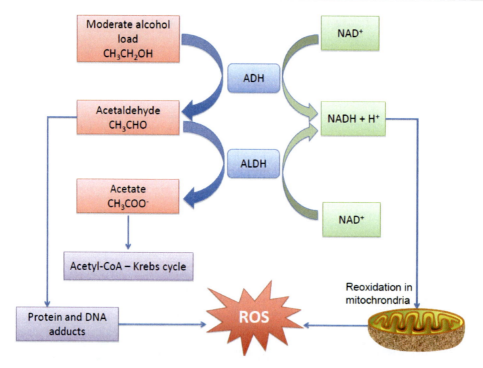

Figure 7. Metabolism of alcohol during moderate, short-term consumption. ADH, alcohol dehydrogenase; ALDH, aldehyde dehydrogenase; NAD, nicotinamide adenine dinucleotide; acetyl-CoA, acetyl-coenzyme A; ROS, reactive oxygen species.

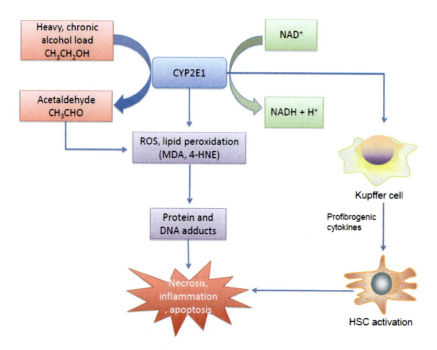

Figure 8. Metabolism of alcohol during heavy, chronic exposure. CYP2E1, cytochrome P450 2E1; NAD, nicotinamide adenine dinucleotide; ROS, reactive oxygen species; MDA, malondialdehyde; 4-HNE, 4-hydroxynonenal; HSC, hepatic stellate cell.

Oxidative Stress in Liver Diseases 79

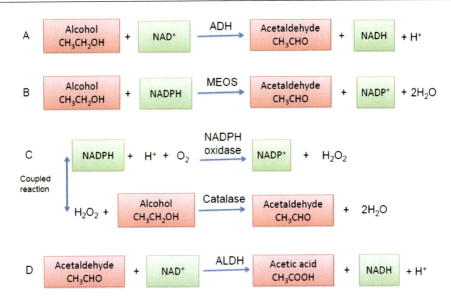

Figure 9. Alcohol and acetaldehyde oxidation reactions. Alcohol is converted into acetaldehyde through several chemical reactions: in reaction A, by ADH and NAD+; in reaction B by MEOS, which involves cytochrome P450 2E1 and NADPH; in reaction C by a combination of NADPH oxidase and catalase. In reaction D acetaldehyde is further oxidized to acetic acid by ALDH. ADH, alcohol dehydrogenase; NAD, nicotinamide adenine dinucleotide; MEOS, microsomal ethanol oxidizing system; NADP, nicotinamide adenine dinucleotide phosphatase; ALDH, aldehyde dehydrogenase.

For example, young women are unable to process alcohol at the same rate as young men because they do not express the ADH as highly; the inverse is true amongst the middle-aged [70]. The level of activity may not strictly correlate to the level of expression due to allelic diversity among the population. Epidemiologically, these allelic differences have been linked to region of origin. Populations from Europe express an allele for the ADH that makes it much more active than those found in populations from Asia or the Americas. For example, the ADH1B2 allele is expressed most commonly in Asian populations whereas those of Caucasian descent rarely carry it and more commonly express the ADH1C alleles [68, 71].

In the setting of a sustained, heavy and chronic alcohol consumption, the main pathway for alcohol oxidation shifts from ADH to cytochrome P450 2E1 (CYP2E1) [68]. CYP2E1 is the central component of the microsomal ethanol oxidizing system and it is predominantly located in hepatocytes and in the gastrointestinal mucosa (see Chapter 16 in this Volume). The induction of CYP2E1 leads to 10 to 20-fold increase over basal activity [72]. Following induction, CYP2E1 becomes the primary pathway for alcohol metabolism and, together with ADH-dependent alcohol metabolism, contributes to hepatic acetaldehyde production. Moreover, *CYP2E1 also leads to increased oxidative stress due to generation of ROS, including hydroxyethyl radicals (HERs)* [68, 73]. *Ethanol is a hydroxyl radical scavenger and HER represents the product of the interaction of ethanol with hydroxyl radical.* HER binds rapidly to proteins to produce alcohol-derived protein adducts. *Interaction of HER with cellular antioxidants could contribute to mechanisms by which alcohol produces a state of oxidative stress* [74]. Once ROS have formed, they can promote DNA and protein adducts directly, or they can cause lipid peroxidation leading to the formation of biologically reactive aldehyde molecules, including 4-HNE and malondialdehyde (MDA) (Figure 8) [72, 75]. An overview of alcohol and acetaldehyde oxidation reactions is presented in Figure 9.

6.2. The Role of Intestinal Endotoxemia, TNFα and Kupffer Cells

Gut-derived bacterial endotoxin has been implicated as an important cofactor in the progression of ALD. In patients with ALD, plasma endotoxin levels are high compared with those in normal subjects and in patients with non-alcoholic cirrhosis [76, 77]. Endotoxemia also correlates with serum levels of both TNFα and TNF receptors, with an association with the stage of liver disease [78]. Interestingly, patients with the highest serum cytokine concentrations showed the highest rate of in-hospital mortality [79]. The mechanism underlying these observations may be an increased intestinal permeability from chronic ethanol exposure [77].

An important role of hepatic Kupffer cells in the pathogenesis of ALD and the related oxidative stress has also been hypothesized. Indeed, *chronic alcohol consumption stimulates Kupffer cells to produce free radicals and cytokines, especially TNFα, which plays a central role in ALD*. This stimulation seems to be mediated by bacterial-derived endotoxin [80]. Experimental studies showed that chemical inactivation of Kupffer cells prevents ALD [81]. Moreover, anti-TNFα antibodies protect against ALD [82]. *In vivo, NADPH oxidase was found to play a key role for generating ROS in Kupffer cells after treatment of rats with alcohol* [83]. The essential role of TNFα in alcohol-induced liver injury was further demonstrated in TNFα receptor 1 knockout mice, because in this model the alcohol-induced pathology is blocked [84]. NF-κB is also involved in the regulation of TNFα. A close temporal association among endotoxemia, Kupffer cells activation, increased transcription of TNFα and hepatic inflammation and damage can be hypothesized. Endotoxin activates Kupffer cells and subsequent production of free radicals, which induce NF-κB. NF-κB increases TNFα levels, followed eventually by tissue damage [80] (Figure 10).

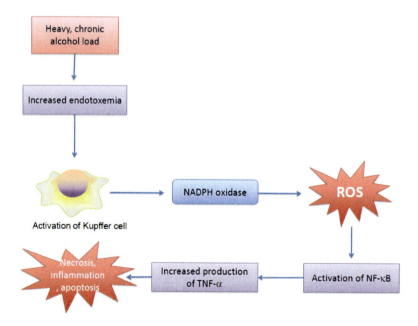

Figure 10. Schematic representation of the role of Kupffer cells in ALD. NADPH, nicotinamide adenine dinucleotide phosphatase; ROS, reactive oxygen species; TNFα, tumor necrosis factor alpha; NF-κB, nuclear factor-κB.

6.3. Oxidative Stress and Mitochondria

Chronic alcohol consumption depresses mitochondrial function causing production of ROS and cell toxicity [85]. An increase in lipid peroxidation-derived products, superoxide ($O_2^{\bullet}$), hydrogen peroxide (H_2O_2) and hydroxyl radical ($OH^{\bullet}$) has been observed in mitochrondria of rats fed alcohol [67].

ROS generation is further elevated after chronic alcohol consumption because of the decreased activity of the respiratory chain in mitochrondria. Interestingly, a single dose of alcohol had no effect on nuclear DNA integrity of mouse liver, whereas it led to extensively damage of hepatic mitochondrial DNA [86].

Moreover, alcohol caused a decline in the mitochondrial membrane potential and triggered opening of the mitochondrial permeability pore; these effects could be blocked by an inhibitor of alcohol metabolism and an antioxidant [87].

6.4 The Role of Adiponectin and PPARα

A pathophysiological link among TNFα, adiponectin and PPARα was recently described, bringing new insight to the complex regulation of ALD. Decreased circulating adiponectin levels have been repeatedly associated with various disease states, including inflammation and ALD.

Moreover, hypoadiponectinemia were reported to enhance hepatic oxidative stress [88-90]. In mouse studies, chronic consumption of alcohol associated with a high-fat diet significantly reduced plasma adiponectin concentrations, and the decreased adiponectin levels correlated with the degree of liver injury [89].

Interestingly, when mice are treated with recombinant adiponectin they show less inflammation, elevation of transaminases and fatty liver. This last finding could be related to the restoration of hepatic fatty acid oxidation disrupted by chronic alcohol feeding [89]. Two adiponectin receptors have been identified, one mostly expressed in skeletal muscle, the other expressed in the liver.

The effects of adiponectin are very likely facilitated by an increase in fatty acid oxidation associated with activation of adenosine monophosphate-activated protein (AMP) kinase and PPARα pathways downstream of adiponectin receptors in the liver [91]. A strong association between AMP-activated protein kinase activation and PPARα signaling pathways that are downstream of adiponectin receptors has been revealed [92].

A link between adiponectin and TNFα in the pathogenesis of ALD was also recently hypothesized. Indeed, moderate alcohol intake significantly increased plasma adiponectin levels both in healthy and insulin-resistant individuals without affecting plasma TNFα concentrations [93].

Moreover, adiponectin and TNFα regulate each other's production and antagonize each other's biological effects in target tissues. Both hepatic expression and plasma concentrations of TNFα increase after alcohol intake, and adiponectin treatment suppresses both plasma and hepatic levels of TNFα [89]. Alcohol may suppress adiponectin through activation of TNFα. An important relationship linking alcohol, adiponectin, PPARα and TNFα may be hypothesized.

6.5. Mechanisms of Protection against Free Radical Toxicity in ALD

Since free radical production is a process that occurs naturally, a number of mechanisms have evolved to protect cells against ROS [80, 94]. It has been shown that these mechanisms may be impaired after long-term alcohol consumption. A list of the main antioxidant systems involved in the elimination of ROS is shown in Table 3. Mitochondrial superoxide dismutases (SODs) catalyze removal of $O_2^{\bullet-}$ radicals (Vol. II, Chapter 5). These enzymes are critical for prevention of ROS-induced toxicity [95]. Studies employing the intragastric administration of alcohol in rats found decreases in SOD activity in the liver, but this finding remains controversial [96]. Catalase, a peroxisomal enzyme, is involved in the removal of H_2O_2 (Vol. II, Chapter 7). It catalyzes a reaction between two H_2O_2 molecules, resulting in the formation of water and O_2. Moreover, it also shows a peroxidative activity by promoting the interaction of H_2O_2 with hydrogen donors so that the H_2O_2 is converted to water and the reduced donor becomes oxidized [80]. The glutathione peroxidase system (GPx; see Vol. II, Chapter 8) consists of several components: the enzymes GPx and GSH reductase, and the cofactors GSH (Vol. II, Chapter 1) and NADPH. The main result of this complex system is the removal of H_2O_2. GSH is a cofactor for GSH transferase and it is an essential component of the GPx system. It acts as an endogenous mitochondrial antioxidant [97].

However, in the setting of chronic alcohol consumption, mitochondrial GSH is depleted, at least in part due to inhibition of GSH uptake [98]. Interestingly, depletion of mitochondrial GSH by chronic alcohol intake occurs especially in pericentral hepatocytes, where most of the liver injury originates [99]. S-adenosyl-L-methionine (SAM) is the main biological methyl donor and, in the liver, is a precursor of GSH through its conversion to cysteine via the trans-sulfuration pathway [100]. SAM is particularly important in opposing the toxicity of free radicals generated by toxins, including alcohol. It has been shown that liver injury of various etiologies causes a decrease in SAM levels [101].

Another important nonenzymatic antioxidant is vitamin E (α-tocopherol; see Vol. II, Chapter 3), which acts as a powerful terminator of lipid peroxidation. Patients with ALD show reduced levels of vitamin E [102]. Several *in vivo* studies revealed that administration of antioxidants, such as ebselen, vitamin E, SOD, or reduced GSH-replenishing agents can ameliorate or prevent the toxicity of alcohol in rats [103]. Chronic alcohol intake in baboons resulted in significant depletion of GSH and hepatic SAM concentrations. These depletions were corrected with SAM administration [104]. Moreover, in rats treated with alcohol, concomitant SAM administration prevented alcoholic liver steatosis [105].

Table 3. Main antioxidant systems involved in the cellular protection against free radicals

Involved system	Mechanism
Superoxide dismutase	Removal of $O_2^{\bullet-}$ radicals
Catalase	Removal of H_2O_2
Glutathione peroxidase	Removal of H_2O_2
S-adenosyl-L-methionine	Precursor of glutathione
Vitamin E	Termination of lipid peroxidation

6.6. Alcoholism and Oxidative Stress

In various studies, parameters of oxidative stress were elevated in patients with chronic alcohol consumption. Levels of an isomer of linoleic acid were elevated in patients with chronic alcoholism immediately after withdrawal, while those still suffering from alcoholism presented with increased free radical activity [106]. Products of lipid peroxidation were significantly higher in alcohol abusers than in controls and decreased during abstinence [107, 108]. Strong 4-HNE-protein adduct staining has been observed by immunohistochemistry in patients with ALD compared with those with chronic viral hepatitis [109]. Similarly to 4-HNE, HER can react with proteins to generate HER-protein adducts. In contrast to controls and non-alcoholic cirrhotic patients, antibodies against HER-protein adducts have been found in patients with alcoholic cirrhosis. In patients with ALD, formation of HER from alcohol HER-protein adducts may lead to the development of immunological reactions [110]. Similarly, other studies have reported the presence of antibodies against MDA, 4-HNE and oxidized phospholipids in the sera of patients with ALD but not in those with fatty liver only [111].

7. Oxidative Stress and Non-Alcoholic Fatty Liver Disease

Considering the increasing prevalence of NAFLD, in the past years many efforts have been dedicated to identify risk factors and mechanisms underlying the development of hepatic steatosis and its possible evolution towards NASH and end-stage liver complications. Hepatic steatosis is considered a manifestation of metabolic syndrome, which is defined as an association of at least 3 of the following disturbances: insulin resistance, central obesity, arterial hypertension, and dyslipidemia (hypertriglyceridemia or low HDL-cholesterol levels) [112, 113]. Only a proportion of individuals with liver steatosis progress to more advanced stages of the hepatic disease [10, 11, 14].

The pathogenesis of NAFLD and the reasons why some patients with fatty liver develop NASH and have progressive liver disease are not entirely understood. The most widely supported theory implicates insulin resistance as the key mechanism in NAFLD, leading to hepatic steatosis and perhaps also to NASH. Obesity, type 2 diabetes, hyperlipidemia and other conditions associated with insulin resistance are generally present in patients with NAFLD [112, 113].

A "two-hit" hypothesis has been proposed, involving the accumulation of fat in the liver ("first hit"), together with a "second hit" that produces oxidative stress. Hepatic steatosis has been recognized as the first of two hits in the pathogenesis of NASH, since the presence of oxidizable fat within the liver is enough to trigger lipid peroxidation [114].

However, many patients with fatty liver do not progress to steatohepatitis. Potential second hits for the evolution towards NASH include all mechanisms contributing to the development of inflammation and fibrosis. The presumed factors initiating second hits are oxidative stress and subsequent lipid peroxidation, proinflammatory cytokines (principally TNFα), and hormones derived from adipose tissue (adipocytokines) [113]. *Oxidative stress due to ROS, gut-derived lipopolysaccharide and soluble mediators synthesized from cells of the adipose tissue and of the immune system have been invoked as risk factors responsible for the "second hit" [115, 116] (Figure 11). The main potential etiologic mechanisms that link NASH with oxidative stress include lipid peroxidation, hyperinsulinemia and hepatic iron (Table 4).*

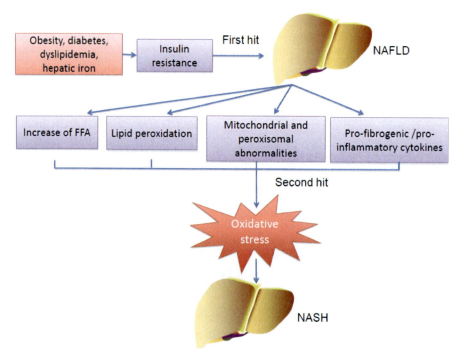

Figure 11. Mechanisms underlying the pathogenesis of hepatic steatosis and non-alcoholic steatohepatitis (NASH). NAFLD, non-alcoholic fatty liver disease.

Table 4. Pathways for oxidative stress involved in NASH pathogenesis.

Involved pathway	Mechanism
Lipid peroxidation	Mitochondrial damage with reduction of respiratory chain activity, production of ROS, reduction of antioxidants, production of TNFα, TGFβ, IL-8 with consequent damage to hepatocytes and liver fibrosis; overexpression of CYP2E1 with free fatty acid lipo-oxygenation
Hyperinsulinemia	Production of ROS, profibrogenic role, ER stress, impaired glucose metabolism
Iron	Link with insulin resistance, increased oxidative stress
Heme oxygenase-1	Antioxidant activity
PPARα	Activation of peroxisomal oxidation, production of ROS

Legend: ROS, reactive oxygen species; TNFα, tumor necrosis factor alpha; IL-8, interleukin 8; TGFβ, transforming growth factor beta; CYP2E1, cytochrome P450 2E1; ROS, reactive oxygen species; ER, endoplasmic reticulum; PPARα, peroxisome proliferator-activated receptor alpha.

7.1. Mechanisms of Lipid Peroxidation

Increased lipid peroxidation has been demonstrated in both animal models of fatty liver and in patients with NAFLD [117, 118]. Products of lipid peroxidation were significantly increased among patients with NAFLD as compared with chronic viral hepatitis [119]. NASH patients have increased levels of oxidative stress as compared with patients with simple steatosis [117]. In these patients, free fatty acids are the likely source of oxidative stress. Patients with NAFLD show increased lipolysis and augmented delivery of free fatty acids to the liver. Moreover, in these subjects the concentration of free fatty acids is associated with more severe liver disease [117, 120]. Indeed, appropriate fat oxidation is necessary to prevent its accumulation in the liver, whereas excessive fatty acid oxidation leads to oxidative stress. The ROS imbalance triggers NASH by lipid peroxidation [117]. *In experimental steatohepatitis, hepatocytes are the major site of lipid peroxidation due to the generation of pro-oxidants from mitochondria and CYP2E1 lipid oxidases* [121]. In NASH patients more than 40% of mitochondria have an abnormal structure, which is associated with impaired electron transport chain enzyme activity and ROS formation, impaired ATP generation and depletion of mitochondrial GSH [122]. Interestingly, *patients with NASH present with damaged antioxidant activities including GSH enzymes, SOD, catalase and NO* [123]. The decreased activities of the mitochondrial respiratory chain increase TNFα expression, which causes additional lipid peroxidation of mitochondrial membranes with further reduction of mitochondrial function. It is noteworthy that administration of anti-TNFα antibody ameliorated liver damage in animal models [124]. In addition to TNFα production, lipid peroxidation induces production of other cytokines which cause additional damage such as TGFβ and IL-8, the former being involved in production of collagen and fibrosis, the latter stimulating neutrophil chemotaxis [121]. Interestingly, CYP2E1, implicated in the lipo-oxygenation of free fatty acids, has been reported to be over-expressed in the liver of patients with NASH [125]. Overall, these molecular mechanisms contribute to the enhancement of lipid peroxidation, liver cell injury and hepatic fibrosis, leading to the development and progression of steatohepatitis. In clinical studies, the use of lipid-lowering agents such as fibrates and statins as a potential therapeutic strategy for NASH led to encouraging results [121]. Fibrates affect lipid oxidation, reduce trygliceride levels and increase serum HDL. It has been shown that fibrates may lead to normalization of liver function tests and lipid metabolism, and improvement of hepatic steatosis. Moreover, they inhibit HSC activation and fibrogenesis in animal models of NASH [126, 127]. Statins decrease transaminases and serum lipid levels and reduce liver steatosis [128].

7.2. Hyperinsulinemia

Hyperinsulinemia is a frequent finding in patients with NAFLD. Insulin can damage the liver through direct and indirect mechanisms [51, 55]. The liver is an important regulator of glucose homeostasis, which is controlled by insulin signaling that acts through binding to its receptor. The insulin binding to its receptor activates the phosphorylation of insulin receptor substrates, which are the main mediators of insulin signaling in the liver [129]. As already mentioned for HCV, *insulin may have a direct effect on the liver through its ability to produce* ROS [51]. Insulin seems to possess a direct profibrogenic role by stimulating CTGF production from HSCs and the synthesis of ECM, especially in the presence of hyperglycemia [55, 130]. Evidences indicate that insulin may also be directly involved in causing ER stress along with the unfolding protein response and apoptosis. This stress in turn leads to suppression of insulin receptor signaling through hyperactivation of c-Jun N-terminal kinase and subsequent serine phosphorylation of insulin receptor substrate-1. Indeed, mice deficient in X-box-binding protein-1, a transcription factor that modulates the ER stress response, develop insulin resistance [131]. An important mechanism underlying the role of insulin resistance in NAFLD is represented by a reduced insulin-suppressing effect in hepatic glucose production, which aggravates peripheral insulin resistance and contributes to hepatic lipogenesis [132]. Therefore, hyperinsulinemia causes an increased synthesis of free fatty acids, with accumulation of triglycerides in the liver. On the other hand, free fatty acids induce hepatic insulin resistance through translocation of the protein kinase C isoforms from the cytosol to the membrane, resulting in impairment of phosphatidylinositol-3-kinase activity [121]. The possible therapeutic application of insulin-sensitizing agents has been proposed for the clinical management of NAFLD. The principal agents that belong to this class of drugs include thiazolidinediones and metformin. Thiazolidinediones improve insulin sensitivity by stimulating adipocytes to increase the uptake of free fatty acids and induce redistribution of hepatic fat to peripheral tissues. However, contrasting results have been obtained in clinical trials [133, 134]. Metformin ameliorates insulin resistance by enhancing insulin signaling. This results in improved hepatic steatosis and decreased TNFα levels [135].

7.3. Iron Overload

Hyperferritinemia has been frequently observed in patients with metabolic syndrome and NAFLD [35]. Hepatic siderosis is also a frequent finding in patients with NAFLD but in most cases hepatic iron deposition is mild. It appears rational that iron causes oxidative stress in NAFLD. It has been proposed that iron, even in relatively low concentrations may synergize with other risk factors such as lipid peroxidation and hyperinsulinemia to increase oxidative stress in the liver [35]. *A frequent association between hepatic steatosis, insulin resistance and hepatic iron overload was found by Mendler and colleagues who coined the term insulin-resistance associated hepatic iron overload (IR-HIO) to describe this syndrome.* In Mendler's study, liver steatosis and NASH were present in 25% and 27% of IR-HIO cases, respectively [136]. A subsequent study confirmed the high prevalence of NAFLD (59.7%) in patients with IR-HIO [137]. Moreover, as in NASH, phlebotomy allows for normalization of body iron stores in IR-HIO [138]. Indeed, IR-HIO shares some features with NASH, such as hyperferritinemia with mostly normal transferrin saturation. However, not all patients with IR-HIO have hepatic steatosis. It is likely that NASH and IR-HIO share some pathogenetic mechanisms. Conceivably, IR-HIO may represent one end of the spectrum of NASH in which hepatic iron concentration is increased. Alternatively, IR-HIO may represent a coincidental convergence of hepatic iron overload with a very common liver disorder in the general population [139]. Recently Aigner and colleagues studied the molecular pathways that potentially underlie iron accumulation in NAFLD. According to their study, iron accumulation in NAFLD may result from an impaired iron export due to down-regulation of ferroportin and ineffective hepatic iron sensing, as indicated by low hemojuvelin expression. Increased hepcidin formation in iron-overloaded NAFLD patients, however, results in decreased ferroportin expression, whereas a reduction in liver ferroportin may perpetuate hepatic iron retention [140]. In recent years it has been proposed that iron overload in the context of NASH may be associated with HFE mutations [35]. However, other studies on this area yielded controversial results. Clinical evidence that supports the role of iron in NAFLD comes from studies on iron-depletion therapy, which improved both transaminase levels and insulin sensitivity [141].

7.4. Other Mechanisms of Oxidative Stress in NASH

Heme oxygenase-1 (HO-1), a heme-degrading enzyme with antioxidant activity (see Vol. II, Chapter 11), is significantly upregulated in animal models of NASH and is over-expressed in patients with NASH [121]. It is inducible by various stimuli, including, ROS, cytokines and metals. HO-1 may also be activated by exposure to products of lipid peroxidation, that is common in NASH. Therefore, steatosis/lipid peroxidation may be followed by liver injury, inflammation, upregulation of HO-1 and finally fibrosis. Notably, HO-1 reactions release iron (Fe^{2+}), which is involved in the pathogenesis of NASH.

Another important pathway that may be altered in NASH involves SAMmetabolism. SAM is formed from methionine and ATP in a reaction catalyzed by methionine adenosyl transferase. In the trans-methylation pathway, SAM is converted to S-adenosylhomocysteine, the levels of which tend to be high in most forms of liver disease [142]. Homocysteine, a known inducer of fatty liver, also tends to be elevated in liver diseases. Abnormal hepatic activity of methionine adenosyl transferase, an enzyme sensitive to oxidative stress, has been described. Knockout mice for an isoform of methionine adenosyl transferase develop steatohepatitis with hepatic SAM deficiency [143]. It has been shown that treatment with SAM replenishes cellular GSH levels and exerts anti-apoptotic and anti-inflammatory effect by decreasing TNFα [121]. PPARα is a transcription factor that controls genes involved in fatty acid oxidation and transport. Activated PPARα governs the expression of both peroxisomal and microsomal lipid oxidation pathways and becomes particularly relevant when CYP2E1 levels are low and free fatty acids accumulate. Activation of peroxisomal oxidation occurs when mitochondrial oxidation is saturated, with peroxisomal proliferation and increased production of ROS (Vol. II, Chapter 17). This results in activation of lipid peroxidation and progression from simple steatosis to NASH [144].

8. Oxidative Stress and Hepatocellular Carcinoma

Primary tumors of the liver represent the fifth most common type of cancer in the world and the third leading cause of cancer-related death. It is currently estimated that 500,000 to 1,000,000 new cases of primary liver tumors are diagnosed each year [145-147]. HCC represents 80% of all primary liver tumors.

Table 5. Mechanisms for oxidative stress-induced hepatocarcinogenesis in chronic liver diseases

Etiology of chronic liver disease	Mechanism
HCV	Oxidative stress induced by HCV core protein, HCV NS5A, iron, steatosis
HBV	Oxidative stress induced by HBsAg, HBx
Alcohol	Production of hepatocarcinogens (aldehydes, nitrosamines) via induction of CYP2E1, neoangiogenesis, iron
NAFLD	Oxidative stress due to insulin resistance, iron

Legend: HCV, hepatitis C virus; HBV, hepatitis B virus; NAFLD, non-alcoholic fatty liver disease; NS5A, non-structural protein 5A; HBsAg, hepatitis B surface antigen; HBx, hepatitis B protein x; CYP2E1, cytochrome P450 2E1.

The incidence is highly related to specific risk factors that include chronic infection with hepatitis viruses, aflatoxin ingestion and prolonged heavy alcohol consumption [68]. Chronic hepatitis and liver cirrhosis associated with either HBV or HCV infection represent major risk factors for HCC development, being implicated in more than 80% of HCC cases worldwide [3, 6, 7]. Alcohol is also a strong primary cause when HCC develops in patients who are heavy alcoholics, most of whom have alcohol-induced cirrhosis. In addition, alcohol is a cofactor when associated with other causative factors including HCV, HBV, and diabetes mellitus. Importantly, combination of two or more of these risk factors has a synergistic effect for HCC development [68]. Regardless of the underlying etiology, the prognosis of patients with HCC is generally poor, despite new treatment strategies that have emerged in recent years. *Oxidative stress is recognized to play an important role in the initiation and promotion of the events of carcinogenesis. Indeed, oxidative stress has emerged as a key player in the pathogenesis of chronic liver diseases and precancerous lesions, induced by HBV or HCV infection, alcoholic and nonalcoholic steatohepatitis.* Polymorphonuclear neutrophils in these inflamed livers are a major source of ROS [55] (Table 5). Moreover, nonparenchymal cells, including Kupffer cells and other macrophages, which release cytokines, are another cause of ROS induction in hepatocytes. In addition, virus proteins and conditions that are frequently associated with chronic liver diseases, such as iron overload and steatosis, may also generate oxidative stress. Oxidative stress is suggested to promote hepatocarcinogenesis through multiple pathways including induction of mutations in the p53 tumor suppressor gene [148].

8.1. Oxidative Stress and HCV-Induced Carcinogenesis

Oxidative stress produced by ROS and RNS has been implicated in HCV-induced hepatic cancer. The induction of NO synthase by HCV core protein generates RNS that may cause DNA damage and mutagenesis within immunoglobulin and tumor suppressor genes [32, 55, 149, 150]. These genotoxic effects of ROS and RNS may contribute to the development of B-cell lymphoma and HCC during HCV chronic infection. Recent evidence for the causal role of HCV in HCC development derives from studies using mouse models. Transgenic mice expressing HCV core protein show an increased accumulation of ROS, which correlates with

HCC development, and transient expression of NS5A alters intracellular calcium levels leading to oxidative stress and activity of STAT3 and NF-κB [150]. Other mechanisms by which the core protein of HCV may induce HCC include modulation of tumor suppressor genes and proto-oncogenes, and inhibition of apoptosis. *Oxidative DNA damage increases chromosomal aberrations associated with cell transformation, which may account, in part, for the mechanism by which oxidative stress promotes the development of HCV-associated HCC [55, 151]. On the other hand, iron overload, which is a common feature of chronic HCV infection, may also participate in liver injury.* The causative role of iron in the pathogenesis of HCC comes from clinical studies demonstrating that patients with hereditary hemochromatosis exhibit a very high risk for HCC [152]. In experimental studies, iron overload induced mitochondrial injury and increased the risk of HCC development in transgenic mice expressing the HCV polyprotein [153]. In contrast, iron reduction therapy by repeated phlebotomy ameliorated hepatocyte injury in patients with HCV infection. Steatosis is another common feature of HCV-infected hepatocytes. It has been shown that steatosis in hepatocytes of patients with HCV infection may also contribute to hepatocarcinogenesis, through mitochondrial dysfunction and ROS generation [55, 151]. Overall, these facts suggest that *ROS production associated with HCV infection may cooperate with other factors and promote HCC development. In this view, adjunctive therapy with antioxidants has been proposed in chronic hepatitis C.*

8.2. Oxidative Stress and HBV-Induced Carcinogenesis

Transgenic mice expressing the HBV surface antigen exhibit oxidative stress and DNA damage, leading to development of HCC [154]. Moreover, HBx protein has drawn considerable attention owing to its role in viral replication and possibly in HCC. It is well established that HBx induces oxidative stress via its direct association with mitochondria leading to elevation of ROS. Although the oncogenic property of HBx remains controversial, it has been established that HBx protein contributes to HCC development, in conjunction with genotoxic stresses and/or oncogene activation [155, 156]. Consequently, the association of HBx protein with mitochondria induces the activation of transcriptional factors, including STAT3 and NF-κB, which is prevented by antioxidants [58]. Taken together, these observations indicate that *HBx protein participates in the development of HCC via ROS generation.*

8.3. Oxidative Stress and Alcohol-Induced Carcinogenesis

Alcohol is nowadays considered a carcinogen [68]. Indeed, some of its metabolites, mainly aldehydes (acetaldehyde, MDA and 4-HNE), have been indentified as toxic compounds with mutagenic properties and several carcinogenic effects both *in vitro* and *in vivo*. Aldehydes can form DNA adducts and adducts with a wide range of cellular proteins, including those involved in DNA repair. The precise mechanism(s) through which aldehyde-protein adducts affect hepatic responses and mediate alcohol-induced hepatocarcinogenesis is not fully understood. Aldehydes are able to interact with lysine residues on proteins that are critical for cell function, including calmodulin and tubulin. Moreover, they stimulate collagen synthesis by HSCs, thus contributing to progressive hepatic scarring leading to cirrhosis and, ultimately, HCC [157]. Also ROS generated in the setting of chronic alcohol abuse are capable of stimulating protein and DNA peroxidation directly, and these molecular events affect DNA and protein integrity and function. Alcohol may also have a hepatocarcinogenic effect via induction of CYP2E1. During chronic alcohol consumption CYP2E1 induction leads to increased acetaldehyde and ROS production that, as already described, can compromise cell integrity through formation of protein and DNA adducts. However, alcohol is not the exclusive substrate for CYP2E1. CYP2E1 is important for the metabolism of acetone and fatty acids under physiological conditions but it can also metabolize several small hydrophic substrates, including solvents, aromatic hydrocarbons, nitrosamines, drugs and tobacco smoke. Therefore, the conversion of several procarcinogens (including nitrosamines) to carcinogenic derivates occurs via CYP2E1, an enzyme inducible by chronic alcohol intake [68]. In summary, alcohol has not only the ability of promoting hepatocarcinogenesis through its proper CYP2E1-dependent metabolism (with production of aldehydes), but also through the effect that CYP2E1 induction has on the metabolism of xenobiotics and other substrates [158].

Another proposed mechanism for alcohol hepatocarcinogenesis includes a possible effect on neoangiogenesis. HCC is a highly vascularized tumor in which neoangiogenesis plays a central role [159]. Currently, little is understood concerning the potential involvement of alcohol during angiogenesis within dysplastic hepatic nodules. However, it has been shown that alcohol causes and imbalance in ET-1 and NO signaling, resulting in increased vasoconstriction and portal hypertension [160]. These changes in the microcirculation in close proximity to dysplastic cells may contribute to angiogenesis within the dysplastic nodules.

Iron has also been proposed as a possible mechanism for hepatocarcinogenesis in ALD. Patients with ALD commonly have elevation of transferrin saturation and serum ferritin concentration; and significant hepatic iron deposition is not infrequent [35, 161, 162]. Most patients with ALD have normal or slightly elevated hepatic iron concentrations [35, 163]. However, there is growing evidence that a mild degree of iron overload is sufficient to enhance alcohol-induced liver injury. Indeed, patients with hereditary haemochromatotis and significant alcohol consumption have a higher incidence of cirrhosis and HCC than those without heavy alcohol consumption [164, 165]. *There are several potential causes for hepatic iron overload in alcoholics, including increased ingestion of iron, increased intestinal iron absorption, up-regulation of hepatic transferrin receptor 1 (TfR1), secondary anemia due to haemolysis, hypersplenism, ineffective erythropoiesis, hypoxemia due to intrapulmonary shunts and portosystemic shunts* [166]. A strong link between hepatic iron overload, HFE mutations and development of HCC in alcoholic cirrhosis has been recently shown in a prospective, large-scale study [167].

8.4. Oxidative Stress and Non-Alcoholic Fatty Liver Disease Carcinogenesis

Numerous studies link the known risk factors for NAFLD to HCC. Obesity is recognized as a significant risk factor for the development of various types of cancer, including HCC. Indeed, among obese males liver cancer showed the highest relative risk of all neoplasms surveyed. Obesity also represents a risk factor for HCC in cirrhosis of other etiologies. It has been suggested that the increased risk for HCC conferred by obesity may be related to two factors: the increased risk for NAFLD, which affects up to 90% of obese individuals, and the carcinogenic potential exerted by obesity *per se* [168, 169]. Similarly, it has been reported that patients with type 2 diabetes mellitus present with an increased risk of HCC [170]. The risk of HCC was found elevated in several cohort studies, including prospective studies [168, 171, 172]. As already described, the main causative factor for the pathogenesis of NASH is insulin resistance with subsequent hyperinsulinemia, which is believed to be a risk factor for several types of cancer including HCC [51, 55, 169]. Insulin resistance may induce HCC by up-regulating multiple growth factors. Insulin induces IGF-1, which stimulates growth through cellular proliferation and inhibition of apoptosis. Insulin also mediates growth by activation of mitogen-activated kinases and phosphorylation of insulin receptor substrate 1. Human hepatoma cells over-express both IGF-1 and insulin receptor substrate 1 [168] and over-expression of insulin receptor substrate 1 may prevent TGFβ mediated apoptosis [173]. There is also evidence that hepatocarcinogenesis in NASH may be partially mediated by increased release of free fatty acids and adipokines secreted by adipose tissue, which alter the immune response and modulate the release of inflammatory and inhibitory cytokines, such as TNFα, NF-κB and IL-6 [174]. This mechanism is associated with reduced release of adiponectin and activation of HSCs, resulting in increased production of ECM and proinflammatory and profibrogenic cytokines. Interestingly, in an insulin-resistant obese mouse model, mitochondrial dysfunction and hepatic lipid peroxidation generate excess ROS, resulting in hepatic hyperplasiaand oxidative stress. Oxidative stress is further implicated in blocking expression of transcription factors that regulate gene transcription encoding enzymatic antioxidants, resulting in steatohepatitis and development of HCC in animal models [175]. As already described, iron overload is a common feature in patients with NAFLD and it may be linked to oxidative stress [35, 121]. Interestingly, clinical evidence suggests a causative role of iron in the development of HCC in patients with NASH-related cirrhosis [176].

9. Oxidative Stress and Paracetamol-Induced Liver Damage

Paracetamol (acetaminophen) is a widely available, safe and effective analgesic and antipyretic drug when used at therapeutic doses. However, an overdose can induce severe liver injury both in experimental *in vivo* models and in humans. Mainly causing liver injury, paracetamol toxicity is one of the most common causes of poisoning worldwide, either for suicidal intent or by unintentional overdose. It accounts for most drug overdoses and cases of acute liver failure in the United States, the United Kingdom, Australia and New Zealand [177]. Many individuals with paracetamol toxicity may have no symptoms in the first 24 hours following overdose. Others may initially have nonspecific complaints such as vague abdominal pain and nausea. With progressive disease, signs of liver failure may develop, including hypoglycemia, acidosis, hemorrhagic diathesis and hepatic encephalopathy. Some will spontaneously resolve, although untreated cases may result in death. N-acetylcysteine can prevent hepatic injury if given within 12 hours of a single ingestion [178]. However, unintentional overdosing is usually recognized after symptoms have developed. Risk factors for enhanced toxicity may include alcohol intake, fasting or anorexia nervosa, and the use of certain drugs such as isoniazid. *Hepatotoxicity results not from paracetamol itself, but from one of its metabolites, N-acetyl-p-benzoquinoneimine (NAPQI). NAPQI depletes the liver's natural antioxidant GSH and directly damages cells in the liver, leading to liver failure.* In the past, the main mechanism for paracetamol toxicity was attributed to metabolic activation of the drug through CYP2E1, depletion of GSH and covalent binding of NADQI to cellular proteins as the main cause of hepatic cell death [179]. More recently, it was proposed that covalent binding is not sufficient for hepatic cell death but it triggers a signal that requires amplification in the cell. *Reactive metabolite formation, GSH depletion and alkylation of proteins, especially mitochondrial proteins, seem to be the critical initiating events for the toxicity* [180]. *Mitochondrial dysfunction, due to covalent binding, leads to formation of ROS and peroxynitrite, which trigger the membrane permeability transition and the collapse of the mitochondrial membrane potential (Figure 12).* The consequences include depletion of ATP, extensive DNA fragmentation and modification of intracellular proteins. All these events contribute to the development of oncotic necrotic cell death [55]. *The rationale for the clinical use of N-acetylcysteine as antidote against paracetamol toxicity is that it is a precursor of GSH, which is depleted during paracetamol hepatotoxicity. Indeed, GSH can effectively protect the liver both by scavenging NADQI and by detoxifying ROS and peroxinitrite* [178]. Antioxidants, such as sylimarin, were also found to protect the liver against paracetamol toxicity in animal models [181].

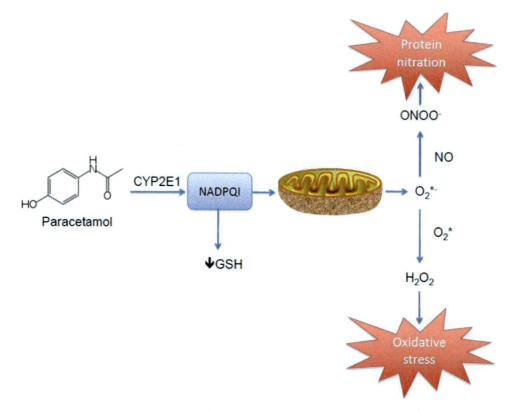

Figure 12. The role of free radicals and oxidative stress in paracetamol toxicity. CYP2E1, cytochrome P450 2E1; NADQI, N-acetyl-p-benzoquinone imine; O_2^{*-}, superoxide anion; NO, nitric oxide; $ONOO^-$, peroxynitrite; GSH, glutathione.

10. Oxidative Stress and Ischemia/Reperfusion Liver Injury

During various surgical procedures, interruption of an organ's blood flow, with consequent lack of oxygen and nutrient supply, is an intrinsic phenomenon that may lead to hepatocellular damage.

The main procedures in liver surgery that can lead to prolonged ischemic periods include resection of large hepatic tumors, management of hepatic trauma, vascular reconstructions and liver transplantation. When the flow of blood and oxygen is re-established, reperfusion increases the damage induced during the ischemic period, thus aggravating injury to hepatic cells [182].

Table 6. Main events, cells and mediators involved in hepatic ischemia-reperfusion injury

Event/cell/mediator	Mechanism
Microcirculatory failure	Ischemic phase: disequilibrium between NO and ET, vasoconstriction, compromised blood flow; leukocytes chemotaxis, platelet aggregation and neutrophil adhesion lead to occlusion of capillaries. Reperfusion phase: the collapse of the microcirculation maintains areas of ischemic liver parenchyma (no-reflow).
Kupffer cells	Major source of ROS and oxidative stress during the reperfusion phase via release of many proinflammatory mediators, including TNFα, interleukins and prostaglandins.
Neutrophils	Contribution to oxidative stress through ROS release, especially superoxide and peroxides.
Platelets	Release of proinflammatory interleukins (IL-1, IL-6), TGFβ, serotonin; production of NO that leads to peroxynitrite formation, which contributes to oxidative stress and is a potent inducer of apoptosis in endothelial cells.
TNFα	Induction of leukocytes chemotaxis, activation of Kupffer cells with ROS production.
Interleukins	Initiation, perpetuation and modulation of inflammatory response
ROS	Transformation of xanthine dehydrogenase into xanthine oxidase, with release of $O_2^{\bullet-}$ and H_2O_2; production of ROS through induction of NADPH oxidase by activated Kupffer cells and neutrophils.
RNS	NO production via nitric oxide synthase and conversion of NO to peroxynitrite.
Reduced oxidative phosphorylation	ATP depletion and loss of calcium homeostasis

Legend: TNFα, tumor necrosis factor alpha; ROS, reactive oxygen species; RNS, reactive nitrogen species; NO, nitric oxide; ET, endothelin; ROS, reactive oxygen species; IL-1, interleukin 1; IL-6, interleukin 6; TGFβ, transforming growth factor beta; NADPH, nicotinamide adenine dinucleotide phosphate; ATP, adenosine triphosphate.

This process is known as ischemia-reperfusion injury and impacts directly on liver viability. The pathophysiology of ischemia-reperfusion includes various events, which are summarized in Table 6.

During the ischemic phase, the lack of nutrients and oxygen produces edema in Kupffer cells and endothelial cells. The balance between NO and endothelins induces a disequilibrium towards endothelins, with consequent vasoconstriction and further compromise of the blood flow. This promotes leukocytes chemotaxis, platelet aggregation and neutrophil adhesion [183, 184].

The capillaries then result partially occluded by cells and platelets. During the reperfusion phase, the collapse of the microcirculation maintains areas of ischemic liver parenchyma (no-reflow) [185]. The microcirculatory failure is indeed the main event in the pathogenesis of ischemia-reperfusion damage.

In addition, *activation of Kupffer cells and neutrophils increases the synthesis of inflammatory cytokines and aggravates hepatic ischemic damage by increasing oxidative stress* [182]. *Kupffer cells release many proinflammatory mediators, including TNFα, interleukins and prostaglandins and also contribute to increase the oxidative stress through ROS production. Indeed, activated Kupffer cells are the main source of ROS during the reperfusion period* [186].

Neutrophils also contribute to increased oxidative stress observed during ischemia-reperfusion damage through ROS release, especially superoxide and peroxide species [182]. Platelets release several factors that play an important role in the ischemia-reperfusion liver damage, including interleukins (IL-1, IL-6), TGFβ and serotonin. Moreover, platelets produce NO that leads to the production of peroxynitrite, which contribute to oxidative stress and acts as a potent inducer of endothelial apoptosis [187, 188].

As in many other conditions, during ischemia-reperfusion liver damage the balance between ROS and antioxidants shifts towards the former [182]. The augmentation of oxidative stress that occurs during ischemia-reperfusion liver injury includes several events:

1) transformation of xanthine dehydrogenase into xanthine oxidase, an oxygen dependant process that produces uric acid, releasing $O_2^{\bullet-}$ and H_2O_2 [189];
2) decline in oxidative phosphorylation, with consequent ATP depletion and loss of calcium homeostasis [182];
3) induction of NADPH oxidase by activated Kupffer cells and neutrophils, with subsequent ROS production;
4) NO production and its conversion to peroxynitrite [190].

The hepatic cellular consequences of these events include nitrosylation of iron-sulfur groups and tyrosine residues, inactivation of heme groups and lipid peroxidation. The critical role of oxidative stress in ischemia-reperfusion induced damage is indicated by evidence that endogenous antioxidant levels decrease significantly during the reperfusion phase [191]. Moreover, the administration of exogenous antioxidants may reduce the severity of ischemia-reperfusion liver injury [182].

Acknowledgments

GS is funded by an unrestricted grant from Roche-Italia.

References

[1] de Franchis R, Hadengue A, Lau G, et al. EASL International Consensus Conference on Hepatitis B. 13-14 September, 2002 Geneva, Switzerland. Consensus statement (long version). *J. Hepatol.* 2003;39 Suppl 1:S3-25.

[2] Lavanchy D. Hepatitis B virus epidemiology, disease burden, treatment, and current and emerging prevention and control measures. *J. Viral. Hepat.* 2004;11:97-107.

[3] Beasley RP. Hepatitis B virus. The major etiology of hepatocellular carcinoma. *Cancer,* 1988;61:1942-56.

[4] Fattovich G, Brollo L, Giustina G, et al. Natural history and prognostic factors for chronic hepatitis type B. *Gut,* 1991;32:294-8.

[5] Global surveillance and control of hepatitis C. Report of a WHO Consultation organized in collaboration with the Viral Hepatitis Prevention Board, Antwerp, Belgium. *J. Viral. Hepat.* 1999;6:35-47.

[6] Alberti A, Chemello L, Benvegnu L. Natural history of hepatitis C. *J. Hepatol.* 1999;31 Suppl 1:17-24.

[7] Ikeda K, Saitoh S, Suzuki Y, et al. Disease progression and hepatocellular carcinogenesis in patients with chronic viral hepatitis: a prospective observation of 2215 patients. *J. Hepatol.* 1998;28:930-8.

[8] Tsukamoto H. Conceptual importance of identifying alcoholic liver disease as a lifestyle disease. *J. Gastroenterol.* 2007;42:603-9.

[9] Day CP, Bassendine MF. Genetic predisposition to alcoholic liver disease. *Gut,* 1992;33:1444-7.

[10] Matteoni CA, Younossi ZM, Gramlich T, Boparai N, Liu YC, McCullough AJ. Nonalcoholic fatty liver disease: a spectrum of clinical and pathological severity. *Gastroenterology,* 1999;116:1413-9.

[11] Clark JM, Diehl AM. Nonalcoholic fatty liver disease: an underrecognized cause of cryptogenic cirrhosis. *JAMA,* 2003;289:3000-4.

[12] Angulo P. Nonalcoholic fatty liver disease. *N. Engl. J. Med.* 2002;346:1221-31.

[13] Cave M, Deaciuc I, Mendez C, et al. Nonalcoholic fatty liver disease: predisposing factors and the role of nutrition. *J. Nutr. Biochem.* 2007;18:184-95.

[14] Caldwell SH, Oelsner DH, Iezzoni JC, Hespenheide EE, Battle EH, Driscoll CJ. Cryptogenic cirrhosis: clinical characterization and risk factors for underlying disease. *Hepatology,* 1999;29:664-9.

[15] Clark JM. The epidemiology of nonalcoholic fatty liver disease in adults. *J. Clin. Gastroenterol.* 2006;40 Suppl 1:S5-10.

[16] McCullough AJ. Pathophysiology of nonalcoholic steatohepatitis. *J. Clin. Gastroenterol.* 2006;40 Suppl 1:S17-29.

[17] Friedman SL. Liver fibrosis -- from bench to bedside. *J. Hepatol.* 2003;38 Suppl 1:S38-53.

[18] Friedman SL. Mechanisms of hepatic fibrogenesis. *Gastroenterology,* 2008;134:1655-69.

[19] Rippe RA, Brenner DA. From quiescence to activation: Gene regulation in hepatic stellate cells. *Gastroenterology,* 2004;127:1260-2.

[20] Li JT, Liao ZX, Ping J, Xu D, Wang H. Molecular mechanism of hepatic stellate cell activation and antifibrotic therapeutic strategies. *J. Gastroenterol.* 2008;43:419-28.

[21] Cubero FJ, Urtasun R, Nieto N. Alcohol and liver fibrosis. *Semin. Liver Dis.* 2009;29:211-21.

[22] Borkham-Kamphorst E, van Roeyen CR, Ostendorf T, Floege J, Gressner AM, Weiskirchen R. Pro-fibrogenic potential of PDGF-D in liver fibrosis. *J. Hepatol.* 2007;46:1064-74.

[23] Adachi T, Togashi H, Suzuki A, et al. NAD(P)H oxidase plays a crucial role in PDGF-induced proliferation of hepatic stellate cells. *Hepatology,* 2005;41:1272-81.

[24] Rockey DC. Vascular mediators in the injured liver. *Hepatology,* 2003;37:4-12.

[25] Inagaki Y, Okazaki I. Emerging insights into Transforming growth factor beta Smad signal in hepatic fibrogenesis. *Gut,* 2007;56:284-92.

[26] Shek FW, Benyon RC. How can transforming growth factor beta be targeted usefully to combat liver fibrosis? *Eur. J. Gastroenterol. Hepatol.* 2004;16:123-6.

[27] Bethanis SK, Theocharis SE. Leptin in the field of hepatic fibrosis: a pivotal or an incidental player? *Dig. Dis. Sci.* 2006;51:1685-96.

[28] Hazra S, Xiong S, Wang J, et al. Peroxisome proliferator-activated receptor gamma induces a phenotypic switch from activated to quiescent hepatic stellate cells. *J. Biol. Chem.* 2004;279:11392-401.

[29] Robertson B, Myers G, Howard C, et al. Classification, nomenclature, and database development for hepatitis C virus (HCV) and related viruses: proposals for standardization. International Committee on Virus Taxonomy. *Arch. Virol.* 1998;143:2493-503.

[30] Lindenbach BD, Rice CM. Unravelling hepatitis C virus replication from genome to function. *Nature,* 2005;436:933-8.

[31] Choi J, Ou JH. Mechanisms of liver injury. III. Oxidative stress in the pathogenesis of hepatitis C virus. *Am. J. Physiol. Gastrointest. Liver Physiol.* 2006;290:G847-51.

[32] Mahmood S, Kawanaka M, Kamei A, et al. Immunohistochemical evaluation of oxidative stress markers in chronic hepatitis C. *Antioxid. Redox. Signal.* 2004;6:19-24.

[33] Di Bisceglie AM, Axiotis CA, Hoofnagle JH, Bacon BR. Measurements of iron status in patients with chronic hepatitis. *Gastroenterology,* 1992;102:2108-13.

[34] Bonkovsky HL, Banner BF, Rothman AL. Iron and chronic viral hepatitis. *Hepatology,* 1997;25:759-68.

[35] Sebastiani G, Walker AP. HFE gene in primary and secondary hepatic iron overload. *World J. Gastroenterol.* 2007;13:4673-89.

[36] Riggio O, Montagnese F, Fiore P, et al. Iron overload in patients with chronic viral hepatitis: how common is it? *Am. J. Gastroenterol.* 1997;92:1298-301.

[37] Sebastiani G, Vario A, Ferrari A, Pistis R, Noventa F, Alberti A. Hepatic iron, liver steatosis and viral genotypes in patients with chronic hepatitis C. *J. Viral. Hepat.* 2006;13:199-205.

[38] Lecube A, Hernandez C, Genesca J, et al. Diabetes is the main factor accounting for the high ferritin levels detected in chronic hepatitis C virus infection. *Diabetes Care,* 2004;27:2669-75.

[39] Sebastiani G, Vario A, Alberti A. Diabetes is the main factor accounting for the high ferritin levels detected in chronic hepatitis C virus infection: response to Lecube et al. *Diabetes Care,* 2005;28:1838; author reply -9.

[40] Van Thiel DH, Friedlander L, Fagiuoli S, Wright HI, Irish W, Gavaler JS. Response to interferon alpha therapy is influenced by the iron content of the liver. *J. Hepatol.* 1994;20:410-5.

[41] Olynyk JK, Reddy KR, Di Bisceglie AM, et al. Hepatic iron concentration as a predictor of response to interferon alfa therapy in chronic hepatitis C. *Gastroenterology,* 1995;108:1104-9.

[42] Pietrangelo A. Metals, oxidative stress, and hepatic fibrogenesis. *Semin. Liver Dis.* 1996;16:13-30.

[43] Fujita N, Sugimoto R, Motonishi S, et al. Patients with chronic hepatitis C achieving a sustained virological response to peginterferon and ribavirin therapy recover from impaired hepcidin secretion. *J. Hepatol.* 2008;49:702-10.

[44] Nishina S, Hino K, Korenaga M, et al. Hepatitis C virus-induced reactive oxygen species raise hepatic iron level in mice by reducing hepcidin transcription. *Gastroenterology,* 2008;134:226-38.

[45] Miura K, Taura K, Kodama Y, Schnabl B, Brenner DA. Hepatitis C virus-induced oxidative stress suppresses hepcidin expression through increased histone deacetylase activity. *Hepatology,* 2008:1420-9.

[46] Wang T, Weinman SA. Causes and consequences of mitochondrial reactive oxygen species generation in hepatitis C. *J. Gastroenterol. Hepatol.* 2006;21 Suppl 3:S34-7.

[47] Okuda M, Li K, Beard MR, et al. Mitochondrial injury, oxidative stress, and antioxidant gene expression are induced by hepatitis C virus core protein. *Gastroenterology,* 2002;122:366-75.

[48] Machida K, Cheng KT, Sung VM, Lee KJ, Levine AM, Lai MM. Hepatitis C virus infection activates the immunologic (type II) isoform of nitric oxide synthase and thereby enhances DNA damage and mutations of cellular genes. *J. Virol.* 2004;78:8835-43.

[49] Sheikh MY, Choi J, Qadri I, Friedman JE, Sanyal AJ. Hepatitis C virus infection: molecular pathways to metabolic syndrome. *Hepatology,* 2008;47:2127-33.

[50] Scherer PE, Williams S, Fogliano M, Baldini G, Lodish HF. A novel serum protein similar to C1q, produced exclusively in adipocytes. *J. Biol. Chem.* 1995;270:26746-9.

[51] Goldstein BJ, Mahadev K, Wu X. Redox paradox: insulin action is facilitated by insulin-stimulated reactive oxygen species with multiple potential signaling targets. *Diabetes,* 2005;54:311-21.

[52] Riordan SM, Skinner NA, Kurtovic J, et al. Toll-like receptor expression in chronic hepatitis C: correlation with pro-inflammatory cytokine levels and liver injury. *Inflamm. Res.* 2006;55:279-85.

[53] Gong G, Waris G, Tanveer R, Siddiqui A. Human hepatitis C virus NS5A protein alters intracellular calcium levels, induces oxidative stress, and activates STAT-3 and NF-kappa B. *Proc. Natl. Acad. Sci. U S A,* 2001;98:9599-604.

[54] Bureau C, Bernad J, Chaouche N, et al. Nonstructural 3 protein of hepatitis C virus triggers an oxidative burst in human monocytes via activation of NADPH oxidase. *J. Biol. Chem.* 2001;276:23077-83.

[55] Muriel P. Role of free radicals in liver diseases. *Hepatol. Int.* 2009.

[56] Brechot C, Hadchouel M, Scotto J, et al. State of hepatitis B virus DNA in hepatocytes of patients with hepatitis B surface antigen-positive and -negative liver diseases. *Proc. Natl. Acad. Sci. U S A, 1981*;78:3906-10.

[57] Meyer M, Caselmann WH, Schluter V, Schreck R, Hofschneider PH, Baeuerle PA. Hepatitis B virus transactivator MHBst: activation of NF-kappa B, selective inhibition by antioxidants and integral membrane localization. *EMBO J.*1992;11:2991-3001.

[58] Waris G, Huh KW, Siddiqui A. Mitochondrially associated hepatitis B virus X protein constitutively activates transcription factors STAT-3 and NF-kappa B via oxidative stress. *Mol. Cell Biol.* 2001;21:7721-30.

[59] Siddiqui A, Jameel S, Mapoles J. Expression of the hepatitis B virus X gene in mammalian cells. *Proc. Natl. Acad. Sci. U S A, 1987*;84:2513-7.

[60] Doria M, Klein N, Lucito R, Schneider RJ. The hepatitis B virus HBx protein is a dual specificity cytoplasmic activator of Ras and nuclear activator of transcription factors. *EMBO J.* 1995;14:4747-57.

[61] Rahmani Z, Huh KW, Lasher R, Siddiqui A. Hepatitis B virus X protein colocalizes to mitochondria with a human voltage-dependent anion channel, HVDAC3, and alters its transmembrane potential. *J. Virol.* 2000;74:2840-6.

[62] Twu JS, Chu K, Robinson WS. Hepatitis B virus X gene activates kappa B-like enhancer sequences in the long terminal repeat of human immunodeficiency virus 1. *Proc. Natl. Acad. Sci. U S A, 1989*;86:5168-72.

[63] Darnell JE, Jr. STATs and gene regulation. *Science, 1997*;277:1630-5.

[64] Carballo M, Conde M, El Bekay R, et al. Oxidative stress triggers STAT3 tyrosine phosphorylation and nuclear translocation in human lymphocytes. *J. Biol. Chem.* 1999;274:17580-6.

[65] Xu Z, Jensen G, Yen TS. Activation of hepatitis B virus S promoter by the viral large surface protein via induction of stress in the endoplasmic reticulum. *J. Virol.* 1997;71:7387-92.

[66] Nordmann R, Ribiere C, Rouach H. Implication of free radical mechanisms in ethanol-induced cellular injury. *Free Radic. Biol. Med.* 1992;12:219-40.

[67] Wu D, Cederbaum AI. Oxidative stress and alcoholic liver disease. *Semin. Liver Dis.* 2009;29:141-54.

[68] McKillop IH, Schrum LW. Role of alcohol in liver carcinogenesis. *Semin. Liver Dis.* 2009;29:222-32.

[69] Jornvall H, Hoog JO. Nomenclature of alcohol dehydrogenases. *Alcohol Alcohol,* 1995;30:153-61.

[70] Parlesak A, Billinger MH, Bode C, Bode JC. Gastric alcohol dehydrogenase activity in man: influence of gender, age, alcohol consumption and smoking in a caucasian population. *Alcohol Alcohol,* 2002;37:388-93.

[71] Day CP. Genes or environment to determine alcoholic liver disease and non-alcoholic fatty liver disease. *Liver Int.* 2006;26:1021-8.

[72] Lu Y, Cederbaum AI. CYP2E1 and oxidative liver injury by alcohol. *Free Radic. Biol.Med.* 2008;44:723-38.

[73] Koop DR. Oxidative and reductive metabolism by cytochrome P450 2E1. *FASEB J.* 1992;6:724-30.

[74] Reinke LA. Spin trapping evidence for alcohol-associated oxidative stress. *Free Radic. Biol. Med.* 2002;32:953-7.

[75] Brooks PJ, Theruvathu JA. DNA adducts from acetaldehyde: implications for alcohol-related carcinogenesis. *Alcohol,* 2005;35:187-93.

[76] Parlesak A, Schafer C, Schutz T, Bode JC, Bode C. Increased intestinal permeability to macromolecules and endotoxemia in patients with chronic alcohol abuse in different stages of alcohol-induced liver disease. *J. Hepatol.* 2000;32:742-7.

[77] Fukui H, Brauner B, Bode JC, Bode C. Plasma endotoxin concentrations in patients with alcoholic and non-alcoholic liver disease: reevaluation with an improved chromogenic assay. *J. Hepatol.* 1991;12:162-9.

[78] Hanck C, Rossol S, Bocker U, Tokus M, Singer MV. Presence of plasma endotoxin is correlated with tumour necrosis factor receptor levels and disease activity in alcoholic cirrhosis. *Alcohol Alcohol,* 1998;33:606-8.

[79] Bird GL, Sheron N, Goka AK, Alexander GJ, Williams RS. Increased plasma tumor necrosis factor in severe alcoholic hepatitis. Ann Intern Med 1990;112:917-20.

[80] Cederbaum AI, Lu Y, Wu D. Role of oxidative stress in alcohol-induced liver injury. *Arch. Toxicol.* 2009;83:519-48.

[81] Adachi Y, Bradford BU, Gao W, Bojes HK, Thurman RG. Inactivation of Kupffer cells prevents early alcohol-induced liver injury. *Hepatology,* 1994;20:453-60.

[82] Iimuro Y, Gallucci RM, Luster MI, Kono H, Thurman RG. Antibodies to tumor necrosis factor alfa attenuate hepatic necrosis and inflammation caused by chronic exposure to ethanol in the rat. *Hepatology,* 1997;26:1530-7.

[83] Kono H, Rusyn I, Uesugi T, et al. Diphenyleneiodonium sulfate, an NADPH oxidase inhibitor, prevents early alcohol-induced liver injury in the rat. *Am. J. Physiol. Gastrointest Liver Physiol.* 2001;280:G1005-12.

[84] Yin M, Wheeler MD, Kono H, et al. Essential role of tumor necrosis factor alpha in alcohol-induced liver injury in mice. *Gastroenterology*, 1999;117:942-52.

[85] Cunningham CC, Coleman WB, Spach PI. The effects of chronic ethanol consumption on hepatic mitochondrial energy metabolism. *Alcohol Alcohol*, 1990;25:127-36.

[86] Mansouri A, Gaou I, De Kerguenec C, et al. An alcoholic binge causes massive degradation of hepatic mitochondrial DNA in mice. *Gastroenterology*, 1999;117:181-90.

[87] Higuchi H, Adachi M, Miura S, Gores GJ, Ishii H. The mitochondrial permeability transition contributes to acute ethanol-induced apoptosis in rat hepatocytes. *Hepatology*, 2001;34:320-8.

[88] Ouchi N, Kihara S, Funahashi T, Matsuzawa Y, Walsh K. Obesity, adiponectin and vascular inflammatory disease. *Curr. Opin. Lipidol.* 2003;14:561-6.

[89] Xu A, Wang Y, Keshaw H, Xu LY, Lam KS, Cooper GJ. The fat-derived hormone adiponectin alleviates alcoholic and nonalcoholic fatty liver diseases in mice. *J. Clin.Invest.* 2003;112:91-100.

[90] You M, Considine RV, Leone TC, Kelly DP, Crabb DW. Role of adiponectin in the protective action of dietary saturated fat against alcoholic fatty liver in mice. *Hepatology,* 2005;42:568-77.

[91] Yamauchi T, Kamon J, Ito Y, et al. Cloning of adiponectin receptors that mediate antidiabetic metabolic effects. *Nature,* 2003;423:762-9.

[92] Yamauchi T, Nio Y, Maki T, et al. Targeted disruption of AdipoR1 and AdipoR2 causes abrogation of adiponectin binding and metabolic actions. *Nat. Med.* 2007;13:332-9.

[93] Sierksma A, Patel H, Ouchi N, et al. Effect of moderate alcohol consumption on adiponectin, tumor necrosis factor-alpha, and insulin sensitivity. *Diabetes Care,* 2004;27:184-9.

[94] Halliwell B. Antioxidant defence mechanisms: from the beginning to the end (of the beginning). *Free Radic. Res.* 1999;31:261-72.

[95] Fridovich I. Superoxide anion radical (O2-.), superoxide dismutases, and related matters. *J. Biol. Chem.* 1997;272:18515-7.

[96] Polavarapu R, Spitz DR, Sim JE, et al. Increased lipid peroxidation and impaired antioxidant enzyme function is associated with pathological liver injury in experimental alcoholic liver disease in rats fed diets high in corn oil and fish oil. *Hepatology,* 1998;27:1317-23.

[97] Garcia-Ruiz C, Fernandez-Checa JC. Mitochondrial glutathione: hepatocellular survival-death switch. *J. Gastroenterol. Hepatol.* 2006;21 Suppl 3:S3-6.

[98] Fernandez-Checa JC, Ookhtens M, Kaplowitz N. Effects of chronic ethanol feeding on rat hepatocytic glutathione. Relationship of cytosolic glutathione to efflux and mitochondrial sequestration. *J. Clin. Invest.* 1989;83:1247-52.

[99] Garcia-Ruiz C, Morales A, Colell A, et al. Feeding S-adenosyl-L-methionine attenuates both ethanol-induced depletion of mitochondrial glutathione and mitochondrial dysfunction in periportal and perivenous rat hepatocytes. *Hepatology,* 1995;21:207-14.

[100] Avila MA, Garcia-Trevijano ER, Martinez-Chantar ML, et al. S-Adenosylmethionine revisited: its essential role in the regulation of liver function. *Alcohol,* 2002;27:163-7.

[101] Avila MA, Berasain C, Torres L, et al. Reduced mRNA abundance of the main enzymes involved in methionine metabolism in human liver cirrhosis and hepatocellular carcinoma. *J. Hepatol.* 2000;33:907-14.

[102] Nanji AA, Hiller-Sturmhofel S. Apoptosis and necrosis: two types of cell death in alcoholic liver disease. *Alcohol Health Res. World,* 1997;21:325-30.

[103] Iimuro Y, Bradford BU, Yamashina S, et al. The glutathione precursor L-2-oxothiazolidine-4-carboxylic acid protects against liver injury due to chronic enteral ethanol exposure in the rat. *Hepatology,* 2000;31:391-8.

[104] Lieber CS, Casini A, DeCarli LM, et al. S-adenosyl-L-methionine attenuates alcohol-induced liver injury in the baboon. *Hepatology,* 1990;11:165-72.

[105] Feo F, Pascale R, Garcea R, et al. Effect of the variations of S-adenosyl-L-methionine liver content on fat accumulation and ethanol metabolism in ethanol-intoxicated rats. *Toxicol. Appl. Pharmacol.* 1986;83:331-41.

[106] Fink R, Clemens MR, Marjot DH, et al. Increased free-radical activity in alcoholics. *Lancet,* 1985;2:291-4.

[107] Letteron P, Duchatelle V, Berson A, et al. Increased ethane exhalation, an in vivo index of lipid peroxidation, in alcohol-abusers. *Gut.* 1993;34:409-14.

[108] Adachi J, Matsushita S, Yoshioka N, et al. Plasma phosphatidylcholine hydroperoxide as a new marker of oxidative stress in alcoholic patients. *J. Lipid. Res.* 2004;45:967-71.

[109] Ohhira M, Ohtake T, Matsumoto A, et al. Immunohistochemical detection of 4-hydroxy-2-nonenal-modified-protein adducts in human alcoholic liver diseases. *Alcohol. Clin. Exp.Res.* 1998;22:145S-9S.

[110] Clot P, Bellomo G, Tabone M, Arico S, Albano E. Detection of antibodies against proteins modified by hydroxyethyl free radicals in patients with alcoholic cirrhosis. *Gastroenterology*, 1995;108:201-7.

[111] Rolla R, Vay D, Mottaran E, et al. Antiphospholipid antibodies associated with alcoholic liver disease specifically recognise oxidised phospholipids. *Gut*, 2001;49:852-9.

[112] Bugianesi E, Manzini P, D'Antico S, et al. Relative contribution of iron burden, HFE mutations, and insulin resistance to fibrosis in nonalcoholic fatty liver. *Hepatology*, 2004;39:179-87.

[113] Duvnjak M, Lerotic I, Barsic N, Tomasic V, Virovic Jukic L, Velagic V. Pathogenesis and management issues for non-alcoholic fatty liver disease. *World J. Gastroenterol.* 2007;13:4539-50.

[114] Day CP, James OF. Steatohepatitis: a tale of two "hits"? *Gastroenterology*, 1998;114:842-5.

[115] Day CP. From fat to inflammation. *Gastroenterology*, 2006;130:207-10.

[116] Lalor PF, Faint J, Aarbodem Y, Hubscher SG, Adams DH. The role of cytokines and chemokines in the development of steatohepatitis. *Semin. Liver Dis.* 2007;27:173-93.

[117] Sanyal AJ, Campbell-Sargent C, Mirshahi F, et al. Nonalcoholic steatohepatitis: association of insulin resistance and mitochondrial abnormalities. *Gastroenterology*, 2001;120:1183-92.

[118] George J, Pera N, Phung N, Leclercq I, Yun Hou J, Farrell G. Lipid peroxidation, stellate cell activation and hepatic fibrogenesis in a rat model of chronic steatohepatitis. *J. Hepatol.* 2003;39:756-64.

[119] Madan K, Bhardwaj P, Thareja S, Gupta SD, Saraya A. Oxidant stress and antioxidant status among patients with nonalcoholic fatty liver disease (NAFLD). *J. Clin. Gastroenterol.* 2006;40:930-5.

[120] Marchesini G, Brizi M, Bianchi G, et al. Nonalcoholic fatty liver disease: a feature of the metabolic syndrome. *Diabetes,* 2001;50:1844-50.

[121] Malaguarnera M, Di Rosa M, Nicoletti F, Malaguarnera L. Molecular mechanisms involved in NAFLD progression. *J. Mol. Med.* 2009;87:679-95.

[122] Pessayre D, Berson A, Fromenty B, Mansouri A. Mitochondria in steatohepatitis. *Semin. Liver Dis.* 2001;21:57-69.

[123] Baskol G, Baskol M, Kocer D. Oxidative stress and antioxidant defenses in serum of patients with non-alcoholic steatohepatitis. *Clin. Biochem.* 2007;40:776-80.

[124] Li Z, Yang S, Lin H, et al. Probiotics and antibodies to TNF inhibit inflammatory activity and improve nonalcoholic fatty liver disease. *Hepatology,* 2003;37:343-50.

[125] Weltman MD, Farrell GC, Hall P, Ingelman-Sundberg M, Liddle C. Hepatic cytochrome P450 2E1 is increased in patients with nonalcoholic steatohepatitis. *Hepatology,* 1998;27:128-33.

[126] Perkins JD. Saying "Yes" to obese living liver donors: short-term intensive treatment for donors with hepatic steatosis in living-donor liver transplantation. *Liver Transpl.* 2006;12:1012-3.

[127] Nakano S, Inada Y, Masuzaki H, et al. Bezafibrate regulates the expression and enzyme activity of 11beta-hydroxysteroid dehydrogenase type 1 in murine adipose tissue and 3T3-L1 adipocytes. *Am. J. Physiol. Endocrinol. Metab.* 2007;292:E1213-22.

[128] Ekstedt M, Franzen LE, Mathiesen UL, Holmqvist M, Bodemar G, Kechagias S. Statins in non-alcoholic fatty liver disease and chronically elevated liver enzymes: a histopathological follow-up study. *J. Hepatol.* 2007;47:135-41.

[129] Virkamaki A, Ueki K, Kahn CR. Protein-protein interaction in insulin signaling and the molecular mechanisms of insulin resistance. *J. Clin. Invest.* 1999;103:931-43.

[130] Svegliati-Baroni G, Ridolfi F, Di Sario A, et al. Insulin and insulin-like growth factor-1 stimulate proliferation and type I collagen accumulation by human hepatic stellate cells: differential effects on signal transduction pathways. *Hepatology,* 1999;29:1743-51.

[131] Ozcan U, Cao Q, Yilmaz E, et al. Endoplasmic reticulum stress links obesity, insulin action, and type 2 diabetes. *Science,* 2004;306:457-61.

[132] Bugianesi E, McCullough AJ, Marchesini G. Insulin resistance: a metabolic pathway to chronic liver disease. *Hepatology,* 2005;42:987-1000.

[133] Ratziu V, Giral P, Jacqueminet S, et al. Rosiglitazone for nonalcoholic steatohepatitis: one-year results of the randomized placebo-controlled Fatty Liver Improvement with Rosiglitazone Therapy (FLIRT) Trial. *Gastroenterology,* 2008;135:100-10.

[134] Vuppalanchi R, Chalasani N. Nonalcoholic fatty liver disease and nonalcoholic steatohepatitis: Selected practical issues in their evaluation and management. *Hepatology,* 2009;49:306-17.

[135] Kumar N, Dey CS. Metformin enhances insulin signalling in insulin-dependent and-independent pathways in insulin resistant muscle cells. *Br. J. Pharmacol.* 2002;137:329-36.

[136] Mendler MH, Turlin B, Moirand R, et al. Insulin resistance-associated hepatic iron overload. *Gastroenterology*, 1999;117:1155-63.

[137] Turlin B, Mendler MH, Moirand R, Guyader D, Guillygomarc'h A, Deugnier Y. Histologic features of the liver in insulin resistance-associated iron overload. A study of 139 patients. *Am. J. Clin. Pathol.* 2001;116:263-70.

[138] Guillygomarc'h A, Mendler MH, Moirand R, et al. Venesection therapy of insulin resistance-associated hepatic iron overload. *J. Hepatol.* 2001;35:344-9.

[139] Lauret E, Rodriguez M, Gonzalez S, et al. HFE gene mutations in alcoholic and virus-related cirrhotic patients with hepatocellular carcinoma. *Am. J. Gastroenterol.* 2002;97:1016-21.

[140] Aigner E, Theurl I, Theurl M, et al. Pathways underlying iron accumulation in human nonalcoholic fatty liver disease. *Am. J. Clin. Nutr.* 2008;87:1374-83.

[141] Facchini FS, Hua NW, Stoohs RA. Effect of iron depletion in carbohydrate-intolerant patients with clinical evidence of nonalcoholic fatty liver disease. *Gastroenterology,* 2002;122:931-9.

[142] Duce AM, Ortiz P, Cabrero C, Mato JM. S-adenosyl-L-methionine synthetase and phospholipid methyltransferase are inhibited in human cirrhosis. *Hepatology,* 1988;8:65-8.

[143] Lu SC, Alvarez L, Huang ZZ, et al. Methionine adenosyltransferase 1A knockout mice are predisposed to liver injury and exhibit increased expression of genes involved in proliferation. *Proc. Natl. Acad. Sci. U S A,* 2001;98:5560-5.

[144] Rao MS, Reddy JK. Peroxisomal beta-oxidation and steatohepatitis. *Semin Liver Dis.* 2001;21:43-55.

[145] Parkin DM. Global cancer statistics in the year 2000. *Lancet Oncol.* 2001;2:533-43.

[146] Shibuya K, Mathers CD, Boschi-Pinto C, Lopez AD, Murray CJ. Global and regional estimates of cancer mortality and incidence by site: II. Results for the global burden of disease 2000. *BMC Cancer,* 2002;2:37.

[147] McGlynn KA, London WT. Epidemiology and natural history of hepatocellular carcinoma. *Best Pract. Res. Clin. Gastroenterol.* 2005;19:3-23.

[148] Hu W, Feng Z, Eveleigh J, et al. The major lipid peroxidation product, trans-4-hydroxy-2-nonenal, preferentially forms DNA adducts at codon 249 of human p53 gene, a unique mutational hotspot in hepatocellular carcinoma. *Carcinogenesis,* 2002;23:1781-9.

[149] Sumida Y, Nakashima T, Yoh T, et al. Serum thioredoxin levels as an indicator of oxidative stress in patients with hepatitis C virus infection. *J. Hepatol.* 2000;33:616-22.

[150] Moriya K, Fujie H, Shintani Y, et al. The core protein of hepatitis C virus induces hepatocellular carcinoma in transgenic mice. *Nat. Med.* 1998;4:1065-7.

[151] Sasaki Y. Does oxidative stress participate in the development of hepatocellular carcinoma? *J. Gastroenterol.* 2006;41:1135-48.

[152] Dragani TA. Risk of HCC: Genetic heterogeneity and complex genetics. *J. Hepatol.* 2009.

[153] Furutani T, Hino K, Okuda M, et al. Hepatic iron overload induces hepatocellular carcinoma in transgenic mice expressing the hepatitis C virus polyprotein. *Gastroenterology,* 2006;130:2087-98.

[154] Hagen TM, Huang S, Curnutte J, et al. Extensive oxidative DNA damage in hepatocytes of transgenic mice with chronic active hepatitis destined to develop hepatocellular carcinoma. *Proc. Natl. Acad. Sci. U S A,* 1994;91:12808-12.

[155] Madden CR, Finegold MJ, Slagle BL. Hepatitis B virus X protein acts as a tumor promoter in development of diethylnitrosamine-induced preneoplastic lesions. *J. Virol.* 2001;75:3851-8.

[156] Terradillos O, Billet O, Renard CA, et al. The hepatitis B virus X gene potentiates c-myc-induced liver oncogenesis in transgenic mice. *Oncogene,* 1997;14:395-404.

[157] Freeman TL, Tuma DJ, Thiele GM, et al. Recent advances in alcohol-induced adduct formation. *Alcohol Clin. Exp. Res.* 2005;29:1310-6.

[158] Badger TM, Ronis MJ, Seitz HK, Albano E, Ingelman-Sundberg M, Lieber CS. Alcohol metabolism: role in toxicity and carcinogenesis. *Alcohol Clin. Exp. Res.* 2003;27:336-47.

[159] Ribatti D, Vacca A, Nico B, Sansonno D, Dammacco F. Angiogenesis and anti-angiogenesis in hepatocellular carcinoma. *Cancer Treat Rev.* 2006;32:437-44.

[160] Bauer M, Paquette NC, Zhang JX, et al. Chronic ethanol consumption increases hepatic sinusoidal contractile response to endothelin-1 in the rat. *Hepatology,* 1995;22:1565-76.

[161] Ludwig J, Hashimoto E, Porayko MK, Moyer TP, Baldus WP. Hemosiderosis in cirrhosis: a study of 447 native livers. *Gastroenterology,* 1997;112:882-8.

[162] Milman N, Ovesen L, Byg K, Graudal N. Iron status in Danes updated 1994. I: prevalence of iron deficiency and iron overload in 1332 men aged 40-70 years. Influence Of blood donation, alcohol intake, and iron supplementation. *Ann. Hematol.* 1999;78:393-400.

[163] Gleeson D, Evans S, Bradley M, et al. HFE genotypes in decompensated alcoholic liver disease: phenotypic expression and comparison with heavy drinking and with normal controls. *Am. J. Gastroenterol.* 2006;101:304-10.

[164] Fargion S, Fracanzani AL, Piperno A, et al. Prognostic factors for hepatocellular carcinoma in genetic hemochromatosis. *Hepatology,* 1994;20:1426-31.

[165] Adams PC, Agnew S. Alcoholism in hereditary hemochromatosis revisited: prevalence and clinical consequences among homozygous siblings. *Hepatology,* 1996;23:724-7.

[166] Alla V, Bonkovsky HL. Iron in nonhemochromatotic liver disorders. *Semin. Liver Dis.* 2005;25:461-72.

[167] Nahon P, Sutton A, Rufat P, et al. Liver iron, HFE gene mutations, and hepatocellular carcinoma occurrence in patients with cirrhosis. *Gastroenterology,* 2008;134:102-10.

[168] Bugianesi E. Non-alcoholic steatohepatitis and cancer. *Clin. Liver Dis.* 2007;11:191-207, x-xi.

[169] Siegel AB, Zhu AX. Metabolic syndrome and hepatocellular carcinoma: two growing epidemics with a potential link. *Cancer,* 2009;115:5651-61.

[170] Calle EE, Rodriguez C, Walker-Thurmond K, Thun MJ. Overweight, obesity, and mortality from cancer in a prospectively studied cohort of U.S. adults. *N. Engl. J. Med.* 2003;348:1625-38.

[171] Fassio E, Alvarez E, Dominguez N, Landeira G, Longo C. Natural history of nonalcoholic steatohepatitis: a longitudinal study of repeat liver biopsies. *Hepatology,* 2004;40:820-6.

[172] Adams LA, Lymp JF, St Sauver J, et al. The natural history of nonalcoholic fatty liver disease: a population-based cohort study. *Gastroenterology,* 2005;129:113-21.

[173] Tanaka S, Mohr L, Schmidt EV, Sugimachi K, Wands JR. Biological effects of human insulin receptor substrate-1 overexpression in hepatocytes. *Hepatology,* 1997;26:598-604.

[174] Page JM, Harrison SA. NASH and HCC. *Clin. Liver Dis.* 2009;13:631-47.

[175] Xu Z, Chen L, Leung L, Yen TS, Lee C, Chan JY. Liver-specific inactivation of the Nrf1 gene in adult mouse leads to nonalcoholic steatohepatitis and hepatic neoplasia. *Proc. Natl. Acad. Sci. U S A,* 2005;102:4120-5.

[176] Sorrentino P, D'Angelo S, Ferbo U, Micheli P, Bracigliano A, Vecchione R. Liver iron excess in patients with hepatocellular carcinoma developed on non-alcoholic steato-hepatitis. *J. Hepatol.* 2009;50:351-7.

[177] Larson AM, Polson J, Fontana RJ, et al. Acetaminophen-induced acute liver failure: results of a United States multicenter, prospective study. *Hepatology,* 2005;42:1364-72.

[178] Polson J, Lee WM. AASLD position paper: the management of acute liver failure. *Hepatology,* 2005;41:1179-97.

[179] Nelson SD. Molecular mechanisms of the hepatotoxicity caused by acetaminophen. *Semin. Liver Dis.* 1990;10:267-78.

[180] Jaeschke H, Bajt ML. Intracellular signaling mechanisms of acetaminophen-induced liver cell death. *Toxicol. Sci.* 2006;89:31-41.

[181] Muriel P, Garciapina T, Perez-Alvarez V, Mourelle M. Silymarin protects against paracetamol-induced lipid peroxidation and liver damage. *J. Appl. Toxicol.* 1992;12:439-42.

[182] Montalvo-Jave EE, Escalante-Tattersfield T, Ortega-Salgado JA, Pina E, Geller DA. Factors in the pathophysiology of the liver ischemia-reperfusion injury. *J. Surg. Res.* 2008;147:153-9.

[183] Vollmar B, Glasz J, Leiderer R, Post S, Menger MD. Hepatic microcirculatory perfusion failure is a determinant of liver dysfunction in warm ischemia-reperfusion. *Am. J. Pathol.* 1994;145:1421-31.

[184] Vollmar B, Menger MD, Glasz J, Leiderer R, Messmer K. Impact of leukocyte-endothelial cell interaction in hepatic ischemia-reperfusion injury. *Am. J. Physiol.* 1994;267:G786-93.

[185] Pretto EA, Jr. Reperfusion injury of the liver. *Transplant Proc.* 1991;23:1912-4.

[186] Shiratori Y, Kiriyama H, Fukushi Y, et al. Modulation of ischemia-reperfusion-induced hepatic injury by Kupffer cells. *Dig. Dis. Sci.* 1994;39:1265-72.

[187] Sindram D, Porte RJ, Hoffman MR, Bentley RC, Clavien PA. Platelets induce sinusoidal endothelial cell apoptosis upon reperfusion of the cold ischemic rat liver. *Gastroenterology,* 2000;118:183-91.

[188] Lesurtel M, Graf R, Aleil B, et al. Platelet-derived serotonin mediates liver regeneration. *Science,* 2006;312:104-7.

[189] McCord JM. Oxygen-derived radicals: a link between reperfusion injury and inflammation. *Fed. Proc.* 1987;46:2402-6.

[190] Selzner N, Rudiger H, Graf R, Clavien PA. Protective strategies against ischemic injury of the liver. *Gastroenterology,* 2003;125:917-36.

[191] Marubayashi S, Dohi K, Ochi K, Kawasaki T. Protective effects of free radical scavenger and antioxidant administration on ischemic liver cell injury. *Transplant Proc.* 1987;19:1327-8.

In: Principles of Free Radical Biomedicine, Volume III
Editors: K. Pantopoulos and H. M. Schipper

ISBN 978-1-61324-184-4
©2012 Nova SciencePublishers, Inc.

Chapter 5

Reactive Oxygen Species in Renal Glomerular Diseases

Andrey V. Cybulsky[*]

Department of Medicine, McGill University Health Centre, McGill University, Montreal, Quebec, Canada

1. Introduction

The clinical manifestations of immune glomerular diseases range from isolated albuminuria or hematuria, to nephrotic syndrome, nephritic syndrome and/or rapidly progressive glomerulonephritis [1]. The immunohistology of lesions responsible for various human glomerular diseases is well described, and investigation of animal models of these pathological entities has provided significant insight into the pathogenic mechanisms, which involve antibodies, complement, and inflammatory and immune cells [2]. Several mediator systems are activated, and result in glomerular injury. This Chapter focuses on reactive oxygen species (ROS) as mediators of glomerular damage.

2. Anatomy and Function of the Glomerulus

The filtering unit of the kidney, the glomerulus, contains a tuft of capillaries situated between the afferent and efferent arterioles [3]. The glomerulus is enclosed by an epithelial cell capsule (Bowman's capsule) that is continuous with the cells of the proximal tubule. The glomerular capillary loops are supported by the mesangium, a structure consisting of mesangial cells and mesangial matrix. Glomerular filtrate, principally containing water and solutes, passes through the glomerular capillary wall, which consists of three layers, including

---

[*]Tel: (514) 398-8148. Fax: (514) 843-2815. E-mail: andrey.cybulsky@mcgill.ca

the fenestrated endothelial cells, the glomerular basement membrane (GBM), and the visceral epithelial cells, also known as podocytes.

In contrast to solute, glomerular capillary wall permeability decreases for macromolecules, such that passage of albumin and IgG is almost entirely restricted. The function of the GBM is to maintain normal glomerular architecture and anchor the adjacent cells. In addition, the GBM acts as a barrier to the filtration of macromolecules. Type IV collagen provides the basic superstructure of the GBM. Laminin and nidogen form a complex, whose major function is to mediate cell adhesion to the GBM. Heparan sulfate proteoglycans are another component of the GBM, although it is unclear whether these anionic molecules play a significant role in maintaining the charge barrier to filtration. Glomerular endothelial cells contain large fenestrae, which are coated with a glycocalyx. The visceral glomerular epithelial cells are attached to the GBM by discrete foot processes. The pores between the foot processes (filtration slits) are closed by a thin membrane (the slit diaphragm), which is believed to function as a modified adherens junction. Glomerular endothelial cells, and in particular, the podocytes, contribute to the maintenance of the permselectivity of the glomerular capillary wall.

3. Mechanisms of Glomerular Injury and Relationship with ROS

Several intersecting and complementary mediator systems may be involved in glomerular injury [2]. Antibodies can produce glomerular injury independently or via activation of complement. In addition, antibodies can interact directly with inflammatory leukocytes through Fc–Fc receptor association. Complement can injure glomerular cells directly (via assembly of the C5b-9 membrane attack complex), or may lead to recruitment of inflammatory leukocytes. Furthermore, appropriately primed T cells may identify glomerular antigens and initiate a local delayed type hypersensitivity-like reaction. These pathways have been integrated into a working model, which includes a potential role for ROS (Figure 1). The role of ROS in glomerular injury has also been addressed in several previous reviews [4-7].

4. Sources of ROS in the Glomerulus

The sources of ROS in the glomerulus may include infiltrating inflammatory leukocytes, and intrinsic glomerular cells (Figure 1). Neutrophils and monocytes can generate ROS in response to numerous stimuli. This process is referred to as the respiratory burst, is associated with a large increase in oxygen uptake, and it is catalyzed by the assembly of a multi-component enzyme complex (the NADPH oxidase), which in the presence of NADPH, reduces molecular oxygen to the superoxide anion ($O_2^{\bullet-}$). Superoxide can then be metabolized to H_2O_2 via superoxide dismutase (SOD; see Vol. II, Chapter 5), and to other ROS, such as the hydroxyl radical ($OH^{\bullet}$) via the Haber-Weiss reaction (in the presence of iron; see Vol. I, Chapter 5).

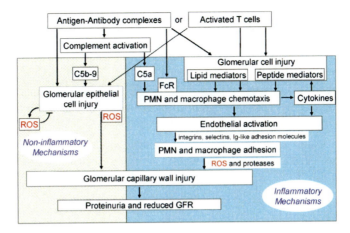

Figure 1. Mediation of glomerular injury. Pathways and mediators that have been shown experimentally to induce glomerular injury are illustrated. The role of ROS as inducers of injury and as signaling molecules is highlighted. Adapted from reference [2]. FcR, Fc receptor; GFR, glomerular filtration rate; Ig, immunoglobulin; PMN, polymorphonuclear leukocyte.

Alternatively, in the presence of a halide, H_2O_2 may be metabolized via myeloperoxidase to hypohalous acids. In experimental models of leukocyte-mediated, proliferative glomerulonephritis, stimulated leukocytes may produce ROS [2, 4-7]. In such leukocyte-dependent models, neutrophils and/or monocytes are recruited and activated at the site of antibody deposition (Figure 1, inflammatory mechanisms). *A number of distinct experimental models of glomerulonephritis, which feature infiltrating glomerular leukocytes and/or macrophages (discussed below), demonstrate involvement of $O_2^{\bullet-}$, H_2O_2, the myeloperoxidase-H_2O_2 halide system in glomerular capillary wall damage.*

Intrinsic glomerular cells under stimulated conditions may produce ROS independently of leukocyte infiltration [2, 4-7]. Normal glomeruli isolated from experimental animals produce ROS after stimulation with phorbol ester. Mesangial cells in culture can generate $O_2^{\bullet-}$ and H_2O_2 following stimulation with immune complexes, zymosan, complement C5b-9 membrane attack complex, or platelet activating factor. Glomerular epithelial cells in culture produce H_2O_2 and/or $O_2^{\bullet-}$ in response to puromycin aminonucleoside or to C5b-9 (Figure 1, non-inflammatory mechanisms). Moreover, mesangial cells and glomerular epithelial cells express all the components of the NADPH oxidase, and studies in the passive Heymann nephritis (PHN) model of human membranous nephropathy (discussed below) demonstrate that expression of the cytochrome b_{558} component is induced in podocytes injured by complement [8-10].

5. ROS Induce Glomerular Injury

ROS may damage glomerular structural proteins by various mechanisms [2, 4, 5]. In conjunction with proteinases, ROS can induce degradation of extracellular matrix proteins by increasing the susceptibility of the GBM to proteolytic damage, or alternatively, by involvement in the activation of latent proteinases, including neutrophil metalloproteinases. ROS have been shown to decrease the synthesis of glomerular proteoglycans in an isolated perfused rat kidney model, and increase albumin permeability in isolated glomeruli. In glomerular cells, ROS can alter cyclic nucleotide content, which may in turn modulate inflammatory responses. ROS may be directly cytotoxic to cultured glomerular cells, including mesangial cells. Another mechanism by which ROS may modulate inflammation is by affecting production of prostaglandins. Thus, ROS can induce production of glomerular prostaglandins via cyclooxygenase, or inhibit the production of prostaglandins stimulated by other agonists. ROS can induce peroxidation of cell membrane lipids (Vol. I, Chapter 7), resulting in the generation of reactive aldehyde groups, which can then complex with lysine residues of proteins (Vol. I, Chapter 6). Peroxidation of polyunsaturated free fatty acids, including arachidonic acid, can also lead to the generation of isoprostanes. These prostaglandin-like compounds are formed without the direct action of cyclooxygenase, and they have potent vasoactive properties.

6. Effects of ROS Relevant to Glomerular Pathophysiology

Several studies have examined the effects of ROS on renal function, glomerular permselectivity and glomerular ultrastructure. In rats, infusion of phorbol myristate acetate into the renal artery resulted in development of proteinuria, a reduction in the glomerular filtration rate, and morphologic glomerular cell injury [11].

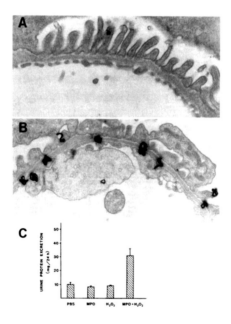

Fig. 2. The myeloperoxidase-hydrogen peroxide-halide system induces glomerular injury. A) Electron microscopy autoradiograph of a glomerular capillary wall from a control rat that was perfused with H_2O_2 and Na[^{125}]I. Essentially no silver grains were demonstrated. B) Electron microscopy autoradiograph of a rat that was perfused with myeloperoxidase followed by H_2O_2 and Na[^{125}]I. Numerous silver grains are present along the capillary wall. Endothelial cell swelling and focal epithelial cell foot process effacement are also prominent. C) Perfusion with myeloperoxidase (MPO) followed by H_2O_2 in a chloride-containing solution resulted in development of proteinuria. Reprinted from reference [13] with permission.

The latter included neutrophil infiltration, glomerular endothelial cell blebbing and separation from the GBM, as well as enlargement of podocytes and widespread foot process effacement. These changes were dependent on neutrophils, and were prevented by co-administration of catalase, which metabolizes H_2O_2 (Vol. II, Chapter 7).

By analogy, infusion of H_2O_2 into the renal artery of rats induced proteinuria, which was prevented by catalase, although in this study, proteinuria was not associated with glomerular morphologic changes [12]. Perfusion of the renal artery with myeloperoxidase, followed by H_2O_2 in a chloride-containing solution, resulted in development of proteinuria, which was associated with glomerular endothelial cell injury and focal effacement of podocyte foot processes (Figure 2) [13]. Proteinuria and glomerular cell injury did not, however, develop in control perfusions (i.e. myeloperoxidase alone or H_2O_2 alone). Moreover, in the presence of free radio-iodine, myeloperoxidase-H_2O_2-perfused kidneys incorporated radio-iodine into the GBM and mesangium (Figure 2). Myeloperoxidase-mediated glomerular disease was associated with endothelial and mesangial cell injury, activation of platelets, and a subsequent proliferative response [14]. Together, these studies demonstrate that *ROS can impair glomerular permselectivity*, and that *the myeloperoxidase-H_2O_2-halide system can induce proteinuria by halogenation of the glomerular capillary wall.*

7. ROS in Experimental Animal Models of Primary Non-Inflammatory Glomerular Diseases

Most of our understanding of mechanisms involved in the pathogenesis of human glomerular disease is based on work carried out in animal models [15, 16]. A number of studies in experimental animals indicate that ROS can mediate proteinuria (Figure 3). Minimal change disease is the most common cause of nephrotic syndrome in children, while focal segmental glomerulosclerosis (FSGS) is an important cause of nephrotic syndrome and end stage kidney failure in adults. In humans, minimal change disease and FSGS are non-inflammatory forms of glomerulopathy, which manifest proteinuria, and are most likely associated with podocyte injury [1]. Podocytes can respond to injury by producing ROS, and releasing eicosanoids, matrix-degrading proteases and GBM matrix components. Minimal change disease and the acquired forms of FSGS in humans are believed to involve T cells, which produce factors that induce podocyte injury and enhance glomerular capillary wall permeability [17]. Puromycin aminonucleoside is a glomerular epithelial cell toxin that when administered to rats, induces a lesion resembling experimental minimal change disease or FSGS. The pathogenesis involves podocyte injury and possibly apoptosis; the latter may contribute to the formation of glomerular sclerotic lesions. Puromycin aminonucleoside nephrosis is associated with production of $O_2^{\bullet-}$, H_2O_2 and hydroxyl radical [18]. In this model, allopurinol (an inhibitor of xanthine oxidase) and SOD reduced proteinuria, and blunted morphological changes of podocyte injury [19]. Other studies in puromycin aminonucleoside nephrosis also demonstrated protective effects of SOD, as well as catalase, hydroxyl radical scavengers, and deferoxamine [20, 21]. Together, these studies confirm a *functional role for xanthine oxidase-generated $O_2^{\bullet-}$, H_2O_2, and hydroxyl radicals in the puromycin aminonucleoside model of glomerular epithelial injury*. Another study demonstrated that administration of methylprednisolone to rats with puromycin aminonucleoside nephrosis increased glomerular SOD, catalase and glutathione peroxidase (GPx; Vol. II, Chapter 8) activities, and reduced proteinuria [22]. While glucocorticoids most likely exert therapeutic effects on multiple targets, this study suggests that protection from ROS-induced damage may be an important action. Conversely, feeding rats a selenium-deficient diet reduced GPx and increased proteinuria [23]. Another experimental model of human FSGS is produced by the administration of adriamycin to mice [24]. *Adriamycin provokes podocyte injury and glomerulosclerosis, which in part involves advanced glycation end products (AGE) and a ROS pathway.* AGE, perhaps best known for their association with diabetic complications (see section 11 and Chapter 9 in this Volume), are generated by the sequential nonenzymatic glycation of protein amino groups and by oxidation reactions [25]. Activation of the renin-angiotensin system might also contribute to AGE formation. While AGE bind nonspecifically to basement membranes and modify their properties, *AGE also induce specific cellular responses, including oxidative stress, by interacting with the receptor for AGE (RAGE), a multiligand member of the immunoglobulin superfamily.* RAGE is expressed in podocytes at low levels, but is upregulated in glomerular diseases [26]. In contrast to wild-type mice, adriamycin-treated RAGE-null mice were protected significantly from effacement of podocyte foot processes, proteinuria, and glomerulosclerosis [24]. Administration of adriamycin to wild-type mice also increased NADPH oxidase activity in the renal cortex and induced generation of RAGE ligands, including AGE, while treatment with soluble RAGE protected against podocyte injury and glomerulosclerosis. Incubation of RAGE-expressing cultured mouse glomerular epithelial cells with adriamycin stimulated AGE formation, and treatment with RAGE ligands activated the NADPH oxidase. *Thus, signaling via RAGE in part accounts for modulation of cellular properties by adriamycin, and RAGE and ROS may contribute to the pathogenesis of podocyte injury in FSGS.*

Animal model	Human disease	Role of ROS
Puromycin aminonucleoside nephrosis Adriamycin nephrosis	Minimal change disease and focal segmental glomerulosclerosis	• Increased production of superoxide, hydrogen peroxide and hydroxyl radical. • Superoxide dismutase, catalase, allopurinol and deferoxamine reduced proteinuria. • Glucocorticoids enhanced superoxide dismutase, catalase, and glutathione peroxidase and reduced proteinuria. • Selenium deficiency reduced glutathione peroxidase and enhanced proteinuria. • ROS production via receptor for advanced glycation end products (RAGE) and reduction in proteinuria in RAGE-null mice.
Passive Heymann nephritis	Membranous nephropathy	• Increased production of superoxid and hydrogen peroxide. • Induction of NADPH oxidase and xanthine oxidase. • Dimethylsulfoxide, dimethylthiourea, sodium benzoate, deferoxamine, probucol and tungsten reduced proteinuria. • Selenium deficiency reduced glutathione peroxidase and enhanced proteinuria.
Anti-GBM nephritis	Goodpasture's nephritis	• Catalase, dimethylthiourea and deferoxamine reduced proteinuria.
Concanavalin A anti-concanavalin A nephritis Anti-Thy 1 nephritis Bovine gamma globulin	Membrano-proliferative glomerulonephritis and IgA nephropathy	• Myeloperoxidase-hydrogen peroxide-halide system was activated. • Increased production of superoxide, hydrogen peroxide and hydroxyl radicals. • Superoxide dismutase, glutathione peroxidase and catalase were reduced. • α-lipoic acid and α-tocopherol reduced proteinuria.

Figure 3. Evidence for the role of ROS in experimental models of human glomerular diseases.

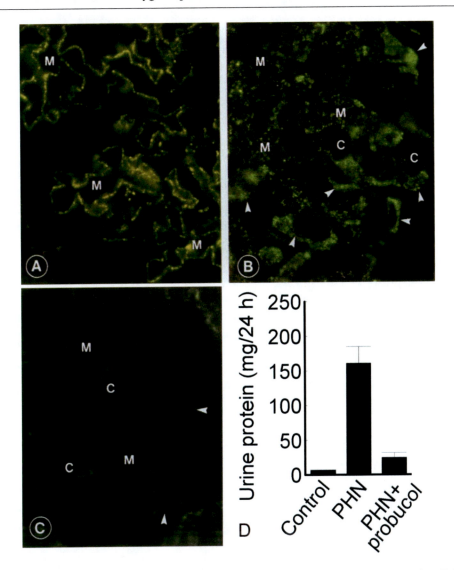

Figure 4. Role of ROS in glomerular injury in PHN. A) Localization of nephritogenic sheep anti-rat FxlA antibody in glomerular immune deposits (immunofluorescence microscopy). Granular deposits of IgG are seen around the peripheral glomerular capillary loops (M, mesangium). B) Malondialdehyde adducts in glomeruli from proteinuric rats with PHN on day 7. Adducts are shown prominently in glomerular epithelial cells in a finely granular pattern extending around the glomerular capillary (C) loops, within the GBM, and throughout the mesangium. C) Malondialdehyde adducts in glomeruli from PHN rats pretreated with probucol (day 7). In the probucol-pretreated rats, there is a marked reduction in glomerular staining for malondialdehyde adducts. D) Treatment of PHN with probucol reduces proteinuria on day 7. Panels A-C are reprinted from reference [29] with permission. Panel D is based on reference [29].

Membranous nephropathy is an important cause of nephrotic syndrome and end stage kidney failure in adults [1]. The understanding of mechanisms involved in the pathogenesis of membranous nephropathy has come from studies carried out in Heymann nephritis in the rat, which closely resembles the clinical and pathologic features of the human disease [10]. Membranous nephropathy involves the *in situ* formation of subepithelial immune deposits as a result of circulating antibodies binding to podocyte antigens. Complement activation leads to assembly of C5b-9 on podocyte plasma membranes, and results in sublethal podocyte injury and proteinuria. *In the PHN model of membranous nephropathy, complement C5b-9-mediated injury of glomerular epithelial cells causes activation of the NADPH oxidase, resulting in formation of ROS* [8]. Proteinuria in PHN was reduced by administration of dimethylsulfoxide, dimethylthiourea, sodium benzoate (hydroxyl radical scavenger), and deferoxamine [27, 28]. SOD and catalase did not, however, affect proteinuria, suggesting a role for the hydroxyl radical in PHN. Furthermore, lipid peroxidation and modification of podocyte membranes and GBM components by malondialdehyde adducts were demonstrated in PHN in association with development of proteinuria. These modifications and the proteinuria were reversed with the antioxidant drug, probucol (Figure 4), and the reduction in proteinuria was independent of the cholesterol-lowering effect of probucol [29]. The results indicate that *C5b-9-mediated podocyte injury and proteinuria are associated with induction of ROS-generating enzymes and production of hydroxyl radicals, with damage to structures of the glomerular capillary wall.* Another study showed that xanthine oxidase activity and $O_2^{\bullet-}$ generation were enhanced in glomeruli isolated from rats with PHN, compared with controls [30]. Rats receiving drinking water supplemented with tungsten showed significant decreases in xanthine oxidase activity and proteinuria. Since treatment with antioxidants prevents lipid peroxidation and the development of proteinuria in PHN, it is *conceivable that podocyte-derived matrix-degrading proteases and ROS released into the cell-matrix interface might alter cell attachment of podocytes to the GBM and lead to foot process effacement and proteinuria.* By analogy to puromycin aminonucleoside nephrosis, feeding rats with PHN a selenium-deficient diet reduced GPx and increased proteinuria [23].

8. ROS in Experimental Animal Models of Primary Inflammatory Glomerulonephritis

Human anti-GBM glomerulonephritis (Goodpasture's glomerulonephritis) is a rare, but severe rapidly progressive kidney disease associated with inflammation, formation of glomerular crescents and loss of renal function [1]. The disease is mediated by antibodies directed to the α3 chain of type IV collagen, which bind to the GBM, activate complement, and induce leukocyte infiltration and a severe inflammatory reaction. In experimental anti-GBM nephritis in the rat (neutrophil-dependent nephrotoxic serum nephritis), treatment with catalase reduced proteinuria and glomerular cell injury, while dimethylsulfoxide (a hydroxyl radical scavenger) and SOD were not effective [31]. In rabbit neutrophil-dependent anti-GBM glomerulonephritis, dimethylthiourea (a hydroxyl radical scavenger), and deferoxamine (an iron chelator) reduced proteinuria [32]. These studies indicate that *mediation of injury in anti-GBM nephritis may involve H_2O_2 and hydroxyl radical, but that there may be species differences.*

Membranoproliferative glomerulonephritis type I (MPGN) is associated with hematuria, proteinuria, and in some cases renal insufficiency [1]. Glomeruli show presence of antibody deposits, complement activation, an inflammatory cell infiltrate, mesangial expansion and cell proliferation. MPGN is typically associated with glomerular deposition of IgG; however, deposition of IgA, i.e. in IgA nephropathy may lead to a histological pattern ranging from mesangial expansion to MPGN. One experimental model of MPGN involves perfusion of the kidney via the renal artery with concanavalin A, which binds to the glomerular endothelial cells. Rats are then given anti-concanavalin A antibody, which binds to the planted antigen, and leads to subendothelial immune deposit formation, complement activation, and neutrophil infiltration. To examine if ROS were generated in this model of immune glomerular injury, rat kidneys were perfused with concanavalin A followed by either non-immune IgG or anti-concanavalin A antibody. A third group underwent neutrophil depletion prior to receiving concanavalin A and anti-concanavalin A antibody. Following administration of radio-iodine, incorporation of radio-iodine into the glomerular capillary wall was observed only in neutrophil-replete rats who received concanavalin A and anti-concanavalin A antibody [33]. These results imply that the *myeloperoxidase-H_2O_2-halide system was activated in this experimental MPGN model.*

Another experimental disease resembling human MPGN and IgA nephropathy is anti-Thy 1 glomerulonephritis in the rat. Glomeruli from rats with anti-Thy 1 nephritis showed enhanced production of H_2O_2, $O_2^{\bullet-}$ and hydroxyl radicals. In parallel there were increases in NADH-dependent and NADPH-dependent oxidative activities. In contrast, glomerular antioxidative activities (SOD, GPx, and catalase) were reduced, thereby potentially amplifying ROS-mediated glomerular damage [34]. In another study of anti-Thy 1 nephritis, treatment of rats with the antioxidant, α-lipoic acid, reduced glomerular ROS production. In addition, α-lipoic acid reduced glomerular cell proliferation, reversed an increase in expression of glomerular transforming growth factor-β (TGF-β), and prevented transformation of mesangial cells into myofibroblasts [35].

The pathogenesis of IgA nephropathy has been studied in an experimental model where rats were immunized orally with bovine gamma globulin. These rats developed glomerular mesangial deposition of IgA and proteinuria [36]. Treatment of these rats with α-tocopherol (vitamin E) was associated with a significant reduction in the severity of proteinuria.

The studies in these experimental glomerulonephritis models indicate that glomerular injury results from induction of oxidative enzymes in resident glomerular cells and/or infiltrating leukocytes. Furthermore, activity of antioxidative enzymes appears to be decreased. Nevertheless, further studies are required, as the understanding of mechanisms that account for the changes is incomplete.

9. ROS in Human Primary Glomerulonephritis

There is now considerable understanding of the mechanisms for generation of ROS by intrinsic glomerular cells and infiltrating glomerular leukocytes, and of the role of ROS in experimental glomerular injury. An important question is whether analogous mechanisms participate in human glomerular disease, but so far, information on the role of ROS in human glomerulonephritis is limited. Expression of antioxidant enzymes was studied by immunohistochemistry in kidney biopsies of patients with various glomerular diseases. Glomerular antioxidant enzymes, including SOD and catalase, were localized in mesangial regions or along the epithelial surface of the glomerular capillary wall. There were no significant differences in expression among minimal change disease, IgM nephropathy, FSGS, and membranous glomerulonephritis. However, expression was increased in IgA nephropathy, as well as lupus nephritis [37].

Leukocytes are not implicated in the PHN model of membranous nephropathy, but there is some evidence to implicate the activation of the myeloperoxidase-H_2O_2-halide pathway in idiopathic human membranous nephropathy [38]. By immunohistochemical staining, a small number of monocytes/macrophages and myeloperoxidase-positive cells were detected in kidney biopsies of patients with membranous nephropathy, while there was negligible presence in minimal change disease, and an abundance in MPGN. Similarly, some staining for HOCl-modified proteins was present in glomeruli of membranous nephropathy, with negative staining in minimal change disease, and prominent staining in MPGN. The study suggests that oxidative modification of the glomerular capillary wall by phagocyte-derived HOCl may contribute to glomerular injury in humans [38].

In human IgA nephropathy associated with chronic renal insufficiency and proteinuria, the presence of advanced oxidation protein products in plasma was associated with disease progression [39]. Advanced oxidation protein products are a class of di-tyrosine-containing protein products formed during oxidative stress and are carried mainly by albumin in vivo [40] An explanation for this finding in IgA nephropathy may be provided by a recent study, which showed that in cultured glomerular epithelial cells, advanced oxidation protein products triggered production of $O_2^{\bullet-}$ by activating the NADPH oxidase, and this led to an upregulation of p53, Bax, caspase-3 activity, and apoptosis. Treatment of normal rats with advanced oxidation protein product-modified rat serum albumin induced loss of podocytes and proteinuria [41].

Based on studies in PHN, showing that treatment with the cholesterol-lowering antioxidant drug, probucol, reduced proteinuria in rats, a study using probucol was conducted in humans with drug-resistant idiopathic membranous nephropathy [42]. Fifteen patients were treated with probucol for three months, followed by a washout period, and then three months of lovastatin (a cholesterol-lowering drug without antioxidant effects). A significant reduction in proteinuria was seen during the probucol treatment with partial remission in four patients. Median protein excretion increased to pretreatment values during the washout period. There was a tendency to decreased proteinuria after lovastatin, although none of the patients achieved partial remission. The authors concluded that proteinuria can be reduced by probucol in some patients with idiopathic membranous nephropathy.

10. ROS as Signaling Molecules in the Glomerulus

$O_2^{\bullet-}$ and H_2O_2 are classically considered to be toxic, and are associated with cell or tissue damage; however, more recent evidence suggests that production of ROS (particularly at low concentrations) may be an important component of cell signaling [43]; see also Vol. I, Chapter 2. In mammalian cells, a large array of intracellular stimuli has been reported to induce ROS production, and inhibition of ROS generation blocks stimulant-dependent signaling. For example, growth factor-mediated ROS generation may be necessary for downstream mitogenic and antiapoptotic signals. As discussed above, significant amounts of ROS are produced in the complement-mediated PHN model of membranous nephropathy, and ROS were associated with induction of glomerular injury and proteinuria. ROS may, however, also mediate complement signaling. In glomerular epithelial cells in culture and in vivo, complement-induced $O_2^{\bullet-}$ production resulted in the activation of the c-Jun N-terminal kinase (JNK) [44]. This activation was dependent on the complement-induced release of arachidonic acid by cytosolic phospholipase A_2. Free arachidonic acid stimulated JNK activity via the NADPH oxidase and production of ROS. Activation of JNK in glomerular epithelial cells in culture was associated with cytoprotection [44]. Thus, *in PHN, ROS may potentially play a dual role, both facilitating signal transduction and contributing to cell damage.* The relative importance of these functions to the pathogenesis of membranous nephropathy will require further study.

There are a number of other examples of ROS-mediated signaling in glomerular cells. For example, in cultured mesangial cells, growth factors stimulated phosphorylation of extracellular signal-regulated kinase in a ROS-dependent manner. Oxidative stress may mediate mesangial cell proliferation [45]. $O_2^{\bullet-}$ was reported to induce ceramide formation in glomerular endothelial cells [46]. Ischemia-reperfusion injury (which is associated with ROS production in the reperfusion phase) activated the Ste20-like kinase, SLK, in glomerular epithelial cells in vitro, and enhanced apoptosis [47]. Additional effects of ROS signaling in podocytes have been reported [48].

Recently, production of ROS has been reported to trigger endoplasmic reticulum (ER) stress, and there is evidence for crosstalk between ER stress and oxidative stress [49-51]; see also Vol. II, Chapter 18. ER stress refers to physiological or pathological states that result in accumulation of misfolded proteins in the ER. Activation of the unfolded protein response (UPR) in the ER upregulates the capacity of the ER to process abnormal proteins. Induction of ER stress in glomerular cells has been described in experimental models of membranous nephropathy and MPGN, and exogenous induction of ER stress (so-called "preconditioning") reduced proteinuria, suggesting that ER stress, possibly together with oxidative stress, may be cytoprotective [51-53].

11. ROS in Diabetic Nephropathy

Diabetic nephropathy is presently the most common cause of nephrotic syndrome and end stage kidney disease. Although the pathogenesis of diabetic nephropathy is complex, a large body of evidence supports a role for ROS in the pathogenesis of diabetic complications [54, 55] (see also Chapter 9 in this Volume). *In diabetic nephropathy, production of ROS may potentially mediate signaling and enhance tissue damage (Figure 5).* Accumulation of plasma and renal AGE and advanced oxidation protein products is a common pathologic finding in patients with diabetes and metabolic syndrome. Studies in glomerular cell culture and isolated glomeruli have shown that high glucose concentration in the culture medium, AGE or advanced oxidation protein products can stimulate production of ROS [7, 40, 41, 56]. Glomeruli isolated from diabetic rats showed increased production of $O_2^{\bullet-}$ and H_2O_2. *The pathways by which hyperglycemia stimulates ROS may involve protein kinase C and NADPH oxidase, as well as mitochondrial dysfunction (Figure 5). In turn, ROS can activate protein kinase C and transcriptional pathways (e.g. AP-1 and NF-κB) leading to production of profibrogenic substances, including cytokines and TGF-β, endothelin-1, as well as extracellular matrix components (e.g. fibronectin)* [7, 56]. These responses are reported to be inhibited by antioxidant drugs. In cultured glomerular epithelial cells, high glucose and advanced oxidation protein products stimulated ROS production and apoptosis. Loss of podocytes, presumably due to apoptosis, is a feature of diabetic nephropathy *in vivo*, and there is a growing appreciation that podocyte loss is related to increasing proteinuria and contributes to the progression of kidney disease. By analogy to podocytes, high glucose stimulated ROS-dependent apoptosis in cultured mesangial cells [7]. Kidneys from rats with experimental diabetes exhibit lipid peroxidation [7]. Diabetic kidney lesions in humans revealed malondialdehyde adducts by immunostaining in expanded glomerular mesangial areas in early diabetic nephropathy and in nodular lesions in advanced diabetic nephropathy, as well as in the thickened intima of arteries with perivascular sclerosis [57].

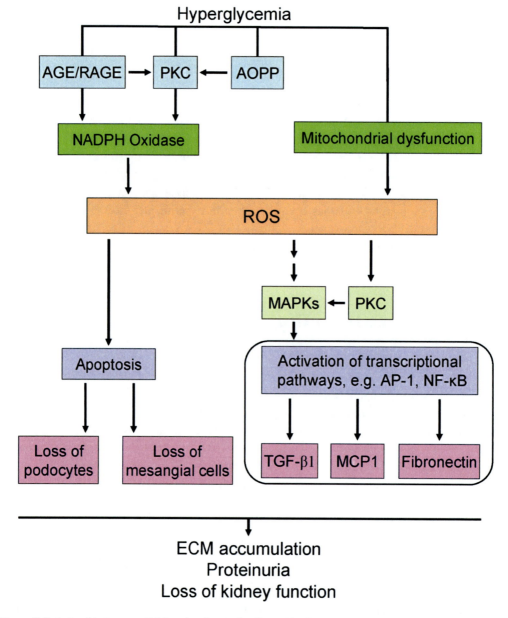

Figure 5. Relationship between ROS and pathways implicated in diabetic nephropathy (based on references [7, 40, 56]). AOPP, advanced oxidation protein products; MAPK, mitogen-activated protein kinase; MCP1, monocyte chemotactic protein-1; PKC, protein kinase C; TGF, transforming growth factor.

Conclusions

ROS may be produced in the glomerulus by infiltrating inflammatory leukocytes, or by intrinsic glomerular cells. Mesangial cells and glomerular epithelial cells express all the components of the NADPH oxidase. Various experimental models of glomerulonephritis, which feature infiltrating glomerular leukocytes and macrophages or which are leukocyte-independent, demonstrate involvement of ROS in glomerular capillary wall damage, as manifested by changes in glomerular cell ultrastructure and proteinuria. More recent studies suggest that besides inducing tissue injury, production of ROS (particularly at low concentrations) may be an important component of glomerular cell signaling. ROS play an important role in the pathogenesis of diabetic nephropathy. So far, information on the role of ROS in the pathogenesis of glomerulonephritis in humans is limited, and further study is essential. A greater understanding of the mechanisms by which ROS may mediate glomerular disease will eventually lead to novel therapeutic approaches.

Acknowledgments

This work was supported by research grants from the Canadian Institutes of Health Research (MOP-53264, MOP-84213) and the Kidney Foundation of Canada, and the Catherine McLaughlin Hakim Chair.

References

[1]   Beck LH, Jr., Salant DJ. Glomerular and tubulointerstitial diseases. *Prim. Care.* 2008; 35:265-96.

[2]   Cybulsky AV, Foster MH, Quigg RJ, Salant DJ. Immunologic mechanisms of glomerular disease. In: Seldin DW, Giebisch G, eds. *The Kidney: Physiology and Pathophysiology*. Philadelphia: Lippincott-Raven Publishers, 2000:2645-2697.

[3]   Tryggvason K, Patrakka J, Wartiovaara J. Hereditary proteinuria syndromes and mechanisms of proteinuria. *N. Engl. J. Med.* 2006; 354:1387-401.

[4]   Gwinner W, Grone HJ. Role of reactive oxygen species in glomerulonephritis. *Nephrol. Dial. Transplant.* 2000; 15:1127-32.

[5]   Kaushal GP, Mayeux PR, Shah SV. Proteases and oxidants in glomerular injury. In: Neilson EG, Couser WB, eds. *Immunologic Renal Diseases*. Philadelphia: Lippincott Williams and Wilkins, 2001:395-414.

[6]   Shah SV. Oxidants and iron in chronic kidney disease. Kidney Int Suppl 2004:S50-5.

[7]   Shah SV, Baliga R, Rajapurkar M, Fonseca VA. Oxidants in chronic kidney disease. *J. Am. Soc. Nephrol.* 2007; 18:16-28.

[8]   Neale TJ, Ullrich R, Ojha P, Poczewski H, Verhoeven AJ, Kerjaschki D. Reactive oxygen species and neutrophil respiratory burst cytochrome b558 are produced by kidney glomerular cells in passive Heymann nephritis. *Proc. Natl. Acad. Sci. USA,* 1993; 90:3645-9.

[9] Greiber S, Munzel T, Kastner S, Muller B, Schollmeyer P, Pavenstadt H. NAD(P)H oxidase activity in cultured human podocytes: effects of adenosine triphosphate. *Kidney Int.* 1998; 53:654-63.

[10] Cybulsky AV, Quigg RJ, Salant DJ. Experimental membranous nephropathy redux. Am *J. Physiol. Renal. Physiol.* 2005; 289:F660-71.

[11] Rehan A, Johnson KJ, Kunkel RG, Wiggins RC. Role of oxygen radicals in phorbol myristate acetate-induced glomerular injury. *Kidney Int.* 1985; 27:503-11.

[12] Yoshioka T, Ichikawa I, Fogo A. Reactive oxygen metabolites cause massive, reversible proteinuria and glomerular sieving defect without apparent ultrastructural abnormality. *J. Am. Soc. Nephrol.* 1991; 2:902-12.

[13] Johnson RJ, Couser WG, Chi EY, Adler S, Klebanoff SJ. New mechanism for glomerular injury. Myeloperoxidase-hydrogen peroxide-halide system. *J. Clin. Invest.* 1987; 79:1379-87.

[14] Johnson RJ, Guggenheim SJ, Klebanoff SJ, et al. Morphologic correlates of glomerular oxidant injury induced by the myeloperoxidase-hydrogen peroxide-halide system of the neutrophil. *Lab. Invest.* 1988; 58:294-301.

[15] Salant DJ, Cybulsky AV. Experimental glomerulonephritis. *Methods Enzymol.* 1988; 162:421-61.

[16] Pippin JW, Brinkkoetter PT, Cormack-Aboud FC, et al. Inducible rodent models of acquired podocyte diseases. *Am. J. Physiol. Renal. Physiol.* 2009; 296:F213-29.

[17] Sellier-Leclerc AL, Duval A, Riveron S, et al. A humanized mouse model of idiopathic nephrotic syndrome suggests a pathogenic role for immature cells. *J. Am. Soc. Nephrol.* 2007; 18:2732-9.

[18] Ricardo SD, Bertram JF, Ryan GB. Reactive oxygen species in puromycin aminonucleoside nephrosis: in vitro studies. *Kidney Int.* 1994; 45:1057-69.

[19] Diamond JR, Bonventre JV, Karnovsky MJ. A role for oxygen free radicals in aminonucleoside nephrosis. *Kidney Int.* 1986; 29:478-83.

[20] Thakur V, Walker PD, Shah SV. Evidence suggesting a role for hydroxyl radical in puromycin aminonucleoside-induced proteinuria. *Kidney Int.* 1988; 34:494-9.

[21] Ricardo SD, Bertram JF, Ryan GB. Antioxidants protect podocyte foot processes in puromycin aminonucleoside-treated rats. *J. Am. Soc. Nephrol.* 1994; 4:1974-86.

[22] Kawamura T, Yoshioka T, Bills T, Fogo A, Ichikawa I. Glucocorticoid activates glomerular antioxidant enzymes and protects glomeruli from oxidant injuries. *Kidney Int.* 1991; 40:291-301.

[23] Baliga R, Baliga M, Shah SV. Effect of selenium-deficient diet in experimental glomerular disease. *Am. J. Physiol.* 1992; 263:F56-61.

[24] Guo J, Ananthakrishnan R, Qu W, et al. RAGE mediates podocyte injury in adriamycin-induced glomerulosclerosis. *J. Am. Soc. Nephrol.* 2008; 19:961-72.

[25] Bohlender JM, Franke S, Stein G, Wolf G. Advanced glycation end products and the kidney. *Am. J. Physiol. Renal. Physiol.* 2005; 289:F645-59.

[26] Tanji N, Markowitz GS, Fu C, et al. Expression of advanced glycation end products and their cellular receptor RAGE in diabetic nephropathy and nondiabetic renal disease. *J. Am. Soc. Nephrol.* 2000; 11:1656-66.

[27] Shah SV. Evidence suggesting a role for hydroxyl radical in passive Heymann nephritis in rats. *Am. J. Physiol.* 1988; 254:F337-44.

[28] Lotan D, Kaplan BS, Fong JS, Goodyer PR, de Chadarevian JP. Reduction of protein excretion by dimethyl sulfoxide in rats with passive Heymann nephritis. *Kidney Int.* 1984; 25:778-88.

[29] Neale TJ, Ojha PP, Exner M, et al. Proteinuria in passive Heymann nephritis is associated with lipid peroxidation and formation of adducts on type IV collagen. *J. Clin.Invest.* 1994; 94:1577-84.

[30] Gwinner W, Plasger J, Brandes RP, et al. Role of xanthine oxidase in passive Heymann nephritis in rats. *J. Am. Soc. Nephrol.* 1999; 10:538-44.

[31] Rehan A, Johnson KJ, Wiggins RC, Kunkel RG, Ward PA. Evidence for the role of oxygen radicals in acute nephrotoxic nephritis. *Lab. Invest.* 1984; 51:396-403.

[32] Boyce NW, Holdsworth SR. Hydroxyl radical mediation of immune renal injury by desferrioxamine. *Kidney Int.* 1986; 30:813-7.

[33] Johnson RJ, Klebanoff SJ, Ochi RF, et al. Participation of the myeloperoxidase-H2O2-halide system in immune complex nephritis. *Kidney Int.* 1987; 32:342-9.

[34] Gaertner SA, Janssen U, Ostendorf T, Koch KM, Floege J, Gwinner W. Glomerular oxidative and antioxidative systems in experimental mesangioproliferative glomerulonephritis. *J. Am. Soc. Nephrol.* 2002; 13:2930-7.

[35] Budisavljevic MN, Hodge L, Barber K, et al. Oxidative stress in the pathogenesis of experimental mesangial proliferative glomerulonephritis. *Am. J. Physiol. Renal. Physiol.* 2003; 285:F1138-48.

[36] Kuemmerle NB, Krieg RJ, Jr., Chan W, Trachtman H, Norkus EP, Chan JC. Influence of alpha-tocopherol over the time course of experimental IgA nephropathy. *Pediatr. Nephrol.* 1999; 13:108-12.

[37] Wang JS, Ger LP, Tseng HH. Expression of glomerular antioxidant enzymes in human glomerulonephritis. *Nephron.* 1997; 76:32-8.

[38] Grone HJ, Grone EF, Malle E. Immunohistochemical detection of hypochlorite-modified proteins in glomeruli of human membranous glomerulonephritis. *Lab. Invest.* 2002; 82:5-14.

[39] Descamps-Latscha B, Witko-Sarsat V, Nguyen-Khoa T, et al. Early prediction of IgA nephropathy progression: proteinuria and AOPP are strong prognostic markers. *Kidney Int.* 2004; 66:1606-12.

[40] Liu Y. Advanced oxidation protein products: a causative link between oxidative stress and podocyte depletion. *Kidney Int.* 2009; 76:1125-7.

[41] Zhou LL, Hou FF, Wang GB, et al. Accumulation of advanced oxidation protein products induces podocyte apoptosis and deletion through NADPH-dependent mechanisms. *Kidney Int.* 2009; 76:1148-60.

[42] Haas M, Mayer G, Wirnsberger G, et al. Antioxidant treatment of therapy-resistant idiopathic membranous nephropathy with probucol: a pilot study. *Wien. Klin. Wochenschr.* 2002; 114:143-7.

[43] Thannickal VJ, Fanburg BL. Reactive oxygen species in cell signaling. *Am. J. Physiol. Lung Cell Mol. Physiol.* 2000; 279:L1005-28.

[44] Peng H, Takano T, Papillon J, Bijian K, Khadir A, Cybulsky AV. Complement activates the c-Jun N-terminal kinase/stress-activated protein kinase in glomerular epithelial cells. *J. Immunol.* 2002; 169:2594-601.

[45] Dentelli P, Rosso A, Zeoli A, et al. Oxidative stress-mediated mesangial cell proliferation requires Rac-1/reactive oxygen species production and beta4 integrin expression. *J. Biol. Chem.* 2007; 282:26101-10.

[46] Huwiler A, Boddinghaus B, Pautz A, et al. Superoxide potently induces ceramide formation in glomerular endothelial cells. *Biochem. Biophys. Res. Commun.* 2001; 284:404-10.

[47] Cybulsky AV, Takano T, Papillon J, et al. Renal expression and activity of the germinal center kinase SK2. *Am. J. Physiol. Renal. Physiol.* 2004; 286:F16-25.

[48] Chuang PY, He JC. Signaling in regulation of podocyte phenotypes. *Nephron Physiol.* 2009; 111:9-15.

[49] Zhang K, Kaufman RJ. From endoplasmic-reticulum stress to the inflammatory response. *Nature,* 2008; 454:455-62.

[50] Kitamura M. Biphasic, bidirectional regulation of NF-kappaB by endoplasmic reticulum stress. *Antioxid. Redox. Signal.* 2009; 11:2353-64.

[51] Cybulsky AV. Endoplasmic reticulum stress in proteinuric kidney disease. *Kidney Int.* 2010; 77:187-93.

[52] Cybulsky AV, Takano T, Papillon J, Khadir A, Liu J, Peng H. Complement C5b-9 membrane attack complex increases expression of endoplasmic reticulum stress proteins in glomerular epithelial cells. *J. Biol. Chem.* 2002; 277:41342-51.

[53] Inagi R, Kumagai T, Nishi H, et al. Preconditioning with endoplasmic reticulum stress ameliorates mesangioproliferative glomerulonephritis. *J. Am. Soc. Nephrol.* 2008; 19:915-22.

[54] Nishikawa T, Edelstein D, Brownlee M. The missing link: a single unifying mechanism for diabetic complications. *Kidney Int. Suppl.* 2000; 77:S26-30.

[55] Brownlee M. Biochemistry and molecular cell biology of diabetic complications. *Nature,* 2001; 414:813-20.

[56] Ha H, Lee HB. Reactive oxygen species as glucose signaling molecules in mesangial cells cultured under high glucose. *Kidney Int. Suppl.* 2000; 77:S19-25.

[57] Horie K, Miyata T, Maeda K, et al. Immunohistochemical colocalization of glycoxidation products and lipid peroxidation products in diabetic renal glomerular lesions. Implication for glycoxidative stress in the pathogenesis of diabetic nephropathy. *J. Clin. Invest.* 1997; 100:2995-3004.

In: Principles of Free Radical Biomedicine, Volume III
Editors: K. Pantopoulos and H. M. Schipper

ISBN 978-1-61324-184-4
©2012 Nova SciencePublishers, Inc.

Chapter 6

Carcinogenesis

Undurti N. Das[*]

UND Life Sciences, 13800 Fairhill Road, #321, Shaker Heights, OH 44120, USA
School of Biotechnology, Jawaharlal Nehru Technological University,
Kakinada-533 003, India

1. Introduction

It is desired that anti-cancer agents preferentially attack tumor cells without exerting adverse effects on normal cells. However, currently available drugs and radiation are not selective in their action on tumor cells. *Radiation and anti-cancer drugs such as anthracyclines and bleomycin, produce free radicals [1-3] which contribute to their tumoricidal actions.* However, free radicals are also responsible for adverse effects seen with these agents.

Free radicals have direct effects on cell growth, developmentand survival, and play a significant role in various diseases including cancer [4-6]. During the electron-transport steps of ATP production, due to the leakage of electrons from mitochondria, reactive oxygen species, e.g. superoxide anion (O_2^-) and hydroxyl (OH^-) radicals, are generated (Vol. II, Chapter 15). Some of these species lead to the production of hydrogen peroxide (H_2O_2), from which further hydroxyl radicals are generated in a reaction that depends on the presence of Fe^{2+} ions [7]; see also Vol. I, Chapter 5. Free radicals have both beneficial and harmful actions (reviewed in [4]). They are needed for signal-transduction pathways that regulate cell growth [8, 9], reduction-oxidation (redox) status [7], and as a first line of defense by polymorphonuclear leukocytes against infections [4]. Excessive amounts of free radicals start lethal chain reactions that inactivate vital enzymes, proteins and other important subcellular elements needed for cell survival and lead to cell death [4, 10-12]. Thus, free radicals are like a double-edged sword.

---

[*]Ph: 001-216-231-5548; Fax: 001-928-833-0316, E-mail: undurti@hotmail.com

2. Lipid Peroxidation in Tumor Cells

An inverse relationship exists between the concentrations of lipid peroxides and the rate of cell proliferation, i.e. the higher the rate of lipid peroxidation (see Vol. I, Chapter 7) in the cells the lower the rate of cell division (reviewed in [13]). This is supported by the observation that tumor cells are more resistant to lipid peroxidation than normal cells [14, 15]. Studies directed at eliciting the relationship between tumor mitochondrial membrane peroxidation and the tumor cell proliferation revealed that lipid peroxidation decreases with increasing growth rate [16]. Indeed, it was shown that in hepatomas, the higher the growth rate of the tumor, the lower the microsomal phospholipid content and the degree of fatty acid unsaturation [13, 17]. Examination of fatty acyl compositions of phospholipids derived from mitochondria and microsomes isolated from Morris hepatoma with slow (9618A), intermediate (7794A) and fast (7777) growth rates showed that the faster the growth rate of the tumor, the larger the sum of the amounts of 16:1, 18:1 and 18:2 fatty acids and the smaller the sum of the contents of all polyunsaturated fatty acids (PUFAs) with four or more double bonds per molecule [18]. The former content was generally higher, and the PUFA contents lower, in hepatoma organelles than in the corresponding host liver organelles. In addition, the reduced rates of lipid peroxidation observed in Yoshida hepatoma cells and their microsomes when compared with control (normal liver) tissue under the same pro-oxidant conditions was found to be due to the much reduced levels of NADPH-cytochrome c reductase and the NADPH-cytochrome P-450 electron transport chain in the Yoshida hepatoma cells [19]. Cheeseman et al. [20] have also reported that in the Novikoffhepatoma cells, the low rate of lipid peroxidation seems to be due to a combination of factors: low levels of PUFAs and cytochrome P-450 and elevated levels of the lipid-soluble anti-oxidant α-tocopherol. Tumor plasma membranes tested for their abilities to undergo lipid peroxidation using xanthine and xanthine oxidase as the free radical generating system had extremely low rates of malondialdehyde accumulation, and LOOH was practically undetectable in the hepatoma cell membranes compared to the normal rat liver membranes [21]. Such a high degree of resistance to peroxidation in the tumor cells has been attributed to a marked decrease in lipid content [21]. These results are very similar to those obtained by Cheeseman et al. [20].

In our studies, it was observed that incubation of cells with PUFAs augmented free radical generation and formation of lipid peroxidation products selectively in the tumor cells compared to normal cells. This increase in free radical generation and lipid peroxidation occurred despite the fact that the uptake of fatty acids was at least 2 to 3 times higher in the normal cells compared to tumor cells [22, 23]. Based on these studies, it can be suggested that there is a close correlation between the rate of lipid peroxidation and degree of malignant deviation of the tumor cell, and the susceptibility of the tumor cell to free radical-induced cytotoxicity, viz: *the higher the degree of malignant nature of the tumor cell, the lower the rate of lipid peroxidation and higher the degree of susceptibility to free radical-induced toxicity*. It may be mentioned here that resistance to lipid peroxidation appears to occur at the premalignant stage of the carcinogenesis process, since administration of diethylnitrosamine and 2-acetylaminofluorene leads to inhibition of peroxidation in normal liver and in preneoplastic nodules as well as in the neoplasms that result from this treatment [24].

The low content of PUFAs in the tumor cells can be attributed to the loss or decreased activity of δ-6- and δ-5-desaturases [25-27]. This results in decreased metabolism of dietary linoleic acid (LA, 18:2, n-6) and alpha-linolenic acid (ALA, 18:3 n-3) to longer chain fatty acids such as gamma-linolenic acid (GLA, 18:3 n-6), dihomo-gamma-linolenic acid (DGLA, 20:3 n-6), arachidonic acid (AA, 20:4 n-6) and eicosapentaenoic acid (EPA, 20:5 n-3) and docosahexaenoic acid (DHA, 22:6 n-3) respectively. In addition, tumor cells have elevated levels of α-tocopherol [20]. For instance, poorly differentiated, fast-growing hepatomas have a microsomal vitamin E to PUFA ratio markedly higher than the corresponding normal liver membranes, while in the highly differentiated, slow-growing hepatomas this ratio is consistently lower (reviewed in [13-16, 20]). The higher vitamin E to PUFA ratio in rapidly growing tumors is due to markedly decreased content of PUFA, while the vitamin E quantified on a per mg protein basis is virtually unchanged. On the other hand, tumor cells have low or almost no superoxide dismutase (SOD), glutathione peroxidase (GPx) and catalase enzymes [28-30]. The relatively high content of vitamin E contributes to the low rate of lipid peroxidation observed in the tumor cells (reviewed in [13]). Thus *both substrate (i.e. PUFAs) deficiency and a relatively high content of vitamin E are responsible for the low rate of lipid peroxidation seen in tumor cells.*

3. Superoxide Dismutase, Free Radicals and Tumor Cells

There are two forms of superoxide dismutase (SOD) in human cells, a mitochondrial isoform (manganese-containing SOD, MnSOD, also known as SOD2) and a copper-zinc containing SOD (CuZnSOD, also known as SOD1); for details see Vol. II, Chapter 5. CuZnSOD is primarily localized in the cytosol in mammalian cells, although some may be present in the nucleus, mitochondrial intermembrane space, lysosomes and peroxisomes. Huang et al [31] showed that transgenic mice lacking MnSOD do not survive due to severe lung damage and neurodegeneration. On the other hand, phenotypic defects in CuZnSOD-negative knockout mice are more subtle [31, 32] and do not result in death. But both types of SOD are essential for healthy aerobic life.

3.1. Superoxide and Other Free Radicals Cause Cell Death by Apoptosis

When the generation of excess radicals occurs or if the oxidative stress is severe, necrosis may result [32, 33]. Many death stimuli also increase formation of free radicals and trigger apoptosis (Vol. II, Chapters 25 and 26). Free radical scavengers often, but not always, delay apoptosis [33, 34]. For example, edelfosine (1-O-octadecyl-2-O-methyl-rac-glycero-3-phosphocholine), a membrane-targeting anti-cancer ether lipid drug, induced cytotoxicity in human leukemia cells (HL-60 and K562) correlating with the production of free radicals [35]. Hepatocyte growth factor (HGF), which can suppress the growth of sarcoma 180 and Meth A cells, enhanced the generation of intracellular reactive oxygen species as judged by flow cytometric analysis using 2', 7'-dichloro-fluorescein diacetate [36]. N-acetylcysteine, a precursor of glutathione and an intracellular free radical scavenger, and the reduced form of glutathione (GSH), prevented HGF-suppressed growth of the tumor cells. This lends support to the involvement of free radicals in the growth suppressive action of HGF. *Tumor necrosis factor α (TNFα) induced tumor cell death and host toxicity that may be related to its ability to generate free radicals* [37]. High intracellular glutathione levels induce tumor cell resistance to recombinant human TNF (rhTNF), whereas low glutathione levels enhance sensitivity to rhTNF. Conversely, pretreatment of the tumor-bearing hosts with DL-buthionine-(S,R)-sulfoximine, an inhibitor of GSH biosynthesis, resulted in an increased sensitivity of tumor cells to rhTNF [37]. Induction of apoptosis by AA in human retinoblastoma cells and other PUFAs was found to be accompanied by increased formation of the lipid peroxidation end products, such as malondialdehyde and 4-hydroxynonenal, suggesting a role for free radicals [22, 38].

Bize et al [39] showed that both total SOD and MnSOD specific activities were lower in the tumor cell homogenates compared to normal liver: the lowest activity was associated with the fastest growing tumors. MnSOD activity was decreased in the fast- and medium-growth rate hepatomas but was slightly increased in the tumor with the slowest growth rate compared to normal liver. This suggests that decreased MnSOD specific activity is not a characteristic of all tumors. In addition, it was observed that antimycin A (an inhibitor of the electron transport chain) stimulated the production of O_2^- in normal rat liver and slow-growth-rate tumor cells but not in the submitochondrial particles of fast-growth-rate tumor cells [39], lending support to the concept that the rate of lipid peroxidation is generally low in tumor cells.

Cheeseman et al. [40] observed a significant decrease in the PUFA content of Novikoff cells or Novikoffmicrosomes, especially AA (20:4 n-6) and eicosapentaenoic acid (EPA, 20:5 n-3). There was also a marked reduction in NADPH-cytochrome c reductase. A substantial increase in α-tocopherol relative both to total lipid and to methylene-interrupted double bonds in fatty acids was noted. Thus both Novikoff rat liver and Yoshida liver tumors showed similar biochemical changes and decreased rates of lipid peroxidation [19, 40]. However, reduced SOD activity has not been found in all tumors. In fact, in certain tumors SOD activities were found to be higher than in normal tissues [41, 42]; and paradoxically in some human gliomas, the malignant phenotype could be suppressed by overexpressing MnSOD [43]. In gastric and colorectal adenocarcinomas, overexpression of MnSOD may correlate with aggressiveness of the tumor [44]. Similarly, in both esophageal and gastric cancers, the levels of MnSOD mRNA were significantly elevated compared to normal tissue [45]. But it is not known whether there is any relationship between the aggressiveness of tumors and the levels of SOD. In some studies, it was observed that the activities of MnSOD and CuZnSOD varied greatly among both human and rat glioma cells [46]. On the other hand, Huang et al. [47] noted that the lower levels of MnSOD in SV40-transformed cells was related to increased cytosine methylation of the SOD2 intron region (the SOD2 gene contains a large CpG island spanning > 3.5 kb that starts near the 5' edge of the promoter and extends into intron 2).

The SH groups of the caspases are essential for their catalytic activity. On exposure to free radicals, these SH groups may be inactivated. In M14 melanoma cells, O_2^- and H_2O_2 may promote tumor cell survival via the inactivation of caspases [48]. Similar to O_2^- and H_2O_2, nitric oxide (NO) may also have a role both in cancer suppression and progression [6]. *In general, it can be said that the majority of the tumors have low SOD concentrations, relatively high amounts of vitamin E, and low PUFA content and lipid peroxides, which may render them more sensitive to free radical attack. A useful therapeutic strategy make be to devise methods or chemicals that can lower SOD, catalase and glutathione and vitamin E concentrations, and at the same time enhance free radical generation and lipid peroxidation in the tumor cells.*

4. Free Radicals, Lipid Peroxides and Cell Proliferation

It is believed that there is a negative correlation between cell proliferation and lipid peroxidation. For example, cells that proliferate rapidly such as spermatozoa show low rates of lipid peroxidation whereas neurons, which seldom divide, have high concentrations of lipid peroxides. Cornwell et al. [49-51] showed that in primary cultures of smooth muscle cells, cell proliferation is controlled, at least in part, by general peroxidation reactions rather than the specific peroxidation reactions involved in prostanoid synthesis when these cells were supplemented with various PUFAs. In particular, they observed that the inhibition of proliferation of primary cultures of smooth muscle cells was related to the structures of different PUFA families decreasing in the order n-9 > n-6 > n-3. As the inhibition of cell proliferation did not correlate with stimulated or inhibited prostaglandin synthesis in these studies, it was concluded that fatty acids themselves modulate cell proliferation. The growth inhibitory actions of PUFAs could be blocked by antioxidants such as vitamin E, butylatedhydroxytoluene (BHT), α-naphthol, 6-hydroxy-2,5,7,8-tetramethyl-chrom-2-carboxylic acid and dipyridamole [49] indicating a role for free radicals and lipid peroxides.

Cheeseman et al. [52] reported that reduced rates of lipid peroxidation could be related, in part, to increased levels of α-tocopherol at times of maximum DNA synthesis [52, 53]. This led to the conclusion that lipid peroxidation is decreased prior to cell division. These results suggest that tilting cellular redox balance towards higher antioxidant capacity may be responsible for the decreased rates of cell death and increased rates of cell proliferation.

5. Free Radicals, Lipid Peroxides, p53, Caspases and Apoptosis

Many of the gene products that control apoptosis are also regulators of cell cycle progression (Vol. II, Chapters 25 and 26). Thus, cell cycle control and cell death are linked. p53 protein is an example of a gene product that affects both cell cycle progression and apoptosis [54]. The ability of p53 overexpression to induce apoptosis may be a major reason why tumor cells, more often than not, disable p53 during the transformation process. At the same time, the same genetic changes that cause loss of apoptosis during tumor development may also result in tumor cell resistance to anti-cancer therapies that kill tumor cells by apoptosis. Hence, elucidation of the genetic and biochemical controls of these cellular processes may provide insights into induction of apoptosis and thus, hopefully, suggest new therapeutic modalities for the management of cancer. In view of this, it is important to delineate the relationships between free radicals, lipid peroxides, Bcl-2, p53 and caspases.

The p53 tumor suppressor is a transcription factor that regulates several gene expression pathways that function collectively to maintain the integrity of the genome. Its nuclear localization is critical to this regulation. Martinez et al [55] reported that ionizing radiation caused a biphasic p53 translocation response: p53 entered the nucleus 1-2 hours post-irradiation, subsequently emerged from the nucleus, and then again entered the nucleus 12-24 hours post-irradiation. These changes in the subcellular localization of p53 could be completely blocked by the free radical scavenger WR 1065. It was also noted that mitomycin C and doxorubicin, two DNA-damaging agents that do not generate free radicals, caused translocation of p53 only after 12-24 hours of exposure to the drugs, and this effect could not be blocked by WR 1065. These results indicate that although all three DNA-damaging agents induced delocalization of p53 to the nucleus, only trans-localization caused by irradiation was sensitive to free radical scavenging. Thus, free radicals have the ability to signal p53 translocation to the nucleus. This free radical-induced translocation of p53 could be an indication that free radicals damage DNA and that p53 may be involved (by inducing DNA repair) in maintaining the integrity of the genome following translocation to the nucleus. This is supported by the observation that brief exposure of the oligodendroglia-type cell line (OLN 93) to H_2O_2 produced a marked translocation of p53 from the cytosolic to the nuclear compartment within 20 minutes of exposure [56]. By 48 hours of exposure to H_2O_2, nearly 60% of the cells exhibited p53 in the nuclei, at which time a large proportion of the cells underwent apoptosis. The genotoxic-induced p53 relocalization appeared to be cell cycle-specific, because cells in the G0/G1 stage had more abundant nuclear-associated p53 and were more susceptible to H_2O_2-induced apoptosis than cells in G1/S phase. It was observed that the p21 and mdm2 genes were upregulated following p53 nuclear translocation, and mdm2 enhancement accelerated the exit of p53 from the nucleus to the cytosol [56]. These results suggest that *following exposure to H_2O_2, cells are induced to undergo p53-dependent apoptosis, an event that coincides with p53 nuclear translocation and that is cell cycle-related.* Kitamura et al. [57] also reported that H_2O_2-induced apoptosis is mediated by p53 protein in glial cells. It was noted that in human A172 glioblastoma cells, H_2O_2 caused cell death in a time- and concentration-dependent manner, accompanied by nucleosomal DNA fragmentation and chromatin condensation [57]. Exposure of A172 cells to H_2O_2 led to increased expression of p53 and enhancement in the protein levels of Bak, p21WAF1/CIP1 and GADD45 with no change in the protein levels of Bcl-2 and Bax. On the other hand, primary cultured astrocytes from p53-deficient mouse brain grew faster than wild-type and heterozygous astrocytes and were also more resistant to H_2O_2-induced apoptosis than wild-type and heterozygous astrocytes. Thus, glial proliferation and the repair of damaged DNA is regulated by p53, and glial apoptosis caused by H_2O_2-induced oxidative stress is also mediated by p53 [56]. In summary, these results [55-57] suggest that free radicals are powerful inducers of p53 activity and that they play a role in the execution of p53-dependent apoptosis.

In this context, it is interesting to note that transformed mouse fibroblasts lacking p53 are significantly more resistant than wild-type controls to the cytotoxic effect of a number of pro-oxidants [58]. Further, it was noted that MnSOD activity was increased in liver tissue from p53-deficient mice in comparison with wild type. Transient transfection of HeLa cells with p53 led to a significant reduction in steady-state MnSOD mRNA levels and enzymatic activity, suggesting that expression of the antioxidant enzyme MnSOD is negatively regulated by p53. Increased expression of MnSOD rendered HeLa cells resistant to p53-dependent cytotoxic treatments and, in co-transfection experiments, counteracted the growth inhibitory effect of p53 [58]. These results indicate that p53 inhibits the expression of MnSOD, a protein known to protect cells from the oxidative injury induced by various cytokines and anti-cancer drugs. They also imply that normally a balance is maintained between p53 and SOD levels and that overexpression of p53 can lead to a decrease in the levels of SOD. On the other hand, in some, if not all, tumor cells that have impaired p53 activity, the SOD activity is likely to be high, imparting increased antioxidant capacity to these cells. This suggests that p53 has a pro-oxidant type of activity. Thus, when tumor cells are exposed to free radicals such as $O_2^{\cdot-}$, H_2O_2 or NO, SOD present in the cells/tissues is not only utilized to quench these free radicals but will also engender an increase in the expression of p53 due to free radical-induced stress [56, 57]. This, in turn, suppresses the expression of SOD, tilting the balance more towards a more pro-oxidant state which, in turn, may promote apoptosis. Further, both free radicals and lipid peroxides can induce damage to a variety of enzymes, proteins and deplete ATP levels in the cells and thus cause cell death [13, 59]. Another mechanism by which reactive species, especially H_2O_2, can cause ATP depletion in the cells is by activating PARP (poly-ADP-ribose-polymerase), the substrate of caspase-3 [38], though there is some controversy about this [60]. But it should be remembered that H_2O_2 induces apoptosis at low concentrations, whereas at higher concentrations causes necrosis. Necrosis is known to occur if oxidative stress is severe [6, 33]. Hence, the final effect of H_2O_2 on tumor cell death, whether it is by apoptosis or necrosis, is dependent on the concentration of H_2O_2 present.

6. Oxidant Stress and Telomeres

Telomeres of human somatic cells shorten with each cell division but are stabilized at constant length in tumors by the enzyme telomerase [61]. *Oxidative stress can shorten telomeres* as evidenced by the observation that H_2O_2 plus Cu(II) caused predominant DNA damage at the site of 5'-GGG-3' in the telomere sequence [62]. H_2O_2 plus Cu(II) induced 8-oxo-7,8-dihydro-2'-deoxyguanosine (8-oxodG) formation in telomere sequences more efficiently than that in non-telomere sequences. NO plus $O_2^{\cdot-}$ caused base alterations at the 5' site of 5'-GGG-3' in the telomere sequence [62]. These results suggest that free radicals play a significant role in telomere shortening. The preferential vulnerability of telomeres to oxidative stress was also reported by von Zglinicki et al [63]; for details see Vol. II, Chapter 24. It was observed that treatment of non-proliferating human MRC-5 fibroblasts with H_2O_2 increased the sensitivity to S1 nuclease in telomeres preferentially and accelerated the shortening of telomeres by a corresponding amount as soon as the cells were allowed to proliferate. On the other hand, a reduction in the activity of intracellular peroxides using the spin trap, alpha-phenyl-t-butyl-nitrone reduced the telomere shortening rate and increased the replicative life span. Telomere shortening rate and the rate of replicative aging can be either accelerated or decelerated by changing the amount of oxidative stress [63], indicating that free radical mediated telomere damage contributes to telomere shortening.

7. Oxidant Stress, Bcl-2 and Apoptosis

The antioxidant activity ofBcl-2 opposes the pro-oxidant action of p53 [64] and its ability to suppress SOD activity. This suggests that a balance exists between the levels of p53, which induces a pro-oxidant status in cells, and the expression and antioxidant activity of Bcl-2. It is possible that increased expression of p53 that occurs during exposure to radiation and free radicals may lead to inhibition of Bcl-2 expression that, in turn, augments free radical generation and apoptosis. This is supported by the observation that Bcl-2 is down-regulated by p53 [65, 66].

Bcl-2 is known to block lipid peroxidation that induces apoptosis [67]. Following an apoptotic signal, progressive lipid peroxidation occurs in the cells, whereas over-expression of Bcl-2 suppresses lipid peroxidation [67]. Thus, a close association exists between lipid peroxidation, Bcl-2 and apoptosis [68]. We observed that when tumor cells are treated with PUFAs, there is not only an increase in the formation of lipid peroxides but also an increase in protein phosphorylation [69]. Thus, it is likely that enhanced lipid peroxidation in the tumor cells may lead to phosphorylation of Bcl-2 and a reduction in its anti-apoptosis potential, and hence, apoptosis would be stimulated. This possible interaction between lipid peroxidation and Bcl-2 is understandable as Bcl-2 is localized at intracellular sites of oxygen free radical generation including mitochondria, endoplasmic reticulum and nuclear membranes.

Thus, optimal expression of Bcl-2 and the presence of adequate amounts of the anti-oxidants SOD, catalase, glutathione, and vitamin E prevent apoptosis, whereas activation of p53, excess production of free radicals, and an increase in the levels of lipid peroxides in the cells trigger apoptosis. This delicate balance between pro-apoptotic and anti-apoptotic signals and chemicals is further complicated by the interactions among them such as the regulatory role of pro-apoptotic signal p53 on Bcl-2 and SOD, the ability of anti-apoptotic signal Bcl-2 to control free radical generation and lipid peroxidation, and finally the role of lipid peroxidation in the promotion of Bcl-2 phosphorylation and inactivation.

In Burkitt's lymphoma cells, increased availability of mitochondrial NAD(P)H was detected in Bcl-2 expressing cells that was correlated with an elevated constitutive mitochondrial production of H_2O_2 [70]. Although production of H_2O_2 was increased by TNFα in Bcl-2- negative lymphoma cells commensurate with the early phases of apoptosis, this increase was not seen in Bcl-2 expressing cells, suggesting that Bcl-2 allows cells to adapt to an increased state of oxidative stress, thereby fortifying cellular antioxidant defenses [70].

It is evident from the preceding discussion that methods designed to augment free radical generation specifically in tumor cells can induce their apoptosis. 2-methoxy-estradiol (2-ME), PUFAs and thalidomide seem to possess such ability [71-75]. Although cytokines, such as TNFα, interleukins (ILs) and some anti-cancer drugs, radiation and protoporphyrin derivatives (used in photodynamic therapy; see Chapter 12 in this Volume) do have the capacity to augment free radical generation and lipid peroxidation in the tumor cells, they have many undesirable side-effects. Of all, PUFAs seem to have fewest sideeffects, significant cytotoxic action on tumor cells and anti-angiogenic properties, and have the ability to augment free radical generation specifically in the tumor cells. In addition, PUFAs, especially n-3 fatty acids, showed promise in animal tumor models and our studies revealed that GLA (γ-linolenic acid, an n-6 fatty acid) inhibited the growth of human gliomas with few adverse effects [76-80].

8. Polyunsaturated Fatty Acids, Cell Proliferation, and Lipid Peroxidation

PUFAs (especially GLA, AA, EPA and DHA) when used at appropriate doses inhibited proliferation of tumor cells in vitro, whereas antioxidants blocked this inhibitory action [49-51], indicating that free radicals and lipid peroxides could be the mediators of their (PUFAs) cytotoxic action.

Prostaglandins (PGs) derived from PUFAs also inhibited the proliferation of human and animal tumor cells in vitro [81-83] but their effects were variable. When used at appropriate concentrations, GLA, AA, EPA and DHA were toxic to tumor cells with little or no effect on normal cells in vitro [84-91]. This selective tumoricidal action of fatty acids was not blocked by cyclo-oxygenase and lipoxygenase inhibitors, suggesting that prostaglandins and leukotrienes do not participate in this process [84-88].

Furthermore, GLA, AA and EPA-treated tumor cells (irrespective of the form in which these fatty acids are delivered), but not normal cells, exhibited 2 - 3 fold increases in free radicals and lipid peroxidation products [22, 23, 86-88]. These results suggest that the low rates of lipid peroxidation observed in tumor cells are, at least in part, due to deficiency of PUFAs and to a relative increase in their antioxidant content [19-21, 25-30, 89-91]. As there is a direct correlation between the rate of lipid peroxidation and the degree of deviation in hepatomas [13-16, 20, 92], and as the rate of lipid peroxidation is low in several tumors, it is suggested that lipid peroxidation might act as a physiological inhibitor of mitosis and thereby regulate cell multiplication [49-53, 93-96].

Tumor cell death caused by TNFα is associated with release of endogenous AA [97, 98], whereas TNFα-induced apoptosis can be prevented by the removal of unesterified AA [97]. Thus, the cellular level of unesterified AA may be a general mechanism by which apoptosis is induced in colon and other tumor cells.

Since other PUFAs, such as GLA, DGLA, EPA and DHA, also induce apoptosis of tumor cells, it is likely that methods designed to enhance the cellular content of unesterified PUFAs may trigger apoptosis in tumor cells [68]. This may explain the beneficial action of EPA- and DHA-rich fish oils in the prevention of colon cancer [99, 100].

Further, tumor cells exposed to PUFAs show low levels of various antioxidants [90, 91], which may cause an increase in oxidant stress and an enhancement in cytotoxicity. PUFAs, especially n-3 fatty acids, suppress carcinogen-induced *ras* activation [101], Bcl-2 expression, and inhibit the activity of cyclo-oxygenase enzyme. Thus PUFAs have several activities that contribute to their anti-cancer actions [68].

9. Free Radicals and Angiogenesis

PUFAs have also been shown to possess anti-angiogenic action [102]. GLA inhibited *in vitro* tube formation of human vascular endothelial cells and produced a significant reduction in the motility of vascular endothelial cells. DHA, which can suppress the growth of tumors both *in vitro* and *in vivo*, also showed anti-angiogenic activity [103].

Conclusions and Clinical Implications

Tumor cells have relatively higher antioxidant capacity and low rates of lipid peroxidation that favor tumor cell proliferation. In the nude mouse model, LA-rich diet enhanced breast cancer progression, whereas n-3 fatty acids (rich in EPA and DHA) exerted suppressive effects [104, 105]. In cell culture studies, LA-stimulated growth of tumor cells [106]. These studies led to the suggestion that n-6 fatty acids augment tumor growth. It should be noted that in these studies oils rich in LA were used. These LA-rich oils did not contain any GLA or AA, which are also n-6 fatty acids but are metabolites of LA. On the other hand, studies performed with oils, which contain both LA and GLA (such as primrose oil), showed suppression of tumor growth [107-109]. This suggests that LA may promote, whereas other n-6 fatty acids such as GLA, DGLA and AA suppress, tumor growth [99, 110]. So a cautious approach is needed while extrapolating results obtained with LA-rich oils to all n-6 fatty acids. This is supported by the observation that GLA, salts of GLA and a chemical formulation containing both GLA and EPA inhibit tumor growth *in vitro* and *in vivo* [111-115].

PUFAs modulate the immune response, inhibit the adhesion of tumor cells to endothelium [116, 117], and suppress tumor cell growth. It is likely that different tumor cells may have different response rates to various PUFAs. Several studies showed that GLA and other PUFAs enhance tumor cell chemosensitivity [118-120]. PUFAs modulate G-protein–mediated signal transduction [121], mobilize Ca^{++} from intracellular stores [122], which may induce apoptosis [123], activate PKC and enhance NADPH oxidase in macrophages [124] thereby enhancing O_2^- generation. EPA decreases Bcl-2 while increasing Bax in tumor cells 125. DHA increased p27, inhibited cyclin-associated kinase, reduced pRb phosphorylation and caused melanoma cells to undergo apoptosis [126, 127]. PUFAs (especially EPA) inhibited cell division by inhibiting translation initiation, preferentially reducing the synthesis and expression of G1 cyclins both in vitro and in vivo [128]. In addition, reactive species, especially H_2O_2, directly activated purified heterodimeric G_i and G_0 (small G proteins) [129], which are important signaling molecules. Thus, PUFAs target several intracellular second messenger molecules and genes either directly or indirectly to enhance free radical generation and induce tumor cell death. In a limited open label clinical study, we showed that *intra-tumoral injection of GLA regresses human brain gliomas without any significant sideeffects* [76-80]. GLA when injected into normal brain tissue of healthy dogs did not show any untoward effects, suggesting that it is non-toxic to normal cells. More studies are needed to confirm these findings. These and other studies suggest that efforts made to augment free radial generation selectively in tumor cells could represent a novel strategy to eliminate cancer. In a recent study, we showed that modified GLA (in the form of lithium GLA coupled to iodized salt solution) when injected intra-arterially can occlude tumor-feeding vessels (see Figures 1-2) thereby inducing tumor necrosis, without any effect on normal blood vessels [130, 131]. This suggests that modified GLAmay act on endothelial cells of tumor-feeding blood vessels and induce their occlusion. Differences in endothelial cell biology may explain the differential impact of GLA-induced free radicals on tumor-feeding and blood vessels. Exposure of endothelial cells of tumor-feeding vessels to PUFAs (such as lithium GLA coupled to iodized salt) enhances free radical generation that, in turn, oxidizes the PUFAs to produce hydroperoxy fatty acids and blocks the production of cytoprotectivelipoxins, resolvins and protectins. These hydroperoxy fatty acids and the formation of other vasoactive PGs, LT and TXs may produce intense vasospasm and occlusion of tumor-feeding vessels. These hydroperoxy fatty acids may also be generated by tumor cells exposed to PUFAs. In addition, there is evidence to suggest that the way PUFAs are handled by normal and tumor cells could be entirely different. For example, DHA that is toxic to tumor cells protects normal neural cells from stress-induced apoptosis. DHA induces apoptosis in neuroblastoma cells. Neuroblastoma cells metabolized DHA to 17-hydroxydocosahexaenoic acid (17-HDHA) via 17-hydroperoxydocosahexaenoic acid (17-HpDHA) through 15-lipoxygenase and autoxidation and did not produce the anti-inflammatory and protective lipid mediators, resolvins and protectins. 17-HpDHA exhibited potent cytotoxic action on tumor cells. DHA inhibited secretion of PGE$_2$. These results suggest that the cytotoxic effect of DHA in neuroblastoma is mediated through production of hydroperoxy fatty acids that accumulate to toxic intracellular levels with restricted production of its cytoprotective products, resolvins and protectins [73, 79, 68, 86, 96, 132, 133]. In a similar fashion, it is possible that when normal cells are exposed to AA and EPA, significant amounts of lipoxins and resolvin are formed, whereas tumor cells would accumulate respective prostanoids, leukotrienes, thromboxanes and cyclopentanone prostaglandins. Thus, *normal cells when exposed to PUFAs produce cytoprotective lipids such as lipoxins, resolvins and protectins while tumor cells generate toxic hydroperoxy fatty acids*. This differential metabolism of PUFAs by normal and tumor cells may explain why PUFAs are toxic to tumor but not normal cells (see Figure 3).

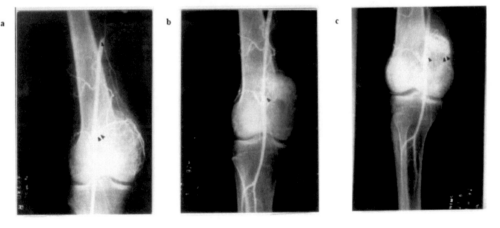

Figure 1. (A) Angiogram of a patient with giant cell tumor of the right femur performed just prior to injection of lithium-GLA coupled with iodized salt. Single arrowhead shows the tip of the catheter in the popliteal artery and the site of injection. Double arrowheads denote the origin of the tumor-feeding vessels. (B) Angiogram performed immediately after the injection of lithium-GLA coupled with iodized salt. Arrowhead shows the site of complete occlusion of the tumor-feeding vessel. Normal blood vessels, which were distal, in the path of the blood flow, and much smaller than the main tumor-feeding vessel, remained patent. (C) Angiogram performed 10 days after the injection of lithium-GLA. Single arrowhead shows the site of occlusion of the main tumor-feeding vessel. Double arrowheads depict the accumulation of lithium-GLA coupled with the iodized salt in the tumor.

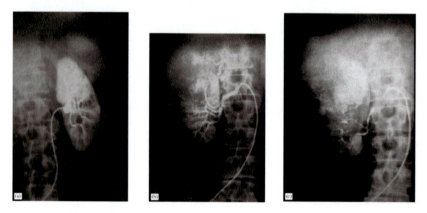

Figure 2. (A) Angiogram of the normal right kidney. (B) Angiogram of the left kidney of the same patient. The kidney is enlarged and distorted due to the presence of a tumor in the upper pole. The lateral margin of the kidney is not clear and an increase in blood supply to the tumor can be seen. (C) Angiogram of the left kidney performed immediately after injection of lithium GLA coupled to iodized salt. There is occlusion of the tumor-feeding vessels but not of the two apparently normal blood vessels feeding the normal lower pole. Figures are from [130].

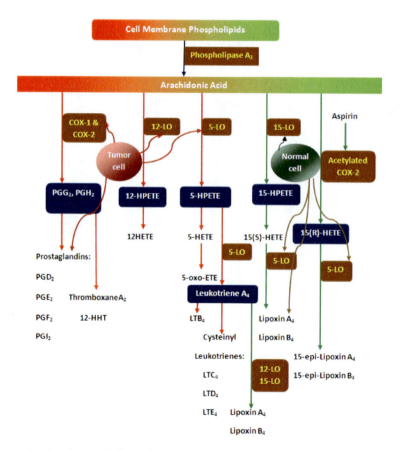

Figure 3. Scheme showing the metabolism of AA in normal and tumor cells. Tumor cells produce more prostaglandins, leukotrienes, thromboxanes, HETEs and HHTs, while normal cells generate lipoxins, resolvins, and protectins that are cytoprotective. Normal cells produce lipoxins from AA, lipoxins and resolvins from EPA, and protectins from DHA.

References

[1] Casppary W J, Niziak C, Lanzo D A, Friedman R, Bachur N R. Bleomycin A2: a ferrous oxidase. *Mol. Pharmacol.* 1979;16: 256-260.

[2] Young, R C, Ozols R F, and Myers C E. The anthracycline antineoplastic drugs. *N. Engl. J. Med.* 1981; 305: 139-153.

[3] Gajewski E, Rao G, Nackerdien Z, Dizdaroglu M Modification of DNA bases in mammalian chromatin by radiation-generated free radicals. *Biochemistry*, 1990; 29: 7876-7882.

[4] Das U N. Oxy radicals and their clinical implications. *Curr. Sci.* 1993; 65: 964-968.

[5] Das U N. Free radicals: Biology and relevance to disease. *J. Assoc. Physicians India,* 1990; 38: 495-498.

[6] Halliwell B A. Superway to kill cancer cells? *Nature Med.* 2000; 6: 1105-1106.

[7] Cleveland J L, Kastan M B. A radical approach to treatment. *Nature*, 2000; 407: 309-311.

[8] Sunderesan M, Yu Z X, Ferrans V J, Irani K, Finkel T. Requirement for generation of H_2O_2 for platelet-derived growth factor signal transduction. *Science* 1995; 270: 296-299.

[9] Suderesan M, Yu Z X, Ferrans V J, Sulciner D J, Gutkind J S, Irani K, Goldschmidt-Clermont P J, Finkel T. Regulation of reactive-oxygen-species generation in fibroblasts by Rac1. *Biochem. J.* 1996; 318: 379-382.

[10] Jayanthi S, Ordonez S, McCoy M T, Cadet J L. Dual mechanism of Fas-induced cell death in neuroglioma cells: a role for reactive oxygen species. *Brain Res. Mol. Brain Res.* 1999; 72: 158-165.

[11] Wang S, Leonard S S, Ye J, Ding M, Shi X. The role of hydroxyl radical as a messenger in Cr(VI)-induced p53 activation. *Am. J. Physiol. Cell Physiol.* 2000; 279: C868-C875.

[12] Das U N. Tuning free radical metabolism to kill tumor cells selectively with emphasis on the interaction(s) between essential fatty acids, free radicals, lymphokines and prostaglandins. *Ind. J. Pathol. Microbiol.* 1990;33: 94-103.

[13] Das U N. Cis-unsaturated fatty acids as potential anti-mutagenic, tumoricidal and anti-metastatic agents. *Asia Pacific J. Pharmacol.* 1992;7: 305-327.

[14] Galeotti T, Borrello S, Masoti L. Oxy radical sources, scavenger systems and membrane damage in cancer cells. In: Das, D. K.; Essman, R., eds. *Oxygen radicals: systemic events and disease processes.* Basel; S. Karger; 1990, 129-148.

[15] Dianzani M U, Rossi M A. Lipid peroxidation in tumors. In: Pani, P.; Feo, F.; Columbano, A.; Cagliari, E. S. A. eds. Recent trends in chemical carcinogenesis. Italy; *Cagliari*; vol 1: 243-257; 1981.

[16] Bartoli G M, Galeotti T. Growth-related lipid peroxidation in tumor microsomal membranes and mitochondria. *Biochim. Biophys. Acta,* 1979; 574: 537-541.

[17] Hostetler K Y, Zenner B D, Morris H P. Phospholipid content of mitochondrial and microsomal membranes from Morris hepatomas of varying growth rates. *Cancer Res.* 1979; 39: 2978-2983.

[18] Hartz J W, Morton R E, Waite M M, Morris H P. Correlation of fatty acyl composition of mitochondrial and microsomal phospholipid with growth rate of rat hepatomas. *Lab. Invest,* 1982; 46: 73-78.

[19] Cheeseman K H, Emery S, Maddix S P, Slater T F, Burton G W, Ingold K. Studies on lipid peroxidation in normal and tumour tissue. The Yoshida rat liver tumour. *Biochem. J.* 1988; 250: 247-252.

[20] Cheeseman K H, Burton G W, Ingold K U, Slater T F. Lipid peroxidation and lipid antioxidants in normal and tumor cells. *Toxicol. Pathol.* 1984;12: 235-239.

[21] Borrello S, Minotti G, Galeotti T. Factors influencing O_2 and t-Bu OOH-dependent lipid peroxidation of tumor microsomes. In: Rotilio, G., ed. *Superoxide and Superoxide dismutase in Chemistry, Biology and Medicine.* Amsterdam: Elsevier; 1988, 323-324.

[22] Das U N, Begin M E, Ells G, Huang Y S, Horrobin D F. Polyunsaturated fatty acids augment free radical generation in tumor cells in vitro. *Biochem. Biophys. Res. Commun.* 1987;145: 15-24.

[23] Das U N, Huang Y S, Begin M E, Ells G, Horrobin D F.Uptake and distribution of cis-unsaturated fatty acids and their effect on free radical generation in normal and tumor cells in vitro. *Free Radical. Biol. Med.* 1987; 3: 9-14.

[24] Bendetti A. Loss of lipid peroxidation as anhistochemical marker for preneoplastic hepatocellular foci of rats. *Cancer Res.* 1984; 44: 5712-5717.

[25] Dunbar L M, Bailey J M. Enzyme deletions and essential fatty acid metabolism in cultured cells. *J. Biol. Chem.* 1975; 250: 1152-1153.

[26] Morton R E, Hartz J W, Reitz R C, Waite B M, Morris H . The acyl-CoA desaturases of microsomes from rat liver and the Morris 7777 hepatoma. *Biochim. Biophys. Acta,*1979; 573: 321-331.

[27] Nassar B A, Das U N, Huang Y S, Ells G, Horrobin D F. The effect of chemical hepatocarcinogenesis on liver phospholipid composition in rats fed n-6 and n-3 fatty acid-supplemented diets. *Proc. Soc. Exp. Biol. Med.* 1992; 199: 365-368.

[28] Oberley L W, Buettner G. Role of SOD in cancer. A review. *Cancer Res.* 1979; 39: 1141-1149.

[29] Tisdale M J, Mahmoud M D. Activities of free radical metabolizing enzymes in tumours. *Br. J. Cancer,* 1983; 47: 809-812.

[30] Bize I B, Oberley L W, Morris H P. Superoxide dismutase and superoxide radical in Morris hepatomas. *Cancer Res.* 1980; 40: 3686-3693.

[31] Huang T T, Carlson E J, Raineri I, Gillespie A M, Kozy H, Epstein C J. The use of transgenic and mutant mice to study oxygen free radical metabolism. *Ann. NY Acad. Sci.* 1999; 893: 95-112.

[32] Halliwell B, Gutteridge J M C. *Free Radicals in Biology and Medicine.*, 3rd edition. Oxford University Press, UK, 1999.

[33] Hampton M B, Fadeel B, Orrenius S. Redox regulation of the caspases during apoptosis. *Ann. N Y Acad. Sci.* 1998; 854: 328-335.

[34] Jacobson M D, Raff M C. Programmed cell death and Bcl-2 protection in very low oxygen. *Nature*1995; 374: 814-816.

[35] Wagner B A, Buettner G R, Oberley L W, Burns C P. Sensitivity of K562 and HL-60 cells to edelfosine, an ether lipid drug, correlates with production of reactive oxygen species. *Cancer Res.* 1998; 58: 2809-2816.

[36] Arakaki N, Kajihara T, Arakaki R, Ohnishi T, Kazi J A, Nakashima H, Daikuhara Y. Involvement of oxidative stress in tumor cytotoxic activity of hepatocyte growth factor/scatter factor. *J. Biol. Chem.* 1999; 274: 13541-13546.

[37] Zimmerman R J, MarafinoJr B J, Chan A, Landre P, Winkelhake J L. The role of oxidant injury in tumor cell sensitivity to recombinant human tumor necrosis factor in vivo. Implications for mechanisms of action. *J. Immunol.* 1989;142: 1405-1409.

[38] Vento R, D'Alessandro N, Giuliano M, Lauricella M, Carabillo M, Tesoriere G Induction of apoptosis by arachidonic acid in human retinoblastoma Y79 cells: involvement of oxidative stress. *Exp. Eye Res.*2000; 70: 503-517.

[39] Bize I B, Oberley L W, Morris H P. Superoxide dismutase and superoxide radical in Morris hepatomas. *Cancer Res.* 1980; 40: 3686-3693.

[40] Cheeseman K H, Collins M, Proudfoot K, Slater T F, Burton G W, Webb A C, Ingold K U. Studies on lipid peroxidation in normal and tumour tissues. The Novikoff rat liver tumour. *Biochem. J.* 1986; 235: 507-514.

[41] Malafa M, Margenthaler J, Webb B, Neitzel L, Christophersen M. MnSOD expression is increased in metastatic gastric cancer. *J. Surg. Res.*2000; 88: 130-134.

[42] Westman N G, Marklund S L. Copper-and zinc-containing superoxide dismutase and manganese-containing superoxide dismutase in human tissues and human malignant tumors. *Cancer Res.* 1981; 41: 2962-2966.

[43] Zhong W, Oberley L W, Oberley T D, St Clair D K. Suppression of the malignant phenotype of human glioma cells by overexpression of manganese superoxide dismutase. *Oncogene*, 1997; 14: 481-490.

[44] Toh Y, Kuninaka S, Oshiro T, Ikeda Y, Nakashima H, Baba H, Kohnoe S, Okamura T, Mori M, Sugimachi K. Overexpression of manganese superoxide dismutase mRNA may correlate with aggressiveness in gastric and colorectal adenocarcinomas. *Int. J. Oncol.* 2000;17: 107-112.

[45] Izutani R, Asano S, Imano M, Kuroda D, Kato M, Ohyanagi H. Expression of manganese superoxide dismutase in esophageal and gastric cancers. *J. Gastroenterol.*1998;33: 816-822.

[46] Zhong W, Yan T, Lim R, Oberley L W. Expression of superoxide dismutases, catalase, and glutathione peroxidase in glioma cells. *Free Rad. Biol. Med.* 1999;27: 1334-1345.

[47] Huang Y, He T, Domann F E. Decreased expression of manganese superoxide dismutase in transformed cells is associated with increased cytosine methylation of the SOD2 gene. *DNA Cell Biol.* 1999; 18: 643-652.

[48] Clement M V, Pervaiz S. Reactive oxygen intermediates regulate cellular apoptosis response to apoptotic stimuli: an hypothesis. *Free Rad. Biol. Med.* 1999;30: 247-252.

[49] Morisaki N, Lindsey J A, Stitts J M, Zhang H, Cornwell D G. Fatty acid metabolism and cell proliferation. V. Evaluation of pathways for the generation of lipid peroxides. *Lipids,*1984; 19: 381-394.

[50] Morisaki N, Sprecher H, Milo G E, Cornwell D G. Fatty acid specificity in the inhibition of cell proliferation and its relationship to lipid peroxidation and prostaglandin biosynthesis. *Lipids,* 1982; 17: 893-899.

[51] Liepkalns V A, Icard-Liepkalns C, Cornwell D G. Regulation of cell division in a human glioma cell clone by arachidonic acid and alpha-tocopherolquinone. *Cancer Lett.* 1982;15: 173-178.

[52] Cheeseman K H, Collins M, Maddix S, Milia A, Proudfoot K, Slater T F, Burton G W, Webb A, Inglod K U. Lipid peroxidation in regenerating rat liver. *FEBS Lett.*1986;209: 191-196.

[53] Slater T F, Cheeseman K H, Benedetto C, Collins M, Emery S, Maddix S, Nodes J T, Proudfoot K, Burton G W, Ingold K U. Studies on the hyperplasia ('regeneration') of the rat liver following partial hepatectomy. Changes in lipid peroxidation and general biochemical aspects. *Biochem. J.* 1990; 265: 51-59.

[54] Kastan M B, Canman C E, Leonard C J. P53, cell cycle control and apoptosis: implications for cancer. *Cancer Metastasis. Rev.* 1995; 14: 3-15.

[55] Martinez J D, Pennington M E, Craven M T, Warters R L, Cress A E. Free radicals generated by ionizing radiation signal nuclear translocation of p53. *Cell Growth Differ.*1997;8: 941-949.

[56] Uberti D, Yavin E, Gil S, Ayasola K R, Goldfinger N, Rotter V. Hydrogen peroxide induces nuclear translocation of p53 and apoptosis in cells of oligodendroglia origin. *Brain Res. Mol. Brain Res.* 1999; 65: 167-175.

[57] Kitamura Y, Ota T, Matsuoka Y, Tooyama I, Kimura H, Shimohama S, Nomura Y, Gebicke-Haerter P J, Taniguchi T. Hydrogen peroxide-indcued apoptosis mediated by p53 protein in glial cells. *Glia*, 1999; 25: 154-164.

[58] Pani G, Bedogni B, Anzevino R, Colavitti R, Palazzotti B, Borrello S, Galeotti T. Deregulated manganese superoxide dismutase expression an resistance to oxidative injury in p53-deficient cells. *Cancer Res.* 2000; 60: 4654-4660.

[59] Hilf R, Murant R S, Narayana U, Gibson S L. Relationship of mitochondrial function and cellular adensine triphosphate levels to hematoporphyrin derivative-induced photosensitization in R 3230 AC mammary tumors. *Cancer Res.* 1986; 46: 211-217.

[60] Lee Y, Shacter E. Hydrogen peroxide inhibits activation, not activity, of cellular caspase-3 in vivo. *Free Radic. Biol. Med.* 2000; 29: 684-692.

[61] Saretzki G, von Zglinicki T. Replicative senescence as a model of aging: the role of oxidative stress and telomere shortening-an overview. *Z. Gerontol. Geriatr.* 1999;32: 69-75.

[62] Oikawa S, Kawanishi S. Site-specific DNA damage at GGG sequence by oxidative stress may accelerate telomere shortening. *FEBS Lett.* 1999;453: 365-368.

[63] vonZglinicki T, Pilger R, Sitte N. Accumulation of single-strand breaks is the major cause of telomere shortening in human fibroblasts. *Free Radic. Biol. Med.* 2000; 28: 64-74.

[64] Tyurina Y Y, Tyurina V A, Certa G, Quinn P J, Schor N F, Kagan V E. Direct evidence for antioxidant effect of BCL-2 in PC 12 rat pheochromocytoma cells. *Arch. Biochem. Biophys.*1997;344: 413-423.

[65] Haldar S, Negrini M, Monne M, Sabbioni S, Croce C M. Down regulation of bcl-2 by p53 in breast cancer cells. *Cancer Res.* 1994; 54: 2095-2097.

[66] Haldar S, Jena N, Croce C M. Inactivation of Bcl-2 by phosphorylation. *Proc. Natl. Acad. Sci. USA,*1995; 92: 4507-4511.

[67] Hockenbery D M, Oltvai Z N, Yin X M, Milliman C L, Korsmeyer S J. Bcl-2 functions in an antioxidant pathway to prevent apoptosis. *Cell*, 1993; 75: 241-251.

[68] Das U N. Essential fatty acids, lipid peroxidation and apoptosis. *Prostaglandins Leukotrienes Essen Fatty Acids,* 1999; 61: 157-163.

[69] Padma M, Das U N. Effect of cis-unsaturated fatty acids on the activity of protein kinases and protein phosphorylation in macrophage tumor (AK-5) cells in vitro. *Prostaglandins Leukotrienes Essen Fatty Acids*, 1999; 60: 55-63.

[70] Esposti M D, Hatzinisiriou I, McLennan H, Ralph S. Bcl-2 and mitochondrial oxygen radicals. New approaches with reactive oxygen species-sensitive probes. *J. Biol. Chem.* 1999; 274: 29831-29837.

[71] Lin HL, Liu TY, Chau GY, Lui WY, Chi CW. Comparison of 2-methoxyestradiol-induced, docetaxel-induced, and paclitaxel-induced apoptosis in hepatoma cells and its correlation with reactive oxygen species. *Cancer* 2000; 89: 983-994.

[72] Huang P, Feng L, Oldham E A, Keating M J, Plunkett W. Superoxide dismutase as a target for the selective killing of cancer cells. *Nature* 2000; 407: 390-395.

[73] Das UN. A radical approach to cancer. *Med. Sci. Monit.* 2002; 8: RA79-RA92.

[74] Ge Y, Byun JS, De Luca P, Gueron G, Yabe IM, Sadiq-Ali SG, Figg WD, Quintero J, Haggerty CM, Li QQ, De Siervi A, Gardner K. Combinatorial antileukemic disruption of oxidative homeostasis and mitochondrial stability by the redox reactive thalidomide 2-(2,4-difluoro-phenyl)-4,5,6,7-tetrafluoro-1H-isoindole-1,3(2H)-dione (CPS49) and flavopiridol.*Mol. Pharmacol.* 2008; 74: 872-883.

[75] Colquhoun A. Mechanisms of action of eicosapentaenoic acid in bladder cancer cells in vitro: alterations in mitochondrial metabolism, reactive oxygen species generation and apoptosis induction. *J. Urol.* 2009; 181: 1885-1893.

[76] Naidu MR, Das UN, Kishan A.Intratumoral gamma-linoleic acid therapy of human gliomas. *Prostaglandins Leukot. Essent. Fatty Acids,* 1992; 45: 181-184.

[77] Das UN, Prasad VV, Reddy DR.Local application of gamma-linolenic acid in the treatment of human gliomas.*Cancer Lett.* 1995; 94: 147-155.

[78] Bakshi A, Mukherjee D, Bakshi A, Banerji AK, Das UN. Gamma-linolenic acid therapy of human gliomas. *Nutrition*, 2003; 19: 305-309.

[79] Das UN. Gamma-linolenic acid therapy of human glioma-a review of in vitro, in vivo, and clinical studies. *Med. Sci. Monit.* 2007; 13: RA119-RA31.

[80] Reddy DR, Prassad VS, Das UN.Intratumoural injection of gamma linolenic acid in malignant gliomas.*J. Clin. Neurosci.* 1998; 5: 36-39.

[81] Smith D L, Willis A L, Mahmud I. Eicosanoid effects on cell proliferation in vitro: relevance to atherosclerosis. *Prostaglandins Leukotrienes Med.* 1984; 16: 1-10.

[82] Sakai T, Yamaguchi N, Shiroko Y, Sekiguchi M, Fujii G, Nishino H. Prostaglandin D_2 inhibits the proloferation of human malignant tumor cells. *Prostaglandins*, 1984; 27: 17-26.

[83] Booyens J, Englebrecht P, Le Roux S, Louwrens C C, Van der Merwe C F, Katzeff I E. Some effects of the essential fatty acids linoleic acid, alpha-linolenic acid, and of their metabolites gamma-linolenic acid, arachidonic acid, eicosapentaenoic acid, and docosahexaenoic acid and of prostaglandins A and E on the proliferation of human osteogenic sarcoma cells in culture. *Prostaglandins Leukotrienes Med.*1984; 15: 15-33.

[84] Begin ME, Das U N, Ells G, Horrobin D F. Selective killing of human cancer cells by polyunsaturated fatty acids. *ProstaglandinsLeukotrienes Med.* 1985; 19: 177-186.

[85] Begin ME, Ells G, Das U N, Horrobin D F. Differential killing of human carcinoma cells supplemented with n-3 and n-6 polyunsaturated fatty acids. *J. Natl. Cancer Inst.*1986; 77: 1053-1062.

[86] Das U N. Tumoricidal action of cis-unsaturated fatty acids and their relationship to free radicals and lipid peroxidation. *Cancer Lett.* 1991;56: 235-243.

[87] Sagar P S, Das U N, Koratkar R, Ramesh G, Padma M, Kumar G S. Cytotoxic action of cis-unsaturated fatty acids on human cervical carcinoma (HeLa) cells: relationship to free radicals and lipid peroxidation and its modulation by calmodulin antagonists. *Cancer Lett.* 1992;63: 189-198.

[88] Kumar G S, Das U N. Free radical-dependent suppression of growth of mouse myeloma cells by α-linolenic and eicosapentaenoic acids in vitro. *Cancer Lett.* 1995;92: 27-38.

[89] Padma M, Das U N. Effect of cis-unsaturated fatty acids on cellular oxidant stress in macrophage tumor (AK-5) cells in vitro. *Cancer Lett.* 1996;109: 63-75.

[90] Seigel I, Liu T L, Yaghoubzadeh E, Kaskey T S, Gleicher N. Cytotoxic effects of free fatty acids on ascites tumor cells. *J. Natl. Cancer Inst.*1987; 78: 271-277.

[91] Tolnai S, Morgan J F. Studies on the in vitro anti-tumor activity of fatty acids. V. Unsaturated fatty acids. *Can. J. Biochem. Physiol.* 1962; 40: 869-875.

[92] Rossi M A, Cecchini G. Lipid peroxidation in hepatomas of different degrees of deviation. *Cell Biochem. Function,* 1983; 1: 49-54.

[93] Burlakova E B, Palmina N P. On the possible role of free radical mechanism on the regulation of cell replication. *Biofizika*, 1967; 12: 82-88.

[94] Gonzalez M, Schemmel R, Dugan L, Gray J, Welsch C. Dietary fish oil inhibits human breast carcinoma growth: A function of increased lipid peroxidation. *Lipids,* 1993; 28: 827-832.

[95] Das UN. Can essential fatty acids reduce the burden of disease(s)? *Lipids Health Dis.* 2008; 7: 9.

[96] Das UN. Tumoricidal and anti-angiogenic actions of gamma-linolenic acid and its derivatives. *Current Pharmaceut. Biotech.* 2006;7: 457-466.

[97] Cao Y, Pearman A T, Zimmerman G A, McIntyre T M, Prescott S M. Intracellular unesterifiedarachidonic acid signals apoptosis. *Proc. Natl. Acad. Sci. USA,*2000; 97: 11280-11285.

[98] Brekke O L, Sagen E, Bjerve K S. Specificity of endogenous fatty acid release during tumor necrosis factor-induced apoptosis in WEHI 164 fibrosarcoma cells. *J. Lipid. Res.* 1999; 40: 2223-2233.

[99] Ramesh G, Das U N. Effect of free fatty acids on two stage skin carcinogenesis in mice. *Cancer Lett.* 1996;100: 199-209.

[100] Calviello G, Palozza O, Piccioni E, Maggiano N, Frattucci A, Franceschelli P, Bartoli G M. Supplementation with eicosapentaenoic and docosahexaenoic acid inhibits growth of Morris hepatocarcinoma 3924A in rats: Effects on proliferation and apoptosis. *Int. J. Cancer,* 1998; 75: 699-705.

[101] Chapkin R S, Jiang Y H, Davidson L A, Lupton J R. Modulation of intracellular second messengers by dietary fat during colonic tumor development. *Adv. Exp. Med. Biol.* 1997; 422: 85-96.

[102] Cai J, Jiang W G, Mansel R E. Inhibition of angiogenic factor- and tumor-induced angiogenesis by gamma linolenic acid. *Prostaglandins Leukotrienes Essen Fatty Acids,* 1999; 60: 21-29.

[103] Rose D P, Connolly J M. Antiangiogenicity of docosahexaenoic acid and its role in the suppression of breast cancer cell growth in nude mice. *Int. J. Oncol.* 1999;15: 1011-1015.

[104] Rose DP, Hatala MA, Connolly JM, Rayburn J. Effect of diets containing different levels of linoleic acid on human breast cancer growth and lung metastasis in nude mice. *Cancer Res.* 1993; 53: 4686-4690.

[105] Rose DP, Connolly JM, Liu X-H. Dietary fatty acids and human breast cancer cell growth, invasion, and metastasis. *Adv. Exp. Med. Biol.* 1994; 364: 83-91.

[106] Rose DP, Connolly JM, Liu X-H. Effects of linoleic acid on the growth and metastasis of two human breast cancer cell lines in nude mice and the invasive capacity of these cell lines in vitro. *Cancer Res,* 1994; 54: 6557-6562.

[107] El-Ela SHA, Prasse KW, Carroll R. Effects of dietary primrose oil on mammary tumorigenesis induced by 7, 12-dimethyl bez(a)anthracene. *Lipids,* 1987; 22: 1041-1044.

[108] El-Ela SHA, Prasse KW, Carroll R, Wade AE, Dharwadkar S, Bunce OR. Eicosanoids synthesis in 7, 12-dimethylbenz(a)anthracene-induced mammary carcionomas in Sprague-Dawley rats fed primrose oil, menhaden oil or corn oil diet. *Lipids,* 1988; 23: 948-954.

[109] Cameron E, Bland J, Marcuson R. Divergent effects of omega-6 and omega-3 fatty acids on mammary tumor development in C3H/Heston mice treated with DMBA. *Nutrition Res.* 1989; 9: 383-393.

[110] Ramesh G, Das U N, Koratkar R, Padma M, Sagar P S. Effect of essential fatty acids on tumor cells. *Nutrition,* 1992; 8: 343-347.

[111] Menendez JA, del Mar Barbacid M, Montero S, Sevilla E, Escrich E, Solanas M, Cortes-Funes H, Colomer R. Effects of gamma-linolenic acid and oleic acid on paclitaxel cytotoxicity in human breast cancer cells. *Eur. J. Cancer,* 2001; 37: 402- 413.

[112] Ravichandran D, Cooper A, Johnson CD. Growth inhibitory effect of lithium gammalinolenate on pancreatic cancer cell lines: Influence of albumin and iron. *Eur. J. Cancer,* 1998; 34: 188-192.

[113] Ravichandran D, Cooper A, Johnson CD. Effect of 1-γlinolenyl-3-eicosapentaenoyl propane diol on the growth of human pancreatic carcinoma in vitro and in vivo. *Eur. J. Cancer,* 2000; 36:423-427.

[114] Kenny FS, Gee JM, Nicholson RI, Morris T, Watson S, Bryce RP, Hartley J, Robertson JFR. Effect of dietary GLA +/- tamoxifen on growth and ER in a human breast cancer xenograft model. *Eur. J. Cancer,* 1998; 34: S20.

[115] Kenny FS, Pinder S, Ellis IO, Bryce RP, Hartley J, Robertson JFR. Gamma linolenic acid with tamoxifen as primary therapy in breast cancer. *Eur. J. Cancer.* 1998;34: S18-S19.

[116] Jiang WG, Bryce RP, Mansel RE. Gamma linolenic acid regulates gap junction communication in endothelial cells and their interaction with tumour cells. *Prostaglandins Leukot Essen Fatty Acids,* 1997; 56: 307-316.

[117] Sethi S, Eastman AY, Eaton JW. Inhibition of phagocyte-endothelium interactions by oxidized fatty acids: a natural anti-inflammatory mechanism? *J. Lab. Clin. Med.* 1996; 128: 27-38.

[118] Germain E, Chajes V, Cognault S, Lhuillery C, Bougnoux P. Enhancement of doxorubicin cytotoxicity by polyunsaturated fatty acids in the human breast tumor cell line MDA-MB-231; relationship to lipid peroxidation. *Int. J. Cancer,* 1998; 75: 578-583.

[119] Shao Y, Pardini L, Pardini RS. Dietary menhaden oil enhances mitomycin C antitumor activity toward human mammary carcinoma MX-1. *Lipids,*1995; 30: 1035-1045.

[120] Sagar P S, Das U N. Gamma-linolenic acid and eicosapentaenoic acid potentiate the cytotoxicity of anti-cancer drugs on human cervical carcinoma (HeLa) cells in vitro. *Med. Sci. Res.* 1993; 21: 457-459.

[121] Chow SC and Jondal M. Ca^{2+} entry in T cells is activated by emptying the inositol 1,4,5-triphosphate sensitive Ca^{2+} pool. *Cell Calcium,* 1990; 11: 641-646.

[122] Nakagawa T, Zhu H, Morishima N, Li E, Xu J, Yanker BA, Yuan J. Caspase-12 mediates endoplasmic reticulum-specific apoptosis and cytotoxicity by amyloid-beta. *Nature,* 2000; 403: 98-103.

[123] Huang ZH, Hii CS, Rathjen DA, Poulos A, Murray AW, Ferrante A. N-6 and N-3 polyunsaturated fatty acids stimulate translocation of protein kinase Calpha, betaI, beta II and –epsilon and enhance agonist-induced NADPH oxidase in macrophages. *Biochem. J.* 1997: 325 (pt 2): 553-557.

[124] Peterson DA, Mehta N, Butterfield J, Husak M, Christopher MM, Jagarlapudi S, Eaton JW. Polyunsaturated fatty acids stimulate superoxide formation in tumor cells: a mechanism for specific cytotoxicity and a model for tumor necrosis factor? *Biochem. Biophys. Res. Commun.* 1988;155: 1033-1037.

[125] Chiu LC and Wan JM. Induction of apoptosis in HL-60 cells by eicosapentaenoic acid (EPA) is associated with downregulation of bcl-2 expression. *Cancer Lett.* 1999;145: 17-27.

[126] Albino AP, Juan G, Traganos F, Reinhart L, Connolly J, Rose DP, Darzynkiewicz Z. Cell cycle arrest and apoptosis of melanoma cells by docosahexaenoic acid: association with decreased pRb phosphorylation. *Cancer Res.* 2000; 60: 4139-4145.

[127] Chen ZY andIstfan NW. Docosahexaenoic acid, a major constitutent of fish oil diets, prevents activation of cyclin-dependent kinases and S-phase entry by serum stimulation in HT-29 cells. *Prostaglandins Leukot. Essen Fatty Acids,* 2001; 64: 67-73.

[128] 128. Palakurthi SS, Fluckiger R, Aktas H, Changlokar AK, Shahsafaei A, Harneit S, Kilic E, Halperin JA. Inhibition of translation initiation mediates the anticancer effect of the n-3 polyunsaturated fatty acid eicosapentaenoic acid. *Cancer Res.* 2000; 60: 2919- 2925.

[129] Nishida M, Maruyama Y, Tanaka R, Kontani K, Nagao T, Kurose H. $G\alpha_i$and $G\alpha_o$ are target proteins of reactive oxygen species. *Nature,* 2000; 408: 492-495.

[130] Das UN. Abrupt and complete occlusion of tumor-feeding vessels by gamma-linolenic acid. *Nutrition* 2002; 18: 662-664.

[131] Das UN. Occlusion of infusion vessels on gamma-linolenic acid infusion. *ProstaglandinsLeukotrienes Essential Fatty Acids* 2004; 70; 23-32.

[132] Gleissman H, Yang R, Martinod K, Lindskog M, Serhan CN, Johnsen JI, Kogner P.Docosahexaenoic acid metabolome in neural tumors: identification of cytotoxic intermediates.*FASEB J.* 2010; 24: 906-915.

[133] Madhavi N and Das UN. Effect of n-6 and n-3 fatty acids on the survival of vincristine sensitive and resistant human cervical carcinoma cells in vitro. *Cancer Lett.* 1994; 84: 31-41.

In: Principles of Free Radical Biomedicine, Volume III
Editors: K. Pantopoulos and H. M. Schipper

ISBN 978-1-61324-184-4
©2012 Nova SciencePublishers, Inc.

Chapter 7

Cancer Chemotherapy

Zuanel Diaz and Wilson Miller[*]

Lady Davis Institute for Medical Research, Departments of Medicine and Physiology,
McGill University, 3755 Cote Sainte-Catherine Road, Montreal, Quebec,
Canada, H3T 1E2

1. Introduction

Cancer is a leading cause of death worldwide. It has been estimated that 12 million new cancer diagnoses will be made and more than 7 million deaths worldwide will occur this year. The projected numbers for 2030 are 20-26 million new diagnoses and 13-17 million deaths. Although cancer is a devastating disease, many cancers are preventable and new effective therapeutic strategies have been developed in the last years. Nevertheless, what we know about how cancer can be prevented and treated is limited and frequently contradictory. *It is well documented that reactive oxygen species (ROS) operate in various signaling cascades related to different behaviors in cancer cells, including tumor initiation, development, progression survival, proliferation, invasion, angiogenesis and metastasis* (see also Chapter 6 in this Volume). On the other hand, *ROS production is also a mechanism shared by the majority of cancer therapeutic approaches, including chemotherapy and radiotherapy, due to its role in promoting cell death.* Because of the dichotomous property of ROS in determining cell fate, both pro- or anti-oxidant therapies have been proposed for cancer treatment and prevention. However, due to the particular complexity of the role of ROS in tumor and normal cells, it is often difficult to determine which aspect is predominant and to decide which strategy is more appropriate for the treatment of a specific patient. In general, antioxidants have been proposed as chemopreventive, and oxidant-enhancing strategies as treatment for established cancers. However, several trials of antioxidants in chemoprevention have failed to exhibit any benefit or even showed harm in some groups of patients [1-2], while evidence is accumulating that persistent high ROS concentrations may support

---

[*]E-mail: wmiller@ldi.jgh.mcgill.ca

malignant growth of established tumors. We attempt to describe herein our current appreciation of approaches aimed at modulation of oxidative stress in cancer and their essential mechanisms. Special emphasis is placed on the development of two opposed strategies aimed at manipulating ROS levels.

2. One Side of the Coin: ROS as Tumor Promoters

Over the last decade, an association between cancer risk and oxidative stress has been recognized, and epidemiological, experimental, and clinical studies have suggested a role for oxidative stress in the development and progression of this disease. The correlation between redox state and malignancy is based on the observations that cancer cell lines exhibiting different degrees of aggressiveness also present significant differences in redox status during cell growth [3-4]. An increasing body of evidence demonstrates that ROS are generated in tumors. Serum ROS levels are elevated in proportion to tumor invasion and show a significant positive correlation with tumor size in a variety of cancers [5]. The source of endogenous ROS can be the tumor cells themselves [6], infiltrating inflammatory phagocytes [7-11], tumor-surrounding stroma [12-13] and/or hypoxic conditions [14]. Although the specific mechanisms leading to oxidative stress in cancer cells are presently unknown, different intrinsic and extrinsic processes have being acknowledged to be responsible for generating oxidative stress in cancer initiation and progression. *Activation of oncogenes, growth factor receptors, intracellular signaling pathway and specific transcription factors related to proliferation are intrinsic factors known to create oxidative stress in cancer cells (Figure 1).*

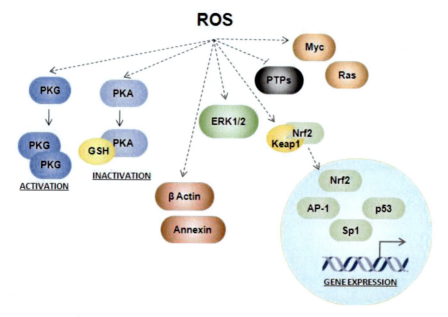

Figure 1. Activation of cell growth regulatory pathways. ROS are implicated in cancer initiation and progression. The expression of specific tumor-promoting genes such as Ras, Bcr-Abl and c-Myc, has been associated with chronic increases in intracellular ROS. ROS function as messengers in cellular signaling

Cancer Chemotherapy

transduction pathways. Redox-sensitive transcription factors are the downstream targets of signaling pathways that modulate the expression of specific genes related to cell proliferation.

2.1. Activation of Oncogenes

The expression of specific tumor-promoting genes such as Ras, Bcr-Abl and c-Myc, has been associated with the generation of ROS in cells and animal models. In transformed fibroblasts, Ras and Rac have being demonstrated to be directly linked to ROS generation through the activation of the enzyme NADPH oxidase (NOX), and the tumorigenic function of these oncogenes is dependent on this ROS formation, as it can be suppressed by antioxidant treatment [15-16].

In addition of the activation of NOX, it was recently demonstrated that introduction of oncogenic Ras in human and rat fibroblast cells is accompanied by a decrease in expression of mRNAs derived from the sestrin family genes SESN1 and SESN3, which encode antioxidant modulators of peroxiredoxins. Thus, *ROS generation and concomitant inhibition of antioxidant defences may both be involved in oncogenic transformation* [17]. In addition, transformation of hematopoietic cells by the oncogenic tyrosine kinase Bcr-Abl is associated with a chronic increase of intracellular ROS [18]. The origin of ROS associated with Bcr-Abl transformation is linked to the mitochondrial electron transport chain [18-19] and PI3K pathway activation [19].

2.2. Activation of Growth Factor Receptors

Accumulation of ROS has been shown to activate growth factor receptors. Although the mechanism of activation remains unclear for several receptors, a ligand-independent mechanism for activation of the epidermal growth factor receptor (EGFR) has been elucidated. In contrast to the phosphorylation induced by its ligand, ROS generate a receptor with negligible phosphorylation at Tyr1045, the major docking site for the ubiquitin ligase c-Cbl. Consequently, EGFR fails to recruit c-Cbl, and thus is not ubiquitinylated, not internalized, and not degraded, conferring prolonged receptor signaling at the plasma membrane [20]. This aberrant phosphorylation coincides with enhanced cell proliferation and has a key role in tumorigenesis. In addition, ROS leads to maintenance of Src oxidation and activation, which results in a sustained ligand-independent phosphorylation of EGFR, activation of EGFR-related pro-survival signals and inhibition of the apoptotic pathway [21-22]. Another receptor found to be activated by ROS is the keratinocyte growth factor receptor (KGFR). Exposure of NIH3T3 cells to oxidant stimuli induces a rapid intracellular production of ROS, which triggers KGFR activation and internalization, in a manner similar to those induced by KGF [23]

2.3. Activation of Intracellular Signaling Pathways

ROS function as messengers in cellular signaling transduction pathways related to proliferation [24-26]. Redox-regulated proteins include protein tyrosine phosphatases (PTP1B, SHP-2, LMW-PTP) [27-28], Src [29-30], the MAP kinases [31-32], focal adhesion kinase [33], PKB [34], G-proteins [35], Cdc25 phosphatases [36-37], and cytoskeletal proteins such as β-actin, annexin [38], and beta-catenin [39]. The ability of ROS to directly modify key proteins of the intracellular signaling pathways suggests that a large amount of the effects of ROS results from their actions on signaling pathways. Although the exact mechanism(s) by which ROS stimulate cell proliferation or death, and how redox imbalance can induce tumorigenesis, are still under investigation, recent studies on the regulation of protein phosphatases and kinases have convincingly demonstrated the biochemical mechanism and the functional relevance of oxidative modifications during cell signaling.

Upon ROS generation, the highly reactive Cys199 located in the activation loop of cAMP-dependent protein kinase (PKA) forms a mixed disulfide with glutathione or an internal disulfide with Cys343 located in the C terminus. This disulfide bond formation results in dephosphorylation of Thr197 and the loss of enzyme activity [40]. Interestingly, guanosine 3',5'-monophosphate (cGMP)-dependent protein kinase (PKG) has been found to function as a redox sensor. In cells treated with H_2O_2, an inter-protein disulfide bond is formed between its two subunits, which activates the kinase activity by increasing its affinity for its specific substrates [41].

Protein Tyrosine Phosphatases (low-molecular mass PTP (LMW-PTP) [42], tensin homologue (PTEN) [43], and kinase-associated phosphatase (KAP) [44] have been also found to be rapidly and reversibly inactivated upon mild treatment with H_2O_2 by forming stable disulfides between active site cysteines. Similarly, treatment with tumor necrosis factor (TNF) induces oxidative inactivation of the mitogen-activated protein kinase phosphatase 3 (MKP3), and consequential sustained activation of Jun N-terminal kinase (JNK) [45].

Reversible oxidation of cysteine and methionine residues has a profound impact on protein function and metabolic processes. Some catalytic cysteines containing proteins are particularly sensitive to changes in the cellular redox state. These proteins act as cellular redox sensors, mediating the initial response to changes in redox state following stimulus-induced ROS production. The activation of these redox sensors mediates the activation or repression of key ROS-induced signaling pathways. There is considerable interest in identifying direct redox sensors and understanding what enables some but not other proteins to directly respond to redox regulation [46].

2.4. Modulation of Transcription Factors

Redox-sensitive transcription factors are the downstream targets of signaling pathways that modulate the expression of specific genes, and are considered immediate-response genes that are activated following a wide variety of environmental agents inducing oxidative stress [47-48]. Redox modulation of transcription factor activity includes the oxidative modification of the DNA-binding motif or posttranslational modifications (phosphorylation or dephosphorylation) that result from the activation of ROS-regulated signaling pathways [49]. Transcription factors that are extremely sensitive to oxidative stress include p53, NF-E2–related factor 2 (Nrf2), nuclear factor kappa-B (NF-κB), AP-1 family (Jun, Fos, Maf, and ATF), signal protein 1 (Sp1), glucocorticoid receptor (GR), and early growth response 1 (Egr1) [50-52]; see also Vol. II, Chapters 12-14.

p53 is a tumor suppressor involved in the regulation of cell-cycle arrest and apoptosis and is considered a redox-sensitive transcriptional factor. p53 protein has 10 cysteine residues, all of which, interestingly, are located within the DNA binding domain, between amino acids 100-300 [53]. p53 oxidation inhibits site-specific p53 binding and p53 transactivation ability [53-58]. After mild stress, low levels of p53 drive the expression of some antioxidant genes that reduce ROS levels and protect cells against DNA damage. However, after severe or extended stress, p53 oxidation and deactivation result in elevated ROS levels, DNA damage and cell death. Studies on p53 redox regulation and adaptive responses are still very active.

In response to oxidative stress, Nrf2 mediates the transcriptional upregulation of antioxidant response element (ARE)-containing genes, including those encoding for endogenous antioxidants and phase II detoxifying enzymes (Vol. II, Chapter 13). While Nrf2 is normally sequestered in the cytoplasm by an inhibitor molecule, Keap-1, oxidative stress can stimulate its release and translocation to the nucleus [59]. Once there, a critical cysteine residue (Cys506) must be in a reduced state for efficient DNA binding to occur [60]. Regulation of Nrf2 function is controlled by numerous factors, but the dissociation of the Nrf2/Keap-1 complex is largely a result of the modification of cysteine residues in Keap-1 (Cys 151, 273 and 288) in the cytoplasm through either electrophilic adduction or oxidative modification [61].

2.5. Contribution to Metastatic Disease

Metastatic tumor cells are a specialized subset of cells capable of completing the multistep metastasis cascade. The process is divided into two stages. First, tumor cells detach from the primary lesion, migrate, degrade the surrounding extracellular matrix, and intravasate into blood and/or lymph vessels. Second, in the circulation, where they escape immunological attack, tumor cells adhere to endothelial cells and extravasate from blood and/or lymph vessels through the endothelium. Then, tumor cells proliferate at sites distant from the primary tumor, and new blood vessels supplying the metastatic tumor are formed [62-63]. Cancer cells do not act alone in these stages, but interact with surrounding tissues, extracellular matrix, immune cells, blood cells, and endothelial cells. *Upon interaction, ROS and other molecules, including cytokines, growth factors, proteases, and angiogenic factors, are released, and most such responses can accelerate tumor metastasis* [63].

Although ROS have been specifically correlated to the initiation and progression of the metastatic process [64-67], the cellular mechanisms induced and the phases of tumor dissemination at which ROS exert their pro-metastatic effects are not well explored. Some studies revealed that low-dose radiation, at levels comparable to those used in radiotherapy, increase the surface expression of $\alpha II\beta 3$ integrin receptors in melanoma cells, conferring upon these cells an enhanced capacity to adhere to endothelial cells that may be crucial for tumor-cell extravasation [68]. It was shown that W256 cells degrade subendothelial matrices by a process involving both the generation of H_2O_2 and the secretion of a matrix metalloproteinase (MMP) [64]. ROS also stimulate MMP expression and influence the remodeling of vascular basement membranes by endothelial cells [67]. These data are supported by experiments showing that inhibition of ROS reduces malignant growth. For example, in mice, treatment with catalase derivatives significantly reduced hepatic metastasis of colon carcinoma cells due to the inhibition of MMP-9, which was highly expressed in the tumor-bearing liver [69]. In addition, PEG-catalase [70] and PEG-superoxide dismutase (SOD) [71], long-lived circulating analogues of these antioxidant enzymes, significantly reduced the number of cells detected in the lung 24 hours after tumor injection, suggesting that the early steps of tumor metastasis, including the adhesion of tumor cells to endothelial cells, could be induced by ROS. Scavenging of ROS has also been effective in reducing metastatic growth in different animal models of pulmonary metastasis [72].

Other studies suggest a critical role of inflammation in the induction of ROS and subsequent increased malignancy. For example, the weakly tumorigenic and nonmetastatic QR-32 cells, derived from a fibrosarcoma in C57BL6 mouse, converted to malignant cells and acquired invasive capacity after being co-implanted with a gelatin sponge to induce inflammation, an effect that was inhibited by an orally active SOD derivative [73]. Another study showed that minisatellite somatic mutations occur at a high frequency when QR-32 cells were co-cultured with inflammatory cells, and the frequency was reduced by addition of a ROS scavenger [74]. The contribution of the nicotinamide adenine dinucleotide phosphate oxidase (NOX)-derived superoxide ($O_2^-\cdot$) to the acquisition of the metastatic phenotype has been recently established. NOX-deficient mice exhibit a reduced number of metastases as compared to wild type mice after implanting cells with high metastatic capacity [75].

Another line of evidence in support of the association between ROS and metastasis comes from clinical findings. In one important study, the steady-state levels of intracellular ROS in a diverse set of tumors positively correlated with the metastatic potential of tumor cells [76]. In another study, oxidative stress-induced enzymes and oxidative damage to DNA were relatively more abundant in metastatic prostatic adenocarcinomas compared with primary tumors and normal human prostate tissues [77]. Lipid peroxidation products such as malondialdehyde, and nitric oxide products, including nitrite (NO_2^-) and nitrate (NO_3^-), are significantly elevated, whereas enzymatic antioxidants (glutathione peroxidase (GPx) and CuZnSOD) are significantly lower in the circulation of prostate cancer patients when compared to healthy controls or patients with benign prostatic hyperplasia subjects [78-79]. Finally, the level of lysyl oxidase, an H_2O_2-producing enzyme that regulates in vitro motility, migration, and cell-matrix adhesion, is increased in distant metastatic human breast cancer tissues as compared with primary tumors, and levels are in both cases greater than in normal breast tissue [80].

Interestingly, a correlation between surgical trauma and locoregional tumor recurrence has been demonstrated [81-83], and there is clinical and preclinical evidence that the removal of a primary tumor can aggravate the growth of micrometastases [84]. In mice where B16 melanoma cells were inoculated, metastatic burden increased by as much as 52 to 181% when excision of local tumor was conducted [85]. In patients with primary cutaneous melanomas, surgery of primary tumors may have enhanced tumor growth at metastatic sites [86]. In addition, the numbers of metastases have been demonstrated to be enhanced in proportion to the degree of surgical stress [87], as well the production of MMP-9, membrane type IBMMP, and urokinase-type plasminogen activator. Although a variety of possible explanations have been postulated for this phenomenon, debates on the mechanism as well as its clinical relevance are still inconclusive.

Interestingly, direct evidence to validate the causal association between ROS and tumor metastasis has been recently provided. Using cytoplasmic hybrid technology, Ishikawa and colleagues described how replacing the endogenous mitochondrial DNA (mtDNA) in a poorly metastatic mouse tumor cell line with mtDNA from a highly metastatic cell line potentiated tumor progression. The transferred mtDNA carried a deficiency in respiratory complex I activity, which caused an overproduction of ROS [88].

In a spontaneous metastatic model of melanoma, the surgical removal of a footpad tumor significantly increased plasma ROS levels [89]. This increase was also observed in mice following removal of a non-tumor-bearing footpad, clearly indicating that surgery itself generates ROS, irrespective of the removal of the footpad tumor. The surgical removal of the tumor and ROS production were linked to a robust proliferation of metastatic tumor cells. Importantly, a single injection of PEG-catalase just before the removal significantly suppressed not only the plasma ROS level but also the metastatic tumor growth. Although there are no ongoing clinical studies on the effects of PEG-catalase, investigation of this approach in humans would be appropriate.

2.6. Changes in Antioxidant Capacities

Increased ROS stress in cancer cells modulates the expression of antioxidant enzymes, such as SODs, catalase, GPx, glutathione-S-transferase (GST), amongst others. Decreased MnSOD activity was observed in H6 hepatoma cells compared to normal mouse liver, and reduced MnSOD activity was also observed in colorectal carcinomas [90]. Low activities of CuZnSOD, catalase and GPx1 are also often reported in transformed cell lines [91]. However, it is still uncertain whether the decreased antioxidant capacity is a major cause of increased oxidative stress in tumors, and caution must be taken when extrapolating results from cell lines to clinical samples. In fact, there is no evidence of significant decreases in ROS-scavenging enzymes in primary cancer tissues. Indeed, SOD expression and activity have been found to be *elevated* in mesothelioma, neuroblastoma, melanoma, stomach, ovarian and breast cancer [92-94], most likely as a result of an adaptive response to intrinsic oxidative stress. These apparently conflicting findings illustrate the limits of our evolving knowledge of the complex redox regulation in tumor cells.

3. Therapeutic Implications and Antioxidant Strategies

Constitutively elevated levels of cellular oxidative stress and dependence on mitogenic and anti-apoptotic ROS signaling represent a specific vulnerability of malignant cells that can be selectively targeted by novel antioxidant approaches.

3.1. Increasing Extracellular ROS Scavenging Systems (Antioxidant Supplementation)

Because ROS have been widely implicated in neoplastic transformation, it is intuitive to think that antioxidants may protect against cancer and inhibit tumor cell proliferation via suppression of the malignant phenotype. In fact, *evidence has accrued fromexperimental studies using animal models and cancer cell lines that antioxidants may decrease oxidative damage and prevent cancer* [95-96]. Observational studies suggest that high intake of fruits and vegetables is associated with reduced cancer incidence and mortality [97-98]. The high levels of antioxidants (particularly β-carotene and vitamin E) in fruits and vegetables are alleged to contribute toward cancer prevention, probably by inhibiting oxidative stress.

However, results from several cancer prevention trials (also called chemoprevention studies), have not conclusively demonstrated such effects in clinical settings. The Nutritional Prevention of Cancer trial reported that selenium supplementation decreased the risk of lung, colon, prostate, and total cancers but increased the risk of non-melanoma skin cancer [99]. The ATBC (Alpha-Tocopherol, Beta-Carotene) Cancer Prevention Trial found no evidence for a beneficial effect of supplemental vitamin E or β-carotene for the prevention of lung cancer. In fact, male smokers who received β-carotene were found to have lung cancer more frequently than those who did not receive it [1]. Two decades later, results from two other major trials, the SELECT (Selenium and Vitamin E Cancer Prevention Trial) by Lippman and colleagues, and the Physicians' Health Study (PHS) II by Gaziano and colleagues, found that neither selenium nor vitamin E supplementation, alone or in combination, mediated any reductions in any type of cancer [2, 100].

Several systematic reviews of randomized controlled trials have been performed leading to the conclusion that there are insufficient data to support the use of multivitamin and/or mineral supplements in primary prevention of cancer and chronic disease in the general population [101]. In addition, analysis of 47 low-bias randomized trials that determined the effects of antioxidant supplements (β-carotene, vitamin A and vitamin E) on all-cause mortality have shown that the antioxidant supplements significantly increased mortality [102]. Another meta-analysis of randomized controlled trials also showed that antioxidant supplements do not exert any significant effects against the development of gastrointestinal cancers and that they increase all-cause mortality [103]. Recently, in another meta-analysis on primary prevention, Bardia et al. reported that antioxidant supplementation did not significantly decrease total cancer incidence or mortality of any site-specific cancer [104].

The results of studies with supplemental antioxidants have also been quite disappointing in other diseases. A compelling amount of evidence has led to the "oxidative hypothesis" of atherosclerosis [105] (see Vol. III, Chapter 8), yet randomized, double-blind, placebo-controlled studies such as the HOPE and HOPE-TOO trials have concluded that vitamin E supplementation does not prevent major cardiovascular events and may, in fact, increase the risk for heart failure [106-107]. A similar situation exists for diabetes mellitus (see Vol. III, Chapter 9): Despite the undeniable presence of substantial oxidative stress in diabetes, attempts to treat the disease by supplementation with antioxidants have failed to produce any significant improvements [108].

Therefore, reasonable intakes of non-specific exogenous scavengers of oxidants fail to inhibit disease onset and progression. It is of note that carcinogenesis, as well as the other aforementioned pathologies, is not uniform across all anatomic sites, so specific antioxidant compounds could be associated with different effects depending on the target organ under study [109]. Perhaps a more appealing strategy might be the targeted delivery of endogenous antioxidant enzymes.

3.2. Targeting ROS-Producing Mechanisms

A molecular approach to target the specific pathways associated with oxidative stress modulation seems a good strategy to effectively regulate redox changes critical to cancer initiation and progression. The benefits of new target-specific therapies such as Trastuzumab, Rituximab, and Imatinib have in fact illustrated the potential of targeting pivotal molecules and genes.

The NOX system is a major source of $O_2^-\cdot$ generation in the cell. Using pharmacologic and genetic approaches, de Carvalho and collegues blocked Nox1-induced ROS production during cell spreading, and observed a reduced mitogenic effect on colon cancer cells [110]. Jajoo *et al.* using similar strategies reduced both the generation of ROS and the invasion of prostate cancer cells on Matrigel [111]. In addition, small interference RNAs (siRNAs) directed at NOX suppressed oncogenic Ras transformation and limited anchorage-independent growth and tumor formation [112]. Furthermore, NOX inhibition appeared to control cell survival of malignant melanoma, pancreatic carcinoma and prostate cancer cells [113-115]. These results suggest that manipulation of NOX activity in human cancers may suppress the malignant phenotype. New NOX inhibitors are being developed with potential future clinical application.

3.3. Enhancing Endogenous ROS Scavenging Systems

The approach of inducing endogenous antioxidant enzymes is based on studies showing that MnSOD overexpression in pancreatic cancer cell lines decreased cell growth and potentiated tumor growth suppression and increased animal survival [116]. The same effects were obtained by overexpression of glutathione peroxidase-1 (GPx1) by means of an adenoviral vector carrying the GPx1 [117] or phospholipid glutathione peroxidase (PhGPx) [118] genes, and by induction of catalase [119]. Interestingly, strategies to prolong the plasma half-life of catalase, SOD and GPx by conjugation with PEG were found to augment its antimetastatic activity in experimental pulmonary metastasis [69], and to prevent the growth of metastatic tumors after surgical removal [71]. Sustained release of PEG-catalase from a gelatin hydrogel sheet significantly inhibits the metastasis of melanoma cells in mice [120].

4. The Other Side of the Coin: ROS as Tumor Therapy

Although treating ROS-inducing tumors with antioxidants appears reasonable, ironically, the production of ROS leading to irreversible oxidative stress has long been known to be a common mechanism of most non-surgical anticancer therapies. It is also known that further elevation of cellular ROS effectively potentiates cancer cell killing.

4.1. Activation of Cell Death Pathways

Excessive ROS can lead to cell death through several mechanisms, including apoptosis, necrosis, and autophagy (see Vol. II, Chapters 16, 23, 25 and 26). Studies focused on apoptosis have shown that ROS mediate the activation of both the extrinsic and the intrinsic apoptotic pathways (Figure 2). In the extrinsic pathway, Fas ligand induces a rapid formation of ROS upon binding to the Fas receptor. This FasL-induced ROS response is required for Fas-tyrosine phosphorylation and subsequent recruitment of Fas-associated death domains, caspase-8 activation, and apoptosis induction. Additionally, FasL-induced ROS mediate the ubiquitination and subsequent degradation by proteasomes of FLICE inhibitory protein (FLIP), which further enhances Fas activation [121].

ROS induce the intrinsic apoptotic pathway by triggering the opening of the permeability transition (PT) pore complex, through both activation of signaling pathways and through direct oxidative damage to PT components. This results in mitochondrial membrane rupture, release of pro-apoptotic proteins, apoptosome formation, caspase activation and apoptosis [122]. Oxidative stress stimulates multiple MAPK signaling pathways, and specifically the c-Jun NH2-teminal Kinase (JNK) mediates key cellular responses to oxidative stress. As with all MAPK family members, activation of JNK occurs as a result of its phosphorylation by the upstream kinases SEK1 (MKK4) and SEK2 (MKK7), which are phosphorylated and activated by ubiquitously expressed MAPKKK such as ASK1.

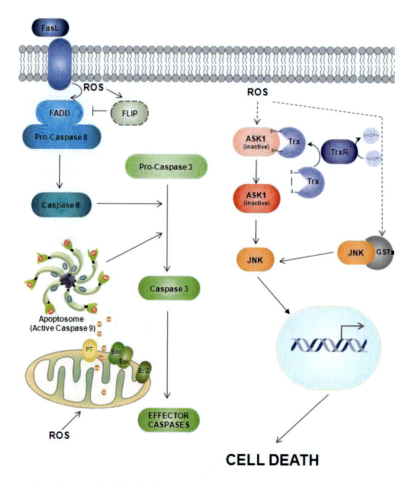

Figure 2. Apoptotic pathways of cell death. The extrinsic pathway is mediated by different death receptors. For example, Fas activation induces the rapid generation of ROS that target FLIP for degradation and induce caspase-8 activation. ROS induce the intrinsic apoptotic pathway by triggering the opening of the permeability transition (PT) pore complex, which results in release of cytochrome c, apoptosome formation, caspase activation and apoptosis. JNK signaling pathway is activated upon oxidative stress through the activation of upstream kinases ASK and SEK and/or through GSTπ oxidation.

The activity of ASK1 depends on the redox status of thioredoxin, as only the reduced form of thioredoxin is capable of binding to ASK1 and blocking its kinase activity. ROS activate the JNK signal cascade through the oxidation of thioredoxin and consequent activation of ASK, SEK and JNK [123]. Another plausible mechanism for the activation of JNK is through GSTπ-JNK complex. The monomeric form of GSTπ binds to the C-terminal fragment of JNK and suppresses its kinase activity [124]. ROS induce GSTπ oxidation, which leads to oligomerization, loss of JNK binding, and JNK activation. In addition, ROS are known to inhibit the activity of protein tyrosine phosphatase (PTP), which negatively regulates oxidative stress signals [125].

After activation by ROS, JNK translocates to the nucleus where it induces the upregulation of pro-apoptotic genes through the transactivation of specific transcription factors, and to the mitochondrial membrane where it activates pore-destabilizing proteins (Bax/Bak) and/or inhibits pore-stabilizing proteins (Bcl-2 and Bcl-xl), leading to opening of the PT pore complex [126]. Therefore, through the coordinated regulation of nuclear and mitochondrial events, JNK ensures the efficient execution of apoptosis.

It has been postulated that the switch from apoptotic to necrotic cell death involves not only a decrease in cellular ATP, but also a burst of intracellular ROS. This was suggested after Hampton and Orrenius reported that low concentrations of H_2O_2 induced apoptosis in Jurkat cells, whereas at higher concentrations, the cells underwent necrosis [127]. A possible mechanism is that caspases have an active site cysteine whose oxidation blocks catalytic activity. Therefore, at high levels of oxidative stress, impaired caspase function leads to necrotic cell death.

4.2. Modulation of Intracellular Redox Status: Chemo-Resistance

The intracellular redox capacity of a particular cell has been related to its response to ROS-inducing agents. Upon oxidative stress, cells try to maintain intracellular redox homeostasis through different mechanisms. Glutathione reductase activity increases, and the GSSG (oxidized glutathione) excess that is formed upon oxidative stress is extruded from the cell. Concomitantly, γ-glutamyl-cysteine synthase (γ-GCS) is activated to produce newly synthesized glutathione (see Vol. II, Chapter 1), or thioldisulphide exchange is promoted. When cellular systems are no longer able to counteract the ROS-mediated insults, oxidative damage occurs and, if excessive, leads to cell death. Therefore, cells with a high buffering capacity tend to respond less to ROS-generating chemotherapeutic agents than cells with low ability to quench reactive species.

In chronic lymphocytic leukemia patients, the basal $O_2^-\cdot$ content in leukemia cells is positively related to their sensitivity to 2-methoxyestradiol, a new anticancer agent currently in clinical trials that induces apoptosis in leukemia cells through a free radical-mediated mechanism [128]. As another example, our group and others have demonstrated that resistance to arsenic trioxide (As_2O_3) is associated with an upregulation of SOD1 and an increase in intracellular GSH (reduced glutathione) levels [129-130]. Multidrug resistant HL-60 cells have been shown to be resistant to the cytotoxic effects of H_2O_2, presumably due to increased levels of catalase [131]. Likewise, several studies suggest that the resistance to chemotherapeutic agents that induce intracellular ROS production is correlated with an increased antioxidant capacity [132].

5. Therapeutic Implications of Pro-Oxidant Strategies

5.1. Increasing ROS Levels in Cancer Cells

Antineoplastic agents generate oxidative stress in patients who receive these drugs during cancer chemotherapy. This is supported by the increase in lipid peroxidation products, decrease of total antioxidant capacity of blood plasma, and marked reduction of tissue glutathione levels that occur during chemotherapy [133-134]. Agents that generate high levels of ROS include the anthracyclines (doxorubicin, epirubicin, and daunorubicin), alkylating agents (cyclophosphamide, busulfan), platinum coordination complexes (cisplatin, carboplatin, and oxaliplatin), epipodophyllotoxins (etoposide and teniposide), and the camptothecins (topotecan and irinotecan). The anthracyclines generate the highest levels of oxidative stress. This is due to their capability to deflect electrons from the electron transport chain in the mitochondria, resulting in abundant formation of superoxide radicals [135].

Table 1. ROS generation by commonly used chemotherapeutic drugs

Generation of oxidative stress	Antineoplastic agent
Very high levels	Anthracyclines • Doxorubicin • Epirubicin • Daunorubicin
High levels	Alkylating agents • Cyclophosphamide • Busulfan Platinum coordination complexes • Cisplatin • Carboplatin • Oxaliplatin Epipodophyllotoxins • Etoposide • Teniposide Camptothecins • Topotecan • Irinotecan
Low levels	Taxanes • Paclitaxel • Docetaxel Vinca alkaloids • Vincristine • Vinblastine Antimetabolites • Methotrexate

In contrast, taxanes (paclitaxel and docetaxel), vinca alkaloids (vincristine and vinblastine), antimetabolites (antifolates), and nucleoside and nucleotide analogues (AraC) generate low levels of oxidative stress (Table 1). Radiation therapy is commonly used in the management of many types of cancers. It is well established that the lethal effects of ionizing radiation are mainly mediated through ROS generated from the radiolytic decomposition of cellular water [136]. Radiation therapy-induced oxidative stress causes DNA damage and a rapid activation of wild-type p53, ATM, and growth factor receptors, including the ERBB family. This initial response increases the activities of RAS family proteins, which in turn activate several cytosolic signal transduction pathways, such as the MAPK, ERK and PI3K pathways, to regulate cell growth [137]. A handful of other compounds whose mechanism of action is robustly related to ROS induction are in advanced clinical trials. Redox-active agents have been found to induce signature transcription profile of cells under oxidative stress. For example, elesclomol (STA-4783), an investigational drug for the treatment of metastatic melanoma, induces ROS generation and oxidative damage in cell lines [138] and enhances the therapeutic index of paclitaxel against human tumor xenografts of breast cancer, lung cancer, and lymphoma cell lines. Other examples are motexafin gadolinium, a porphyrin-like molecule and fenretinide (4HPR), a synthetic retinoid, that induce apoptosis in many types of cancer cells including neuroblastoma, breast, lung, head and neck, cervical and ovarian cancer cells [139-141]; and KP1019, a Ru(III) complex salt [142], which shows superior activity over that of the standard anticancer drug 5-fluorouracil in experimental therapy of autochthonous colorectal carcinoma of the rat and which caused no serious adverse effects in a clinical phase-I study [143].

5.2. Modulating ROS Metabolism

Strategies to deplete the intracellular GSH pool and modulate ROS detoxification have been found to impact cell survival and drug sensitivity. Various compounds including diterpenes, sesquiterpenes, aziridine compounds such as Imexon and organic isothiocyanates (BITC, PeITC, sulphoraphane), conjugate with GSH and deplete its intracellular pool, inducing oxidative stress and cell death [144-145]. An additional contribution to their biological activity is the simultaneous reaction of the electrophilic moiety of these compounds with cysteine residues in redox-modulating enzymes, such as peroxidases, peroxiredoxins and thiolreductases. Modulation of other antioxidant systems in order to inhibit tumor growth and induce apoptosis has been investigated. The specific inhibitor of thioredoxin 1, PX-12, has demonstrated strong antitumor activity in patients with advanced solid malignancies [146], and phase II clinical trials are currently underway in patients with advanced pancreatic cancer. Inhibition of SOD by 2-methoxyestradiol (2-ME) selectively kills leukemia cells, but not normal lymphocytes [128], and a phase I trial is being conducted in patients who have advanced solid tumors (clinicaltrials.gov).

5.3. Targeting Different Redox-Modulating Mechanisms

To maximize the impact on intracellular redox status, one promising approach is to combine compounds that induce ROS through disparate mechanisms. The ROS-generating agent motexafin gadolinium (MGd) is a metalloporphyrin that selectively inhibits tumor cell growth. This compound has proven to potentiate doxorubicin antineoplastic activity in patients with advanced solid tumors [147], as well as in chronic lymphocytic leukemia and small lymphocytic lymphoma [148]. Another combination tested in leukemic cells is ABT-737, a pan-Bcl-2 inhibitor, and the synthetic retinoid N-(4-hydroxyphenyl)retinamide (4-HPR), an agent known to generate ROS. When both compounds were added simultaneously, synergistic cytotoxicity was observed in ALL cell lines [149]. As another example, the ROS-inducing agent Imexon was synergistic when combined with DNA-binding agents (cisplatin, dacarbazine, melphalan) and pyrimidine-based antimetabolites (cytarabine, xuorouracil, gemcitabine) in human malignant melanoma and multiple myeloma cell lines. A safety study of Imexon plus gemcitabine in untreated pancreatic adenocarcinoma patients is ongoing (clinicaltrials.gov).

Another effective combination therapy recently employed emodin, a natural anthraquinone derivative that induces ROS, which significantly enhances chemosensitivity to cisplatin, carboplatin and oxaliplatin in human cancer cell lines and xenograft models of human tumors [150]. Co-administration of low doses of emodin ($0.5–10\mu M$) with As_2O_3 enhanced As_2O_3-mediated cytotoxicity in leukemic cells [151]. *In vivo*, emodin made the EC/CUHK1 cell-derived tumors more sensitive to As_2O_3 with no additional systemic toxicity or side effects [152].

It is important to underline that many compounds show contradictory behaviors because they can act as antioxidants or pro-oxidants in the biological microenvironment, contingent upon factors such as drug concentration, transition metal ions present, and cellular redox status. The relative importance of the antioxidant and pro-oxidant activities of 'antioxidants' is an area of current research. For example, trolox, a known antioxidant congener of vitamin E (Vol. II, Chapter 3), behaves as a pro-oxidant potentiating As_2O_3-induced ROS generation and cell death in APL, myeloma, and breast cancer cells. *In vivo*, this combination increased the survival time and limited metastatic spread in tumor-bearing mice. However, in normal organs, trolox behaved as an antioxidant protecting hepatic and renal cells from As_2O_3 toxicity [153-154].

Another strategy to exploit the ROS-mediated cell death mechanism is to combine ROS-inducing agents with drugs that repress the cellular antioxidant capacity. For example, the combination of As_2O_3 and the SOD inhibitor 2-Me demonstrated significant synergistic effects in potentiating anticancer activity against primary chronic lymphocytic leukemia cells [155] and enhanced the sensitivity of myeloma cells to Bortezomib [156].

6. Other Considerations

Improving therapeutic activity without excessive toxicity is a key goal in the development of new anticancer drugs. Therefore, numerous studies have been conducted to understand the genetic and metabolic differences between cancer and normal cells.

A unique biochemical alteration frequently seen in cancer cells of various tissue origins is the increase in aerobic glycolysis and the dependency on the glycolytic pathway for ATP generation, known as the Warburg effect [157]. Growing evidence also suggests that cancer cells have increased levels of ROS compared with normal cells. Interestingly, a recent study established a critical role of cellular oxidative stress in the Warburg effect [158]. Specifically, it was found that increasing the level of ROS stress in hepatoma cells may directly upregulate HIF-1α, a key transcription factor that activates a series of genes involved in glucose transport, glycolysis, angiogenesis and rate of cellular respiration [159-160]; see also Vol. II, Chapter 22. Based on this evidence, it is *suggested that the dependency on glycolysis in cancer cells may be related to ROS. This altered energy metabolism, common to many types of cancer but not normal cells, is an attractive target for therapeutic development.* For example, Cornerstone Pharmaceutical Inc. has used its Altered Energy Metabolism-Directed (AEMD) technology platform to develop CPI-613, a synthetic alpha-lipoic acid analogue. CPI-613 is the first drug in a new chemical class that, through a novel mechanism, inhibits metabolic and regulatory processes required for cell growth in solid tumors but not in normal cells according to preclinical studies. Studies of CPI-613 are now being conducted at clinical trial sites in both the US and Canada. It is important to mention that whereas low levels of ROS are central for normal cell function and survival signaling, excessive ROS can lead to cell death. Therefore, it is reasonable to speculate that further ROS insults induced by exogenous agents or impairment of the cellular capacity to eliminate ROS might push the cancer cells beyond a cellular tolerability threshold, which could lead to oxidative cell death. Consequently, redox modulation has been considered as an approach to selectively kill cancer cells without causing severe toxicity to normal cells (Figure 3).

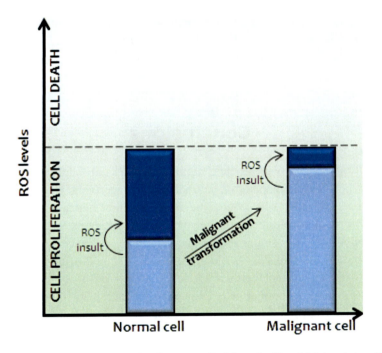

Figure 3. Redox differences between normal and cancer cells. Normal cells exhibit low intracellular ROS levels (light blue bar). These cells have a high ability (dark blue bar) to adapt and cope with free radicals, probably due to their high antioxidant capacity, which prevent the ROS levels from reaching the cell-death threshold (dotted line) and consequently from undergoing cell death. If ROS are gradually increased malignant transformation may result. Cancer cells are under increased oxidative stress due to the activation of oncogenes, growth factor receptors, intracellular signaling pathways and specific transcription factors related to proliferation. Therefore, ROS insults will readily increase intracellular ROS levels above threshold, resulting in irreversible oxidative stress and cell death.

However, it is important to take into consideration that redox adaptation occurs within the cancer cell (acquisition of a resistant phenotype) [161] and that the redox alterations found in cancer cells are particularly complex because multiple factors are involved in redox regulation and oxidative stress control. Therefore, the simple addition of a ROS-inducing agent might not always result in the selective killing of cancer cells.

To develop effective therapeutic strategies for both prevention and treatment of malignant disorders, it is crucial to understand the advantages and disadvantages of the redox-modulating approaches.

An in-depth analysis of the intracellular cellular redox status should be performed to predict the sensitivity of a tumor cell to a specific redox modulating strategy. Indeed, levels of gene expression for antioxidant enzymes, transcription factors, and other proteins involved in cellular redox modulation have been claimed to represent a *redox signature score* that is predictive of outcome in patients with diffuse large B-cell lymphoma [162]. A common signature characteristic of breast cancer cell immortalization have been recently identified and showed significant expression changes of genes involved in oxidoreductase activity [163]. Therefore, the *use of this signature may predict the response of patients to redox modulators and improve disease outcome.*

In the future, microarray-based technologies to characterize tumors, both at the genomic and proteomic levels, may help delineate oxidative response expression patterns that could be related to disease outcome and drug resistance.

The generation of tumor-predictive biomarkers based on combining parameters of oxidative damage with those of cellular proliferation, DNA-repair and antioxidant capacity may provide a unique opportunity to define an effective therapeutic approach, monitor therapeutic efficacy at early time points and improve patient outcomes.

Conclusions

Paradoxically, ROS can both promote tumor initiation and induce tumor cell death. In addition to this dichotomy, compared to normal cells, cancer cells have higher basal ROS levels, which are associated with oncogenic transformation and alterations in metabolic activity. Therefore, the key roles of oxidative stress in this setting provide disparate rationales for two opposed therapeutic strategies for the treatment of cancer. One approach is to potentiate antioxidant mechanisms to eliminate ROS. Using this approach, ROS-induced signaling pathways that promote proliferation and cell survival are repressed, obviating malignant transformation in normal cells or leading to growth inhibition of an established tumor. Unfortunately, several antioxidants tested in clinical trials have not demonstrated beneficial effects and have, in some cases, been associated with increased cancer incidence. In addition, antioxidants may reduce systemic effectiveness of certain chemotherapeutic agents, including bortezomib [164] and paclitaxel [165], which could hinder patients' clinical responses and long-term survival. The reverse approach is to treat cancer cells with compounds that either induce ROS or decrease the cellular antioxidant capacity, or with a combination of both. Several preclinical models and clinical studies have demonstrated a therapeutic advantage when adopting this strategy in cancer patients. Considering that the intracellular redox status may predict whether an increase in oxidative stress can induce death in a given cell, analyses of oxidative response expression patterns and redox predictive biomarkers of tumors will become increasingly important to guide the manipulation of ROS in cancer prevention and treatment.

References

[1] The effect of vitamin E and beta carotene on the incidence of lung cancer and other cancers in male smokers. The Alpha-Tocopherol, Beta Carotene Cancer Prevention Study Group. *The New England Journal of Medicine* 1994;330:1029-35.

[2] Lippman SM, Klein EA, Goodman PJ, et al. Effect of selenium and vitamin E on risk of prostate cancer and other cancers: the Selenium and Vitamin E Cancer Prevention Trial (SELECT). *JAMA,* 2009;301:39-51.

[3] Ceccarelli J, Delfino L, Zappia E, et al. The redox state of the lung cancer microenvironment depends on the levels of thioredoxin expressed by tumor cells and affects tumor progression and response to prooxidants. *Int. J. Cancer,* 2008;123:1770-8.

[4] Chaiswing L, Bourdeau-Heller JM, Zhong W, Oberley TD. Characterization of redox state of two human prostate carcinoma cell lines with different degrees of aggressiveness. *Free Radic. Biol. Med.* 2007;43:202-15.

[5] Inokuma T, Haraguchi M, Fujita F, Tajima Y, Kanematsu T. Oxidative stress and tumor progression in colorectal cancer. *Hepatogastroenterology* 2009;56:343-7.

[6] Szatrowski TP, Nathan CF. Production of large amounts of hydrogen peroxide by human tumor cells. *Cancer Research,* 1991;51:794-8.

[7] Babior BM, Kipnes RS, Curnutte JT. Biological defense mechanisms. The production by leukocytes of superoxide, a potential bactericidal agent. *J. Clin. Invest.* 1973;52:741-4.

[8] Weissmann G, Smolen JE, Korchak HM. Release of inflammatory mediators from stimulated neutrophils. *The New England Journal of Medicine* 1980;303:27-34.

[9] Vakkila J, Lotze MT. Inflammation and necrosis promote tumour growth. *Nat. Rev. Immunol.* 2004;4:641-8.

[10] Fukasawa M, Bryant SM, diZerega GS. Superoxide anion production by postsurgical macrophages. *J. Surg. Res.* 1988;45:382-8.

[11] Zallen G, Moore EE, Johnson JL, et al. Circulating postinjury neutrophils are primed for the release of proinflammatory cytokines. *J. Trauma,* 1999;46:42-8.

[12] Meier B, Radeke HH, Selle S, et al. Human fibroblasts release reactive oxygen species in response to interleukin-1 or tumour necrosis factor-alpha. *Biochem. J.* 1989;263:539-45.

[13] Shaughnessy SG, Buchanan MR, Turple S, Richardson M, Orr FW. Walker carcinosarcoma cells damage endothelial cells by the generation of reactive oxygen species. *Am. J. Pathol.* 1989;134:787-96.

[14] Chandel NS, Maltepe E, Goldwasser E, Mathieu CE, Simon MC, Schumacker PT. Mitochondrial reactive oxygen species trigger hypoxia-induced transcription. *Proc. Natl. Acad. Sci. U S A,* 1998;95:11715-20.

[15] Irani K, Xia Y, Zweier JL, et al. Mitogenic signaling mediated by oxidants in Ras-transformed fibroblasts. *Science,* 1997;275:1649-52.

[16] Kissil JL, Walmsley MJ, Hanlon L, et al. Requirement for Rac1 in a K-ras induced lung cancer in the mouse. *Cancer Research,* 2007;67:8089-94.

[17] Kopnin PB, Agapova LS, Kopnin BP, Chumakov PM. Repression of sestrin family genes contributes to oncogenic Ras-induced reactive oxygen species up-regulation and genetic instability. *Cancer Research,* 2007;67:4671-8.

[18] Sattler M, Verma S, Shrikhande G, et al. The BCR/ABL tyrosine kinase induces production of reactive oxygen species in hematopoietic cells. *J. Biol. Chem.* 2000;275:24273-8.

[19] Kim JH, Chu SC, Gramlich JL, et al. Activation of the PI3K/mTOR pathway by BCR-ABL contributes to increased production of reactive oxygen species. *Blood,* 2005;105:1717-23.

[20] Ravid T, Sweeney C, Gee P, Carraway KL, 3rd, Goldkorn T. Epidermal growth factor receptor activation under oxidative stress fails to promote c-Cbl mediated down-regulation. *J. Biol. Chem.* 2002;277:31214-9.

[21] Frisch SM, Screaton RA. Anoikis mechanisms. *Curr. Opin. Cell Biol.* 2001;13:555-62.

[22] Zhu Z, Sanchez-Sweatman O, Huang X, et al. Anoikis and metastatic potential of cloudman S91 melanoma cells. *Cancer Research,* 2001;61:1707-16.

[23] Marchese C, Maresca V, Cardinali G, et al. UVB-induced activation and internalization of keratinocyte growth factor receptor. *Oncogene,* 2003;22:2422-31.

[24] Burdon RH, Gill V, Alliangana D. Hydrogen peroxide in relation to proliferation and apoptosis in BHK-21 hamster fibroblasts. *Free Radic. Res.* 1996;24:81-93.

[25] Schimmel M, Bauer G. Proapoptotic and redox state-related signaling of reactive oxygen species generated by transformed fibroblasts. *Oncogene,* 2002;21:5886-96.

[26] Behrend L, Henderson G, Zwacka RM. Reactive oxygen species in oncogenic transformation. *Biochem. Soc. Trans.* 2003;31:1441-4.

[27] Meng TC, Fukada T, Tonks NK. Reversible oxidation and inactivation of protein tyrosine phosphatases in vivo. *Mol. Cell,* 2002;9:387-99.

[28] Tonks NK. Redox redux: revisiting PTPs and the control of cell signaling. *Cell,* 2005;121:667-70.

[29] Chiarugi P. Src redox regulation: there is more than meets the eye. *Mol. Cells,* 2008;26:329-37.

[30] Giannoni E, Buricchi F, Raugei G, Ramponi G, Chiarugi P. Intracellular reactive oxygen species activate Src tyrosine kinase during cell adhesion and anchorage-dependent cell growth. *Mol. Cell. Biol.* 2005;25:6391-403.

[31] Mehdi MZ, Pandey NR, Pandey SK, Srivastava AK. H2O2-induced phosphorylation of ERK1/2 and PKB requires tyrosine kinase activity of insulin receptor and c-Src. *Antioxid. Redox. Signal,* 2005;7:1014-20.

[32] Lee M, Kim JY, Anderson WB. Src tyrosine kinase inhibitor PP2 markedly enhances Ras-independent activation of Raf-1 protein kinase by phorbol myristate acetate and H2O2. *J. Biol. Chem.* 2004;279:48692-701.

[33] Chiarugi P, Pani G, Giannoni E, et al. Reactive oxygen species as essential mediators of cell adhesion: the oxidative inhibition of a FAK tyrosine phosphatase is required for cell adhesion. *J. Cell Biol.* 2003;161:933-44.

[34] Esposito F, Chirico G, Montesano Gesualdi N, et al. Protein kinase B activation by reactive oxygen species is independent of tyrosine kinase receptor phosphorylation and requires SRC activity. *J. Biol. Chem.* 2003;278:20828-34.

[35] Nishida M, Maruyama Y, Tanaka R, Kontani K, Nagao T, Kurose H. G alpha(i) and G alpha(o) are target proteins of reactive oxygen species. *Nature,* 2000;408:492-5.

[36] Buhrman G, Parker B, Sohn J, Rudolph J, Mattos C. Structural mechanism of oxidative regulation of the phosphatase Cdc25B via an intramolecular disulfide bond. *Biochemistry,* 2005;44:5307-16.

[37] Sohn J, Rudolph J. Catalytic and chemical competence of regulation of cdc25 phosphatase by oxidation/reduction. *Biochemistry,* 2003;42:10060-70.

[38] Wang J, Chen L, Li D, et al. Intrauterine growth restriction affects the proteomes of the small intestine, liver, and skeletal muscle in newborn pigs. *J. Nutr.* 2008;138:60-6.

[39] Funato Y, Michiue T, Asashima M, Miki H. The thioredoxin-related redox-regulating protein nucleoredoxin inhibits Wnt-beta-catenin signalling through dishevelled. *Nat. Cell Biol.* 2006;8:501-8.

[40] Humphries KM, Deal MS, Taylor SS. Enhanced dephosphorylation of cAMP-dependent protein kinase by oxidation and thiol modification. *J. Biol. Chem.* 2005;280:2750-8.

[41] Burgoyne JR, Madhani M, Cuello F, et al. Cysteine redox sensor in PKGIa enables oxidant-induced activation. *Science,* 2007;317:1393-7.

[42] Caselli A, Marzocchini R, Camici G, et al. The inactivation mechanism of low molecular weight phosphotyrosine-protein phosphatase by H_2O_2. *J. Biol. Chem.* 1998;273:32554-60.

[43] Lee SR, Yang KS, Kwon J, Lee C, Jeong W, Rhee SG. Reversible inactivation of the tumor suppressor PTEN by H2O2. *J. Biol. Chem.* 2002;277:20336-42.

[44] Song H, Hanlon N, Brown NR, Noble ME, Johnson LN, Barford D. Phosphoprotein-protein interactions revealed by the crystal structure of kinase-associated phosphatase in complex with phosphoCDK2. *Mol. Cell,* 2001;7:615-26.

[45] Seth D, Rudolph J. Redox regulation of MAP kinase phosphatase 3. *Biochemistry,* 2006;45:8476-87.

[46] den Hertog J, Groen A, van der Wijk T. Redox regulation of protein-tyrosine phosphatases. *Arch. Biochem. Biophys.* 2005;434:11-5.

[47] Karin M, Takahashi T, Kapahi P, et al. Oxidative stress and gene expression: the AP-1 and NF-kappaB connections. *Biofactors,* 2001;15:87-9.

[48] Surh YJ, Kundu JK, Na HK, Lee JS. Redox-sensitive transcription factors as prime targets for chemoprevention with anti-inflammatory and antioxidative phytochemicals. *J. Nutr.* 2005;135:2993S-3001S.

[49] Esposito F, Ammendola R, Faraonio R, Russo T, Cimino F. Redox control of signal transduction, gene expression and cellular senescence. *Neurochem. Res.* 2004;29:617-28.

[50] Lluis JM, Buricchi F, Chiarugi P, Morales A, Fernandez-Checa JC. Dual role of mitochondrial reactive oxygen species in hypoxia signaling: activation of nuclear factor-{kappa}B via c-SRC and oxidant-dependent cell death. *Cancer Research,* 2007;67:7368-77.

[51] Abate C, Patel L, Rauscher FJ, 3rd, Curran T. Redox regulation of fos and jun DNA-binding activity in vitro. *Science,* 1990;249:1157-61.

[52] Webster KA, Prentice H, Bishopric NH. Oxidation of zinc finger transcription factors: physiological consequences. *Antioxid. Redox. Signal.* 2001;3:535-48.

[53] Rainwater R, Parks D, Anderson ME, Tegtmeyer P, Mann K. Role of cysteine residues in regulation of p53 function. *Mol. Cell Biol.* 1995;15:3892-903.

[54] Cobbs CS, Whisenhunt TR, Wesemann DR, Harkins LE, Van Meir EG, Samanta M. Inactivation of wild-type p53 protein function by reactive oxygen and nitrogen species in malignant glioma cells. *Cancer Research*, 2003;63:8670-3.

[55] Wu HH, Thomas JA, Momand J. p53 protein oxidation in cultured cells in response to pyrrolidine dithiocarbamate: a novel method for relating the amount of p53 oxidation in vivo to the regulation of p53-responsive genes. *Biochem. J.* 2000;351:87-93.

[56] Verhaegh GW, Richard MJ, Hainaut P. Regulation of p53 by metal ions and by antioxidants: dithiocarbamate down-regulates p53 DNA-binding activity by increasing the intracellular level of copper. *Mol. Cell Biol.* 1997;17:5699-706.

[57] Buzek J, Latonen L, Kurki S, Peltonen K, Laiho M. Redox state of tumor suppressor p53 regulates its sequence-specific DNA binding in DNA-damaged cells by cysteine 277. *Nucleic Acids Res.* 2002;30:2340-8.

[58] Hainaut P, Mann K. Zinc binding and redox control of p53 structure and function. *Antioxid. Redox. Signal.* 2001;3:611-23.

[59] Kaspar JW, Niture SK, Jaiswal AK. Nrf2:INrf2 (Keap1) signaling in oxidative stress. *Free Radic. Biol. Med.* 2009;47:1304-9.

[60] Bloom D, Dhakshinamoorthy S, Jaiswal AK. Site-directed mutagenesis of cysteine to serine in the DNA binding region of Nrf2 decreases its capacity to upregulate antioxidant response element-mediated expression and antioxidant induction of NAD(P)H:quinone oxidoreductase1 gene. *Oncogene*, 2002;21:2191-200.

[61] Sekhar KR, Rachakonda G, Freeman ML. Cysteine-based regulation of the CUL3 adaptor protein Keap1. *Toxicol. Appl. Pharmacol.* 2010;244:21-6.

[62] Engers R, Gabbert HE. Mechanisms of tumor metastasis: cell biological aspects and clinical implications. *J. Cancer Res. Clin. Oncol.* 2000;126:682-92.

[63] Bogenrieder T, Herlyn M. Axis of evil: molecular mechanisms of cancer metastasis. *Oncogene*, 2003;22:6524-36.

[64] Shaughnessy SG, Whaley M, Lafrenie RM, Orr FW. Walker 256 tumor cell degradation of extracellular matrices involves a latent gelatinase activated by reactive oxygen species. *Arch. Biochem. Biophys.* 1993;304:314-21.

[65] Sellak H, Franzini E, Hakim J, Pasquier C. Reactive oxygen species rapidly increase endothelial ICAM-1 ability to bind neutrophils without detectable upregulation. *Blood*, 1994;83:2669-77.

[66] Rajagopalan S, Meng XP, Ramasamy S, Harrison DG, Galis ZS. Reactive oxygen species produced by macrophage-derived foam cells regulate the activity of vascular matrix metalloproteinases in vitro. Implications for atherosclerotic plaque stability. *J. Clin. Invest.* 1996;98:2572-9.

[67] Belkhiri A, Richards C, Whaley M, McQueen SA, Orr FW. Increased expression of activated matrix metalloproteinase-2 by human endothelial cells after sublethal H_2O_2 exposure. *Lab. Invest.* 1997;77:533-9.

[68] Onoda JM, Piechocki MP, Honn KV. Radiation-induced increase in expression of the alpha IIb beta 3 integrin in melanoma cells: effects on metastatic potential. *Radiat. Res.* 1992;130:281-8.

[69] Nishikawa M, Tamada A, Hyoudou K, et al. Inhibition of experimental hepatic metastasis by targeted delivery of catalase in mice. *Clin. Exp. Metastasis,* 2004;21:213-21.

[70] Hyoudou K, Nishikawa M, Umeyama Y, Kobayashi Y, Yamashita F, Hashida M. Inhibition of metastatic tumor growth in mouse lung by repeated administration of polyethylene glycol-conjugated catalase: quantitative analysis with firefly luciferase-expressing melanoma cells. *Clin. Cancer Res.* 2004;10:7685-91.

[71] Hyoudou K, Nishikawa M, Kobayashi Y, Ikemura M, Yamashita F, Hashida M. SOD derivatives prevent metastatic tumor growth aggravated by tumor removal. *Clin. Exp. Metastasis,* 2008;25:531-6.

[72] Nishikawa M, Tamada A, Kumai H, Yamashita F, Hashida M. Inhibition of experimental pulmonary metastasis by controlling biodistribution of catalase in mice. *Int. J. Cancer,* 2002;99:474-9.

[73] Okada F, Shionoya H, Kobayashi M, et al. Prevention of inflammation-mediated acquisition of metastatic properties of benign mouse fibrosarcoma cells by administration of an orally available superoxide dismutase. *Br. J. Cancer,* 2006;94:854-62.

[74] Okada F, Nakai K, Kobayashi T, et al. Inflammatory cell-mediated tumour progression and minisatellite mutation correlate with the decrease of antioxidative enzymes in murine fibrosarcoma cells. *Br. J. Cancer,* 1999;79:377-85.

[75] Okada F, Kobayashi M, Tanaka H, et al. The role of nicotinamide adenine dinucleotide phosphate oxidase-derived reactive oxygen species in the acquisition of metastatic ability of tumor cells. *Am. J. Pathol.* 2006;169:294-302.

[76] Lim SD, Sun C, Lambeth JD, et al. Increased Nox1 and hydrogen peroxide in prostate cancer. *Prostate,* 2005;62:200-7.

[77] Oberley TD, Zhong W, Szweda LI, Oberley LW. Localization of antioxidant enzymes and oxidative damage products in normal and malignant prostate epithelium. *Prostate,* 2000;44:144-55.

[78] Arsova-Sarafinovska Z, Eken A, Matevska N, et al. Increased oxidative/nitrosative stress and decreased antioxidant enzyme activities in prostate cancer. *Clin. Biochem,* 2009;42:1228-35.

[79] Yilmaz MI, Saglam K, Sonmez A, et al. Antioxidant system activation in prostate cancer. *Biol. Trace Elem. Res.* 2004;98:13-9.

[80] Payne SL, Fogelgren B, Hess AR, et al. Lysyl oxidase regulates breast cancer cell migration and adhesion through a hydrogen peroxide-mediated mechanism. *Cancer Research,* 2005;65:11429-36.

[81] Bouvy ND, Marquet RL, Jeekel J, Bonjer HJ. Laparoscopic surgery is associated with less tumour growth stimulation than conventional surgery: an experimental study. *Br. J. Surg.* 1997;84:358-61.

[82] van den Tol PM, van Rossen EE, van Eijck CH, Bonthuis F, Marquet RL, Jeekel H. Reduction of peritoneal trauma by using nonsurgical gauze leads to less implantation metastasis of spilled tumor cells. *Ann. Surg.* 1998;227:242-8.

[83] Kodama M, Kodama T, Nishi Y, Totani R. Does surgical stress cause tumor metastasis? *Anticancer Res.* 1992;12:1603-16.

[84] Demicheli R, Abbattista A, Miceli R, Valagussa P, Bonadonna G. Time distribution of the recurrence risk for breast cancer patients undergoing mastectomy: further support about the concept of tumor dormancy. *Breast Cancer Res. Treat,* 1996;41:177-85.

[85] Arai K, Asakura T, Nemir P, Jr. Effect of local tumor removal and retained oncolysate on lung metastasis. *J. Surg. Res.* 1992;53:30-8.

[86] Smolle J, Soyer HP, Smolle-Juttner FM, Rieger E, Kerl H. Does surgical removal of primary melanoma trigger growth of occult metastases? An analytical epidemiological approach. *Dermatol. Surg.* 1997;23:1043-6.

[87] Tsuchiya Y, Sawada S, Yoshioka I, et al. Increased surgical stress promotes tumor metastasis. *Surgery,* 2003;133:547-55.

[88] Ishikawa K, Takenaga K, Akimoto M, et al. ROS-generating mitochondrial DNA mutations can regulate tumor cell metastasis. *Science,* 2008;320:661-4.

[89] Hyoudou K, Nishikawa M, Kobayashi Y, Umeyama Y, Yamashita F, Hashida M. PEGylated catalase prevents metastatic tumor growth aggravated by tumor removal. *Free Radic. Biol. Med.* 2006;41:1449-58.

[90] Van Driel BE, Lyon H, Hoogenraad DC, Anten S, Hansen U, Van Noorden CJ. Expression of CuZn- and Mn-superoxide dismutase in human colorectal neoplasms. *Free Radic. Biol. Med.* 1997;23:435-44.

[91] Wang M, Kirk JS, Venkataraman S, et al. Manganese superoxide dismutase suppresses hypoxic induction of hypoxia-inducible factor-1alpha and vascular endothelial growth factor. *Oncogene,* 2005;24:8154-66.

[92] Sanchez M, Torres JV, Tormos C, et al. Impairment of antioxidant enzymes, lipid peroxidation and 8-oxo-2'-deoxyguanosine in advanced epithelial ovarian carcinoma of a Spanish community. *Cancer Lett.* 2006;233:28-35.

[93] Lee OJ, Schneider-Stock R, McChesney PA, et al. Hypermethylation and loss of expression of glutathione peroxidase-3 in Barrett's tumorigenesis. *Neoplasia,* 2005;7:854-61.

[94] Soini Y, Kallio JP, Hirvikoski P, et al. Oxidative/nitrosative stress and peroxiredoxin 2 are associated with grade and prognosis of human renal carcinoma. *APMIS* 2006;114:329-37.

[95] Tomita Y, Himeno K, Nomoto K, Endo H, Hirohata T. Augmentation of tumor immunity against syngeneic tumors in mice by beta-carotene. *Journal of the National Cancer Institute,* 1987;78:679-81.

[96] Wright GL, Wang S, Fultz ME, Arif I, Matthews K, Chertow BS. Effect of vitamin A deficiency on cardiovascular function in the rat. *Can. J. Physiol. Pharmacol.* 2002;80:1-7.

[97] Hertog MG, Bueno-de-Mesquita HB, Fehily AM, Sweetnam PM, Elwood PC, Kromhout D. Fruit and vegetable consumption and cancer mortality in the Caerphilly Study. *Cancer Epidemiol Biomarkers Prev.* 1996;5:673-7.

[98] Steinmetz KA, Potter JD. Vegetables, fruit, and cancer prevention: a review. *J. Am. Diet. Assoc* .1996;96:1027-39.

[99] Clark LC, Combs GF, Jr., Turnbull BW, et al. Effects of selenium supplementation for cancer prevention in patients with carcinoma of the skin. A randomized controlled trial. Nutritional Prevention of Cancer Study Group. *JAMA* 1996;276:1957-63.

[100] Gaziano JM, Glynn RJ, Christen WG, et al. Vitamins E and C in the prevention of prostate and total cancer in men: the Physicians' Health Study II randomized controlled trial. *JAMA* 2009;301:52-62.

[101] Huang HY, Caballero B, Chang S, et al. The efficacy and safety of multivitamin and mineral supplement use to prevent cancer and chronic disease in adults: a systematic review for a National Institutes of Health state-of-the-science conference. *Ann. Intern. Med.* 2006;145:372-85.

[102] Bjelakovic G, Nikolova D, Gluud LL, Simonetti RG, Gluud C. Mortality in randomized trials of antioxidant supplements for primary and secondary prevention: systematic review and meta-analysis. *JAMA* 2007;297:842-57.

[103] Bjelakovic G, Nikolova D, Simonetti RG, Gluud C. Antioxidant supplements for prevention of gastrointestinal cancers: a systematic review and meta-analysis. *Lancet,* 2004;364:1219-28.

[104] Bardia A, Tleyjeh IM, Cerhan JR, et al. Efficacy of antioxidant supplementation in reducing primary cancer incidence and mortality: systematic review and meta-analysis. *Mayo Clin. Proc.* 2008;83:23-34.

[105] Walter MF, Jacob RF, Jeffers B, et al. Serum levels of thiobarbituric acid reactive substances predict cardiovascular events in patients with stable coronary artery disease: a longitudinal analysis of the PREVENT study. *J. Am. Coll. Cardiol.* 2004;44:1996-2002.

[106] Lonn E, Bosch J, Yusuf S, et al. Effects of long-term vitamin E supplementation on cardiovascular events and cancer: a randomized controlled trial. *JAMA,* 2005;293:1338-47.

[107] Brown BG, Crowley J. Is there any hope for vitamin E? *JAMA* 2005;293:1387-90.

[108] Wiernsperger NF. Oxidative stress: the special case of diabetes. *Biofactors,* 2003;19:11-8.

[109] Goodman GE, Schaffer S, Omenn GS, Chen C, King I. The association between lung and prostate cancer risk, and serum micronutrients: results and lessons learned from beta-carotene and retinol efficacy trial. *Cancer Epidemiol. Biomarkers Prev.* 2003;12:518-26.

[110] de Carvalho DD, Sadok A, Bourgarel-Rey V, et al. Nox1 downstream of 12-lipoxygenase controls cell proliferation but not cell spreading of colon cancer cells. *Int. J. Cancer.* 2008;122:1757-64.

[111] Jajoo S, Mukherjea D, Watabe K, Ramkumar V. Adenosine A(3) receptor suppresses prostate cancer metastasis by inhibiting NADPH oxidase activity. *Neoplasia,* 2009;11:1132-45.

[112] Mitsushita J, Lambeth JD, Kamata T. The superoxide-generating oxidase Nox1 is functionally required for Ras oncogene transformation. *Cancer Research,* 2004;64:3580-5.

[113] Brar SS, Kennedy TP, Sturrock AB, et al. An NAD(P)H oxidase regulates growth and transcription in melanoma cells. *Am. J. Physiol. Cell Physiol.* 2002;282:C1212-24.

[114] Vaquero EC, Edderkaoui M, Pandol SJ, Gukovsky I, Gukovskaya AS. Reactive oxygen species produced by NAD(P)H oxidase inhibit apoptosis in pancreatic cancer cells. *J. Biol. Chem.* 2004;279:34643-54.

[115] Brar SS, Corbin Z, Kennedy TP, et al. NOX5 NAD(P)H oxidase regulates growth and apoptosis in DU 145 prostate cancer cells. *Am. J. Physiol. Cell Physiol.* 2003;285:C353-69.

[116] \Weydert C, Roling B, Liu J, et al. Suppression of the malignant phenotype in human pancreatic cancer cells by the overexpression of manganese superoxide dismutase. *Mol. Cancer Ther.* 2003;2:361-9.

[117] Liu J, Hinkhouse MM, Sun W, et al. Redox regulation of pancreatic cancer cell growth: role of glutathione peroxidase in the suppression of the malignant phenotype. *Hum. Gene. Ther.* 2004;15:239-50.

[118] Liu J, Du J, Zhang Y, et al. Suppression of the malignant phenotype in pancreatic cancer by overexpression of phospholipid hydroperoxide glutathione peroxidase. *Hum. Gene. Ther.* 2006;17:105-16.

[119] Nelson SK, Bose SK, Grunwald GK, Myhill P, McCord JM. The induction of human superoxide dismutase and catalase in vivo: a fundamentally new approach to antioxidant therapy. *Free Radic. Biol. Med.* 2006;40:341-7.

[120] Hyoudou K, Nishikawa M, Ikemura M, et al. Prevention of pulmonary metastasis from subcutaneous tumors by binary system-based sustained delivery of catalase. *J. Control Release*, 2009;137:110-5.

[121] Wang L, Azad N, Kongkaneramit L, et al. The Fas death signaling pathway connecting reactive oxygen species generation and FLICE inhibitory protein down-regulation. *J. Immunol.* 2008;180:3072-80.

[122] Madesh M, Hajnoczky G. VDAC-dependent permeabilization of the outer mitochondrial membrane by superoxide induces rapid and massive cytochrome c release. *J. Cell Biol.* 2001;155:1003-15.

[123] Ichijo H, Nishida E, Irie K, et al. Induction of apoptosis by ASK1, a mammalian MAPKKK that activates SAPK/JNK and p38 signaling pathways. *Science*, 1997;275:90-4.

[124] Wang T, Arifoglu P, Ronai Z, Tew KD. Glutathione S-transferase P1-1 (GSTP1-1) inhibits c-Jun N-terminal kinase (JNK1) signaling through interaction with the C terminus. *J. Biol. Chem.* 2001;276:20999-1003.

[125] Lee K, Esselman WJ. Inhibition of PTPs by H(2)O(2) regulates the activation of distinct MAPK pathways. *Free Radic. Biol. Med.* 2002;33:1121-32.

[126] Asakura T, Ohkawa K. Chemotherapeutic agents that induce mitochondrial apoptosis. *Curr. Cancer Drug Targets*, 2004;4:577-90.

[127] Hampton MB, Orrenius S. Dual regulation of caspase activity by hydrogen peroxide: implications for apoptosis. *FEBS Lett*, 1997;414:552-6.

[128] Zhou Y, Hileman EO, Plunkett W, Keating MJ, Huang P. Free radical stress in chronic lymphocytic leukemia cells and its role in cellular sensitivity to ROS-generating anticancer agents. *Blood*, 2003;101:4098-104.

[129] Davison K, Cote S, Mader S, Miller WH. Glutathione depletion overcomes resistance to arsenic trioxide in arsenic-resistant cell lines. *Leukemia*, 2003;17:931-40.

[130] Davison K, Mann KK, Miller WH, Jr. Arsenic trioxide: mechanisms of action. *Semin. Hematol.* 2002;39:3-7.

[131] Lenehan PF, Gutierrez PL, Wagner JL, Milak N, Fisher GR, Ross DD. Resistance to oxidants associated with elevated catalase activity in HL-60 leukemia cells that overexpress multidrug-resistance protein does not contribute to the resistance to

daunorubicin manifested by these cells. *Cancer Chemother. Pharmacol.* 1995;35:377-86.

[132] Hoshida Y, Moriyama M, Otsuka M, et al. Gene expressions associated with chemosensitivity in human hepatoma cells. *Hepatogastroenterology,* 2007;54:489-92.

[133] Erhola M, Kellokumpu-Lehtinen P, Metsa-Ketela T, Alanko K, Nieminen MM. Effects of anthracyclin-based chemotherapy on total plasma antioxidant capacity in small cell lung cancer patients. *Free Radic. Biol. Med.* 1996;21:383-90.

[134] Faure H, Coudray C, Mousseau M, et al. 5-Hydroxymethyluracil excretion, plasma TBARS and plasma antioxidant vitamins in adriamycin-treated patients. *Free Radic. Biol. Med.* 1996;20:979-83.

[135] Gille L, Nohl H. Analyses of the molecular mechanism of adriamycin-induced cardiotoxicity. *Free Radic. Biol. Med.* 1997;23:775-82.

[136] Hutchinson F. The molecular basis for radiation effects on cells. *Cancer Research,* 1966;26:2045-52.

[137] Valerie K, Yacoub A, Hagan MP, et al. Radiation-induced cell signaling: inside-out and outside-in. *Mol. Cancer Ther.* 2007;6:789-801.

[138] Kirshner JR, He S, Balasubramanyam V, et al. Elesclomol induces cancer cell apoptosis through oxidative stress. *Mol. Cancer Ther.* 2008;7:2319-27.

[139] Kadara H, Lacroix L, Lotan D, Lotan R. Induction of endoplasmic reticulum stress by the pro-apoptotic retinoid N-(4-hydroxyphenyl)retinamide via a reactive oxygen species-dependent mechanism in human head and neck cancer cells. *Cancer Biol. Ther.* 2007;6:705-11.

[140] Corazzari M, Lovat PE, Oliverio S, et al. Fenretinide: a p53-independent way to kill cancer cells. *Biochem. Biophys. Res. Commun.* 2005;331:810-5.

[141] Evens AM. Motexafin gadolinium: a redox-active tumor selective agent for the treatment of cancer. *Curr. Opin. Oncol.* 2004;16:576-80.

[142] Kapitza S, Jakupec MA, Uhl M, Keppler BK, Marian B. The heterocyclic ruthenium(III) complex KP1019 (FFC14A) causes DNA damage and oxidative stress in colorectal tumor cells. *Cancer Lett.* 2005;226:115-21.

[143] Hartinger CG, Jakupec MA, Zorbas-Seifried S, et al. KP1019, a new redox-active anticancer agent--preclinical development and results of a clinical phase I study in tumor patients. *Chem. Biodivers,* 2008;5:2140-55.

[144] Wang J, Zhao L, Wang R, Lu M, Chen D, Jing Y. Synthesis and anticancer activity of 2-alkylaminomethyl-5-diaryl-methylenecyclopentanone hydrochlorides and related compounds. *Bioorg. Med. Chem.* 2005;13:1285-91.

[145] Xu K, Thornalley PJ. Involvement of glutathione metabolism in the cytotoxicity of the phenethyl isothiocyanate and its cysteine conjugate to human leukaemia cells in vitro. *Biochem. Pharmacol.* 2001;61:165-77.

[146] Ramanathan RK, Kirkpatrick DL, Belani CP, et al. A Phase I pharmacokinetic and pharmacodynamic study of PX-12, a novel inhibitor of thioredoxin-1, in patients with advanced solid tumors. *Clin. Cancer Res.* 2007;13:2109-14.

[147] Traynor AM, Thomas JP, Ramanathan RK, et al. Phase I trial of motexafin gadolinium and doxorubicin in the treatment of advanced malignancies. *Invest New Drugs,* 2009.

[148] Lin TS, Naumovski L, Lecane PS, et al. Effects of motexafin gadolinium in a phase II trial in refractory chronic lymphocytic leukemia. *Leuk. Lymphoma,* 2009;50:1977-82.

[149] Kang MH, Wan Z, Kang YH, Sposto R, Reynolds CP. Mechanism of synergy of N-(4-hydroxyphenyl)retinamide and ABT-737 in acute lymphoblastic leukemia cell lines: Mcl-1 inactivation. *Journal of the National Cancer Institute,* 2008;100:580-95.

[150] Wang W, Sun YP, Huang XZ, et al. Emodin enhances sensitivity of gallbladder cancer cells to platinum drugs via glutathion depletion and MRP1 downregulation. *Biochem. Pharmacol.* 2010;79:1134-40.

[151] Yi J, Yang J, He R, et al. Emodin enhances arsenic trioxide-induced apoptosis via generation of reactive oxygen species and inhibition of survival signaling. *Cancer Research,* 2004;64:108-16.

[152] Yang J, Li H, Chen YY, et al. Anthraquinones sensitize tumor cells to arsenic cytotoxicity in vitro and in vivo via reactive oxygen species-mediated dual regulation of apoptosis. *Free Radic. Biol. Med.* 2004;37:2027-41.

[153] Diaz Z, Laurenzana A, Mann KK, Bismar TA, Schipper HM, Miller WH, Jr. Trolox enhances the anti-lymphoma effects of arsenic trioxide, while protecting against liver toxicity. *Leukemia,* 2007;21:2117-27.

[154] Diaz Z, Colombo M, Mann KK, et al. Trolox selectively enhances arsenic-mediated oxidative stress and apoptosis in APL and other malignant cell lines. *Blood,* 2005;105:1237-45.

[155] Pelicano H, Feng L, Zhou Y, et al. Inhibition of mitochondrial respiration: a novel strategy to enhance drug-induced apoptosis in human leukemia cells by a reactive oxygen species-mediated mechanism. *J. Biol. Chem.* 2003;278:37832-9.

[156] Zhou L, Hou J, Fu W, Wang D, Yuan Z, Jiang H. Arsenic trioxide and 2-methoxyestradiol reduce beta-catenin accumulation after proteasome inhibition and enhance the sensitivity of myeloma cells to Bortezomib. *Leuk. Res.* 2008;32:1674-83.

[157] Warburg O. On the origin of cancer cells. *Science,* 1956;123:309-14.

[158] Shi DY, Xie FZ, Zhai C, Stern JS, Liu Y, Liu SL. The role of cellular oxidative stress in regulating glycolysis energy metabolism in hepatoma cells. *Mol. Cancer,* 2009;8:32.

[159] Semenza GL. Hypoxia-inducible factor 1: master regulator of O_2 homeostasis. *Curr. Opin. Genet. Dev.* 1998;8:588-94.

[160] Wenger RH. Cellular adaptation to hypoxia: O_2-sensing protein hydroxylases, hypoxia-inducible transcription factors, and O_2-regulated gene expression. *FASEB J.* 2002;16:1151-62.

[161] Hwang IT, Chung YM, Kim JJ, et al. Drug resistance to 5-FU linked to reactive oxygen species modulator 1. *Biochem. Biophys. Res. Commun.* 2007;359:304-10.

[162] Tome ME, Johnson DB, Rimsza LM, et al. A redox signature score identifies diffuse large B-cell lymphoma patients with a poor prognosis. *Blood,* 2005;106:3594-601.

[163] \Dairkee SH, Nicolau M, Sayeed A, et al. Oxidative stress pathways highlighted in tumor cell immortalization: association with breast cancer outcome. *Oncogene,* 2007;26:6269-79.

[164] Shah JJ, Kuhn DJ, Orlowski RZ. Bortezomib and EGCG: no green tea for you? *Blood,* 2009;113:5695-6.

[165] Ramanathan B, Jan KY, Chen CH, Hour TC, Yu HJ, Pu YS. Resistance to paclitaxel is proportional to cellular total antioxidant capacity. *Cancer Research,* 2005;65:8455-60.

In: Principles of Free Radical Biomedicine, Volume III
Editors: K. Pantopoulos and H. M. Schipper

ISBN 978-1-61324-184-4
©2012 Nova SciencePublishers, Inc.

Chapter 8

Oxidative Stress in Arterial Hypertension and Atherosclerosis

Ernesto L. Schiffrin[1,*] and Rhian M. Touyz[2]

[1]Lady Davis Institute for Medical Research, Jewish General Hospital, McGill University, Montreal, Quebec, Canada
[2]Kidney Research Centre, University of Ottawa, Ottawa Health Research Institute, Ottawa, Ontario, Canada

1. Introduction

Oxidative stress is an important cause of vascular injury in hypertension and a contributor to the development and progression of atherosclerosis. Among the major reactive oxygen species (ROS) important in these processes are $\bullet O_2^-$, H_2O_2, $\bullet OH$, $HOCl$ and the reactive nitrogen species (RNS), nitric oxide (NO) and peroxynitrite ($ONOO^-$); see Vol. II, Chapters 2 and 3. ROS/RNS are produced under physiological conditions in a highly regulated fashion at low concentrations and function as signaling molecules that control endothelial and vascular smooth muscle cell function [4-7]. In pathological situations increased ROS production leads to endothelial dysfunction, enhanced contractility and growth of vascular smooth muscle cells, lipid peroxidation, inflammation and increased deposition of extracellular matrix proteins, all contributing to vascular injury, triggering atherosclerosis and leading to hypertension [7-9]. Generation of ROS is enhanced in many organs and tissues in experimental models of hypertension [10-13]. Markers of systemic oxidative stress such as plasma and urinary levels of thiobarbituric acid-reactive substances (TBARS) and 8-epi-isoprostane have been reported to be elevated in human hypertension [14, 15]. Treatment with antioxidants or superoxide dismutase (SOD) mimetics (Vol. II, Chapter 6) improved blood pressure and vascular structure and function in experimental and human hypertension [12, 13, 16, 17]. Gene deletion of ROS-generating enzymes, Nox1 or Nox2, in mice results in lower

---

*E-mail: ernesto.schiffrin@mcgill.ca

blood pressure in models of acute Ang II-induced hypertension, but not in models of chronic Ang II-dependent hypertension [18, 19]. *Vascular smooth muscle cells and isolated arteries from hypertensive rats and humans generate more ROS and exhibit reduced antioxidant capacity compared to those from normotensive counterparts* [12, 13, 21-23]. Indeed, there is abundant evidence that vascular oxidative stress participates in mechanisms associated with blood pressure elevation. Enhanced ROS production occurs in hypertension also in the heart, kidney and brain [24-26]. However, discussion in the present Chapter will be limited to the vasculature specifically in hypertension and atherosclerosis.

2. Vascular Production of Reactive Oxygen Species

Production of $•O_2^-$ occurs in blood vessels mainly in the media and adventitia, with small levels of generation in the endothelium [27, 28]. In patients with diabetes mellitus and in atherosclerosis the endothelium may become more important [29]. *ROS is produced from multiple cellular sources in the vessel wall* [30-34], *including leakage from the mitochondrial electron transport chain, small molecules, enzymes, including cyclooxygenase, lipoxygenase, heme oxygenase, uncoupled nitric oxide synthase (NOS), cytochrome P450 monooxygenase, xanthine oxidase, and NADPH (nicotinamide adenine dinucleotide phosphate, reduced form) oxidase (Figure 1)*.

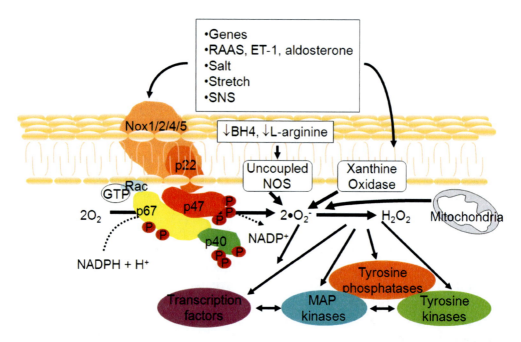

Figure 1. Diagram demonstrating major sources of reactive oxygen species, superoxide ($•O_2^-$) and hydrogen peroxide (H_2O_2), in the vasculature. Activation of ROS-generating enzymes results in intracellular production of $•O_2^-$, which is dismutated by superoxide dismutase (SOD) to form H_2O_2. ROS influence redox-sensitive signaling molecules such as transcription factors, mitogen activated-protein (MAP) kinases, tyrosine phosphatases, which regulate vascular cell function. RAAS, renin-angiotensin-aldosterone system; ET-1, endothelin-1, SNS, sympathetic nervous system, BH4, tetrahydrobiopterin; p, phosphorylation.

Of these, xanthine oxidase, uncoupled NOS, the mitochondrial electron transport chain and NADPH oxidase, are major producers of ROS in the vascular wall.

2.1. Xanthine Oxidase

Xanthine oxidase (XO) and xanthine dehydrogenase (XDH) are interconvertible forms of the same enzyme, known as xanthine oxidoreductase. Physiologically, XO andXDH participate in many biochemical reactions, with the primary role being degradation of purines and theconversion of hypoxanthine to xanthine and xanthine to uricacid. As a byproduct in the purine degradation pathway, XO oxidizes NADH to form $\bullet O_2^-$ and H_2O_2 [3]. In the vascular wall, XO-derived $\bullet O_2^-$ reacts rapidly with NO to form ONOO⁻, which can lead to a negative feedback of the enzyme [36]. Xanthine oxidase is expressed in vascular cells, it circulates in the plasma and it bindsto endothelial cell extracellular matrix. Although xanthine oxidase-derived $\bullet O_2^-$ has been studied mainly in the context of cardiac disease and atherosclerosis, there is also evidence suggesting its involvement in hypertension [37, 38].

2.2.Uncoupled Nitric Oxide Synthase

Under physiological conditions, nitric oxide synthase (NOS), in the presence of substrate L-arginine and cofactortetrahydrobiopterin (BH4), produces NO. In the absence of these, becauseof oxidative destruction or downregulationof GTP cyclohydrolase-1, which is the rate-limiting enzyme in BH4 production, uncoupled NOS produces $\bullet O_2^-$ rather than NO [39, 40]. All three NOS isoforms are capable of 'uncoupling' that leads to the preferential formation of $\bullet O_2-$ [41]. eNOS uncoupling has been demonstrated in DOCA-salt-induced hypertension and in spontaneously-hypertensive rats (SHR) [42, 43]; moreover, it has been implicated in atherosclerosis and endothelial dysfunction in low-density lipoprotein receptor-deficient mice (LDLR-/-) fed a high salt, high fat diet [44].

2.3. Mitochondrial Respiratory Enzymes

More than 95% of O_2 consumed by cells is reduced by four electrons to yield two molecules of H_2O via mitochondrial electron transport chain complexes (I-IV), with 1-2% of the electron flow leaking to O_2 to form $\bullet O_2^-$ under normoxic conditions [45]. Mitochondrial ROS production is modulated by many factors including cytokines and vasoactive agonists [46-48]. Ang II and ET-1 stimulate mitochondrial ROS generation in endothelial and vascular smooth muscle cells and in rat aorta *in vivo* [47-50].

Alterations in mitochondrialbiogenesis are associated with mitochondrial dysfunction and mitochondrial oxidative stress (Vol. II, Chapter 15). Impaired activity and/or decreased expression of mitochondrial electron transport chain complexes I, III and IV have been implicated in vascular aging and cardiovascular disease, and an association between mitochondrial dysfunction and blood pressure has been reported in human and experimental hypertension [50-52].

2.4. ROS-Generating Nox-Family NADPH Oxidases

In endothelial, adventitial and vascular smooth muscle cells, ROS are derived predominantly from NADPH oxidase. This multi-subunit enzyme [34, 53-55] catalyzes generation of $\bullet O_2^-$ by reduction of oxygen with NADPH as the electron donor: $2O_2 + NADPH \rightarrow 2O_2^- + NADPH + H^+$ (Figure 1). The prototypical and best characterized NADPH oxidase is that found in phagocytes and comprises five subunits: p47phox (p47 PHagocyte OXidase), p67phox, p40phox (cytosolic subunits), p22phox and gp91phox (membrane-associated subunits) [56, 57]. Phosphorylation of p47phox upon stimulation is followed by complex formation with the remaining cytosolic subunits, translocation to the membrane and association with cell membrane-bound subunits to generate the active oxidase [58]. NADPH oxidase then transfers electrons from NADPH to O_2 leading to the generation of $\bullet O_2^-$ [56]. Dysfunction of NADPH oxidase due to defects in the genes encoding for either gp91phox, p22phox, p67phox or p47phox is found in chronic granulomatous disease, which is characterized by recurrent infections. These result from deficiency to generate the oxidative burst whereby $\bullet O_2^-$ plays a role in host defense against invading microorganisms [57]. NADPH oxidase is also functionally present and important in non-phagocytic cells and is the main source of $\bullet O_2^-$ in the vasculature [28, 53, 58-61]. In endothelial and adventitial cells p47phox, p67phox, p22phox and gp91phox are present [53, 58, 60-63]. In vascular smooth muscle cells only p47phox and p22phox seem to be consistently expressed [53]. In rat aortic vascular smooth muscle cells, p22phox and p47phox, but not gp91phox, are present, whereas in human resistance arteries, all of the major subunits, including gp91phox, are expressed [31, 54, 58]. The discovery of gp91phox homologues has led to new understanding of the Nox family of NADPH oxidases [61, 64-66] (Table 1). The Nox family includes seven members: Nox1, Nox2 (formerly termed gp91phox), Nox3, Nox4, Nox5, Duox1 and Duox2 that mediate diverse biological functions. Nox1 is found in vascular cells. Nox2 is expressed in vascular, cardiac, renal and neural cells. Nox3 is found in fetal tissue and the adult inner ear. Nox4 was originally called Renox (renal oxidase) but is also found in vascular cells. Nox5 is present in human vascular cells. Duox1 and 2 are thyroid Noxes. Nox1 mRNA is expressed in rat aortic smooth muscle and may be a substitute for gp91phox in these cells [67]. Nox1 requires p47phox and p67phox and is regulated by NOXO1 (Nox organizer 1) and NOXA1 (Nox activator 1) [68]. Nox1 is significantly upregulated in vascular injury [53] and may be important in the pathophysiology of acute, but not chronic, forms of Ang II-induced hypertension [64-71]. Nox1-deficient mice have low blood pressure and respond poorly to the pressor action of Ang II [69]. Overexpression of vascular Nox1 in mice results in an exaggerated blood pressure response to Ang II and enhanced vascular remodeling [70]. Nox4, originally termed Renox (renal oxidase) because of its extensiveabundance in thekidney, is also found in vascularcells, fibroblasts and osteoclasts [71, 72]. In vascular smooth muscle cells, Nox4 and p22phox co-localize with vinculin in focal adhesions. Nox4 has also been found in the endoplasmic reticulum and nucleus of vascular cells [73]. Nox4 produces mainly H_2O_2, while Nox1 generates mostly $\bullet O_2^-$ that is subsequently converted to H_2O_2. The difference in the products generated by Nox1 and Nox4 may contribute to distinct roles of these Noxes in cell signaling. Nox 4 does not seem to require p47phox, p67phox, p40phox or Rac for its activation, although Nox R1, a Nox 4-binding protein was recently identified, which may be important for Nox4 regulation [74, 75]. In cultured vascular smooth muscle and endothelial cells, Nox4 localizes to focal adhesions and the endoplasmic reticulum and has been implicated in cell migration, proliferation, tube formation, angiogenesis and cell differentiation [74-76] and is regulated byPoldip2 (polymerase [DNA-directed]delta-interacting protein) [76]. Nox5 is a Ca^{2+}-dependent homologue, found in testes and lymphoid tissue, but also in vascular cells [77]. While all Nox proteins are present in rodents and man, the mouse and rat genome does not contain thenox5gene. Unlike other vascular Noxes, Nox5 possesses an amino-terminal calmodulin-like domain with four binding sites for Ca^{2+} (EF hands) and does not require p22phox or other subunits for its activation. Nox5 is directly regulated by intracellular Ca^{2+} ($[Ca^{2+}]_i$), the binding of which induces a conformational change leading to enhanced ROS generation [78]. The functional significance of vascular Nox5 is unknown, although it has been implicated in endothelial cell proliferation and angiogenesis, in platelet-derived growth factor (PDGF)-induced proliferation of vascular smooth muscle cells and in oxidative damage in atherosclerosis [79-81]. Vascular Nox5 is activated by thrombin, PDGF, ionomycin, Ang II and ET-1 [82, 83]. Duox1 and duox2 are thyroid Noxes involved in thyroid hormone biosynthesis [84]. Whether they play a role in vascular function is unknown. The activity of vascular NADPH oxidase and expression of oxidase subunits are regulated by cytokines, growth factors and vasoactive agents. Ang II induces activation of NADPH oxidase, increases expression of its subunits and stimulates ROSproduction in cultured vascular cells and intact arteries [31, 58, 60, 62]. Phopholipase D (PLD), protein kinase C (PKC), c-Src, phophoinositide 3kinase (PI3K) and Rac may be important in the signal transduction pathway between the angiotensin AT_1 receptor and NADPH oxidase [62, 63]. PDGF, transforming growth factor-β (TGF-β), tumor necrosis factor (TNF)α and thrombin also activate NADPH oxidase in vascular smooth muscle [64, 85, 86], whereas the antioxidants catalase (Vol. II, Chapter 7) and glutathione (Vol. II, Chapter 1) protect from agonist-induced ROS generation. Activators of peroxisome proliferator-activated receptors (PPARs), statins and antihypertensive drugs such as β-blockers, calcium channel blockers, angiotensin converting enzyme inhibitors and angiotensin receptor blockers, act as antioxidants by downregulating the expression of NADPH oxidase subunits and decrease its activity [87, 88]. Pressure, stretch, pulsatile strain and shear stress also activate NADPH oxidase [53, 89].

Table 1. mRNA Expression of Nox isoforms in cardiovascular cells

Enzyme	VSMC	EC	Fibroblasts	Cardiomyocytes
Nox1	+	+	+	-
Nox2	+	+	+	+
Nox3	-	-	-	-
Nox4	+	+	+	+
Nox5	Human	HUVEC	Human cardiac	-
Duox1	+	-	-	-

VSMC, vascular smooth muscle cells; EC, endothelial cells;

HUVEC, human umbilical vein endothelial cells.

3. Vascular Antioxidant Defense Systems

Enzymatic and nonenzymatic systems have evolved to protect against injurious oxidative stress. Major enzymatic antioxidants found within the vascular system include SOD, catalase, glutathione peroxidase (GPx), thioredoxin (Trx) and peroxiredoxin (Prx) [90-92] (see also Vol. II, Chapters 1-4). Non-enzymatic antioxidants include ascorbate, tocopherols, glutathione, bilirubin and uric acid and scavenge OH· and other free radicals [90-92] (see also Vol. II, Chapters 13-16). Three mammalian SODs have been identified: Cu/ZnSOD (SOD1), mitochondrial MnSOD (SOD2), and extracellular SOD (SOD3) [24]. The concentration of SOD in the extracellular fluid is lower than in the intracellular fluid. Therefore $\bullet O_2^-$ can survive longer and travel further once it gains access to the extracellular space. Arteries contain large amounts of extracellular SOD in the interstitium, which suggests that this SOD isoform may have a special role in the vessel wall [93, 94]. SOD converts $\bullet O_2^-$ to H_2O_2, which is hydrolyzed by catalase and GPx to H_2O and O_2. GPx is the major enzyme protecting the cell membrane against lipid peroxidation, since reduced glutathione (GSH) donates protons to membrane lipids maintaining them in a reduced state [95]. Oxidized glutathione (GSSG) can be recycled by glutathione reductase to reduced GSH utilizing NADPH as a substrate or it can be exported from the cell via active transport by the multidrug resistance protein 1 (MRP1) [96]. Hypertension induced by DOCA-salt or Ang II was attenuated in MRP1-/- mice, and vascular glutathione flux was blunted in MRP1-/- mice allowing recycling of GSSG to reduced glutathione and promoting increased intracellular antioxidant capacity [97]. MRP1inhibitionmay protect against oxidant stress by preventing loss of glutathione from vascular cells. Catalase is an intracellular antioxidant enzyme located primarily in cellular peroxisomes; it catalyzes the reaction of H_2O_2 to water and O_2 [98]. Catalase is very effective in high-level oxidative stress andprotects cells from H_2O_2 produced within the cell. Thioredoxin reductase participates in thiol-dependent cellular reductive processes [99, 100].

Reduced antioxidant bioavailability promotes cellular oxidative stress and has been implicated in cardiovascular and renal oxidative damage associated with hypertension [101-103]. Activity of SOD, catalase and GSH peroxidase is lower, and the GSSG/GSH is higher in plasma and circulating cells from hypertensive patients than normotensive subjects [100-104]. In mice deficient in EC-SOD and in rats in which GSH synthesis is inhibited, blood pressure is significantly elevated, demonstrating that *reduced antioxidant capacity is associated with elevated blood pressure. Failure to upregulate antioxidant genes and reduced antioxidant capacity are also associated with age-accelerated atherosclerosis* [105]. Based on this, it has been suggested that antioxidant supplementation may have beneficial therapeutic effects in reducing oxidative stress in cardiovascular disease.

4. Molecular Targets of Reactive Oxygen Species in Vascular Cells

ROS function as mediators in many signaling pathways [106-108] in association with redox-sensitive molecules that include transcription factors, protein tyrosine phosphatases, protein tyrosine kinases, mitogen-activated protein (MAP) kinases and ion channels (Figure

2). Protein tyrosine phosphatases and transcription factors such as NF-κB (Vol. II, Chapter 12), AP-1 (Vol. II, Chapter 14) and HIF-1 (Vol. II, Chapter 22) appear to be directly regulated by ROS [107-113] whereas other signaling molecules are indirectly regulated by ROS.

The best-established direct targets of ROS signaling are protein tyrosine phosphatases [107-111], which contribute to the tight regulation of tyrosine phosphorylation. ROS inhibit activity of tyrosine phosphatases, resulting in increased tyrosine phosphorylation and activation of several receptor protein tyrosine kinases such as the EGFR and insulin receptor [114-117]. This is particularly important with respect to Ang II, which mediates many of its signaling events in vascular cells through EGFR transactivation [118]. H2O2 has also been shown to regulate non-receptor tyrosine kinases and MAP kinases through inhibition of tyrosine phosphatase activity [118-121].

In hypertension and atherosclerosis activation of vascular MAP kinases is enhanced, which is a major mechanism contributing to vascular damage [103, 104]. MAP kinases are in part activated by ROS [122, 123]. ROS generation mediates Ang II-induced activation of p38MAPK, JNK and ERK5, whereas phosphorylation of ERK1/2 appears to be redox-insensitive [124, 125].

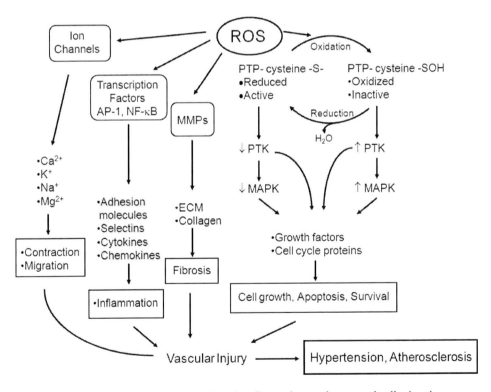

Figure 2. Schematic demonstrating redox-sensitive signaling pathways that control cell migration, growth/apoptosis, contraction/dilation, inflammation and fibrosis. Increased oxidative stress induces activation of ion channels, transcription factors, MMPs, kinases and phosphatases which promotes vascular hypertrophy, reactivity, fibrosis and inflammation leading to vascular injury and remodeling in hypertension and atherosclerosis. PTP, protein tyrosine phosphatases; PTK, protein tyrosine kinases; ECM, extracellular matrix; MMP, matrix metalloproteinase. Other abbreviations as in Figure 1.

Redox-regulation of MAP kinases may be ligand- and cell- specific. Upstream regulators (MEKs, tyrosine kinases and phosphatases) of MAP kinases, rather than the latter themselves, are likely direct targets of $\bullet O_2^-$ and H_2O_2.

ROSalsomodulate intracellular calcium concentration ($[Ca^{2+}]_i$), a major determinant of vascular contraction. Superoxide and H_2O_2 increase $[Ca^{2+}]_i$ in vascular smooth muscle and endothelial cells [127] via redox-dependent inositol-trisphosphate-induced Ca^{2+} mobilization, increased Ca^{2+} influx and decreased activation of Ca^{2+}-ATPase [109, 110].

Plasma membrane K^+ channels in VSMCs that control a hyperpolarization-elicited relaxation are opened by mechanisms associated with thiol oxidation by ROS [127]. These redox-regulated Ca^{2+} processes may play a role in the altered vascular contractility in hypertension, as shown by enhanced contractile responses to H_2O_2 found in arteries from SHR [128, 129].

5. Vascular Mechanisms of Oxidative Stress in Hypertension

Oxidative stress promotes vascular smooth muscle cell proliferation and hypertrophy, collagen deposition and alterations in activity of matrix metalloproteinases (MMP) in hypertension, thereby contributing to remodeling of the vasculature (Figure 2). Superoxide anion and H_2O_2 stimulate growth factor-like cellular responses, such as intracellular alkalinization, MAP kinase phosphorylation, and tyrosine kinase activation. H_2O_2 induces vascular smooth muscle cell DNA synthesis, increases expression of protooncogenes and promotes cell growth [106, 107, 126].

Superoxide anion and H_2O_2 influence activity of vascular MMP2 and MMP9, which promote degradation of basement membrane and elastin, respectively [130]. Redox-sensitive inflammatory processes, including expression of proinflammatory molecules, such as vascular cell adhesion molecule-1 (VCAM-1) and monocyte chemotactic protein-1 (MCP-1), lipid peroxidation and cell migration, further contribute to vascular remodeling in hypertension [131].

5.1. Reactive Oxygen Species Reduce NO Bioavailability

Impaired endothelium-mediated vasodilatation has been linked to reduced NO bioavailability. This may be secondary to decreased synthesis of NO due to uncoupling of NOS and/or decreased bioavailability of NO by interaction with $\bullet O_2^-$ to form $ONOO^-$ [133]. Peroxynitrite is a weak vasodilator compared with NO and is pro-inflammatory [134]. ROS also induce recruitment of inflammatory cells, which worsens vascular injury. Polymorphonuclear leukocytes, which generate $\bullet O_2^-$, participate in oxidative stress and inflammation in patients with hypertension [135, 136].

Many of the redox-sensitive vascular changes that occur in hypertension also exist in atherosclerotic vessels. In fact *oxidative stress-mediated vascular damage and endothelial dysfunction may link hypertension to atherosclerosis* [135, 136].

6. Reactive Oxygen Species in Hypertension

6.1. Oxidative Stress in Experimental Models of Hypertension

The relationship between oxidative stress and increased blood pressure has been demonstrated in many models of hypertension. Increased ROS formation precedes development of hypertension in SHR, and is implicated in fetal programming and development of hypertension later in life, supporting the important role of ROS in the genesis and maintenance of hypertension [137-140]. Markers of oxidative stress, such as TBARS, and $F_{2\alpha}$-isoprostanes (Vol. I, Chapter 7), tissue concentrations of $\bullet O_2^-$ and H_2O_2 and activation of NADPH oxidase and xanthine oxidase are increased, whereas levels of NO and antioxidant enzymes are reduced in experimental hypertension [141, 142].

Ang II-dependent hypertension is particularly sensitive to NADPH oxidase-derived ROS. In rats and mice made hypertensive by Ang II infusion, expression of NADPH oxidase subunits (Nox1, Nox2, Nox4, p22phox), oxidase activity and generation of ROS are increased [143-145]. To support a role for NADPH oxidase-derived ROS generation in the pathogenesis of Ang II-induced hypertension, various mouse models with altered subunit expression of this enzyme have been studied. In p47phox knockout mice and in gp91phox (Nox2) knockout mice, Ang II infusion fails to induce hypertension and these animals do not show the same increases in $\bullet O_2^-$ production, vascular hypertrophy and endothelial dysfunction observed in Ang II-infused wild-type mice [144, 145]. In Ang II-infused mice treated with siRNA targeted to renal p22phox, renal NADPH oxidase activity was blunted, ROS formation was reduced and blood pressure elevation was attenuated suggesting that p22phox is required for Ang II-induced oxidative stress and hypertension [146]. On the other hand, overexpression of vascular p22phox was associated with increased oxidative stress and vascular dysfunction, but no significant increase in blood pressure [147]. Treatment with apocynin or diphenylene iodinium, non-specific pharmacological inhibitors of NADPH oxidase, or gp91dstat, a novel specific inhibitor of NADPH oxidase, reduced vascular $\bullet O_2^-$ production, prevented cardiovascular remodeling and attenuated development of hypertension in Ang II-treated mice [148]. Nox1-deficient mice have reduced vascular $\bullet O_2^-$ production and blood pressure elevation in response to Ang II is blunted [149], whereas in transgenic mice in which Nox1 is overexpressed in the vascular wall, Ang II-mediated vascular hypertrophy and blood pressure elevation are enhanced [150, 151]. In most of these models, Ang II was infused for a short time period (1-3 weeks), inducing an acute hypertensive response. In a model of chronic Ang II-dependent hypertension, where transgenic mice expressing human renin (which exhibit an Ang II-sensitive hypertensive phenotype) were crossed with Nox2-/- or Nox1-/- mice, development of hypertension was not prevented even though oxidative stress was reduced, suggesting that Noxes may be more important in acute than in chronic hypertension [71, 152].

There is also evidence for ROS involvement in the pathogenesis of hypertension independent of direct Ang II actions. In SHR, vascular, renal and cardiac $\bullet O_2^-$ production is enhanced compared with normotensive controls [153, 154]. In stroke-prone SHR, aortic expression of Nox1 and Nox4 is significantly increased compared with normotensive Wistar Kyoto (WKY) controls [155]. In DOCA salt-induced mineralocorticoid hypertension, vascular $\bullet O_2^-$ production is increased via elevated NADPH oxidase activity and uncoupling of endothelial NOS and mitochondrial sources, in part through the endothelin-1 (ET-1)/ETA receptor pathway [156]. Infusion of ET-1 increases NADPH oxidase-dependent $\bullet O_2^-$ production; however, preventing this increase in ROS generation does not inhibit development of hypertension in these animals [157]. Overexpression of human ET-1 in mice also induces vascular remodeling and impairs endothelial function, via activation of NADPH oxidase [158].

Increased activation of vascular xanthine oxidase [159], the electron transport chain of mitochondria, and uncoupling of eNOS [160, 161] may also play a role in oxidative stress-induced hypertension. Inhibition of ROS generation with apocynin or allopurinol, scavenging of free radicals with antioxidants or SOD mimetics or coupling of NOS with tetrahydrobiopterin (BH4), decreases blood pressure and prevents development of hypertension in most models of experimental hypertension [162-164], which may result from improvement in endothelial function, regression of vascular remodeling and reduced vascular inflammation [165].

6.2. Oxidative Stress and Clinical Hypertension

Although studies in humans have not been as convincing as those in experimental models, there is evidence that oxidative stress is increased in patients with essential hypertension, renovascular hypertension, malignanthypertension, salt-sensitive hypertension, cyclosporine-induced hypertension and preeclampsia [166-170]. These findings arebased, in large part, on increased levels of plasma thiobarbituricacid-reactive substances and 8-epi-isoprostanes, biomarkersof lipid peroxidation and oxidative stress (Vol. I, Chapter 7). Polymorphonuclearleukocyte- and platelet- derived $\bullet O_2^-$, which alsoparticipate in vascular oxidative stress and inflammation, are increased inhypertensive patients [171].

Hypertensive patientsexhibit a significantly higher production of plasma H_2O_2 than normotensive subjects [172]. Additionally, normotensive subjects with a family history of hypertension have greater H_2O_2 production than blood pressure–matched normotensiveswithout a family history of hypertension, suggesting that there may be a genetic component that leads to elevatedproduction of H_2O_2 [173]. Plasma levels of asymmetric dimethylarginine (ADMA) (eNOS inhibitor) and the lipid peroxidation product of linoleic acid, 13-hydroxyoctadecadienoic acid (HODE), a marker of ROS production, were inversely correlated with microvascular endothelial dysfunction and elevated blood pressure in hypertensive patients [174].

We showed that ROS production is increased in vascular smooth muscle cells from resistance arteries of hypertensive patients and that this is associated with upregulation of vascular NADPH oxidase [175]. The importance of this oxidase in oxidative stress in human cardiovascular disease is further supported by studies showing that polymorphisms in NADPH oxidase subunits are associated with increased atherosclerosis and hypertension [176]. However, recent clinical evidence questions the role of gp91phox-containing NADPH oxidase in the pathogenesis of hypertension, as patients with chronic granulomatous disease, who are deficient in gp91phox, do not display significant alterations in blood pressure, despite altered vascular function [177].

In addition to excess ROS generation, decreased antioxidant defense mechanisms contribute to oxidative stress in patients with hypertension [178, 179]. Hypertensive patients have reduced activity and decreased content of antioxidant enzymes, including SOD, GPx and catalase [178-180]. Decreased levels of antioxidant vitamins A, C and E have been reported in newly diagnosed, untreated hypertensive patients compared with normotensive controls [180]. Moreover, SOD activity correlates inversely with blood pressure in patients with hypertension [181]. Antioxidant vitamins reduced blood pressure and arterial stiffness in patients with diabetes, but had no effect in postmenopausal women, in healthy subjects or in the prevention of preeclampsia [181-183]. In patients with white coat hypertension, where elevated blood pressure is only observed in a clinical setting but not outside the clinic, serum protein carbonyl (PCO, indicating protein oxidation) was increased and endogenous antioxidant proteins (protein thiol, SOD, glutathione) were decreased compared with normotensive individuals, further supporting a relationship between oxidative stress and hypertension [184].

7. Atherosclerosis

Oxidative stress plays an important role in atherogenesis by promoting lipid and protein oxidation in the vascular wall. Excess ROS and RNS generation has been associated with vascular lesion formation and endothelial dysfunction in atherosclerosis. Common cardiovascular risk factors that promote atherosclerosis, such as hypercholesterolemia, diabetes mellitus, hypertension, smoking, age, nitrate intolerance and activation of the renin-angiotensin-system (RAS), also increase ROS production [185]. The importance of the RAS in redox-sensitive atherogenesis is supported by the findings that: a) Ang II induces upregulation of LOX-1, the human endothelial receptor for oxidized low-density lipoprotein [186]; b) Ang II promotes increased uptake of oxidized LDL by macrophages [187]; c) progression of atherosclerosis is accelerated by Ang II in apoE knockout mice [188]; d) components of the RAS are upregulated in atheromatous plaque [189] and e) the vascular protective response to RAS blockade in experimental and human studies with ACE inhibitors or AT_1 receptor blockers [190].

Mechanisms whereby ROS lead to acceleration of atherosclerosis include incorporation of oxidized LDL to the intima in the vascular wall, proliferation and migration to the intima of smooth muscle cells [191, 192], formation and necrosis of foam cells and fibrosis to form the fibrous cap of the atheromatous plaque. Matrix metalloproteinases (MMPs) are stimulated by Ang II and other agents, and contribute to the progression of plaque formation and their instability [193, 194]. Vascular oxidant stress enhances progression and angiogenesis of experimental atheroma [195].

Overexpression of vascular smooth muscle cell NADPH oxidase (p22phox subunit) in mice was associated with larger arterial lesions than in control mice [196]. Hydrogen peroxide and vascular endothelial growth factor (VEGF) levels were elevated in mice overexpressing the NADPH oxidase subunit, probably because of increased expression of HIF-1α through enhanced oxidative stress, and accordingly, lesions in the transgenic mice were associated with neointimal angiogenesis. Neovascularization has been well described in atheroma, and is considered to play an important role in the progression of atherosclerosis and in plaque instability [197]. Thus, *oxidative stress can trigger an angiogenic switch leading to angiogenesis and atheroma progression*. Further evidence of the role played by NADPH oxidase is the requirement of p47phox for plaque progression in hypercholesterolemic mice [198]. The predominant ROS detected in this study was H_2O_2, which appears to be the one associated with an angiogenic switch [199].

In humans, ROS generation by NADPH oxidase has also been demonstrated in atherectomy specimens [200]. NADPH oxidase catalytic subunits, gp91phox, Nox 1 and Nox4 may contribute to increased oxidative stress in human coronary atherosclerosis in a cell-specific manner [201]. In coronary artery segments from explanted human hearts, $\bullet O_2^-$ production in nonatherosclerotic coronary arteries occurred throughout the intima, media, and adventitia. In atherosclerotic arteries, ROS generation is increased in the plaque shoulder, which is rich in macrophages and α-actin–positive cells. The p22phox subunit of NADPH oxidase colocalized with gp91phox mainly in macrophages, whereas Nox4 was found in nonphagocytic vascular cells. gp91phox and p22phox mRNA expression correlated with the severity of atherosclerosis. gp91phox correlated with the plaque macrophage content, whereas Nox4 correlated with the content of α-actin–positive cells. Nox1 expression was low both in human coronary arteries and isolated vascular cells.

NADPH oxidase is not the only source of ROS that can influence progression of atherosclerosis. Xanthine oxidase, myeloperoxidase [202] and endothelial nitric oxide synthase have also been incriminated. Recently, the role of mitochondrial dysfunctionin ROS productionin endothelial dysfunction and atherosclerosis, which can be stimulated by angiotensin II, has been increasingly recognized. Mitochondria are both sources and targets of reactive oxygen species, and there is growing evidence that mitochondrial dysfunction may be a relevant intermediate mechanism by which cardiovascular risk factors lead to the formation of vascular lesions [203]. Once oxidant mechanisms have generated oxidized LDL, other mechanisms become operational. In atherosclerotic lesions of ApoE-null mice, aldose reductase has been located in macrophage-rich regions in proportion to progression of lesions [204]. Pharmacological inhibition or genetic ablation of aldose reductase increased lesion formation. ApoE null mice accumulated the aldose reductase substrate 4-hydroxy trans-2-nonenal (HNE) in plasma and protein-HNE adducts in arterial lesions less than aldose reductase/apoE double null mice. Thus, aldose reductase was upregulated in atherosclerotic lesions and may protect against early stages of atherogenesis by removing toxic aldehydes generated in oxidized lipids. Antioxidant mechanisms that may contribute to protect from progression of atherosclerosis involve superoxide dismutase and catalase. However, some recent studies implicate other enzymes, such as heme oxygenase (HO)-1, which is the rate-limiting enzyme in the catabolism of heme, leading to generation of the antioxidant biliverdin, iron, and carbon monoxide (see Vol. II, Chapter 11). HO-1 has antioxidant and anti-inflammatory activity that contributes to antiatherogenic effects. Deficiency of HO-1 expression in macrophages of HO-1 null mice was associated with enhanced ROS formation and increased proinflammatory cytokines such as MCP-1 and IL-6 [205]. As well, there was increased foam cell formation when treated with oxLDL. Reconstitution of irradiated LDL receptor null mice with bone marrow of HO-1 null mice was associated with greater progression of atherosclerosis than with bone marrow of wild type mice, confirming the vascular protective role of HO-1.

Oxidized LDL (oxLDL) is more important than native LDL in atherogenesis. Increased ROS in atherosclerotic arteries contributes to endothelial dysfunction and inflammation. oxLDL is internalized through receptor-mediated pathways that include scavenger receptors

(SR) like class A SR, class B SR type I and CD36, and the lectin-like oxLDL receptor-1 (LOX-1) responsible for binding and uptake of oxLDL in endothelial cells, and which is upregulated in proatherogenic conditions, such as diabetes, hypertension and dyslipidemia. Mehta et al. [206] crossed LOX-1 null mice with LDLR null mice and fed them a high cholesterol diet. Aortic atherosclerosis was much more extensive and inflammatory mediator levels higher in LDLR null than double knockout mice. Anti-inflammatory IL-10 expression and SOD activity were low in the LDLR null mice but not in the double knockout mice. These and other data point toward the interaction of oxidant and antioxidant mechanisms in modulation of LOX-1 effects on atherogenesis.

The proteasome is another less appreciated mechanism that may contribute to protect from oxidative stress and progression of atherosclerosis. Chronic proteasome inhibition in pigs is associated with increased coronary artery oxidative stress and early atherosclerosis [207]. Aging and vascular senescence may also contribute to oxidant stress and low-grade inflammation that accelerate atherosclerosis. In human atheroma, vascular smooth muscle fibrous caps expressed markers of senescence such as senescence-associated α-galactosidase (SAαG) and p16 and p21, which are cyclin-dependent kinase inhibitors (cdkis) not found in normal vessels [208]. Plaques and fibrous cap smooth muscle also had shorter telomeres. Telomere shortening correlated with severity of atherosclerosis. Vascular senescence was mediated by changes in cyclins D/E, p16, p21, and retinoblastoma protein (pRB). Levels of telomerase were low. However, telomerase expression alone rescued plaque vascular cell senescence despite short telomeres, normalizing the cdki/pRB changes. Telomere damage appeared secondary to oxidant stress (see Vol. II, Chapter 24). Oxidants induced premature senescence *in vitro*, with accelerated telomere shortening and reduced telomerase activity. *These data bring together aging, telomerase deficiency and shortened telomeres, oxidative stress and exaggerated atherogenesis via oxidative stress-induced DNA damage leading to inhibition of telomerase and marked telomere shortening.*

8. Antioxidant Therapy and Cardiovascular Disease

Since oxidative stress plays a major role in mediating vascular injury, it is not surprising that there has been great interest in targeting ROS to treat or prevent cardiovascular disease, including atherosclerosis and hypertension, by increasing antioxidant bioavailability through diet or supplements and/or reducing ROS generation through decrease in activity of superoxide-generating enzymes. *The ability of antioxidants to treat conditions associated with oxidative stress, such as hypertension and atherosclerosis, is supported by experimental, observational and epidemiological studies in humans [209-225]. Findings have not however been consistent, with most large trials demonstrating negative effects of antioxidants on cardiovascular outcomes.* A recent study investigating effects of vitamins C and E on the development of hypertension in pregnancy also failed to show any benefit of antioxidant vitamins on hypertension outcomes [226]. However, smaller clinical studies, which were well controlled and which investigated effects of antioxidants specifically on blood pressure demonstrated, in large part, beneficial effects [227-230].

Possible reasons for the failure of primary and secondary prevention trials of antioxidants may relate to insufficient dose or duration of therapy, interactions between antioxidant agents, and lack of cellular access to sites of production or action of ROS [220]. Since patients studied had significant or advanced cardiovascular disease, it may at this stage be impossible to reverse the effects of oxidative stress on the cardiovascular system. As well, many patients were taking aspirin, which has anti-oxidant properties, reducing any additional effects of vitamin C or E. It may also be possible that antioxidants are not getting to the site at which ROS are generated, such as the mitochondria. Finally none of these trials had blood pressure or hypertension as a primary end point. *Based on the current data, it is recommended that the general population should consume a balanced diet with emphasis on antioxidant rich fruits and vegetables and whole grains, such as the DASH diet [231-234].*

9. Other Therapeutic Strategies to Reduce ROS Bioavailability

Theoretically, agents that reduce oxidantformation should be more efficacious than non-specific, inefficient antioxidant vitamin scavengers. This is based on experimental evidence whereit has been demonstrated that inhibition of NADPH oxidase–mediated•O_2^- generation, using pharmacological and gene-targetedstrategies, leads to regression of vascular remodeling, improvedendothelial function, lowering of blood pressure and prevention of atherosclerosis. Harrison and colleagues proposed a new strategy to increase antioxidant capacity without the use of exogenous antioxidants [97]. They suggest that drugs that selectively inhibit MRP1 would prevent cellular glutathione loss and thereby protect against oxidative damage, endothelial dysfunction and hypertension [97]. Another interesting approach is targeting glucose-6-phosphate dehydrogenase (G6PD), which is a source of NADPH, the substrate for NADPH oxidase [235]. Inhibition of G6PD has been shown to ameliorate development of pulmonary hypertension, possibly through decreased oxidative stress. To date only investigational G6PD inhibitors are available.

Some of the beneficial effectsof classical antihypertensive agents such as ß-adrenergicblockers, ACE inhibitors, AT_1 receptor antagonists,and Ca^{2+} channel blockers may be mediated, in part, by decreasingvascular oxidative stress [236-240]. These effects have been attributedto direct inhibition of NADPH oxidase activity and to intrinsic antioxidant propertiesof the drugs. In addition to drugs and diet, an important lifestyle modification that may have cardiovascular protective and blood pressure lowering effects by reducing oxidative stress is exercise. *In experimental models of hypertension and in human patients with coronary artery disease, exercise reduced vascular NADPH oxidase activity and ROS production, ameliorated vascular injury and reduced blood pressure [241]*

Conclusions

Until recently it was thought that ROS were byproducts of cellular metabolism, which induced DNA damage, lipid peroxidation and cell death. However, it is now clear that oxygen free radicals are produced in the vessel wall in a controlled and tightly regulated manner and that they have critical signaling functions that maintain vascular integrity. In hypertension and

Oxidative Stress in Arterial Hypertension and Atherosclerosis 183

atherosclerosis, dysregulation of enzymes such as NADPH oxidase, mitochondria, NOS, xanthine oxidase or SOD that generate $\bullet O_2$, H_2O_2 and $\bullet OH$, or reduced scavenging by endogenous antioxidants, results in increased formation of ROS and consequent oxidative damage. Oxidative stress in hypertension and atherosclerosis contribute to vascular injury by promoting VSMC growth, endothelial dysfunction, inflammation, increased vascular tone and matrix metalloproteinases activation. These processes lead to altered vascular contractility, inflammation and structural remodeling, characteristic features of vessels in hypertension and atherosclerosis. Although inconclusive, clinical data suggest that treatment strategies to alter ROS production may have vascular protective actions. With greater understanding of mechanisms that regulate ROS metabolism and identification of processes that tip the balance to states of oxidative stress which cause vascular injury, it should be possible to target therapies more effectively so that detrimental actions of vascular oxygen free radicals can be reduced and beneficial effects of NO can be enhanced. Such therapies would be useful in the prevention and treatment of many disease processes associated with vascular damage, including hypertension and atherosclerosis.

Acknowledgments

Studies from the author's laboratories were supported by grants 37917 and 82790 (ELS) and 44018 and 57886 (RMT), from the Canadian Institutes of Health Research.

References

[1] G. Zalba, G. San Jose, M.U. Moreno, M.A. Fortuno, A. Fortuno, F.J. Beaumont, J. Diez, Oxidative stress in arterial hypertension: role of NAD(P)H oxidase, *Hypertension* 38(6), 1395-1399 (2001).

[2] U. Landmesser, D.G. Harrison, Oxidative stress and vascular damage in hypertension, *Coronary Artery Dis*ease 12(6), 455-61 (2001).

[3] K.K. Griendling, D. Sorescu, B. Lassegue, M. Ushio-Fukai, Modulation of protein kinase activity and gene expression by reactive oxygen species and their role in vascular physiology and pathophysiology, *Arteriosclerosis, Thrombosis, and Vascular Biology* 20, 2175-2183 (2000).

[4] F. Cosentino, J.C. Sill, Z.S. Katusic, Role of superoxide anions in the mediation of endothelium-dependent contractions, *Hypertension* 23, 229-235 (1994).

[5] R.M. Touyz, E.L. Schiffrin, Ang II-stimulated superoxide production is mediated via phospholipase D in human vascular smooth muscle cells, *Hypertension* 34(4), 976-982 (1999).

[6] A.M. Zafari, M. Ushio-Fukai, M. Akers, K. Griendling, Role of NADH/NADPH oxidase-derived H_2O_2 in angiotensin II-induced vascular hypertrophy, *Hypertension* 32, 488-495 (1998).

[7] G.N. Rao, BC. Berk, Active oxygen species stimulate vascular smooth muscle cell growth and proto-oncogene expression, *Circulation Research* 70, 593-599 (1992).

[8] DG. Harrison, Cellular and molecular mechanisms of endothelial cell dysfunction, *Journal of Clinical Investigation* 100, 2153-2157 (1997).

[9] J.H. Chin, S. Azhar, B.B. Hoffman, Inactivation of endothelium derived relaxing factor by oxidized lipoproteins, *Journal of Clinical Investigation* 89, 10-18 (1992).

[10] M.C. Zimmerman, E. Lazartigues, J.A. Lang, P. Sinnayah, I.M. Ahmad, D.R. Spitz, R.L. Davisson, Superoxide mediates the actions of angiotensin II in the central nervous system, *Circulation Research* 91(11), 1038-1045 (2002).

[11] S. Kerr, J. Brosnan, M. McIntyre, J.L. Reid, A.F. Dominiczak, C.A. Hamilton, Superoxide anion production is increased in a model of genetic hypertension. Role of endothelium, *Hypertension* 33, 1353-1358 (1999).

[12] C.G. Schnackenberg, W. Welch, C.S. Wilcox, Normalization of blood pressure and renal vascular resistance in SHR with a membrane-permeable superoxide dismutase mimetic. Role of nitric oxide, *Hypertension* 32, 59-64 (1999).

[13] X. Chen, R.M. Touyz, J.B. Park, E.L. Schiffrin, Antioxidant effects of vitamins C and E are associated with altered activation of vascular NAD(P)H oxidase and superoxide dismutase in stroke-prone SHR, *Hypertension* 38(2), 606-611 (2001).

[14] A. Quinones-Galvan, A. Pucciarelli, A. Fratta-Pasini, U. Garbin, F. Franzoni, F. Galetta, A. Natali, L. Cominacini, E. Ferrannini, Effective blood pressure treatment improves LDL-cholesterol susceptibility to oxidation in patients with essential hypertension, *Journal of Internal Medicine* 250(4), 322-326 (2001).

[15] J.C. Romero, J.F. Reckelhoff, Role of angiotensin and oxidative stress in essential hypertension, *Hypertension* 34(4), 943-949 (1999).

[16] K.M. Hoagland, K.G. Maier, R.J. Roman, Contributions of 20-HETE to the antihypertensive effects of Tempol in Dahl salt-sensitive rats, *Hypertension* 41(3 Pt 2), 697-702 (2003).

[17] R.C. Sharma, H.N. Hodis, W.J. Mack, Probucol suppresses oxidant stress in hypertensive arteries. Immunohistochemical evidence, *American. Journal of Hypertenion* 9, 577-590 (1996).

[18] J.K. Bendall, A.C. Cave, C. Heymes, N. Gall, A.M. Shah, Pivotal role of a gp91(phox)-containing NADPH oxidase in angiotensin II-induced cardiac hypertrophy in mice, *Circulation* 105(3), 293-296 (2002).

[19] J.M. Li, A.M. Shah, Mechanism of endothelial cell NADPH oxidase activation by angiotensin II. Role of the p47phox subunit, *Journal of Biochemical Chemisty* 278(14), 12094-12100. (2003).

[20] C.Berry, C.A. Hamilton, M.J. Brosnan, F.G. Magill, G.A. Berg, J.J. McMurray, A.F. Dominiczak, Investigation into the sources of superoxide in human blood vessels: angiotensin II increases superoxide production in human internal mammary arteries, *Circulation* 101(18), 2206-2212 (2000).

[21] H.E. Lob, P.J. Marvar, T.J. Guzik, S. Sharma, L.A. McCann, C. Weyand, F.J. Gordon, D.G. Harrison. Induction of hypertension and peripheral inflammation by reduction of extracellular superoxide dismutase in the central nervous system. *Hypertension.* 55(2):277-283 (2010).

[22] Priviero, S.M. Zemse, C.E. Teixeira, R.C. Webb, Oxidative stress impairs vasorelaxation induced by the soluble guanylyl cyclase activator BAY 41-2272 in spontaneously hypertensive rats. *American Journal of Hypertension* 22(5), 493-9 (2009).

[23] M.S. Zhou, I.H. Schulman, L. Raij, Role of angiotensin II and oxidative stress in vascular insulin resistance linked to hypertension, *American Journal* of *Physiology, Heart* and *Circulatory Physiology* 296(3), H833-839 (2009).

[24] E.J. Cantor, E.V. Mancini, R. Seth, X.H. Yao, T. Netticadan, Oxidative stress and heart disease: cardiac dysfunction, nutrition, and gene therapy, *Current Hypertension Report* 5(3), 215-220 (2003).

[25] J. Zanzinger, Mechanisms of action of nitric oxide in the brain stem: role of oxidative stress, *Autonomic Neuroscience* 98(1-2), 24-27 (2002).

[26] C.S. Wilcox, Reactive oxygen species: roles in blood pressure and kidney function, *Current Hypertension Report* 4, 160-166 (2002).

[27] J.H. Oak, J.Y. Youn,H. Cai, Aminoguanidine inhibits aortic hydrogen peroxide production, VSMC NOX activity and hypercontractility in diabetic mice. *Cardiovascular Diabetology* 8, 65-69 (2009).

[28] K.M. Channon, T.J. Guzik, Mechanisms of superoxide production in human blood vessels: relationship to endothelial dysfunction, clinical and genetic risk factors, *Journal of Physiology and Pharmacology* 53(4), 515-524 (2002).

[29] H. Cai, D.G. Harrison, Endothelial dysfunction in cardiovascular diseases: the role of oxidant stress, *Circulation Research* 87, 840-844 (2000).

[30] D. Wang, S. Hope, Y. Du, Paracrine role of adventitial superoxide anion in a model of genetic hypertension. Role of endothelium, *Hypertension* 33, 1353-1358 (1999).

[31] D. Sorescu, D. Weiss, B. Lassegue, R.E. Clempus, K. Szocs, G.P. Sorescu, L. Valppu, M.T. Quinn, J.D. Lambeth, J.D. Vega, W.R. Taylor, K.K. Griendling, Superoxide production and expression of nox family proteins in human atherosclerosis, *Circulation* 105(12), 1429-1435 (2002).

[32] J-I. Abe, B.C. Berk, Reactive oxygen species of signal transduction in cardiovascular disease, *Trends* in *Cardiovascular Medicine* 8, 59-64 (1998).

[33] S. Rajagopalan, S. Kurz, T. Munzel, Angiotensin II mediated hypertension in the rat increases vascular superoxide production via membrane NADH/NADPH oxidase activation: contribution to alterations of vasomotor tone, *Journal of Clinical Investigation* 97, 1916-1923 (1996).

[34] S.A. Jones, V.B. O'Donnell, J.D. Wood, Expression of phagocyte NADPH oxidase components in human endothelial cells, *American Journal of Physiology- Heart and Circulatory Physiology* 100, H1626-H1634 (1996).

[35] H. Suzuki, F.A. DeLano, D.A. Parks, N. Jamshidi, D.N. Granger, H. Ishii et al. Xanthine oxidase activity associated with arterial blood pressure in spontaneously hypertensive rats, *Proceedings of the National Academy of Sciences of the United States of America* 95, 4754-4759 (1998).

[36] F.A. Delano, D.A. Parks, J.M., Ruedi, B.M. Babior, G.W. Schmid-Schonbein Microvascular display of xanthine oxidase and NAD(P)H oxidase in the spontaneously hypertensive rat, *Microcirculation* 13(7), 551-566 (2006).

[37] E.M. Mervaala, Z.J. Cheng, I. Tikkanen, R. Lapatto, K. Nurminen, H. Vapaatalo et al. Endothelial dysfunction and xanthine oxidoreductase activity in rats with human renin and angiotensinogen genes, *Hypertension* 37, 414-418 (2001).

[38] J. Laakso, E. Mervaala, J.J. Himberg, T.L. Teravainen, H. Karppanen, H. Vapaatalo et al. Increased kidney xanthine oxidoreductase activity in salt-induced experimental hypertension. *Hypertension* 32, 902-906. (1998).

[39]	Cosentino, J.E. Barker, M.P. Brand, S.J. Heales, E.R. Werner, J.R. Tippins, N. West, K.M. Channon, M. Volpe, T.F. Luscher, Reactive oxygen species mediate endothelium-dependent relaxations in tetrahydrobiopterin-deficient mice, *Arteriosclerosis, Thrombosis, and Vascular Biology* 21(4), 496-502 (2001).

[40]	U. Landmesser, S. Dikalov, S.R. Price, L. McCann, T. Fukai, S.M. Holland, W.E. Mitch, D.G. Harrison, Oxidation of tetrahydrobiopterin leads to uncoupling of endothelial cell nitric oxide synthase in hypertension, *The Journal of Clinical Investigation* 111(8), 1201-1209 (2003).

[41]	P. J. Andrew, B. Mayer. Enzymatic function of nitric oxide synthases. *Cardiovascular Research* 43, 521-531 (1999).

[42]	Y.H. Du, Y.Y. Guan, N.J. Alp, K.M. Channon, A.F. Chen, Endothelium-specific GTP cyclohydrolase I overexpression attenuates blood pressure progression in salt-sensitive low-renin hypertension, *Circulation* 117(8), 1045-54 (2008).

[43]	A.L. Moens, E. Takimoto, C.G. Tocchetti, K. Chakir, D. Bedja, G. Cormaci, E.A. Ketner, M. Majmudar, K. Gabrielson, M.K. Halushka, J.B. Mitchell, S. Biswal, K.M. Channon, M.S. Wolin, N.J. Alp, N. Paolocci, H.C. Champion, D.A. Kass, Reversal of cardiac hypertrophy and fibrosis from pressure overload by tetrahydrobiopterin: efficacy of recoupling nitric oxide synthase as a therapeutic strategy, *Circulation* 117(20), 2626-2636 (2008).

[44]	J. Ketonen, E. Mervaala, Effects of dietary sodium on reactive oxygen species formation and endothelial dysfunction in low-density lipoprotein receptor-deficient mice on high-fat diet, *Heart Vessels* 23(6), 420-429 (2008).

[45]	A. Boveris, B. Chance, The mitochondrial generation of hydrogen peroxide. General properties and effect of hyperbaric oxygen, *Biochemical Journal* 134(3), 707-716 (1973).

[46]	M. Mari, F. Caballero, A. Colell, A. Morales, J. Caballeria, A. Fernandez, C. Enrich, J.C. Fernandez-Checa, C. Garcia-Ruiz,Mitochondrial free cholesterol loading sensitizes to TNF- and Fas-mediated steatohepatitis, *Cell Metabolism* 4(3), 185-198 (2006).

[47]	J. Wosniak, C.X. Santos, A.J. Kowaltowski, F.R. Laurindo, Cross-Talk Between Mitochondria and NAD(P)H Oxidase: Effects of Mild Mitochondrial Dysfunction on Angiotensin II-Mediated Increase in Nox Isoform Expression and Activity in Vascular Smooth Muscle Cells, *Antioxidants and Redox Signaling* 11(6), 1265-78 (2009).

[48]	S. Alvarez, L.B. Valdez, T. Zaobornyj, A. Boveris, Oxygen dependence of mitochondrial nitric oxide synthase activity, *Biochemical and Biophysical Research Communications* 305(3),771-775 (2003).

[49]	G.X. Zhang, X.M. Lu, S. Kimura, A. Nishiyama, Role of mitochondria in angiotensin II-induced reactive oxygen species and mitogen-activated protein kinase activation, *Cardiovasular Research* 76(2), 204-212 (2007).

[50]	V.C. De Giusti, M.V. Correa, M.C. Villa-Abrille, C. Beltrano, A.M. Yeves, G.E. de Cingolani, H.E. Cingolani, E.A. Aiello, The positive inotropic effect of endothelin-1 is mediated by mitochondrial reactive oxygen species, *Life Science* 83(7-8), 264-271 (2008).

[51]	Z.Ungvari, N. Labinskyy, S. Gupte, P.N. Chander, J.G. Edwards, A. Csisz, Dysregulation of mitochondrial biogenesis in vascular endothelial and smooth muscle cells of aged rats, *The American Journal of Physiology - Heartand Circulatory Physiology* 294(5), H2121-2128 (2008).

[52] A.K. Doughan, D.G. Harrison, S.I. Dikalov, Molecular mechanisms of angiotensin II-mediated mitochondrial dysfunction: linking mitochondrial oxidative damage and vascular endothelial dysfunction, *Circulation Research* 102(4), 488-96 (2008).

[53] B. Lassegue, R.E. Clempus, Vascular NAD(P)H oxidases: specific features, expression, and regulation, *American Journal of Physiology - Regulatory, Integrative and Comparative Physiology* 285(2), R277-R297 (2003).

[54] H. Azumimi, N. Inoue, S. Takeshita, Expression of NADH/NADPH oxidase p22phox in human coronary arteries, *Circulation*100, 1494-1498 (1999).

[55] K.K. Griendling, D. Sorescu, M. Ushio-Fukai, NAD(P)H oxidase: role in cardiovascular biology and disease, *Circulation Research*86, 494-501 (2000).

[56] B.M. Babior, J.D. Lambeth, W. Nauseef, The neutrophil NADPH oxidase, *Archives of Biochemistry and Biophysics*397, 342-344 (2002).

[57] M. Geiszt, A. Kapus, E. Ligeti, Chronic granulomatous disease: more than the lack of superoxide? *Journal of Leukocyte Biology* 69(2), 191-196 (2001).

[58] R.M. Touyz, G. Yao, M.T. Quinn, P.J. Pagano, E.L. Schiffrin, p47phox associates with the cytoskeleton through cortactin in human vascular smooth muscle cells: role in NAD(P)H oxidase regulation by angiotensin II. *Arteriosclerosis, Thrombosis, and Vascular Biology* 25(3), 512-518 (2005).

[59] F.E. Rey, P.J. Pagano, The reactive adventitia: fibroblast oxidase in vascular function, *Arteriosclerosis, Thrombosis, and Vascular Biology* 22(12), 1962-1971 (2002).

[60] R.M. Touyz, g. Yao, E.L. Schiffrin, c-Src induces phosphorylation and translocation of p47phox: role in superoxide generation by angiotensin II in human vascular smooth muscle cells. *Arteriosclerosis, Thrombosis, and Vascular Biology* 23, 981-987 (2003).

[61] K.K. Griendling, C.A. Minieri, J.D. Ollerenshaw, R.W. Alexander, Angiotensin II stimulates NADH and NADPH oxidase activity in cultured vascular smooth muscle cells, *Circulation Research* 74(6), 1141-1148 (1994).

[62] P.N. Seshiah, D.S. Weber, P. Rocic, L. Valppu, Y. Taniyama, K.K. Griendling, Angiotensin II stimulation of NAD(P)H oxidase activity. Upstream mediators, *Circulation Research* 91, 406-413 (2002).

[63] R.M. Touyz, G. Yao, E.L. Schiffrin, c-Src Induces Phosphorylation and Translocation of p47phox: Role in Superoxide Generation by Angiotensin II in Human Vascular Smooth Muscle Cells, *Arteriosclerosis, Thrombosis, and Vascular Biology* 23(6), 981-987 (2003).

[64] K. Bedard, K.H Krause.The NOX family of ROS-generating NADPH oxidases: physiology and pathophysiology, *Physiological Review* 87(1), 245-313 (2007)

[65] M. Geiszt, NADPH oxidases: New kids on the block. *Cardiovascular Research* 71, 289-299 (2006).

[66] H. Sumimoto, K. Miyano, R. Takeya. Molecular composition and regulation of the Nox family NAD(P)H oxidases, *Biochemical and Biophysical Research Communications* 338(1), 677-86 (2005)

[67] Y.A. Suh, R.S. Arnold, B. Lassegue, Cell transformation by the superoxide-generating Mox-1, *Nature* 410, 79-82 (1999).

[68] R.M. Touyz, X. Chen, G. He, M.T. Quinn, E.L. Schiffrin, Expression of a gp91phox-containing leukocyte-type NADPH oxidase in human vascular smooth muscle cells – modulation by Ang II, *Circulation Research* 90, 1205-1213 (2002).

[69] T. Ueyama, K. Lekstrom, S. Tsujibe, N. Saito, T.L. Leto, Subcellular localization and function of alternatively spliced Noxo1 isoforms, *Free Radical Biology and Medicine* 42(2), 180-90 (2007).

[70] K. Matsuno, H. Yamada, K. Iwata, D. Jin, M. Katsuyama, M. Matsuki, S. Takai, K. Yamanishi, M. Miyazaki, H. Matsubara, C. Yabe-Nishimura. Nox1 is involved in angiotensin II-mediated hypertension: a study in Nox1-deficient mice, *Circulation* 112(17), 2677-85 (2005).

[71] A. Dikalova, R. Clempus, B. Lassegue, G. Cheng, J. McCoy, S. Dikalov, A. San Martin, A. Lyle, D.S. Weber, D. Weiss, W.R. Taylor, H.H. Schmidt, G.K. Owens, J.D. Lambeth, K.K. Griendling Nox1 overexpression potentiates angiotensin II-induced hypertension and vascular smooth muscle hypertrophy in transgenic mice, *Circulation.* 112(17), 2668-76 (2005).

[72] R.M. Touyz, C. Mercure, Y. He, D. Javeshghani, G. Yao, G.E. Callera, A. Yogi, N. Lochard, T.L. Reudelhuber. Angiotensin II-dependent chronic hypertension and cardiac hypertrophy are unaffected by gp91phox-containing NADPH oxidase, *Hypertension.* 45(4), 530-7(2005).

[73] Gavazzi, B. Banfi, C. Deffert, L. Fiette, M. Schappi, F. Herrmann, K.H. Krause KH, Decreased bloodpressure in NOX1-deficient mice, *FEBS Letters* 580(2), 497-504 (2006).

[74] K. Matsuno, H. Yamada, K. Iwata, D. Jin, M. Katsuyama, M. Matsuki, S. Takai, K. Yamanishi, M. Miyazaki, H. Matsubara, C. Yabe-Nishimura, Nox1 is involved in angiotensin II-mediated hypertension: a study in Nox1-deficient mice, *Circulation* 112(17), 2677-85 (2005).

[75] L.L. Hilenski, Clempus RE, Quinn MT, Lambeth JD, Griendling KK. Distinct subcellular localizations of Nox1 and Nox4 in vascular smooth muscle cells, *Arteriosclerosis, Thrombosis, and Vascular Biology* 24, 677–683 (2004).

[76] R.E. Clempus, D. Sorescu, A.E. Dikalova, L. Pounkova, P. Jo, G.P. Sorescu, H.H. Schmidt, B. Lassegue, K.K. Griendling, Nox4 is required for maintenance of the differentiated vascular smooth muscle cell phenotype. *Arteriosclerosis, Thrombosis, and Vascular Biology* 27, 42–48 (2007).

[77] A.N. Lyle, N.N. Deshpande, Y. Taniyama, B. Seidel-Rogol, L. Pounkova, P. Du, C. Papaharalambus, B. Lassègue, K.K. Griendling, Poldip2, a Novel Regulator of Nox4 and Cytoskeletal Integrity in Vascular Smooth Muscle Cells, *Circulation Research* 105, 249-259 (2009).

[78] L. Serrander, V. Jaquet, K. Bedard, O. Plastre, O. Hartley, S. Arnaudeau, N. Demaurex, W. Schlegel, K.H. Krause, NOX5 is expressed at the plasma membrane and generates superoxide in response to protein kinase C activation, *Biochimie* 89(9), 1159-1167 (2007).

[79] R.S. BelAiba, T. Djordjevic, A. Petry, K. Diemer, S. Bonello, B. Banfi, J. Hess, A. Pogrebniak, C. Bickel, A. Görlach, NOX5 variants are functionally active in endothelial cells, *Free Radical Biology and Medicine* 42(4), 446-459 (2007).

[80] D. Jagnandan, J.E. Church, B. Banfi, D.J. Stuehr, M.B. Marrero, D.J. Fulton, Novel mechanism of activation of NAD(P)H oxidase 5. calcium sensitization via phosphorylation, *Journal of Biological Chemistry* 282(9), 6494-6507 (2007).

[81] Tirone, J.A. Cox, NAD(P)H oxidase 5 (NOX5) interacts with and is regulated by calmodulin. *FEBS Letters* 581(6), 1202-1208 (2007).

[82] D. B. Jay, C.A. Papaharalambus, B. Seidel-Rogol, A.E. Dikalova, B. Lassègue, K.K. Griendling, Nox5 mediates PDGF-induced proliferation in human aortic smooth muscle cells. *Free Radical Biology and Medicine* 45(3), 329-335 (2008).

[83] E. Schulz, T. Münzel, NOX5, a new "radical" player in human atherosclerosis? *Journal of American College of Cardiology* 52(22), 1810-1812 (208).

[84] A.C. Montezano, D. Burger, T.M. Paravicini, A.Z. Chignalia, H. Yusuf, M. Almasri , Y. He, G.E. Callera, G. He, K.H. Krause, D. Lambeth, M.T. Quinn, R.M. Touyz, Nicotinamide adenine dinucleotide phosphate reduced oxidase 5 (Nox5) regulation by angiotensin II and endothelin-1 is mediated via calcium/calmodulin-dependent, rac-1-independent pathways in human endothelial cells, *Circulation Research* 106(8), 1363-1373 (2010).

[85] H. Ohye, M. Sugawara, Dual oxidase, hydrogen peroxide and thyroid diseases. *Experimental biology and medicine (Maywood, N.J.)* 235(4), 424-433 (2010).

[86] R.P. Brandes, F.J. Miller, S. Beer, J. Haendeler, J. Hoffmann, T. Ha, S.M. Holland, A. Gorlach, R. Busse, The vascular NADPH oxidase subunit p47phox is involved in redox-mediated gene expression, *Free Radical Biology and Medicine* 32(11), 1116-1122 (2002).

[87] K.T. Moe, S. Aulia, F. Jiang, Y.L. Chua, T.H. Koh, M.C. Wong, G.J. Dusting. Differential upregulation of Nox homologues of NADPH oxidase by tumor necrosis factor-alpha in human aortic smooth muscle and embryonic kidney cells. *Journal of Cellular and MolecularMedicine* 10(1), 231-239 (2006).

[88] Q.N. Diep, F. Amiri, R.M. Touyz, J.S. Cohn, D. Endemann, M.F. Neves, E.L. Schiffrin, PPARalpha activator effects on Ang II-induced vascular oxidative stress and inflammation, *Hypertension* 40(6), 866-871 (2002).

[89] P. Dandona, R. Karne, H. Ghanim, W. Hamouda, A. Aljada, C.H. Magsino, Carvedilol inhibits reactive oxygen species generation by leukocytes and oxidative damage to amino acids, *Circulation*101, 122-124 (2000).

[90] K. Grote, I. Flach, M. Luchtefeld, E. Akin, S.M. Holland, H. Drexler, B. Schieffer, Mechanical stretch enhances mRNA expression and proenzyme release of matrix metalloproteinase-2 (MMP-2) via NAD(P)H oxidase-derived reactive oxygen species,*Cirulation Research*92(11), e80-e86 (2003).

[91] S. Wassmann, K. Wassmann, G. Nickenig, Modulation of oxidant and antioxidant enzyme expression and function in vascular cells, *Hypertension* 44(4), 381-386 (2004).

[92] R.K. Sindhu, A. Ehdaie,F. Farmand, K.K. Dhaliwal,T. Nguyen, C.D. Zhan, C.K. Roberts, N.D. Vaziri, Expression of catalase and glutathione peroxidase in renal insufficiency, *Biochimica et Biophysica Acta (BBA)* 1743(1-2), 86-92 (2005).

[93] M. Tajima, Y. Kurashima, K. Sugiyama, T. Ogura, H. Sakagami, The redox state of glutathione regulates the hypoxic induction of HIF-1, *The European Journal of Pharmacology* 606(1-3), 45-49 (2009).

[94] P. Stralin, K. Karlsson, B.O. Johannson, S.L. Marklund, The interstitium of the human arterial wall contains very large amounts of extracellular superoxide dismutase, *Arteriosclerosis, Thrombosis, and Vascular Biology* 15, 2032-2036 (1995).

[95] M. McIntyre, D.F. Bohr, A.F. Dominiczak, Endothelial function in hypertension. The role of superoxide anion, *Hypertension* 34, 539-545 (1999).

[96] S.S. Chung, M. Kim, B.S. Youn, N.S. Lee, J.W. Park, I.K. Lee, Y.S. Lee, J.B. Kim, Y.M. Cho, H.K. Lee, K.S. Park, Glutathione peroxidase 3 mediates the antioxidant effect of peroxisome proliferator-activated receptor gamma in human skeletal muscle cells, *Molecular and Cellular Biology* 29(1), 20-30 (2009).

[97] J. D. Widder, T.J. Guzik, C.F. Mueller, R.E. Clempus, H.H. Schmidt, S.I. Dikalov, K.K. Griendling, D.P. Jones, D.G. Harrison, Role of the multidrug resistance protein-1 in hypertension and vascular dysfunction caused by angiotensin II. *Arteriosclerosis, Thrombosis, and Vascular Biology* 27(4), 762-768 (2007).

[98] C.F. Mueller, K. Wassmann, J.D. Widder, S. Wassmann, C.H. Chen, B. Keuler, A. Kudin, W.S. Kunz, G. Nickenig, Multidrug resistance protein-1 affects oxidative stress, endothelial dysfunction, and atherogenesis via leukotriene C4 export. *Circulation* 117(22), 2912-2918 (2008).

[99] M. Zamocky, P.G. Furtmüller, C. Obinger, Evolution of catalases from bacteria to humans, *Antioxidants andRedox Signaling* 10(9), 1527-1548 (2008).

[100] C.S. Wilcox, A. Pearlman, Chemistry and antihypertensive effects of tempol and other nitroxides, *Pharmacological Reviews* 60(4), 418-469 (2008).

[101] S. Chrissobolis, S.P. Didion, D.A. Kinzenbaw, L.I. Schrader, S. Dayal, S.R. Lentz, F.M. Faraci, Glutathione peroxidase-1 plays a major role in protecting against angiotensin II-induced vascular dysfunction, *Hypertension* 51(4), 872-877 (2008).

[102] T. Ebrahimian, R.M. Touyz, Thioredoxin in vascular biology: role in hypertension. *Antioxidants and Redox Signaling* 10(6), 1127-1136 (2008).

[103] J. Redon, M.R. Oliva, C. Tormos, V. Giner, J. Chaves, A. Iradi et a, Antioxidant activities and oxidative stress byproducts in human hypertension, *Hypertension* 41, 1096-1101 (2003).

[104] W.J. Welch, T. Chabrashvili, G. Solis, Y. Chen, P.S. Gill, S. Aslam, X. Wang,H. Ji, K. Sandberg, P, Jose, C.S. Wilcox, Role of extracellular superoxide dismutase in the mouse angiotensin slow pressor response, *Hypertension* 48(5), 934-941 (2006).

[105] D. Javeshghani, E.L. Schiffrin, M.R. Sairam, R.M. Touyz, Potentiation of vascular oxidative stress and nitric oxide-mediated endothelial dysfunction by high-fat diet in a mouse model of estrogen deficiency and hyperandrogenemia, *Journal of American Society of Hypertension* 3(5), 295-305 (2009).

[106] P.R. Augusti, G.M. Conterato, S. Somacal, R. Sobieski, A. Quatrin, L. Maurer, M.P. Rocha, I.T. Denardin, T. Emanuelli, Astaxanthin reduces oxidative stress, but not aortic damage in atherosclerotic rabbits, *Journal ofCardiovascular Pharmacologyand Therapeutics* 14(4), 314-322 (2009).

[107] W. Droge, Free radicals in the physiological control of cell function, *Physiological Reviews* 82, 47-95 (2001).

[108] K.K. Griendling, D.G. Harrison, Dual role of reactive oxygen species in vascular growth, *Circulation Research* 85, 562-563 (1999).

[109] K.T. Turpaev, Reactive Oxygen Species and Regulation of Gene Expression, *Biochemistry* 67(3), 281-292 (2002).

[110] S.R. Lee, K.S. Kwon, S.R. Kim, S.G. Rhee, Reversible inactivation of protein-tyrosine phosphatase 1B in A431 cells stimulated with epidermal growth factor, *Journal of Biological Chem*istry 273(25), 15366-153372 (1998).

[111] T.C. Meng, T. Fukada, N.K. Tonks, Reversible oxidation and inactivation of protein tyrosine phosphatases in vivo, *Molecular Cell* 9(2), 387-399 (2002).

[112] F. Tabet, E.L. Schiffrin, G.E. Callera, Y. He, G. Yao, A. Ostman, K. Kappert, N.K. Tonks, R.M. Touyz, Redox-sensitive signaling by angiotensin II involves oxidative inactivation and blunted phosphorylation of protein tyrosine phosphatase SHP-2 in vascular smooth muscle cells from SHR, *Circulation Research* 103(2), 149-158 (2008).

[113] J.J. Haddad, Antioxidant and prooxidant mechanisms in the regulation of redox(y)-sensitive transcription factors, *Cellular Signaling* 14(11), 879-897 (2002).

[114] Y.R. Seo, M.R. Kelley, M.L. Smith, Selenomethionine regulation of p53 by a refl-dependent redox mechanism, *Proceedings of the National Academy of Sciences of the United States of America* 99(22), 14548-14553 (2002).

[115] G. Fritz, Human APE/Ref-1 protein, *The International Journal of Biochemistry* and *Cell Biology* 32(9), 925-929 (2000).

[116] J.N. Anderson, O.H. Mortensen, G.H. Peters, P.G. Drake, L.F. Iversen, OH Olsen, P.G. Jansen, H.S. Andersen, N.K. Tonks, N.P. Moller, Structural and evolutionary relationships among protein tyrosine phosphatase domains, *Molecular and Cellular Biology* 21, 7117-7136 (2001).

[117] J.M. Denu, K.G. Tanner, Specific and reversible inactivation of protein tyrosine phosphatases by hydrogen peroxide: evidence for a sulfenic acid intermediate and implications for redox regulation, *Biochemistry7*, 5633-5642 (1998).

[118] C. Blanchetot, L.G.J. Tertoolen, J.D. Hertog, Regulation of receptor protein tyrosine phosphatase α by oxidative stress, *EMBO Journal* 21(4), 493-503 (2002).

[119] H. Kamata, Y. Shibukawa, S-I. Oka, H. Hirata, Epidermal growth factor receptor is modulated by redox through multiple mechanisms. Effects of reductants and H_2O_2, *European Journal of Biochemistry* 267, 1933-1944 (2000).

[120] K. Lee, W.J. Esselman, Inhibition of PTPS by H_2O_2 regulates the activation of distinct MAPK pathways, *Free Radical Biology and Medicine* 33(8), 1121-1132 (2002).

[121] R.M. Touyz, X.H. Wu, G. He, S. Salomon, E.L. Schiffrin, Increased angiotensin II-mediated Src signaling via epidermal growth factor receptor transactivation is associated with decreased C-terminal Src kinase activity in vascular smooth muscle cells from spontaneously hypertensive rats, *Hypertension* 39(2 Pt 2), 479-485 (2002).

[122] R.M. Touyz, E.L. Schiffrin, Signal transduction mechanisms mediating the physiological and pathophysiological actions of angiotensin II in vascular smooth muscle cells, *Pharmacological Reviews* 52(4), 639-672 (2000).

[123] G. Pearson, F. Robinson, T. Beers Gibson, Mitogen-activated protein kinase pathways: regulation and physiological functions, *Endocrine Reviews* 22(2), 153-183 (2001).

[124] Q. Xu, Y. Liu, M. Gorospe, Acute hypertension activates mitogen-activated protein kinases in arterial wall, *Journal of Clinical Investigations* 97(2), 508-514 (1996).

[125] R.M. Touyz, C. Deschepper, J.B. Park, E.L. Schiffrin, Inhibition of mitogen-activated protein/extracellular signal-regulated kinase improves endothelial function and attenuates Ang II-induced contractility of mesenteric resistance arteries from spontaneously hypertensive rats, *Journal of Hypertens*ion 20(6), 1127-1134 (2002).

[126] M. Torres. Mitogen-activated protein kinase pathway in redox signaling, *Frontiers in Bioscience* 8, 369-391 (2003).

[127] M. Ushio-Fukai, R.W. Alexander, M. Akers, K.K. Griendling, p38 Mitogen-activated protein kinase is a critical component of the redox-sensitive signaling pathways activated by angiotensin II. Role in vascular smooth muscle cell hypertrophy, *Journal of Biological. Chemistry* 273(24), 15022-15029 (1998).

[128] R.M. Touyz, M. Cruzado, F. Tabet, G. Yao, S. Salomon, E.L. Schiffrin, Redox-dependent MAP kinase signaling by Ang II in vascular smooth muscle cells – role of receptor tyrosine kinase transactivation, *Canadian Journal of Physiology and Pharmacology* 81, 159-167 (2003).

[129] K.M. Lounsbury, Q. Hu, R.C. Ziegelstein, Calcium signaling and oxidant stress in the vasculature, *Free Radical Biology and Medicine* 28(9), 1362-1369 (2000).

[130] Y.J. Gao, R.M. Lee, Hydrogen peroxide induces a greater contraction in mesenteric arteries of spontaneously hypertensive rats through thromboxane A(2) production, *British Journal of Pharmacology* 134(8), 1639-1646 (2001).

[131] F. Tabet, C. Savoia, E.L. Schiffrin, R.M. Touyz, Differential calcium regulation by hydrogen peroxide and superoxide in vascular smooth muscle cells from spontaneously hypertensive rats, *Journal of Cardiovascula Pharmacology* 44(2), 200-208 (2004).

[132] S. Rajagopalan, X.P. Meng, S. Ramasamy, D.G. Harrison, Z.S. Galis, Reactive oxygen species produced by macrophage-derived foam cells regulate the activity of vascular matrix metalloproteinases in vitro, *J. Clin. Invest.* 98, 2572-2579 (1996).

[133] D.N. Muller, R. Dechend, E.M.A. Mervaala, J.K. Park, F. Schmidt, A. Fiebeler et al, NFκB inhibition ameliorates Angiotensin II-induced inflammatory damage in rats, *Hypertension* 35(1 Pt 2), 193-201 (200).

[134] F.C. Luft, Mechanisms and cardiovascular damage in hypertension, *Hypertension* 37, 594-598 (2001).

[135] M. Tschudi, S. Mesaros, T.F. Luscher, T. Malinski, Direct in situ measurement of nitric oxide in mesenteric resistance arteries: increased decomposition by superoxide in hypertension, *Hypertension* 27, 32-35 (1996).

[136] C. Szabo, Multiple pathways of peroxynitrite cytotoxicity, *Toxicology Letters* 140, 105-112 (2003).

[137] B. Kristal, R. Shurta-Swirrski, J. Chezar, Participation of peripheral polymorphonuclear leukocytes in the oxidative stress and inflammation in patiemnts with essential hypertension, *American Journal of Hypertenion* 11, 921-928 (1998).

[138] R.W. Alexander, Hypertension and the pathogenesis of atherosclerosis. Oxidative stress and the mediation of arterial inflammatory response: a new perspective, *Hypertension* 25, 155-161 (1995).

[139] A.M. Nuyt, Mechanisms underlying developmental programming of elevated blood pressure and vascular dysfunction: evidence from human studies and experimental animal models. *Clinical Science (London)* 114(1), 1-17 (2008).

[140] R.S. Friese, P. Mahboubi, N.R. Mahapatra, S. K. Mahata, N. J. Schork, G. W. Schmid-Schönbein, D.T. O'Connor, Common genetic mechanisms of blood pressure elevation in two independent rodent models of human essential hypertension. *American Journal of Hypertension* 18(5 Pt 1), 633-652 (2005).

[141] J. Török, Participation of nitric oxide in different models of experimental hypertension. *Physiological Research* 57(6), 813-825 (2008).

[142] E.C. Viel, K. Benkirane, D. Javeshghani, R.M. Touyz, E.L. Schiffrin, Xanthine oxidase and mitochondria contribute to vascular superoxide anion generation in DOCA-salt hypertensive rats. *The American Journal of Physiology - Heartand Circulatory Physiology* 295(1), H281-288 (2008).

[143] P. Puddu, G.M. Puddu, E. Cravero, M. Rosati, A. Muscari, The molecular sources of reactive oxygen species in hypertension. *Blood Pressure* 17(2), 70-77 (2008).

[144] R.D. Roghair, J.L. Segar, K.A. Volk, M.W. Chapleau, L.M. Dallas, A.R. Sorenson, T. D. Scholz, F.S. Lamb, Vascular nitric oxide and superoxide anion contribute to sex-specific programmed cardiovascular physiology in mice. *American Journal of Physiology - Regulatory, Integrative and Comparative Physiology* 296(3), R651-662 (2009).

[145] R.M. Touyz, Oxidative stress and vascular damage in hypertension, *Current Hypertension Report* 2, 98-105 (2000).

[146] A.Virdis, M.F. Neves, F. Amiri, R. M. Touyz, E. L. Schiffrin, Role of NAD(P)H oxidase on vascular alterations in angiotensin II-infused mice, *Journal of Hypertension* 22, 535-542 (2004).

[147] R. E. Nisbet, A.S. Graves, D.J. Kleinhenz, H.L. Rupnow,A. L. Reed, T. H. Fan, P.O. Mitchell, R.L. Sutliff, C.M. Hart, The role of NAD(P)H oxidase in chronic intermittent hypoxia-induced pulmonary hypertension in mice, *American Journal of Respiratory Cell and MolecularBiology* 40(5), 601-609 (2009).

[148] P. Modlinger, T. Chabrashvili, P.S. Gill, M. Mendonca, D.G. Harrison, K.K. Griendling, M. Li, J. Raggio, A. Wellstein, Y. Chen, W.J. Welch, C.S. Wilcox, RNA silencing in vivo reveals role of p22phox in rat angiotensin slow pressor response, *Hypertension* 47(2), 238-244 (2006).

[149] K. Laude, H. Cai, B. Fink, N. Hoch, D.S. Weber, L. McCann, G. Kojda, T. Fukai, H.H. Schmidt, S. Dikalov, S. Ramasamy, G. Gamez, K.K. Griendling, D.G. Harrison, Hemodynamic and biochemical adaptations to vascular smooth muscle overexpression of p22phox in mice, *The American Journal of Physiology - Heartand Circulatory Physiology* 288(1), H7-12 (2005).

[150] F.E. Rey, M.E. Cifuentes, A. Kiarash, M.T. Quinn, P.J. Pagano, Novel competitive inhibitor of NAD(P)H oxidase assembly attenuates vascular O_2^{-} and systolic blood pressure in mice, *Circulation Research* 89, 408-414 (2001).

[151] K. Matsuno, H. Yamada, K. Iwata,D. Jin, M. Katsuyama, M. Matsuki, S. Takai, K. Yamanishi, M. Miyazaki, H. Matsubara, C. Yabe-Nishimura, Nox1 is involved in angiotensin II-mediated hypertension: a study in Nox1-deficient mice, *Circulation* 112(17), 2677-2685 (2005).

[152] A. Dikalova, R. Clempus, B. Lassegue, G. Cheng, J. McCoy, S. Dikalov et al, Nox1 overexpression potentiates angiotensin II-induced hypertension and vascular smooth muscle hypertrophy in transgenic mice *Circulation* 112, 2668-2676 (2005).

[153] Agarwal D, Haque M, Sriramula S, Mariappan N, Pariaut R, Francis J. Role of proinflammatory cytokines and redox homeostasis in exercise-induced delayed progression of hypertension in spontaneously hypertensive rats. *Hypertension.* 54(6):1393-400. (2009).

[154] A. Yogi, C. Mercure, J. Touyz, G.E. Callera, A.C. Montezano, A.B. Aranha, R.C. Tostes, T. Reudelhuber, R.M. Touy, Renal redox-sensitive signaling, but not blood pressure, is attenuated by Nox1 knockout in angiotensin II-dependent chronic hypertension, *Hypertension* 51(2), 500-506 (2008).

[155] E. Yamamoto, N. Tamamaki, T. Nakamura, K. Kataoka, Y. Tokutomi, Y.F. Dong, M. Fukuda, S. Matsuba, H. Ogawa, S. Kim-Mitsuyam, Excess salt causes cerebral neuronal apoptosis and inflammation in stroke-prone hypertensive rats through angiotensin II-induced NAD(P)H oxidase activation, *Stroke* 39(11), 3049-3056 (2008).

[156] E.B. Peixoto, B.S. Pessoa, S.K. Biswas, J.B. Lopes de Faria, Antioxidant SOD mimetic prevents NAD(P)H oxidase-induced oxidative stress and renal damage in the early stage of experimental diabetes and hypertension. *American Journal of Nephrology* 29(4), 309-318 (2009).

[157] M.U. Somers, K. Mavromatis, Z.S. Galis, D.G. Harrison DG, Vascular superoxide production and vasomotor function in hypertension induced by deoxycorticosterone acetate-salt, *Circulation* 101, 1722-1728 (200).

[158] G.E. Callera, R.M. Touyz, S.A. Teixeira, M.N. Muscara, M. H. Carvalho, Z.B. Fortes et al, ETA receptor blockade decreases vascular superoxide generation in DOCA-salt hypertension, *Hypertension* 42, 811-817 (2003).

[159] G.E. Callera, R.C. Tostes, A. Yogi, A.C. Montezano, R.M. Touyz, Endothelin-1-induced oxidative stress in DOCA-salt hypertension involves NADPH-oxidase-independent mechanisms, *Clinical Science (London)* 110(2), 243-253 (2006).

[160] F. Amiri, A. Virdis, M.F. Neves, M. Iglarz, N.G. Seidah, R.M. Touyz et al, Endothelium-restricted overexpression of human endothelin-1 causes vascular remodeling and endothelial dysfunction, *Circulation* 110, 2233-2240 (2004)

[161] Y. Quiroz, A. Ferrebuz, N.D. Vaziri, B. Rodriguez-Iturbe, Effect of Chronic Antioxidant Therapy with Superoxide Dismutase-Mimetic Drug, Tempol, on Progression of Renal Disease in Rats with Renal Mass Reduction. *Nephron Experimental Nephrology* 112(1), e31-e42 (2009).

[162] M.M. Castro, E. Rizzi, G.J. Rodrigues, C.S. Ceron, L.M. Bendhack,R. F. Gerlach Tanus-Santos JE. Antioxidant treatment reduces matrix metalloproteinase-2-induced vascular changes in renovascular hypertension. *Free Radical Biology and Medicine* 46(9), 1298-1307 (2009).

[163] X. Chen, R,M. Touyz, J.B. Park, E.L. Schiffrin, Antioxidant effects of vitamins C and E are associated with altered activation of vascular NAD(P)H oxidase and superoxide dismutase in stroke-prone SHR, *Hypertension* 38(3 Pt 2),606-611 (2001).

[164] C.J. Wallwork, D.A. Parks, G.W. Schmid-Schonbein, Xanthine oxidase activity in the dexamethasone-induced hypertensive rat, *Microvascular Research* 66(1), 30-37 (2003).

[165] S, Milstien, Z. Katusic, Oxidation of tetrahydrobiopterin by peroxynitrite: implications for vascular endothelial function, *Biochemical and Biophysical Research Communications* 263(3), 681-684 (1999).

[166] J. Vasquez-Vivar, D. Duquaine, J. Whitsett, B. Kalyanaraman, S. Rajagopalan, Altered tetrahydrobiopterin metabolism in atherosclerosis: implications for use of oxidized tetrahydrobiopterin analogues and thiol antioxidants, *Arteriosclerosis, Thrombosis, and Vascular Biology*22(10), 1655-1661 (2002).

[167] C.S. Schnackenberg, Oxygen radicals in cardiovascular-renal disease, *Current Opinion in Pharmacology* 2, 121-125 (2002).

[168] J.M. Frenoux, B. Noirot, E.D. Prost, S. Madani, J.P. Blond, J.L. Belleville, J.L. Prost, Very high alpha-tocopherol diet diminishes oxidative stress and hypercoagulation in hypertensive rats but not in normotensive rats, *Medical Science Monitor* 8(10), BR401-7 (2002).

[169] J.B. Park, R.M. Touyz, X. Chen, E.L. Schiffrin, Chronic treatment with a superoxide dismutase mimetic preventsvascular remodeling and progression of hypertension in salt-loaded stroke-prone spontaneously hypertensive rats, *American Journal of Hypertension* 15, 78-84 (2002).

[170] C. S. Wilcox. Effects of tempol and redox-cycling nitroxides in models of oxidative stress. *Pharmacology and Therapeutics* 126(2), 119-45 (2010).

[171] A. Fortuno, S. Olivan, O. Beloqui, G. San Jose, M.U. Moreno, J. Diez et al, Association of increased phagocytic NAD(P)H oxidase-dependent superoxide production with diminished nitric oxide generation in essential hypertension, *Journal of Hypertension* 22, 2169-2175 (2004).

[172] Y. Higashi, S. Sasaki, K. Nakagawa, H. Matsuura, T. Oshima, K. Chayama, Endothelial function and oxidative stress in renovascular hypertension, *New England Journal of Medicine* 346, 1954-1962 (2002).

[173] G.Y. Lip, E. Edmunds, S.L. Nuttall, M.J. Landray, A.D. Blann, D.G. Beevers, Oxidative stress in malignant and non-malignant phase hypertension. *Journal of Human Hypertension* 16, 333-336 (2002).

[174] V.M. Lee, P.A. Quinn, S.C. Jennings, L.L. Ng, Neutrophil activation and production of reactive oxygen species in pre-eclampsia, *Journal of Hypertension* 21, 395-402 (2003).

[175] N.C. Ward, J.M. Hodgson, I.B. Puddey, T.A. Mori, L.J. Beilin, K.D. Croft, Oxidative stress in human hypertension: association with antihypertensive treatment, gender, nutrition, and lifestyle, *Free Radical Biology and Medicine* 36, 226-232 (2004).

[176] K. Yasunari, K. Maeda, M. Nakamura, J. Yoshikawa, Oxidative stress in leukocytes is a possible link between blood pressure, blood glucose, and C-rreacting protein, *Hypertension* 39, 777-780 (2002).

[177] F. Lacy, M.T. Kailasam, D.T. O'Connor, G.W. Schmid-Schonbein, R.J. Parmer, Plasma hydrogen peroxide production in human essential hypertension: role of heredity, gender, and ethnicity, *Hypertension* 36(5), 878-884 (2000).

[178] F. Lacy, D.T. O'Connor, G.W. Schmid-Schönbein, Plasma hydrogen peroxide production in hypertensives and normotensive subjects at genetic risk of hypertension, *Journal of Hypertension* 16, 291–303 (1998).

[179] D. Wang, S. Strandgaard, J. Iversen, C.S. Wilcox, Asymmetric dimethylarginine, oxidative stress, and vascular nitric oxide synthase in essential hypertension, *American Journal of Physiology - Regulatory, Integrative and Comparative Physiology* 296(2), R195-200 (2009).

[180] R. M. Touyz, E.L. Schiffrin, Increased generation of superoxide by angiotensin II in smooth muscle cells from resistance arteries of hypertensive patients: role of phospholipase D-dependent NAD(P)H oxidase-sensitive pathways, *Journal of Hypertension* 19(7), 1245-1254 (2001).

[181] Y. Kokubo, N. Iwai, N. Tago, N. Inamoto, A. Okayama, H. Yamawaki, H. Naraba, H. Tomoike, Association analysis between hypertension and CYBA, CLCNKB, and KCNMB1 functional polymorphisms in the Japanese population--the Suita Study, *Circulation Journal* 69(2), 138-142 (2005).

[182] G.T. Saez, C. Tormos, V. Giner, J. Chaves, J.V. Lozano, a. Iradi, J. Redon, Factors related to the impact of antihypertensive treatment in antioxidant activities and oxidative stress by-products in human hypertension, *American Journal of Hypertension* 17(9), 809-816 (2004).

[183] D.V. Simic, J. Mimic-Oka, M. Pljesa-Ercegovac, A. Savic-Radojevic, M. Opacic, D. Matic, B. Ivanovic, T. Simic, Byproducts of oxidative protein damage and antioxidant

enzyme activities in plasma of patients with different degrees of essential hypertension, *Journal of Human Hypertension* 20(2), 149-155 (2006).

[184] J. Chen, J. He, L. Hamm, V. Batuman, P.K. Whelton, Serum antioxidant vitamins and blood pressure in the United States population, *Hypertension* 40,810-816 (2002).

[185] B.A. Mullan, I.S. Young, H. Fee, D.R. McCance, *Hypertension* 40(6), 804-809 (2002).

[186] M. Zureik, P. Galan, S. Bertrais, L. Mennen, S. Czernichow, J. Blacher, P. Ducimetière, S. Hercberg, Effects of long-term daily low-dose supplementation with antioxidant vitamins and minerals on structure and function of large arteries. *Arteriosclerosis, Thrombosis, and Vascular Biology* 24(8), 1485-1491 (2004).

[187] H. Xu, R. Perez-Cuevas, X. Xiong, H. Reyes, C. Roy, P. Julien, G. Smith, P. von Dadelszen, L. Leduc, F. Audibert, J.M. Moutquin, B. Piedboeuf, B. Shatenstein, . Parra-Cabrera, P. Choquette, S. Winsor, S. Wood, A. Benjamin, M. Walker, M. Helewa, J. Dubé, G. Tawagi, G. Seaward, A. Ohlsson, L.A. Magee, F. Olatunbosun, R. Gratton, R.Shear, N. Demianczuk, J.P. Collet, S. Wei, W.D. Fraser, INTAPP study group An international trial of antioxidants in the prevention of preeclampsia (INTAPP), *American Journal of Obstetrics and Gynecology* 202(3), 239.e1-239.e10 (2010).

[188] M. Caner, Y. Karter, H. Uzun, A. Curgunlu, S. Vehid, H. Balci, R. Yucel, I. Güner, A. Kutlu, A. Yaldiran, E. Oztürk, Oxidative stress in human sustained and white coat hypertension, *International Journal of Clinical Practice* 60(12, :1565-1571 (2006).

[189] G. Nickenig, D.G. Harrison, The AT$_1$-Type Angiotensin Receptor in Oxidative Stress and Atherogenesis. Part I: Oxidative Stress and Atherogenesis, *Circulation* 105, 393-396 (2002).

[190] H. Morawietz, U. Rueckschloss, B. Niemann et al, Angiotensin II induces LOX-1, the human endothelial receptor for oxidized low-density lipoprotein, *Circulation* 100, 899–902 (1999).

[191] S. Keidar, J. Attias, Angiotensin II injection into mice increases the uptake of oxidized LDL by their macrophages via a proteoglycan-mediated pathway, *Biochemical and Biophysical Research Communications* 239, 63–67 (1997).

[192] D. Weiss, J.J. Kools, W.R. Taylor, Angiotensin II-induced hypertension accelerates the development of atherosclerosis in apoE-deficient mice, *Circulation* 103(3), 448-454 (2001).

[193] S. Yusuf, P. Sleight, J. Pogue, J. Bosch, R. Davies, G. Dagenais, Heart Outcome Prevention Evaluation Study Investigators. Effects of an angiotensin-converting-enzyme, ramipril, on cardiovascular events, *New England Journal of Medicine* 342, 145–153 (2000).

[194] A. Prasad, T. Tupas-Habib, W. H. Schenke et al, Acute and chronic angiotensin-1 receptor antagonism reverses endothelial dysfunction in atherosclerosis, *Circulation* 101, 2349–2354 (2000).

[195] K.K. Griendling, D.G. Harrison, Dual role of reactive oxygen species in vascular growth, *Circultation Research* 85, 562–563 (1999).

[196] R. Ross, Atherosclerosis: an inflammatory disease, *New England Journal of Medicine* 340, 115–126 (1999).

[197] P. Brassard, F. Amiri, E.L. Schiffrin, Combined angiotensin II type 1 and type 2 receptor blockade on vascular remodeling and matrix metalloproteinases in resistance arteries, *Hypertension* 46, 598-606 (2005).

[198] S. Rajagopalan, X.P. Meng, S. Ramasamy et al, Reactive oxygen species produced by macrophage-derived foam cells regulate the activity of vascular matrix metalloproteinases in vitro: implications for atherosclerotic plaque stability, *Journal of Clinical Investigation* 98, 2572–2579 (1996).

[199] K.K. Griendling, R.W. Alexander, Oxidative stress and cardiovascular disease, *Circulation* 96, 3264–3265 (1997).

[200] D. Harrison, K.K. Griendling, U. Landmesser, B. Hornig, H. Drexler, Role of oxidative stress in atherosclerosis, *American Journal of Cardioogy* 91,7A–11A (2003).

[201] J.J. Khatri, C. Johnson, R. Magid, S. M. Lessner, K.M. Laude, S.I. Dikalov, D.G. Harrison, H-J. Sung, Y. Rong, Z.S. Galis, Vascular Oxidant Stress Enhances Progression and Angiogenesis of Experimental Atheroma, *Circulation* 109, 520-525 (2004).

[202] A.N. Tenaglia, K.G. Peters, M.H. Sketch Jr et al, Neovascularization in atherectomy specimens from patients with unstable angina: implications for pathogenesis of unstable angina, *American Heart Journal* 135,10–14 (1998).

[203] P.A. Barry-Lane, C. Patterson, M. van der Merwe et al, p47phox is required for atherosclerotic lesion progression in ApoE(-/-) mice, *Journal of Clinical Investigation* 108,1513–1522 (2001).

[204] Gorlach, I. Diebold, V.B. Schini-Kerth et al, Thrombin activates the hypoxia-inducible factor-1 signaling pathway in vascular smooth muscle cells: role of the p22(phox)-containing NADPH oxidase, *Circulation Research* 89, 47–54 (2001).

[205] Azumi, N. Inoue, Y. Ohashi et al, Superoxide generation in directional coronary atherectomy specimens of patients with angina pectoris: important role of NAD(P)H oxidase, *Arteriosclerosis, Thrombosis, and Vascular Biology* 22,1838–1844 (2002).

[206] D. Sorescu, D. Weiss, B. Lassègue, R.E. Clempus, K. Szöcs, G.P. Sorescu, L. Valppu, M.Y. Quinn, J.D. Lambeth, J.D. Vega, W.R. Taylor, K.K. Griendling, Superoxide Production and Expression of Nox Family Proteins in Human Atherosclerosis, *Circulation* 105, 1429-1435 (2002).

[207] T.S. McMillen, J.W. Heinecke, R.C. LeBoeuf, Expression of Human Myeloperoxidase by Macrophages Promotes Atherosclerosis in Mice, *Circulation* 111, 2798-2804 (2005),

[208] P. Puddu, G.M. Puddu , E. Cravero, S. De Pascalis, A. Muscari, The emerging role of cardiovascular risk factor-induced mitochondrial dysfunction in atherogenesis, *Journal of Biomedical Science* 16(1), 112-120 (2009).

[209] S. Srivastava, E. Vladykovskaya, O.Q. Barski, M. Spite, K. Kaiserova, J.M. Petrash, S.S. Chung, G. Hunt, B. Dawn, A. Bhatnagar, Aldose Reductase Protects Against Early Atherosclerotic Lesion Formation in Apolipoprotein E-Null Mice, *Circulation Research* 105, 793-802 (2009).

[210] L.D. Orozco, M.H. Kapturczak, B. Barajas, X. Wang, M.M. Weinstein, J. Wong, J. Deshane, S. Bolisetty, Z. Shaposhnik, D.M. Shih, A. Agarwal, A.J. Lusis, J.A. Araujo, Heme Oxygenase-1 Expression in Macrophages Plays a Beneficial Role in Atherosclerosis, *Circulation Research* 100, 1703-1711 (2007).

[211] J.L. Mehta, N. Sanada, C.P. Hu, J. Chen, A. Dandapat, F. Sugawara, H. Satoh, K. Inoue, Y. Kawase, K. Jishage, H. Suzuki, M. Takeya, L. Schnackenberg, R. Beger, P.L. Hermonat, M. Thomas, T. Sawamura, *Circulation Research* 100, 1634-1642 (2007).

[212] Herrmann, A.M. Saguner, D. Versari, T.E. Peterson, A. Chade, M. Olson, L.O. Lerman, A. Lerman, Chronic Proteasome Inhibition Contributes to Coronary Atherosclerosis, *Circulation Research* 101(9), 865-874 (2007).

[213] Matthews, I. Gorenne, S. Scott, N. Figg, P. Kirkpatrick, A. Ritchie, M. Goddard, M. Bennett, Vascular Smooth Muscle Cells Undergo Telomere-Based Senescence in Human Atherosclerosis Effects of Telomerase and Oxidative Stress, *Circulation Research* 99, 156-164 (2006).

[214] A.A. Brown, F.B. Hu, Dietary modulation of endothelial function: implications for cardiovascular disease, *American Journal of Clinical Nutrition* 73, 673-686 (2001).

[215] A. Shihabi, W.-G. Li, FJ Miller, N.L. Weintraub, Antioxidant therapy for atherosclerotic vascular disease: the promise and the pitfalls, *American Journal of Physiology* 282, H797-H802 (2002).

[216] D. Salvemini, S. Cuzzocrea, Therapeutic potential of superoxide dismutase mimetics as therapeutic agents in critical care medicine, *Critical Care Medicine* 31(1), S29-S38 (2003).

[217] M.J. Stampfer, C.H. Hennekens, J.E. Manson, G.A. Colditz, B. Rosner, W.C. Willett, Vitamin E consumption and the risk of coronary heart disease in women, *New England. Journal of Medicine* 328(20), 1444-1449 (1993).

[218] E.B. Rimm, M.J. Stampfer, A. Ascherio, E. Giovannucci, G.A. Colditz, W.C. Willett, Vitamin E consumption and the risk of coronary heart disease in men, *New England. Journal of Medicine* 328(20), 1450-1456 (1993).

[219] K.-T. Khaw, S. Bingham, A. Welch, R. Luben, N. Wareham, S. Oakes et al, Relation between plasma ascorbic acid and mortality in men and women in EPIC-Norfolk prospective study: a prospective population study, *Lancet*357, 657-663 (2001).

[220] Chen, J. He, L. Hamm, V. Batuman, P.K. Whelton, Serum antioxidant vitamins and blood pressure in the United States population, *Hypertension* 40(60), 810-816 (2002).

[221] N.G. Stephens, A. Parsons, P.M. Schofield, F. Kelly, K. Cheeseman, Mitchinson MJ. Randomised controlled trial of vitamin E in patients with coronary disease: Cambridge Heart Antioxidant Study (CHAOS), *Lancet* 347(9004), 781-786 (1996).

[222] Jialal, S. Devaraj, B.A. Huet, M. Traber, GISSI-Prevenzione Investigators, Dietary supplementation with n-3 polyunsaturated fatty acids and vitamin E after myocardial infarction: results of the GISSI-Prevenzione trial, Gruppo Italiano per lo Studio della Sopravvivenza nell'Infarto miocardico, *Lancet* 354(9177), 447-455 (1999).

[223] S. Yusuf, G. Dagenais, J. Pogue, J. Bosch, P. Sleight, HOPE Investigators, Vitamin E supplementation and cardiovascular events in high risk patients, *New England Journal of Medicine* 342, 154-160 (2000).

[224] MRC/BHF Heart protection study of antioxidant vitamin supplementation in 20 536 high-risk individuals: a randomized placebo-controlled trial, *Lancet*360, 23-33 (2002)

[225] D.P. Vivekananthan, M.S. Penn, S.K. Sapp, A. Hsu, E.J. Topol, Use of antioxidant vitamins for the prevention of cardiovascular disease: meta-analysis of randomised trials, *Lancet* 361(9374), 2017-2023 (2003).

[226] J.M. Roberts, L. Myatt L, CY. Spong, Thom EA, Hauth JC et al. Vitamins C and E to prevent complications of pregnancy-associated hypertension, *New England Journal of Medicine* 362,1282-1291 (2010).

[227] S.J. Duffy, N. Gokce, M. Holbrook, A. Huang, B. Frei, J.F. Keaney, J.A. Vita, Treatment of hypertension with ascorbic acid, *Lancet* 354, 2048-2049 (1999).

[228] M.D. Fotheby, J.C. Williams, L.A. Forster, P. Craner, G.A. Ferns Effect of vitamin C on ambulatory blood pressure and plasma lipids in older patients, *Journal of Hypertension* 18, 411-415 (2000).

[229] B. Mullan, I.S. Young, H. Fee, D.R. McCance, Ascorbic acid reduces blood pressure and arterial stiffness in type 2 diabetes, *Hypertension* 40, 804-809 (2002).

[230] M. Boshtam, M. Rafiei, K. Sadeghi, N. Sarraf-Zadegan, Vitamin E can reduce blood pressure in mild hypertensives, *International Journal of Vitamins and Nutitional Research* 72(5), 309-314 (2002).

[231] D.L. Tribble, Antioxidant consumption and risk of coronary heart disease: emphasis on vitamin C, vitamin E and β-carotene. A statement for the healthcare professionals from the American Heart Association. *Circulation.* 99, 591-595 (1999).

[232] A. Carr, B. Frei, The role of natural antioxidants in preserving the biological activity of endothelium-derived nitric oxide, *Free Radical Biology and Medicine* 28, 1806-1814 (2000).

[233] F.M. Sacks, L.P. Svetkey, W.M. Vollmer, L.J. Appel, G.A. Bray, D. Harsha, E. Obarzanek, P.R. Conlin, E.R. Miller III, D.G. Simons-Morton, N. Karanja, P.H. Lin, DASH-Sodium Collaborative Research Group. Effects on blood pressure of reduced dietary sodium and the Dietary Approaches to Stop Hypertension (DASH) diet. DASH-Sodium Collaborative Research Group, *New England Journal of Medicine* 344(1), 3-10 (2001).

[234] J.H. John, S. Ziebland, P. Yudkin, L.S. Roe, H.A.W. Neil, Effects of fruit and vegetable consumption on plasma antioxidant concentrations and blood pressure: a randomized controlled trial, *Lancet* 359, 1969-1973 (2002).

[235] Gupte SA. Glucose-6-phosphate dehydrogenase: a novel therapeutic target in cardiovascular diseases. *Curr Opin Investig Drugs* 9(9):993-1000 (2008).

[236] Chen S, Ge Y, Si J, Rifai A, Dworkin LD, Gong R. Candesartan suppresses chronic renal inflammation by a novel antioxidant action independent of AT1R blockade. *Kidney Int.* 74(9):1128-1138. (2008)

[237] Oliveira PJ, Goncalves L, Monteiro P, Providencia LA, Moreno AJ. Are the antioxidant properties of carvedilol important for the protection of cardiac mitochondria? *Curr Vasc Pharmacol.* 3(2):147-158. (2005)

[238] Cifuentes ME, Pagano PJ. Targeting reactive oxygen species in hypertension. *Curr Opin Nephrol Hypertens.* 15(2):179-186. (2006).

[239] Berk BC. Novel approaches to treat oxidative stress and cardiovascular diseases. *Trans Am Clin Climatol Assoc.*118: 209–214. (2007)

[240] Sugiura T, Kondo T, Kureishi-Bando Y, Numaguchi Y, Yoshida O, Dohi Y, Kimura G, Ueda R, Rabelink TJ, Murohara T. Nifedipine improves endothelial function: role of endothelial progenitor cells. *Hypertension.* 52(3):491-498. (2008).

[241] Adams V, Linke A, Krankel N, Erbs S, Gielen S, Mobius-Winkler S, Gummert JF, Mohr FW, Schuler G, Hambrecht R. Impact of regular physical activity on the NAD(P)H oxidase and angiotensin receptor system in patients with coronary artery disease,*Circulation.* 111(5):555-562. (2005).

In: Principles of Free Radical Biomedicine, Volume III
Editors: K. Pantopoulos and H. M. Schipper

ISBN 978-1-61324-184-4
©2012 Nova SciencePublishers, Inc.

Chapter 9

Diabetes Mellitus

Peter Rösen[*]
German Diabetes Research Center,
Düsseldorf, Federal Republic of Germany

1. Introduction

Diabetes mellitus is one of the fastest growing health problems in the world. It is quickly being recognized as one of the major epidemics of the 21st century and is growing most rapidly in developing countries. Its importance lies in the fact that affected people are at very high risk for serious health-related consequences including blindness, kidney failure, amputations, infections, heart attacks and premature death. Even more importantly, it is now clear that many (if not all) consequences of diabetes, and even diabetes itself can be prevented by currently available therapies.

It is expected that in 2025 nearly 33.3 million subjects will be suffering from diabetes mellitus in the United States [1]. According to estimates of the National Health and Nutrition Examination Survey, diabetes mellitus was diagnosed in 2002 in more than 19.3 % of the US American adults (approximately 9.3% of the total population). Moreover, in ~26%, fasting blood glucose levels were elevated or glucose tolerance was clearly impaired; both events are taken as indicators of a pre-diabetic state. 90-95% of the diabetic population has type 2 diabetes; the rest suffer from type 1. It is estimated that in the US about 132 billion dollars (10% of public heath funding) are spent annually for treatment of diabetic patients [2].

Type 2 diabetes mellitus (non-insulin dependent diabetes mellitus, NIDDM) is characterised by resistance to insulin, impaired glucose metabolism in the presence of insulin, and excessive mobilization and utilisation of fatty acids. One of the major reasons for the increased prevalence of type 2 diabetes is the increased number of adipose subjects, especially those with visceral adiposity [3].

---

[*]E-mail: roesen@uni-duesseldorf.de, Tel. +49-234-61583

In the latter, fat is increasingly deposited in ectopic tissues such as skeletal muscle and liver resulting in subclinical, chronic inflammation, altered release of adipokines and, finally, in a diminished efficacy of insulin to enhance glucose disposal, lipoprotein synthesis and reduce rates of lipolysis. Blood glucose levels in the fasting and postprandial states remain normal as long as compensatory secretion of insulin by the β-cells remains adequate. Diabetes mellitus becomes manifest if the β-cell is no longer able to adapt secretion of insulin to the enhanced need. Although type 2 diabetes is predominantly a disease of the elderly, recent years have witnessed increasing affliction of younger individuals.

Type 1 diabetes mellitus is primarily a disease of the β-cells. On the basis of a genetic background, activation of autoimmunological processes leads to depletion of β-cells and insufficient production and secretion of insulin. Most patients are young, with many presenting during or shortly after puberty. Whereas in type 1 diabetics treatment with insulin is inevitable (insulin dependent diabetes mellitus, IDDM), type 2 diabetes may be managed with diet, exercise and a broad spectrum of hypoglycemic compounds. Most oral agents, to date, do not impact the pathophysiological events leading to the development of insulin resistance [4].

There is emerging evidence that reactive oxygen species (ROS) contribute to destruction of β-cells in both types of diabetes and that they additionally play an important role in the complex network of interactions leading to insulin resistance. ROS also contribute to the characteristic complications of diabetes including accelerated ischemic heart disease, nephropathy, neuropathy and retinopathy [5-8]. Development of insulin resistance and diabetes leads to depletion of the cellular antioxidant defense system and increased levels of ROS. This realization may offer unique therapeutic options to treat diabetes and its complications.

The "unifying hypothesis" proposed by Brownlee and co-workers [5] is intriguing and brings together experimental evidence providing an explanation for the basic mechanisms underlying the development of diabetes and its complications. Using antioxidants or nutrients with high antioxidant capacity has been suggested to prevent development of diabetes and to mitigate its complications. Antioxidants have been shown to reduce indices of oxidative stress in experimental disease models. However, the evidence in human studies is not yet convincing.

2. Is Oxidative Stress Increased in Diabetes?

The biomedical literature claims that "reactive oxygen species (ROS)" and "reactive nitrogen species (RNS)" are involved in many human diseases and that the increased formation of those compounds accompanies tissue injury [9, 10].

We will use the term ROS as a collective term that includes both oxygen radicals and non-radicals, which are oxidizing agents and can beeasily converted to radicals; oxidative stress indicates an unbalanced generation of ROS not compensated for by antioxidants. *At present, there seems to be general agreement that the production of free radicals is increased in diabetic conditions; this conclusion results from experimental observations using isolated cells, animals with different types of metabolic defects, and data derived from clinical studies.*

2.1. Assessment of ROS in Isolated Cells and Tissues

Only in isolated cells or tissues it is possible to directly measure the amounts of ROS or RNS. Fluorescence dyes such as DCF and DHT are suitable and sufficiently sensitive to follow ROS generation. With some precautions, the amount of ROS and RNS can also be quantified [11-13]. Using these techniques, increases in ROS, and more specifically in superoxide anions (O_2^-), as a function of the concentrations of glucose and fatty acids have been demonstrated in various cell types which take up glucose via the Glut1 transporter independently of the action of insulin, e.g. endothelial, smooth muscle, neuronal, and isolated β-cells [6-8] (Figure 1). Many questions remain, however, concerning the differentialeffects of acute, short-term (minutes) vs. chronic, long-term (> 24 hours) glucose exposure on ROS generation in these cells. Furthermore, it appears that fluctuating glucose concentrations in culture media may be more detrimental to cells than high, but sustained levels of the sugar.

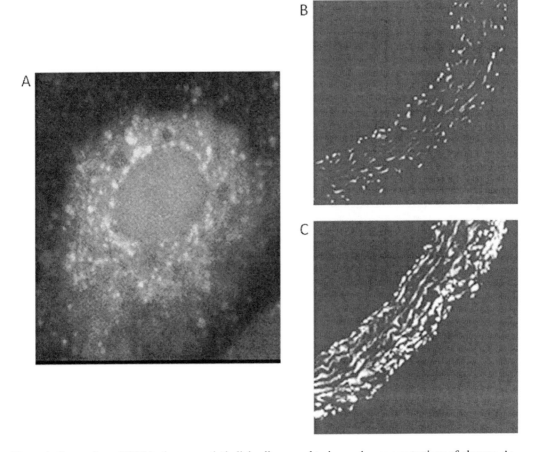

Figure 1. Generation of ROS by human endothelial cell exposed to increasing concentrations of glucose. A: Human endothelial cells were preloaded with DCF (15 min) and then incubated with increasing concentrations of D-glucose. The formation of ROS is indicated by the fluorescence after reaction of DCF with ROS. The generation of ROS in response to glucose is inhibited by antioxidants (vitamin E, ascorbic acid and lipoic acid) as well as by N-nitroarginine, an inhibitor of the endothelial nitric oxide synthase. B and C: Aortae from control (B) and diabetic (C) rats (3 months) were stained with dihydroethidium to detect ROS. Aorta from diabetic rats exhibits intense ROS generation relative to control levels.

2.2. Assessment of ROS *In Vivo*

In human and whole animal studies, the formation of ROS is usually estimated indirectly after reaction of ROS with specific substrates or reporter molecules:

(i) Reaction products of ROS with DNA (Vol. I, Chapter 9): 8-hydroxydeoxyguanosine (8-OHdG), 8-hydroxyadenine and 7-methyl-8-hydroxy-guanine; the most exploited is 8-OHdG.

(ii) Lipid peroxidation [14] (see also Vol. I, Chapter 7): Measurement of malondialdehyde (MDA) by the thiobarbituric acid (TBA) test; ferrous oxidation with xylenol orange; the FOX assay as a marker of hydroperoxides (ROOH); and the arachidonate-derived compound, 8-epi-prostaglandin $F_{2\alpha}$ (8-epi-PGF$_{2\alpha}$) [15-17].

(iii) Protein oxidation [18, 19] (see also Chapter Vol. I, 6); immunochemical or HPLC detection of 3-nitrotyrosine derived from RNS attack on tyrosine residues; other oxidative modifications of amino acid residues including tryptophan hydroxylation and the formation of valine-hydroxides, 8-oxo-histidine, dityrosine, and ortho- and meta-tyrosinesand the carbonyl assay, a widely-used test for oxidative protein damage based on the ability of several ROS to generate carbonyls within amino acid residues [19].

2.3. Experimental Models of Diabetes

Markers of enhanced oxidative stress have been amply demonstrated in animals with type 1-like and type 2-like diabetes (streptozotocin diabetes, ZDF rats, ob/ob mice, db/db mice, etc.). These markers include MDA, 8-epi PGF2a, 8-hydroxyadenosine, 7-methyl-8-hydroxyguanine, 8-oxohistidine, dityrosine, o- and m-hydroxytyrosine, tryptophan hydroxylation and carbonyl formation. In many cases, treatment of animals with insulin or hypoglycemic compounds (metformin, sulfonylureas, acarbose, and glitazones) was able to prevent or attenuate the increase in ROS suggesting a causal relationship between the generation of ROS and the metabolic defect [7, 21-23].

2.4. Clinical Studies

Several clinical studies show increases in levels of oxidative stress markers, for instance ROOH, 8-epi-PGF$_{2\alpha}$ 8-OHdG and oxLDL, in tissues of IDDM and NIDDM patients relative to healthy age-matched control subjects [7, 17, 24] (Table1). Dandona and coworkers showed an approximately four-fold higher median concentration of 8-OHdG in mononuclear cells of diabetic patients compared to corresponding controls [25]. This finding indicated the susceptibility to oxidative DNA damage in diabetic patients.

Clinical studies [17, 24] showed an approximately two-fold increase in the plasma oxidative stress indices, 8-epi PGF$_{2\alpha}$ and ROOH in diabetic patients relative to healthy subjects. The relationship of hydroperoxides and the level of the antioxidant RRR-α-tocopherol (standardised to cholesterol) also suggested a 3-6 fold increase in levels of oxidative stress in the plasma of diabetic patients. In addition, Davi et al. reported that the increased levels of urinary 8-epi-PGF$_{2\alpha}$ observed in type 1 and 2 diabetic patients can be normalized by improved metabolic control [26]. A major hypothesis is that oxidized lipoprotein (oxLDL) contributes to the cardiovascular complications of diabetes. Several studies have demonstrated increased LDL-oxidation in diabetic patients. The concept of imbalance between oxidative stress measures and antioxidant depletion has been applied to the pro-atherogenic LDL oxidation process in diabetic patients. Others reported an imbalance between elevated oxLDL-levels and decreased RRR-α-tocopherol levels (cholesterol-standardised) in LDL particles of diabetic patients when compared to healthy controls. The increase in LDL modification by oxidation may be a function of enhanced ROS production and diminished antioxidant protection [7].

A decrease in antioxidant capacity has been observed in the plasma of diabetic patients by several research groups [7]. In a prospective study, Salonen and coworkers found a decline of plasma RRR-α-tocopherol levels after the onset of type 2 diabetes [27]. Thornalley and coworkers reported decreased levels of the endogenous antioxidant glutathione in erythrocytes of diabetic patients [28]. The decline in the plasma levels of the antioxidants RRR-α-tocopherol or glutathione may be explained as a result of the increased production of free radicals in diabetic patients. However, other explanations need to be taken into considerations. Rosen et al. presented data from two nutritional studies showing a dietary-induced RRR-α-tocopherol deficiency in older subjects and especially in diabetic patients [7]. Dietary recommendations for diabetic patients primarily strive to reduce fat intake in order to decrease body weight. RRR-α-tocopherol is present in the fat-soluble phase of food ingredients and may therefore be underrepresented in a fat-reduced diabetic diet. In addition, the RRR-α-tocopherol content of dietary recommendations for diabetic patients was analysed in food records of 100 diabetic patients and compared with the recommended dietary allowance (RDA) of RRR-α-tocopherol. In about 43% of the eating plans and dietary recommendations, the RRR-α-tocopherol intake was significantly lower than the RDA. A correlation was found between energy intake and RRR-α-tocopherol levels. Furthermore, there was a negative relationship in the energy content of the diabetic diet and the dietary RRR-α-tocopherol intake, resulting in a potentially severe α-tocopherol deficiency in those diabetic patients who were obese and adhering to a slimming diet. Long-term dietary restriction of RRR-α-tocopherol leads to reduced RRR-α-tocopherol plasma levels in men. The contribution of impaired nutritional antioxidant intake to the observed imbalance between increased plasma oxidative stress measures and decreased antioxidant plasma levels in diabetic patients requires further evaluation.

3. What Are the Mechanisms Leading to Enhanced Generation of ROS in Diabetes?

A variety of cellular enzyme systems are potential sources of ROS [29], including NAD(P)H oxidase, xanthine oxidase, uncoupled endothelial nitric oxide (NO) synthase (eNOS), and arachidonic acid-metabolizing enzymes such as the cytochrome P-450 system, lipoxygenases and cyclooxygenases.

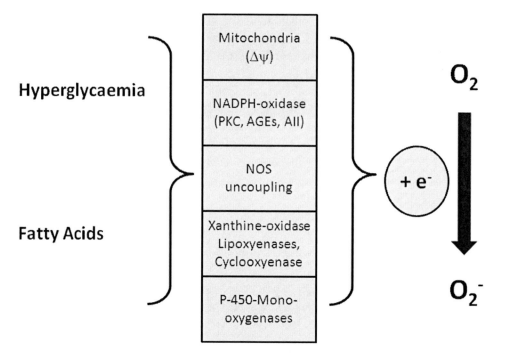

Figure 2. Generation of ROS in response to hyperglycemia and fatty acids. Besides the mitochondria and NADPH-oxidase, nitric oxide synthase contributes significantly to the generation of ROS in response to glucose and fatty acids. Others systems may also contribute to generation of ROS, but their roles have not been precisely defined.

Table 1. Markers of oxidative stress elevated in the blood of diabetic patients. Better metabolic control leads to a reduction of several markers of oxidative stress suggesting a causal relationship between hyperglycemia and oxidative stress

Markers of oxidative stress elevated in the blood of diabetic patients (type1 and 2):
• Lipid hydroperoxides • Malondialdehyde • Oxidized LDL • Hydroxyguanosines • Isoprostanes • Carbonyl residues • Nitrotyrosine • Hydroxylated Amino Acids

Specifically, the mitochondrial respiratory chain may be a major source of ROS in diabetes [6, 30]. However, this source may strongly vary dependent on the tissues and cells involved. The functional significance of mitochondria-derived ROS in vascular endothelial cells has received little attention for a long time, because in general vascular cells exhibit low metabolic activity [31] and the production of ROS in mitochondria (Vol. II, Chapter 15) seem to be less well regulated as compared to other systems (for example like NAD(P)H oxidase)

[32]. New evidence suggests, however, that the mitochondrial respiratory chain is a major source of ROS in most mammalian cells in diabetes including the vasculature endothelium [6, 30]; see also Chapter 8 in this Volume. A simplified scheme of the systems involved in the generation of ROS is shown in Figure 2.

It is assumed that hyperglycemia causes an accelerated flow through the glycolytic pathway and an accumulation of C3- and C6 intermediates if the rate of uptake is higher than the metabolic conversion rate. This metabolic situation has two important consequences:

(i) An excess formation of NADH, which is transported into the mitochondria via either the malate-aspartate or the glycerol phosphate shuttle systems. NADH is the main electron donor to the mitochondrial respiratory chain. It has been hypothesised that the electron transport chain becomes uncoupled if the electrochemical potential provided by the high inflow of NADH exceeds a threshold value; rather than driving ATP production, this would promote the 1-electron reduction of oxygen to $O_2^{\cdot-}$. Similarly, if mitochondria utilize free fatty acids as fuel for oxidation, beta-oxidation and oxidation of free fatty acids in the tricarboxylic acid cycle would generate electron donors (NADH) for oxidative phosphorylation. Thus, an excess of free fatty acids would simulate mitochondrial defects and the generation of ROS akin to the effects of hyperglycaemia [6, 30]. Augmented mitochondrial ROS production has not only be postulated as candidate in the pathogenesis of diabetes and its complications, but has also been implicated in aging and a broad range of degenerative diseases [33, 34].

(ii) On the other hand, C3 intermediates are used to synthesize diacylglycerol (DAG) which is a potent activator of protein kinase C (PKC). The latter, in turn, facilitates the cytoplasmic translocation of NADPH oxidase, which catalyzes the reduction of single molecular oxygen to $O_2^{\cdot-}$. There is also evidence that advanced glycation end-products (AGEs) favoured in diabetes stimulate NADPH oxidase after binding to specific receptors (RAGE) and thereby contribute to the increased generation of ROS [35-37]NADPH oxidase was initially observed in neutrophils where it plays a decisive role in host-pathogen defense via the generation of ROS in millimolar quantities. This enzyme complex is now known to be expressedalso in non-phagocytotic cells such as endothelial cells, fibroblasts, mesangial and tubular cells and smooth muscle cells (see also Chapter 8 in this Volume). It consists of multiple subunits p^{22phox}, p^{47phox}, p^{67phox}, p^{40phox}, Nox01, NoxA1, Rac1 and a unique Nox isoform based on gp91^{phox}. Although the composition of the complex may vary in a tissue-dependant manner, certain subunits are consistently up-regulated in diabetes, in models of the metabolic syndrome, and in rats fed a high carbohydrate diet [35-40].

These observations further implicate oxidative stress in the pathogenesis of diabetes. Inhibition of NADPH oxidase by apocynin prevents the upregulation of p^{47phox} and gp^{91phox} subunits. We demonstrated that in smooth muscle cells, hyperglycaemia-induced ROS generation can be attenuated to a considerable degree by NADPH oxidase blockade (Figure 3). Furthermore, others have adduced evidence that inhibition of NADPH oxidase may prevent complications in experimental diabetes [40, 41].

In addition to generation of ROS, activation of NADPH oxidase consumes NADPH at high rates. As a consequence, the antioxidant potential of cells might be compromised because the recycling of reduced glutathione (GSH) from its oxidized form (GSSG; see Vol. II, Chapter 1) is impaired under those conditions. NADPH is also an essential co-substrate for endothelial nitric oxide synthase (eNOS).

Activation of NADPH oxidase may affect eNOS activity in two ways, by reduction of its co-substrate and directly by interaction with tetrahydrobiopterin in the NOS catalytic centre. Activation of NADPH oxidase is an important reason for impairment of nitric oxide generation and for defects in endothelial function [29].

Another aspect might be of importance: The renin-angiotensin-system is induced in diabetes leading to increased activity of angiotensin II, a potent activator of NADPH oxidase [40, 42]. At least part of the deleterious effects of angiotensin II on the vasculature is mediated by its effect on NADPH oxidase and the production of ROS (Chapter 8 in this Volume). In our hands, uncoupling of NOS is of major relevance in endothelial cells as we could prevent the formation of endothelial ROS under hyperglycemic conditions by inhibiting this enzyme. Similar results were obtained in porcine aortas exposed to L-arginine and specific inhibitors of NOS (Figure 3). NOS and the insulin receptor are topologically associated to the extent that both are expressed in caveolae, tiny invaginations in the plasma membrane [43].

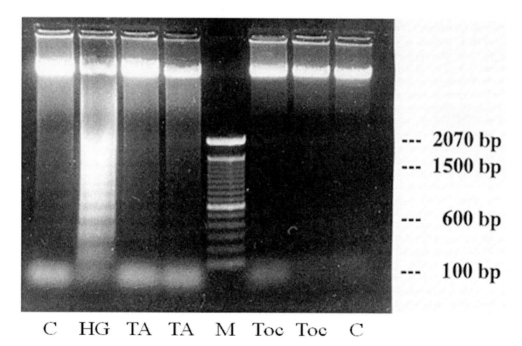

Figure 3. Inhibition of glucose-ROS mediated induction of apoptosis in human endothelial cells by antioxidants. Human endothelial cells were incubated with glucose (30 mM = HG vs. 5 mM = C for 20 hrs) in the presence and absence of antioxidants (Toc = vitamin E, lipoic acid = TA, DNA markers = M). Thereafter, the amount of apoptotic cells was determined by flow cytometry and the DNA was analyzed by gel electrophoresis [44]. DNA is degraded after incubation of cells with high glucose indicating induction of apoptosis. The latter is prevented by pre-incubation of the cells with antioxidants such as vitamin E and lipoic acid.

This colocalization raises the possibility that ROS generation accruing from defects in NOS function may directly damage insulin receptors, glucose transporters and some caveolin isoforms affecting the permeability of the plasma membrane.

We showed that inhibition of eNOS not only prevented ROS production, but also induction of apoptosis and activation of the transcription factor NF-κB. These findings further support the view that eNOS-related ROS production contributes to vascular cell injury and dysfunction in the face of hyperglycemia and elevated fatty acids [11, 13, 44]. Inhibition of eNOS has been shown to prevent defects in endothelium-dependent vessel relaxation in experimental diabetes [12].

It should also be taken into account that the capacity to scavenge ROS may already be compromised in pre-diabetic states. Thus, Ceriello and coworkers have pointed out that both antioxidant enzyme activities and concentrations of antioxidant vitamins are reduced in pre-diabetic humans [45]. This conclusion is buttressed by experimental data indicating diminished expression of superoxide dismutase (SOD) isoenzymes, glutathione peroxidase (GPx) and heme oxygenase-2 (HO-2) in response to high fat and high carbohydrate feeding. Thus the capacity to inactivate ROS in pre-diabetes/diabetes seems to be generally hampered.

Increased concentrations of reduced glutathione reported in some studies may represent an adaptation to chronic or repeated oxidative stress in these conditions. Taken together, the data suggest that diverse systems linked by complex interrelationships cooperate to augment the burden of oxidative stress in states of insulin resistance and the metabolic syndrome.

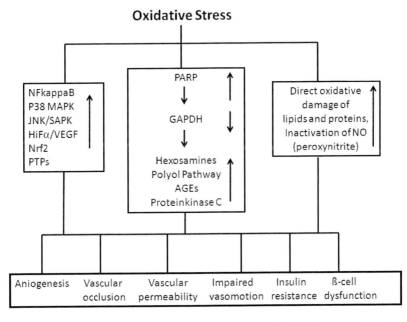

Figure 4. Proposed activation of signaling pathways as consequence of oxidative stress, which may contribute to the pathophysiology of diabetes and its complications. ROS may either directly impact macromolecules (direct action) or activate various signaling pathways (indirect action) such as the stress-sensitive pathways NF-κB, p38 MAPK, JNK/SAPK, HIFα, and Nrf2. Other pathways are invoked following activation of PARP, which leads to ribosylation and inhibition of GAPDH. As consequence, the polyol, hexosamine- and PKC-pathways are activated. In addition, the formation of AGEs is increased leading to further activation of NADPH-oxidase and oxidative stress (vicious cycle). Oxidative stress mediates impairment of β-cell function, insulin resistance and the development of vascular complications.

4. Consequences of the Increased Generation of ROS

In addition to their ability to directly oxidize and damage DNA, proteins and lipids, ROS are important activators of several signaling pathways (NF-κB, JNK/SAPK, p38 MAPK, AP-1, hypoxia inducible factor α (HIFα), NF-E2-related factor 2 (Nrf2) (see Vol. II, Chapters 12-14 and 22). Indirectly, ROS may cause activation of PKC, poly(adenylribose)polymerase (PARP) and the hexosamine pathway [46, 47].

Dysregulation of these signaling pathways by aberrant ROS production may contribute to β-cell dysfunction and the development of diabetic complications [6, 7, 48]. A hypothetical signaling scheme is given in Figure 4.

4.1. NF-κB

There is ample evidence that the transcription factor NF-κB is a target of ROS (see Vol. II, Chapter 12) and is activated by hyperglycemia and free fatty acids [11, 49, 50]. Activation is the consequence of a proteasome-mediated degradation of the inhibitor IκB after phosphorylation by upstream serine kinases (IKKβ).

In endothelial cells, smooth muscle and various other cell types, the ROS-dependent activation of NF-κB can be inhibited by a broad spectrum of antioxidants. The expression of a large number of genes is activated by NF-κB (e.g. VEGF, RAGE, ICAM-1, VCAM-1 etc.).

Activation of NF-κB is associated with pro-inflammatory, pro-adhesive responses and the induction of apoptosis (loss of vascular, muscular and β-cells); it also impairs the stability and number of progenitor cells, which are important for tissue repair mechanisms. Activation of NF-κB further enhances the generation of AGEs and reactive species thereby completing a vicious cycle of oxidative stress amplification in affected tissues.

Activation of IKKβ has also been linked to insulin resistance [51, 52]. Treatment with antioxidants such as vitamin E, glutathione and others prevented activation of NF-κB and its downstream effects [7, 11, 21, 53].

4.2. JNK/SAPK

JNK/SAPK are members of the family of MAP serine/threonine protein kinases [54]. They are stress-activated kinases, which respond to an array of stimuli (oxidative stress, hyperglycemia, osmotic stress, cytokines heat shock, radiation).

They have been implicated in induction of apoptosis and changes in patterns of cell proliferation. High concentrations of vitamin C inhibited hyperglycemia-induced activation of JNK/SAPK in endothelial cells [48].

4.3. p38 MAPK

p38 MAPK is activated in response to hyperglycemia and diabetes (smooth muscle cells). In streptozotocin-diabetic rats, MAPK is augmented in renal glomeruli followed by increased phosphorylation of heat shock protein 25. Levels of total MAPK activity are elevated in nerve tissue of patients with type 1 and 2 diabetes.

4.4. HIF-1α

HIF-1α is implicated in oxygen sensing (Vol. II, Chapter 22). Generation of ROS is associated with an enhanced expression of this transcription factor and the vascular endothelial growth factor (VEGF). Both factors are involved in the up-regulation of genes related to angiogenesis and cell proliferation, processes which are of special importance for development of diabetic vascular complications such as retinopathy (Vol. III, Chapter 11) and nephropathy [40]; see also Vol. III, Chapter 5).

4.5. Nrf2

Enhanced NF-E2-related factor 2 activity (see Vol. II, Chapter 13) may play a role as a compensatory response to mild, transient elevations in tissue ROS. Low concentrations of ROS activate the Nrf2-mediated expression of antioxidant enzymes, which help to maintain redox homeostasis in early states of the metabolic syndrome and diabetes [40].

4.6. Other Factors

In addition to engagement of the aforelisted transcription factors, activation of poly(adenylribose)polymerase (PARP) may be germane to the pathophysiology of diabetes (Figure 4): Brownlee et al. [5] provided evidence that ROS mediate PARP activation under hyperglycemic conditions. This results not only in the breakdown of NADH and depletion of ATP, but also in ribosylation of glyceraldehyde dehydrogenase (GAPDH). Consequently, glycolysis is inhibited at the level of GAPDH leading to accumulation of glyceraldehyde-/dihydroxyacetone-phosophate, which activates PKC-dependent processes. Accumulation of glucose-6-phoshate may further reduce the uptake of glucose and stimulate alternative pathways for the metabolism of glucose, such as the hexosamine pathway, leading to O-glycosylation of transcription factors (SP1) and NOS [46]. The latter elicits further activation of pro-inflammatory processes (plasminogen activator inhibitor-1, transforming growth factor β-1) [55]. Excess NO produced by activated NOS may combine with O_2^- to yield the highlycytotoxic species, peroxytnitrite. Consumption of NO may concomitantly diminish its cytoprotective effects on the vasculature (relaxation, anti-thrombotic and anti-proliferative effects); additionally, it aggravates vascular damage by inactivation of prostacyclin synthase, activation of thromboxane synthase and impairment of the myogenic response.

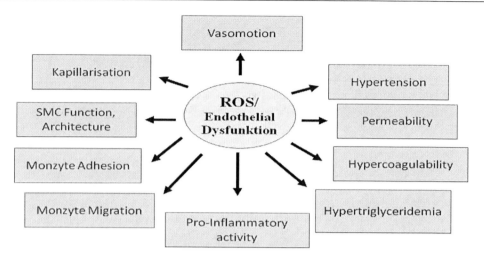

Figure 5. Vascular defects, which are casually linked to oxidative stress and endothelial dysfunction.

In summary, the hyperglycemia and fatty acid-mediated formation of ROS plays a pivotal role in activating a host of signaling and metabolic pathways with downstream deleterious consequences for insulin secretion, insulin resistance (see below) and the vasculature (Figure 5). Impacted mostly are cells taking up glucose in an insulin-independent manner by glucose transporter 1 (Glut1), which may partly explain the predilection of specific tissue targets for development of diabetic complications. These realizations have fuelled interest in the potential use of antioxidants to prevent both diabetes and its complications [6, 7, 47, 56].

5. Does Treatment with Antioxidants Reduce Oxidative Stress and the Complications of Diabetes?

The effects of antioxidant supplementation on oxidative stress measures and diabetic complications provide an indirect way to adduce further support for a role of ROS in the pathophysiology of this condition. It has been shown in several studies that whole plasma and isolated LDL from NIDDM patients are more prone to peroxidation when compared to corresponding controls, and that supplementation with RRR-α-tocopherol decreases these oxidative processes in diabetic patients [57-59]. Supplementation with α-lipoic acid or α-tocopherol decreases ROOH concentrations and LDL-oxidation as well as the imbalance between ROOH and cholesterol-standardised RRR-α-tocopherollevels [21, 26, 60-62].

Despite the arguments that have been raised concerning the validity of some individual biomarkers, the sum of evidence from biomarkers reporting oxidative damage to DNA, lipids and proteins supports the concept of increased oxidative stress in diabetes. More important is the question whether reduction of oxidative stress translates into reduced vascular risk. It is known that vitamins C and E exert significant protective effects on the vasculature and blood cells (Table 2). These vitamins have been shown to improve defective endothelial-dependent relaxation not only in patients with type 2 diabetes, but also in hypertensive and hypercholesterolemic subjects as well as in smokers and patients with coronary artery disease.

4.3. p38 MAPK

p38 MAPK is activated in response to hyperglycemia and diabetes (smooth muscle cells). In streptozotocin-diabetic rats, MAPK is augmented in renal glomeruli followed by increased phosphorylation of heat shock protein 25. Levels of total MAPK activity are elevated in nerve tissue of patients with type 1 and 2 diabetes.

4.4. HIF-1α

HIF-1α is implicated in oxygen sensing (Vol. II, Chapter 22). Generation of ROS is associated with an enhanced expression of this transcription factor and the vascular endothelial growth factor (VEGF). Both factors are involved in the up-regulation of genes related to angiogenesis and cell proliferation, processes which are of special importance for development of diabetic vascular complications such as retinopathy (Vol. III, Chapter 11) and nephropathy [40]; see also Vol. III, Chapter 5).

4.5. Nrf2

Enhanced NF-E2-related factor 2 activity (see Vol. II, Chapter 13) may play a role as a compensatory response to mild, transient elevations in tissue ROS. Low concentrations of ROS activate the Nrf2-mediated expression of antioxidant enzymes, which help to maintain redox homeostasis in early states of the metabolic syndrome and diabetes [40].

4.6. Other Factors

In addition to engagement of the aforelisted transcription factors, activation of poly(adenylribose)polymerase (PARP) may be germane to the pathophysiology of diabetes (Figure 4): Brownlee et al. [5] provided evidence that ROS mediate PARP activation under hyperglycemic conditions. This results not only in the breakdown of NADH and depletion of ATP, but also in ribosylation of glyceraldehyde dehydrogenase (GAPDH). Consequently, glycolysis is inhibited at the level of GAPDH leading to accumulation of glyceraldehyde-/dihydroxyacetone-phosophate, which activates PKC-dependent processes. Accumulation of glucose-6-phoshate may further reduce the uptake of glucose and stimulate alternative pathways for the metabolism of glucose, such as the hexosamine pathway, leading to O-glycosylation of transcription factors (SP1) and NOS [46]. The latter elicits further activation of pro-inflammatory processes (plasminogen activator inhibitor-1, transforming growth factor β-1) [55]. Excess NO produced by activated NOS may combine with O_2^- to yield the highlycytotoxic species, peroxytnitrite. Consumption of NO may concomitantly diminish its cytoprotective effects on the vasculature (relaxation, anti-thrombotic and anti-proliferative effects); additionally, it aggravates vascular damage by inactivation of prostacyclin synthase, activation of thromboxane synthase and impairment of the myogenic response.

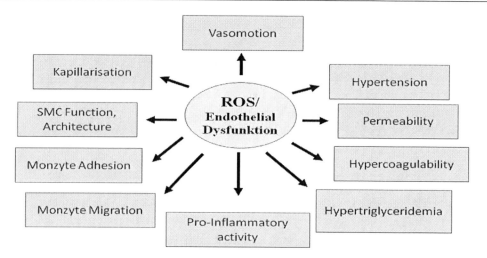

Figure 5. Vascular defects, which are casually linked to oxidative stress and endothelial dysfunction.

In summary, the hyperglycemia and fatty acid-mediated formation of ROS plays a pivotal role in activating a host of signaling and metabolic pathways with downstream deleterious consequences for insulin secretion, insulin resistance (see below) and the vasculature (Figure 5). Impacted mostly are cells taking up glucose in an insulin-independent manner by glucose transporter 1 (Glut1), which may partly explain the predilection of specific tissue targets for development of diabetic complications. These realizations have fuelled interest in the potential use of antioxidants to prevent both diabetes and its complications [6, 7, 47, 56].

5. Does Treatment with Antioxidants Reduce Oxidative Stress and the Complications of Diabetes?

The effects of antioxidant supplementation on oxidative stress measures and diabetic complications provide an indirect way to adduce further support for a role of ROS in the pathophysiology of this condition. It has been shown in several studies that whole plasma and isolated LDL from NIDDM patients are more prone to peroxidation when compared to corresponding controls, and that supplementation with RRR-α-tocopherol decreases these oxidative processes in diabetic patients [57-59]. Supplementation with α-lipoic acid or α-tocopherol decreases ROOH concentrations and LDL-oxidation as well as the imbalance between ROOH and cholesterol-standardised RRR-α-tocopherollevels [21, 26, 60-62].

Despite the arguments that have been raised concerning the validity of some individual biomarkers, the sum of evidence from biomarkers reporting oxidative damage to DNA, lipids and proteins supports the concept of increased oxidative stress in diabetes. More important is the question whether reduction of oxidative stress translates into reduced vascular risk. It is known that vitamins C and E exert significant protective effects on the vasculature and blood cells (Table 2). These vitamins have been shown to improve defective endothelial-dependent relaxation not only in patients with type 2 diabetes, but also in hypertensive and hypercholesterolemic subjects as well as in smokers and patients with coronary artery disease.

Improvement of endothelial-dependent vasodilatation may be particularly relevant here as disturbed endothelium-dependent vasodilatation is a strong indicator of vascular risk and precedes the development of atherosclerotic lesions. Antioxidants also confer protection to pancreatic β-cells and the major organs targeted in diabetes (heart, kidney, eye, nerve). We and others have demonstrated efficacious treatment of diabetic rats and mice with antioxidants such as vitamin E, vitamin C, probucol, α-lipoic acid, N-acetylcysteine [7, 21]. Tissue-specific overexpression of antioxidative enzymes (SOD, GPx, catalase) and metallothionein prevent or delay the development of frank diabetes, insulin resistance and diabetic complications [13, 63]. For example, treatment with high concentrations of vitamin E or probucol prevented nearly completely the impairment of endothelial relaxation, cardiac pathology (hypertrophy, accumulation of collagen-like structures) and degeneration of sympathetic and parasympathetic nerves in diabetic rats (Figure 6). Similarly, overexpression of the metal-binding protein metallothinein obviated the development of cardiomyopathy, attenuated inflammatory processes and nitrosative stress, and normalized cardiac energy metabolism in diabetic animals. Up-regulation of the metalloprotein also normalized fat induced-contractile dysfunction, and levels of calcium-cycling proteins, while reducing the NADPH oxidase activity and PARP cleavage relative to untreated counterparts [63, 64]. Changes in the cytoarchitecture of heavy myosin chains typically seen in hearts of diabetic rats were not detected in rats after overexpression of metallothionein.

Table 2. Protective effects of vitamin E and/or C in diabetic patients (clinical observations)

Protective effects of vitamin E and vitamin C on vasculature (clinicaloberservations)
• Inhibition of NF-κB activation in monocytes
• Inhibition of NF-κB dependent pro-inflammatory processes
• Inhibition of LDL oxidation
• Inhibition of formation of glycated proteins
• Inhibition oflipidperoxidation
• Inhibition of thromboxane A_2 formation
• Reduced fragilbility of erythrocytes (stabilization of plasma membranes)

• Normalisationofendothelialdysfunction
    o   in type 2 diabetic patients and
    o   after acutehyperglycaemia

• Protectionofendothelialpermeability
• Reduction of activity and adhesivity of thrombocytes
• Reduction of the adhesion of monocytes (MCP-1)
• Inhibition of the proliferation of smooth muscle cells
• Improvement of retinal blood flow and creatine clearance
• Increased generation of anti-adhesive, anti-proliferative, and anti-thrombotic mediators (NO and prostacyclin)

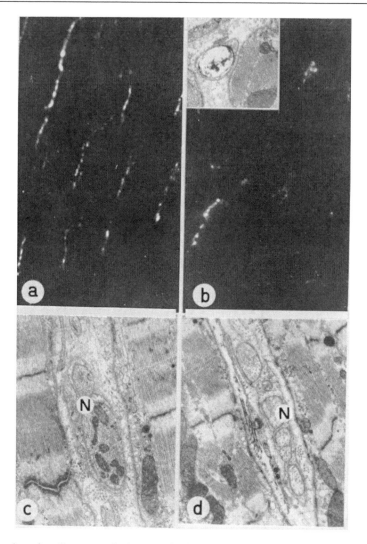

Figure 6. Preservation of cardiac sympathetic nerves in diabetic rats by vitamin E. Diabetic rats (streptozotocin model) were treated with vitamin E for 6 months. Thereafter, the hearts were isolated and the sympathetic nerve fibres were identified by catecholamine-related fluorescence and analysed by microfluorimetry. The amount fluorescent fibres in the diabetic heart (a) was compared to that of diabetic rats treated with vitamin E (n). There were no significant difference between non-diabetic controls and vitamin E-treated diabetic rats. Morphological changes in diabetic (c) and diabetic/vitamin E-treated preparations (d) are contrasted.

Furthermore, diabetic changes in the kidney were largely prevented (reduced podocyte damage, less glomerular cell death, higher density of podocyte foot processes, less expansion of glomerular and mesangial volumes, reduction in albumin excretion [65]. Qualitatively similar results have been reported in diabetic animals after tissue-specific overexpression of SOD and catalase and following administration of SOD mimetics [66, 67]. Of note, antioxidants also inhibit angiotensin II-mediated dysfunctions in heart and kidney. This is of considerable significance because the renin-angiotensin system becomes activated in diabetes and contributes prominently to the development of late complications (see also Chapter 8 in this Volume). Despite fairly compelling experimental and epidemiological studies supporting the salutary effects of antioxidants in diabetes, clinical evidence from randomized clinical trials (RCT) remains inadequate. Specifically, little prospective evidence exists implicating antioxidants in the prevention of diabetes and its major complications. Intervention studies assessing the effects of vitamin C and/or vitamin E have thus far failed to show convincing clinical benefits in diabetic patients [68-79].

6. Paradoxical Role of ROS in Insulin Signaling and Resistance?

With respect to the action of insulin, ROS seem to play an ambivalent role: On the one hand, ROS participate in the signaling pathway of insulin and facilitate the uptake of glucose; on the other hand, ROS may contribute to development of insulin resistance. That oxidant species are potentially involved in insulin signaling was conjectured more than 30 years ago [80]. It was shown that low ROS concentrations facilitate insulin signaling and the insulin-mediated glucose uptake in adipose cells. The insulin action on these cells was also accompanied by oxidation of sulfhydryl groups. Accordingly, blocking of sulfhydryl groups enhanced insulin receptor function and glucose uptake. These observations implicated ROS as 'second messengers' in the insulin signaling cascade [81]. Recent years have witnessed much support for this hypothesis: *In contrast to high chronic levels of ROS ("generalized oxidative stress") which play an important role in the development of diabetes and its complications, transient bursts of small amounts of strictly-localized ROS are triggered by insulin (as well as various growth factors, cytokines and other hormones) which enhance insulin's effects in target tissues.* The underlying mechanism has not yet fully been elucidated, but it is assumed that these small amounts of ROS are generated by a specific family of NADPH oxidases (NOX4) that lead to oxidation of susceptible signaling enzymes containing vicinal thiols essential for catalytic activity [81] (Figure 7).

One group of enzymes receiving considerable attention in this regard are the protein tyrosine phosphatases, especially PTPB1. PTPs are required for receptor dephosphorylation, deactivation and the termination of the cellular response to insulin. *In vivo* dissociation of insulin from its receptor is followed by rapid dephosphorylation and by deactivation of the kinase activity of the insulin receptor, presumably executed by PTPB1. Studies of insulin signaling in PTPB1 knockout mice revealed enhanced insulin-stimulated phosphorylation of the insulin receptor and the insulin receptor substrates in skeletal muscle and in liver, but not in adipose tissue. Knockout mice exhibited decreased adiposity, resistance to weight gain when fed a high fat diet and an increased basal metabolic rate. Taken together, these observations suggest that low levels of ROS are involved in insulin signaling by inhibition of PTPs resulting in a pronounced prolongation of insulin action [81] (Figure 8).

It is also important to consider that physical exercise and weight loss, which exert favorable effects on insulin sensitivity and are able to prevent the development of diabetes type 2, augment ROS generation by skeletal muscles (Chapter 15 in this Volume). Activation of mitochondrial respiration as consequence of physical exercise is strictly linked to mitochondrial production of ROS; ROS are natural by-products of mitochondrial metabolism.

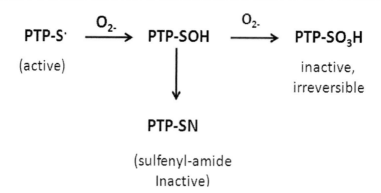

Figure 7. Inhibition of Protein-tyrosine phosphatases (PTPs) by ROS (simplified scheme modified from [81].

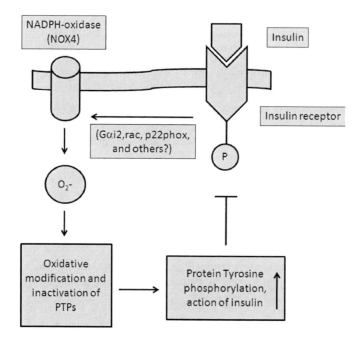

Figure 8. Effects of oxidative modification of PTPs on insulin signaling via inhibition of insulin receptor dephosphorylation (modified from [81]).

These transient bursts of ROS may represent an important adaptation to exercise (metabolic stress) by pre-conditioning the up-regulation of mitochondrial antioxidant defenses (SOD, GPx) [82-84]. The latter may contribute to longevity in flies and mice [85] and attenuate chronic disease processes in humans [86]. It has been suggested that the transient effects of ROS mediate the removal of dysfunctional mitochondria thereby bestowing affected cells with a more resilient network of healthy mitochondria ("mitohormesis") [87].

In contradistinction to the beneficial aspects of ROS-enhanced insulin signaling, "generalized oxidative stress" facilitates the development of insulin resistance. Although precise mechanisms responsible for the latter remain enigmatical, the close link between obesity and insulin resistance has suggested that an adipose-derived factor(s) may be involved (TNFα, leptin, resistin, free fatty acids) [88-90]. The excessive caloric intake and low energy expenditure typical of subjects with the metabolic syndrome are closely associated with an expansion of visceral adipose tissue and a change in the pattern of adipokines released by this tissue (less adiponectin; more TNFα, free fatty acids, resistin etc.). Increased levels of fatty acids are positively correlated with insulin resistance [88, 89]. Steinberg and coworkers [91] and Laasko et al. [92] garnered evidence that fatty acids directly reduce the activation of nitric oxide synthase, diminish skeletal muscle perfusion, and engender some degree of insulin resistance. The surplus of energy substrates may amplify the mitochondrial membrane potential ($\Delta\Psi$) and accelerate the 1-electron reduction of oxygen to superoxide. In support of this formulation, mitochondrial dysfunction is clearly associated with reduced insulin sensitivity [93, 94]. Mitochondrial dysfunction and expression of mitochondrial oxidative phosphorylation genes are related to insulin resistance, and reduced mitochondrial metabolism is functionally associated with type 2 diabetes [95, 96]. Mutations in mitochondrial genes lacking histone protection in the course of aging and cellular stress have also been proposed to explain the reduction of insulin sensitivity with increasing age. It is also noteworthy that mitochondrial biogenesis is impaired in elderly human subjects, and the rate of oxidative phosphorylation is reduced in strong association with developing insulin resistance. The accumulation of fatty acids and other lipid metabolites may contribute further to deterioration of mitochondrial function and ROS production exacerbating defective insulin signaling [97].

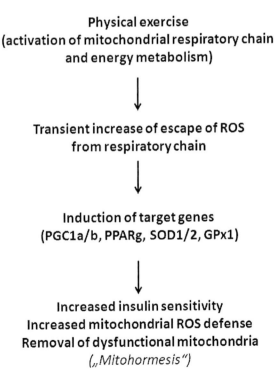

Figure 9. Formation of ROS in response to physical exercise and its consequences for insulin sensitivity and maintenance of a resilient mitochondrial network ("mitohormesis") (modified from [99]). PGC1α, PCG1β, and PPARγ are inducers of insulin sensitivity; superoxide dismutase (SOD) 1 and 2 and glutathione peroxidase 1 (GPx) are key enzymes of antioxidant defense.

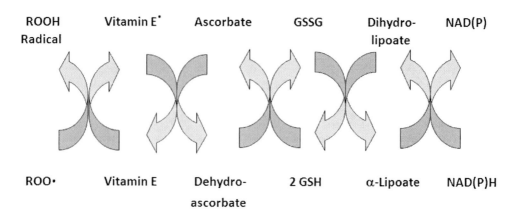

Figure 10. The antioxidant network.

The ambivalent roles of ROS make it difficult to predict whether treatment of diabetes with antioxidant supplements will be beneficial or not. There is evidence that the use of antioxidants such as vitamin E and C inhibits the transient increases in ROS in response to exercise and fasting [98, 99]. Thus, antioxidants may provide some prophylaxis against exercise-induced free radicals. On the other hand, antioxidants may hamper the training-induced adaptations in endurance performance and compensatory increases in antioxidant enzymes and may thereby interfere with the health-promoting effects of exercise [99, 100].

There are several lines of evidence that antioxidants might be protective in metabolic situations where the generation of ROS becomes chronically elevated ("generalized oxidative stress" [48, 101]. If this hypothesis is true, then reversal of the imbalance between ROS and antioxidant capacity should improve insulin resistance. This has been demonstrated with the antioxidant α-lipoic acid [102], which *in vitro*, in animals and in diabetic patients improved glucose utilisation and insulin sensitivity [103]. However, these beneficial effects of α-lipoic acid may be only partly attributable to its anti-oxidative activity, as it also impacts glucose oxidation and the activity of pyruvate dehydrogenase. Salutary effects of other antioxidants, such as vitamin E, acetylcysteine and glutathione, have also been demonstrated. Vitamin E confers anti-inflammatory activity and improves insulin secretion and action *in vitro* [7, 75, 104-106]. In spite of these protective effects, most authors of large intervention trials have concluded that antioxidants are ineffective in delaying the onset of type 2 diabetes [72, 107].

Recent studies suggest that oxidative stress may also participate in the development of IDDM [48, 108]. Non-obese diabetic (NOD) mice develop autoimmune diabetes following the infiltration of inflammatory cells into pancreatic islets. Those infiltrating cells, comprised of T and B lymphocytes, macrophages and natural killer cells, may mediate β-cell cytotoxicity through ROS. Various studies have found increases in ROS (superoxide radical, hydrogen peroxide) in β-cells infiltrated by inflammatory cells. β-cells are especially vulnerable to oxidative stress, likely due their relatively low levels of SOD, catalase, and GPx. Antioxidants such as RRR-α-tocopherol and nicotinamide have been shown to have protective effects against diabetes in NOD mice [109, 110]. In order to prove the concept of oxidative stress-mediated pancreatic β-cell destruction, Miyazaki and coworkers generated a NOD transgenic mouse overexpressing thioredoxin, a small (12 kDa) protein with antioxidant function (see Vol. II, Chapter 9), exclusively in pancreatic β-cells. Spontaneous diabetes was prevented or delayed in the NOD transgenic mice [111]. The results support the hypothesis that ROS play an essential role in the pathogenesis of IDDM and that antioxidant treatment (such as thioredoxin overexpression) protects against the development of this disease. Large, controlled clinical trials will be necessary to establish definitively the protective role of antioxidants in type I diabetes.

Conclusions and Future Aspects

On the basis of available clinical evidence, it is not possible at this juncture to advocate antioxidant treatment to prevent the onset of diabetes or delay its vascular complications. There may be some exceptions. Antioxidant supplementation may be recommended for subjects on a strict slimming diet, for elderly patients whose consumption of fresh fruits and vegetables is inadequate, and for other malnourished subjects.

The apparent ineffectiveness of antioxidant supplementation to prevent the onset of diabetes or its complications in humans does not necessarily undermine the role(s) of ROS in this disorder. Other considerations must be entertained: (i) The type of antioxidant used: it is possible that the compounds administered and their dosing regimens were insufficient. For example, vitamin E and C may acquire pro-oxidant properties in altered redox microenvironments [112] as may occur in diabetic (and other) patients with aberrant antioxidant defense networks (Figure 10). (ii) Orally-administered antioxidants may be inaccessible to sources of ROS generation within specific intracellular compartments or organelles (limited bioavailability). (iii) Administration of high-dose alpha-tocopherol may suppress levels of gamma-tocopherol and thereby limit benefits, which are fairly unique to the latter, e.g. trapping of reactive nitrogen species and detoxification of nitrogen dioxide [113, 114].(iv) In some studies, antioxidant supplements may have been administered late in the course of diabetes when many vascular and other complications of the disease became irreversible. (v) There may be confounding effects of concurrent medication exposure. Many patients enrolled in large clinical trials were taking aspirin prophylactically. Aspirin exhibits some intrinsic antioxidative activity, which could mask benefits accruing from additional exposure to exogenous free radical scavengers ('ceiling effect'). Similarly, inhibition of NADPH oxidase by angiotensin-converting enzyme inhibitors or angiotensin receptor antagonists (used for the treatment of hypertension) may contribute to the reduction of vascular risk and the onset of type 2 diabetes independently of other antioxidant exposure [115].(vi) Certain genetic polymorphisms may influence the responsiveness of individuals to exogenous antioxidants. For example, persons bearing the haptoglobin 2-2 and haptoglobin 1 genotypes exhibit significantly different responses to the antioxidant effects of vitamin E. (vii) The net effects of a given antioxidant on the detrimental and adaptive aspects of ROS generation in diabetes may differ from individual to individual on the basis of undisclosed genetic and environmental factors [116].

In light of available data, the American Heart Association [117] has recommended that the general population consume a diet emphasizing antioxidant-rich fruits, vegetables and grains. The hope remains that more specific antioxidant therapies will be developed which attenuate selectively the detrimental aspects of excess ROS generation in patients with diabetes while sparing or bolstering the manifest adaptive ('physiological') properties of these reactive intermediates. The advent of the latter would address an unmet clinical imperative in the prevention and management of diabetes and its complications.

References

[1] King H, Aubert RE, Herman WH. Global burden of diabetes, 1995-2025: prevalence, numerical estimates, and projections. *Diabetes Care*, 1998; 21(9):1414-1431.

[2] Cowie CC, Rust KF, Byrd-Holt DD, Eberhardt MS, Flegal KM, Engelgau MM et al. Prevalence of diabetes and impaired fasting glucose in adults in the U.S. population: National Health And Nutrition Examination Survey 1999-2002. *Diabetes Care*, 2006; 29(6):1263-1268.

[3] Despres JP, Lemieux I. Abdominal obesity and metabolic syndrome. *Nature*, 2006; 444(7121):881-887.

[4] Porte D, Jr., Schwartz MW. Diabetes complications: why is glucose potentially toxic? *Science*, 1996; 272(5262):699-700.

[5] Baynes JW. Role of oxidative stress in development of complications in diabetes. *Diabetes,* 1991; 40(4):405-412.

[6] Brownlee M. Biochemistry and molecular cell biology of diabetic complications. *Nature,* 2001; 414(6865):813-820.

[7] Rosen P, Nawroth PP, King G, Moller W, Tritschler HJ, Packer L. The role of oxidative stress in the onset and progression of diabetes and its complications: a summary of a Congress Series sponsored by UNESCO-MCBN, the American Diabetes Association and the German Diabetes Society. *Diabetes Metab. Res. Rev.* 2001; 17(3):189-212.

[8] Stirban A, Rosen P, Tschoepe D. Complications of type 1 diabetes: new molecular findings. *Mt. Sinai J. Med.* 2008; 75(4):328-351.

[9] Sies E. *Antioxidants in disease: mechanisms and therapy.* London: Academic Press, 1997.

[10] Halliwell B. Antioxidants: the basics - what they are - how to evaluate them. In: Sies H, editor. *Antioxidants in disease: mechanisms and therapy.* London: Academic Press, 1997: 3-20.

[11] Du X, Stocklauser-Farber K, Rosen P. Generation of reactive oxygen intermediates, activation of NF-kappaB, and induction of apoptosis in human endothelial cells by glucose: role of nitric oxide synthase? *Free Radic. Biol. Med.* 1999; 27(7-8):752-763.

[12] Hink U, Li H, Mollnau H, Oelze M, Matheis E, Hartmann M et al. Mechanisms underlying endothelial dysfunction in diabetes mellitus. *Circ. Res.* 2001; 88(2):E14-E22.

[13] Bellin C, de Wiza DH, Wiernsperger NF, Rosen P. Generation of reactive oxygen species by endothelial and smooth muscle cells: influence of hyperglycemia and metformin. *Horm. Metab. Res.* 2006; 38(11):732-739.

[14] Halliwell B, Chirico S. Lipid peroxidation: its mechanism, measurement, and significance. *Am. J. Clin. Nutr.* 1993; 57(5 Suppl):715S-724S.

[15] Nourooz-Zadeh J, Tajaddini-Sarmadi J, McCarthy S, Betteridge DJ, Wolff SP. Elevated levels of authentic plasma hydroperoxides in NIDDM. *Diabetes,* 1995; 44(9):1054-1058.

[16] Nourooz-Zadeh J, Tajaddini-Sarmadi J, Wolff SP. Measurement of plasma hydroperoxide concentrations by the ferrous oxidation-xylenol orange assay in conjunction with triphenylphosphine. *Anal. Biochem.* 1994; 220(2):403-409.

[17] Gopaul NK, Zacharowski K, Halliwell B, Anggard EE. Evaluation of the postprandial effects of a fast-food meal on human plasma F(2)-isoprostane levels. *Free Radic. Biol. Med.* 2000; 28(5):806-814.

[18] Davis M, Dean R. Radical-mediated protein oxidation. From chemsitry to medicine. Oxford, UK: Oxford University Press, 1997.

[19] Levine RL, Garland D, Oliver CN, Amici A, Climent I, Lenz AG et al. Determination of carbonyl content in oxidatively modified proteins. *Methods Enzymol.* 1990; 186:464-478.

[20] Beckman J, Chen J, Ischiropoulos H, Crow J. *Oxidative damage of peroxinitrite.* 1994: 229-240.

[21] Rosen P, Toeller M. Vitamin E in diabetes. Increased oxidative stress and its prevention as a strategy to prevent vascular complications? *Int. J. Vitam. Nutr. Res.* 1999; 69(3):206-212.

[22] Rosen P, Osmers A. Oxidative stress in young Zucker rats with impaired glucose tolerance is diminished by acarbose. *Horm. Metab. Res.* 2006; 38(9):575-586.

[23] Rosen P, Wiernsperger NF. Metformin delays the manifestation of diabetes and vascular dysfunction in Goto-Kakizaki rats by reduction of mitochondrial oxidative stress. *Diabetes Metab. Res. Rev.* 2006; 22(4):323-330.

[24] Nourooz-Zadeh J, Rahimi A, Tajaddini-Sarmadi J, Tritschler H, Rosen P, Halliwell B et al. Relationships between plasma measures of oxidative stress and metabolic control in NIDDM. *Diabetologia,* 1997; 40(6):647-653.

[25] Dandona P, Thusu K, Cook S, Snyder B, Makowski J, Armstrong D et al. Oxidative damage to DNA in diabetes mellitus. *Lancet,* 1996; 347(8999):444-445.

[26] Davi G, Ciabattoni G, Consoli A, Mezzetti A, Falco A, Santarone S et al. In vivo formation of 8-iso-prostaglandin f2alpha and platelet activation in diabetes mellitus: effects of improved metabolic control and vitamin E supplementation. *Circulation,* 1999; 99(2):224-229.

[27] Salonen JT, Nyyssonen K, Tuomainen TP, Maenpaa PH, Korpela H, Kaplan GA et al. Increased risk of non-insulin dependent diabetes mellitus at low plasma vitamin E concentrations: a four year follow up study in men. *BMJ,* 1995; 311(7013):1124-1127.

[28] Thornalley PJ, McLellan AC, Lo TW, Benn J, Sonksen PH. Negative association between erythrocyte reduced glutathione concentration and diabetic complications. *Clin. Sci.* (Lond) 1996; 91(5):575-582.

[29] Rosen P, Rosen R. Oxidative stress and microvascular function in insulin-resistant states. In: Wiernsperger N, Bouskela E, editors. *Microcirculation and insulin resistance.* Bentham E-Books, 2009.

[30] Nishikawa T, Edelstein D, Brownlee M. The missing link: a single unifying mechanism for diabetic complications. *Kidney Int. Suppl.* 2000; 77:S26-S30.

[31] Pagano PJ, Ito Y, Tornheim K, Gallop PM, Tauber AI, Cohen RA. An NADPH oxidase superoxide-generating system in the rabbit aorta. *Am. J. Physiol.* 1995; 268(6 Pt 2):H2274-H2280.

[32] Droge W. Free radicals in the physiological control of cell function. *Physiol. Rev.* 2002; 82(1):47-95.

[33] Cadenas E, Davies KJ. Mitochondrial free radical generation, oxidative stress, and aging. *Free Radic. Biol. Med.* 2000; 29(3-4):222-230.

[34] Raha S, Robinson BH. Mitochondria, oxygen free radicals, disease and ageing. *Trends Biochem. Sci.* 2000; 25(10):502-508.

[35] Inoguchi T, Li P, Umeda F, Yu HY, Kakimoto M, Imamura M et al. High glucose level and free fatty acid stimulate reactive oxygen species production through protein kinase C--dependent activation of NAD(P)H oxidase in cultured vascular cells. *Diabetes,* 2000; 49(11):1939-1945.

[36] Inoguchi T, Sonta T, Tsubouchi H, Etoh T, Kakimoto M, Sonoda N et al. Protein kinase C-dependent increase in reactive oxygen species (ROS) production in vascular tissues of diabetes: role of vascular NAD(P)H oxidase. *J. Am. Soc. Nephrol.* 2003; 14(8 Suppl 3):S227-S232.

[37] Wautier MP, Chappey O, Corda S, Stern DM, Schmidt AM, Wautier JL. Activation of NADPH oxidase by AGE links oxidant stress to altered gene expression via RAGE. *Am. J. Physiol. Endocrinol. Metab.* 2001; 280(5):E685-E694.

[38] Roberts CK, Barnard RJ, Sindhu RK, Jurczak M, Ehdaie A, Vaziri ND. Oxidative stress and dysregulation of NAD(P)H oxidase and antioxidant enzymes in diet-induced metabolic syndrome. *Metabolism,* 2006; 55(7):928-934.

[39] Gao CL, Zhu C, Zhao YP, Chen XH, Ji CB, Zhang CM et al. Mitochondrial dysfunction is induced by high levels of glucose and free fatty acids in 3T3-L1 adipocytes. *Mol. Cell Endocrinol.* 2010; 320(1-2):25-33.

[40] Gao L, Mann GE. Vascular NAD(P)H oxidase activation in diabetes: a double-edged sword in redox signalling. *Cardiovasc. Res.* 2009; 82(1):9-20.

[41] Forbes JM, Coughlan MT, Cooper ME. Oxidative stress as a major culprit in kidney disease in diabetes. *Diabetes,* 2008; 57(6):1446-1454.

[42] Zhou MS, Hernandez S, I, Pagano PJ, Jaimes EA, Raij L. Reduced NAD(P)H oxidase in low renin hypertension: link among angiotensin II, atherogenesis, and blood pressure. *Hypertension,* 2006; 47(1):81-86.

[43] Venugopal J, Hanashiro K, Yang ZZ, Nagamine Y. Identification and modulation of a caveolae-dependent signal pathway that regulates plasminogen activator inhibitor-1 in insulin-resistant adipocytes. *Proc. Natl. Acad. Sci. U S A,* 2004; 101(49):17120-17125.

[44] Du XL, Sui GZ, Stockklauser-Farber K, Weiss J, Zink S, Schwippert B et al. Introduction of apoptosis by high proinsulin and glucose in cultured human umbilical vein endothelial cells is mediated by reactive oxygen species. *Diabetologia,* 1998; 41(3):249-256.

[45] Ceriello A, Bortolotti N, Crescentini A, Motz E, Lizzio S, Russo A et al. Antioxidant defenses are reduced during the oral glucose tolerance test in normal and non-insulin-dependent diabetic subjects. *Eur. J. Clin. Invest.* 1998; 28(4):329-333.

[46] Du X, Matsumura T, Edelstein D, Rossetti L, Zsengeller Z, Szabo C et al. Inhibition of GAPDH activity by poly(ADP-ribose) polymerase activates three major pathways of hyperglycemic damage in endothelial cells. *J. Clin. Invest.* 2003; 112(7):1049-1057.

[47] Pacher P, Mabley JG, Soriano FG, Liaudet L, Szabo C. Activation of poly(ADP-ribose) polymerase contributes to the endothelial dysfunction associated with hypertension and aging. *Int. J. Mol. Med.* 2002; 9(6):659-664.

[48] Evans, JL, Goldfine I, Maddux B, Grodsky G. Are oxidative stress-acitvatedsignaling pathways mediators of insulin resistance and ß-cell dysfunction? *Diabetes*, 52, 1-8. 2003.

[49] Schulze-Osthoff K, Bauer M, Wesselborg S, Baeuerle P. Reactive oxygen species as primary signals and second messenger in the activation of transcription factors. In: Forman H, Cadenas E, editors. *Oxidative stress and signal transduction*. New York: Chapmann and Hall, 1997: 239-259.

[50] Ho E, Bray TM. Antioxidants, NFkappaB activation, and diabetogenesis. *Proc. Soc. Exp. Biol. Med.* 1999; 222(3):205-213.

[51] Itani SI, Ruderman NB, Schmieder F, Boden G. Lipid-induced insulin resistance in human muscle is associated with changes in diacylglycerol, protein kinase C, and IkappaB-alpha. *Diabetes*, 2002; 51(7):2005-2011.

[52] Ragheb R, Medhat AM, Shanab GM, Seoudi DM, Fantus IG. Links between enhanced fatty acid flux, protein kinase C and NFkappaB activation, and apoB-lipoprotein production in the fructose-fed hamster model of insulin resistance. *Biochem. Biophys.Res. Commun.* 2008; 370(1):134-139.

[53] Rosen P, Ballhausen T, Bloch W, Addicks K. Endothelial relaxation is disturbed by oxidative stress in the diabetic rat heart: influence of tocopherol as antioxidant. *Diabetologia* 1995; 38(10):1157-1168.

[54] Simon A, Fanburg B, Cochran B. STAT activation by oxidative stress. In: Forman H, Cadenas E, editors. *Oxidative stress and signal transduction*. New York: Chapmann and Hall, 1997: 260-271.

[55] Du XL, Edelstein D, Rossetti L, Fantus IG, Goldberg H, Ziyadeh F et al. Hyperglycemia-induced mitochondrial superoxide overproduction activates the hexosamine pathway and induces plasminogen activator inhibitor-1 expression by increasing Sp1 glycosylation. *Proc. Natl. Acad. Sci. U S A*, 2000; 97(22):12222-12226.

[56] Pacher P, Liaudet L, Soriano FG, Mabley JG, Szabo E, Szabo C. The role of poly(ADP-ribose) polymerase activation in the development of myocardial and endothelial dysfunction in diabetes. *Diabetes*, 2002; 51(2):514-521.

[57] Fuller CJ, Chandalia M, Garg A, Grundy SM, Jialal I. RRR-alpha-tocopheryl acetate supplementation at pharmacologic doses decreases low-density-lipoprotein oxidative susceptibility but not protein glycation in patients with diabetes mellitus. *Am. J. Clin. Nutr.* 1996; 63(5):753-759.

[58] Facchini FS, Humphreys MH, DoNascimento CA, Abbasi F, Reaven GM. Relation between insulin resistance and plasma concentrations of lipid hydroperoxides, carotenoids, and tocopherols. *Am. J. Clin. Nutr.* 2000; 72(3):776-779.

[59] Reaven G. Insulin resistance and its consequences: type 2 diabetes and coronary heart disease. In: LeRoith D, Taylor S, Olefsky J, editors. Diabetes mellitus: A fundamental and clinical text. Philadelphia: Lippicott Williams and Wilkins, 2000: 604-615.

[60] Astley S, Langrish-Smith A, Southon S, Sampson M. Vitamin E supplementation and oxidative damage to DNA and plasma LDL in type 1 diabetes. *Diabetes Care*, 1999; 22(10):1626-1631.

[61] Bursell SE, King GL. Can protein kinase C inhibition and vitamin E prevent the development of diabetic vascular complications? *Diabetes Res. Clin. Pract.* 1999; 45(2-3):169-182.

[62] Lee IK, Koya D, Ishi H, Kanoh H, King GL. d-Alpha-tocopherol prevents the hyperglycemia induced activation of diacylglycerol (DAG)-protein kinase C (PKC) pathway in vascular smooth muscle cell by an increase of DAG kinase activity. *DiabetesRes. Clin. Pract.* 1999; 45(2-3):183-190.

[63] Wang Y, Feng W, Xue W, Tan Y, Hein DW, Li XK et al. Inactivation of GSK-3beta by metallothionein prevents diabetes-related changes in cardiac energy metabolism, inflammation, nitrosative damage, and remodeling. *Diabetes,* 2009; 58(6):1391-1402.

[64] Dong F, Li Q, Sreejayan N, Nunn JM, Ren J. Metallothionein prevents high-fat diet induced cardiac contractile dysfunction: role of peroxisome proliferator activated receptor gamma coactivator 1alpha and mitochondrial biogenesis. *Diabetes,* 2007; 56(9):2201-2212.

[65] Zheng S, Carlson EC, Yang L, Kralik PM, Huang Y, Epstein PN. Podocyte-specific overexpression of the antioxidant metallothionein reduces diabetic nephropathy. *J. Am. Soc. Nephrol.* 2008; 19(11):2077-2085.

[66] Ebenezer PJ, Mariappan N, Elks CM, Haque M, Francis J. Diet-induced renal changes in Zucker rats are ameliorated by the superoxide dismutase mimetic TEMPOL. *Obesity,* (Silver Spring) 2009; 17(11):1994-2002.

[67] Fujita H, Fujishima H, Chida S, Takahashi K, Qi Z, Kanetsuna Y et al. Reduction of renal superoxide dismutase in progressive diabetic nephropathy. *J. Am. Soc. Nephrol.* 2009; 20(6):1303-1313.

[68] Fardoun RZ. The use of vitamin E in type 2 diabetes mellitus. *Clin. Exp. Hypertens,* 2007; 29(3):135-148.

[69] Lopes de Jesus CC, Atallah AN, Valente O, Moca T, V. Vitamin C and superoxide dismutase (SOD) for diabetic retinopathy. *Cochrane DatabaseSyst. Rev.* 2008;(1):CD006695.

[70] Madsen-Bouterse SA, Kowluru RA. Oxidative stress and diabetic retinopathy: pathophysiological mechanisms and treatment perspectives. *Rev. Endocr. Metab. Disord.* 2008; 9(4):315-327.

[71] Hamer M, Chida Y. Intake of fruit, vegetables, and antioxidants and risk of type 2 diabetes: systematic review and meta-analysis. *J. Hypertens,* 2007; 25(12):2361-2369.

[72] Liu S, Lee IM, Song Y, Van Denburgh M, Cook NR, Manson JE et al. Vitamin E and risk of type 2 diabetes in the women's health study randomized controlled trial. *Diabetes,* 2006; 55(10):2856-2862.

[73] Song Y, Cook NR, Albert CM, Van Denburgh M, Manson JE. Effects of vitamins C and E and beta-carotene on the risk of type 2 diabetes in women at high risk of cardiovascular disease: a randomized controlled trial. *Am. J. Clin. Nutr.* 2009; 90(2):429-437.

[74] Riccioni G, Bucciarelli T, Mancini B, Corradi F, Di Ilio C, Mattei PA et al. Antioxidantvitaminsupplementation in cardiovasculardiseases. *Ann. Clin. Lab. Sci.* 2007; 37(1):89-95.

[75] Singh U, Jialal I. Alpha-lipoic acid supplementation and diabetes. *Nutr. Rev.* 2008; 66(11):646-657.

[76] Tang J, Wingerchuk DM, Crum BA, Rubin DI, Demaerschalk BM. Alpha-lipoic acid may improve symptomatic diabetic polyneuropathy. *Neurologist*,2007; 13(3):164-167.

[77] Ziegler D, Nowak H, Kempler P, Vargha P, Low PA. Treatment of symptomatic diabetic polyneuropathy with the antioxidant alpha-lipoic acid: a meta-analysis. *Diabet Med.* 2004; 21(2):114-121.

[78] Yim S, Malhotra A, Veves A. Antioxidants and CVD in diabetes: where do we stand now. *Curr. Diab. Rep.* 2007; 7(1):8-13.

[79] Kowluru RA, Chan PS. Oxidative stress and diabetic retinopathy. *Exp. Diabetes, Res.* 2007; 2007:43603.

[80] Czech MP, Lawrence JC, Jr., Lynn WS. Evidence for the involvement of sulfhydryl oxidation in the regulation of fat cell hexose transport by insulin. *Proc. Natl. Acad. Sci. U S A* 1974; 71(10):4173-4177.

[81] Goldstein BJ, Mahadev K, Wu X. Redox paradox: insulin action is facilitated by insulin-stimulated reactive oxygen species with multiple potential signaling targets. *Diabetes*, 2005; 54(2):311-321.

[82] Powers SK, Jackson MJ. Exercise-induced oxidative stress: cellular mechanisms and impact on muscle force production. *Physiol. Rev.* 2008; 88(4):1243-1276.

[83] Higuchi M, Cartier LJ, Chen M, Holloszy JO. Superoxide dismutase and catalase in skeletal muscle: adaptive response to exercise. *J. Gerontol.* 1985; 40(3):281-286.

[84] Holloszy JO, Kohrt WM, Hansen PA. The regulation of carbohydrate and fat metabolism during and after exercise. *Front Biosci.* 1998; 3:D1011-D1027.

[85] Boveris A, Fraga CG. Oxidative stress in aging and disease. *Mol. Aspects Med.* 2004; 25(1-2):1-4.

[86] Warburton DE, Nicol CW, Bredin SS. Health benefits of physical activity: the evidence. *CMAJ,* 2006; 174(6):801-809.

[87] Tapia P. Sublethal mitochondrial stress with attendant stoichiometric augmentation of reactive oxygen species may precipitate many of the beneficial alterations in cellular physiology produced by caloric restriction, intermittent fasting, exercise and dietary phytonutrients: "Mitohormesis" for health and vitality. *Med. Hypothesis,* 2006; 66:832-843.

[88] McGarry JD. Banting lecture 2001: dysregulation of fatty acid metabolism in the etiology of type 2 diabetes. *Diabetes*, 2002; 51(1):7-18.

[89] Boden G. Role of fatty acids in the pathogenesis of insulin resistance and NIDDM. *Diabetes*, 1997; 46(1):3-10.

[90] Steppan CM, Bailey ST, Bhat S, Brown EJ, Banerjee RR, Wright CM et al. The hormone resistin links obesity to diabetes. *Nature,* 2001; 409(6818):307-312.

[91] Steinberg HO, Chaker H, Leaming R, Johnson A, Brechtel G, Baron AD. Obesity/insulin resistance is associated with endothelial dysfunction. Implications for the syndrome of insulin resistance. *J. Clin. Invest.* 1996; 97(11):2601-2610.

[92] Laakso M, Edelman SV, Brechtel G, Baron AD. Decreased effect of insulin to stimulate skeletal muscle blood flow in obese man. A novel mechanism for insulin resistance. *J. Clin. Invest.* 1990; 85(6):1844-1852.

[93] Ritz P, Berrut G. Mitochondrial function, energy expenditure, aging and insulin resistance. *Diabetes Metab.* 2005; 31 Spec No 2:5S67-5S73.

[94] Frisard M, Ravussin E. Energy metabolism and oxidative stress: impact on the metabolic syndrome and the aging process. *Endocrine*, 2006; 29(1):27-32.

[95] Simoneau JA, Kelley DE. Altered glycolytic and oxidative capacities of skeletal muscle contribute to insulin resistance in NIDDM. *J. Appl. Physiol.* 1997; 83(1):166-171.

[96] Petersen KF, Befroy D, Dufour S, Dziura J, Ariyan C, Rothman DL et al. Mitochondrial dysfunction in the elderly: possible role in insulin resistance. *Science,* 2003; 300(5622):1140-1142.

[97] Kim JA, Wei Y, Sowers JR. Role of mitochondrial dysfunction in insulin resistance. *Circ. Res.* 2008; 102(4):401-414.

[98] Davison GW, Ashton T, George L, Young IS, McEneny J, Davies B et al. Molecular detection of exercise-induced free radicals following ascorbate prophylaxis in type 1 diabetes mellitus: a randomised controlled trial. *Diabetologia,* 2008; 51(11):2049-2059.

[99] Ristow M, Zarse K, Oberbach A, Kloting N, Birringer M, Kiehntopf M et al. Antioxidants prevent health-promoting effects of physical exercise in humans. *Proc. Natl. Acad. Sci. U S A,* 2009; 106(21):8665-8670.

[100] Gomez-Cabrera MC, Domenech E, Vina J. Moderate exercise is an antioxidant: upregulation of antioxidant genes by training. *Free Radic. Biol. Med.* 2008; 44(2):126-131.

[101] Houstis N, Rosen ED, Lander ES. Reactive oxygen species have a causal role in multiple forms of insulin resistance. *Nature,* 2006; 440(7086):944-948.

[102] Packer L, Rösen P, Tritschler H, King GL, Azzi A. *Antioxidants in diabetesmanagement.* New York: Marcel Dekker, 2000.

[103] Jacob S, Ruus P, Hermann R, Tritschler HJ, Maerker E, Renn W et al. Oral administration of RAC-alpha-lipoic acid modulates insulin sensitivity in patients with type-2 diabetes mellitus: a placebo-controlled pilot trial. *Free Radic. Biol. Med.* 1999; 27(3-4):309-314.

[104] Barbagallo M, Dominguez LJ, Tagliamonte MR, Resnick LM, Paolisso G. Effects of vitamin E and glutathione on glucose metabolism: role of magnesium. *Hypertension,* 1999; 34(4 Pt 2):1002-1006.

[105] Paolisso G, D'Amore A, Galzerano D, Balbi V, Giugliano D, Varricchio M et al. Daily vitamin E supplements improve metabolic control but not insulin secretion in elderly type II diabetic patients. *Diabetes Care,* 1993; 16(11):1433-1437.

[106] Paolisso G, D'Amore A, Giugliano D, Ceriello A, Varricchio M, D'Onofrio F. Pharmacologic doses of vitamin E improve insulin action in healthy subjects and non-insulin-dependent diabetic patients. *Am. J. Clin. Nutr.* 1993; 57(5):650-656.

[107] Czernichow S, Couthouis A, Bertrais S, Vergnaud AC, Dauchet L, Galan P et al. Antioxidant supplementation does not affect fasting plasma glucose in the Supplementation with Antioxidant Vitamins and Minerals (SU.VI.MAX) study in France: association with dietary intake and plasma concentrations. *Am. J. Clin. Nutr.* 2006; 84(2):395-399.

[108] Brownlee M. A radical explanation for glucose-induced beta cell dysfunction. *J. Clin. Invest.* 2003; 112(12):1788-1790.

[109] Elliott RB, Pilcher CC, Stewart A, Fergusson D, McGregor MA. The use of nicotinamide in the prevention of type 1 diabetes. *Ann. N Y Acad. Sci.* 1993; 696:333-341.

[110] Beales PE, Williams AJ, Albertini MC, Pozzilli P. Vitamin E delays diabetes onset in the non-obese diabetic mouse. *Horm. Metab. Res.* 1994; 26(10):450-452.

[111] Hotta M, Tashiro F, Ikegami H, Niwa H, Ogihara T, Yodoi J et al. Pancreatic beta cell-specific expression of thioredoxin, an antioxidative and antiapoptotic protein, prevents autoimmune and streptozotocin-induced diabetes. *J. Exp. Med.* 1998; 188(8):1445-1451.

[112] Winterbone MS, Sampson MJ, Saha S, Hughes JC, Hughes DA. Pro-oxidant effect of alpha-tocopherol in patients with type 2 diabetes after an oral glucose tolerance test--a randomised controlled trial. *Cardiovasc. Diabetol.* 2007; 6:8.

[113] Gutierrez AD, de Serna DG, Robinson I, Schade DS. The response of gamma vitamin E to varying dosages of alpha vitamin E plus vitamin C. *Metabolism* 2009; 58(4):469-478.

[114] Devaraj S, Leonard S, Traber MG, Jialal I. Gamma-tocopherol supplementation alone and in combination with alpha-tocopherol alters biomarkers of oxidative stress and inflammation in subjects with metabolic syndrome. *Free Radic Biol Med* 2008; 44(6):1203-1208.

[115] Yusuf S, Dagenais G, Pogue J, Bosch J, Sleight P. Vitamin E supplementation and cardiovascular events in high-risk patients. The Heart Outcomes Prevention Evaluation Study Investigators. *N. Engl. J. Med.* 2000; 342(3):154-160.

[116] Milman U, Blum S, Shapira C, Aronson D, Miller-Lotan R, Anbinder Y et al. Vitamin E supplementation reduces cardiovascular events in a subgroup of middle-aged individuals with both type 2 diabetes mellitus and the haptoglobin 2-2 genotype: a prospective double-blinded clinical trial. *Arterioscler. ThrombVasc. Biol.* 2008; 28(2):341-347.

[117] Tribble DL. AHA Science Advisory. Antioxidant consumption and risk of coronary heart disease: emphasison vitamin C, vitamin E, and beta-carotene: A statement for healthcare professionals from the American Heart Association. *Circulation* 1999; 99(4):591-595.

In: Principles of Free Radical Biomedicine, Volume III
Editors: K. Pantopoulos and H. M. Schipper

ISBN 978-1-61324-184-4
©2012 Nova SciencePublishers, Inc.

Chapter 10

Redox Neurology

Hyman M. Schipper[*]

Centre for Neurotranslational Research, Lady Davis Institute for Medical Research,
Jewish General Hospital, McGill University, Montreal
Quebec, Canada, H3T 1E2

1. Introduction

There has been, in recent years, a deluge of information implicating reactive oxygen, nitrogen and sulfur species (ROS, RNS, RSS) and oxidative stress (OS) in virtually every field of biology and medicine. In conditions as diverse as ischemic heart disease, asthma, diabetes mellitus, inflammatory bowel disease, macular degeneration and cataractogenesis, glomerulonephritis, infertility and cancer, OS has been acknowledged as a critical common pathway for cell death and dysfunction, and a salient target for therapeutic intervention.More recently, it has become apparent that, at 'physiological' concentrations, ROS and other reactive intermediates may play beneficial roles as signaling molecules involved in gene regulation, cell growth, differentiation, replicative senescence and apoptosis, and as a pivotal defense mounted by tissue macrophages and leukocytes against invading pathogens.

OS has been implicated in a wide spectrum of disorders affecting the central and peripheral nervous systems. *Redox Neurology* may be defined as *the study of the roles of free radicals, transition metals, oxidative stress and antioxidant defences in diseases of the nervous system.* The prominent rise in numbers of published clinical and experimental reports related to the 'redox neurosciences' over the last couple of decades (Figure 1) underscores the intense interest in this area.

The objectives of this Chapter are to facilitate an appreciation of biological features which render the nervous system uniquely prone to free radical injury, describe major etiopathogenetic mechanisms mediating oxidative neural damage, and discuss select diseases which illustrate key principles of 'redox neurology'.

---

[*]E-mail: hyman.schipper@mcgill.ca

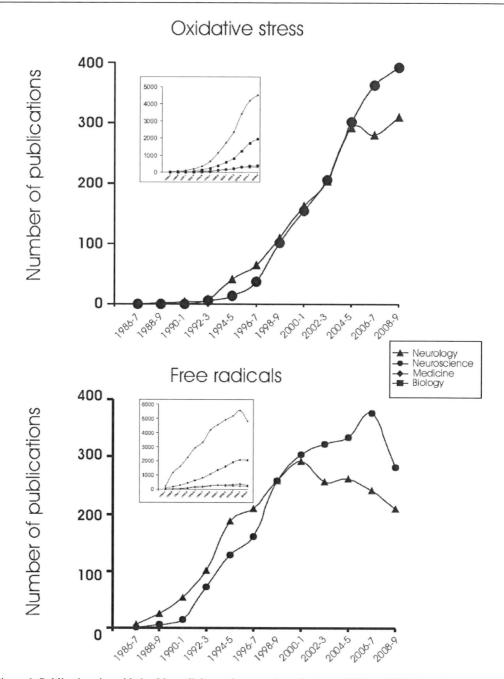

Figure 1. Publications in oxidative biomedicine and neuroscience between 1986 and 2009 based on PUBMED searches of the biological and medical literature. A. Search terms: [FREE RADICAL] and [NEUROLOGY] or [NEUROSCIENCE] or [MEDICINE] or [BIOLOGY]. B. Search terms: [OXIDATIVE STRESS] and [NEUROLOGY] or [NEUROSCIENCE] or [MEDICINE] or [BIOLOGY].

To impress upon the reader the richness and complexity of this burgeoning field, the author's research interest in disorders of brain iron homeostasis is presented with much finer granularity. The hierarchical arrangement of the chapter topics should allow the reader to navigate the text at the desired level of detail. Italics denote general principles and key concepts.

2. The Vulnerable Brain

Various biochemical and physiological factors have been delineated that place the nervous system at particular risk for oxidative damage. Some of the more important of these are discussed in this section.

2.1. Oxygen Consumption

The human brain is responsible for ~20% of total O_2 consumption under basal conditions, although it represents only 2% of total body mass. This *high flux of molecular oxygen in normally-respiring neural tissues provides a substrate for ample ROS generation within mitochondria, the endoplasmic reticulum and other subcellular compartments.* Excessive free radical production may be responsible, at least in part, for iatrogenic central nervous system (CNS) and retinal damage in premature neonates accruing from hyperoxic exposure.

2.2. Free Radicals, Mitochondria and Brain Aging

Under basal conditions, ~1-3% of molecular oxygen taken up by respiring mitochondria is metabolized to O_2^- and then to other, more damaging free radical intermediates (Vol. II, Chapter 15). Mitochondrial ROS generation substantially increases in aging and diseased tissues, particularly in post-mitotic cells such as neurons, cardiomyocytes and skeletal muscle. It is therefore hardly surprising that rare disorders stemming from mutations in the mitochondrial genome, such as MELAS, MERRF and the Kearn-Sayre syndrome, predominantly affect the CNS, heart and skeletal muscle. Mitochondrial free radical production also figures centrally in the development of the far more common, aging-related neurodegenerative disorders. *The "free radical-mitochondrial" theory remains among the most successful conceptualizations of the aging process and may inform the pathogenesis of Alzheimer disease (AD), Parkinson disease (PD) and other late-life human neurodegenerative afflictions.* The theory posits that oxidative mitochondrial damage, initiated by environmental insults and/or intrinsic metabolic processes, results in a self-reinforcing cycle of events characterized by infidelity of electron transport and augmented ROS generation (superoxide, hydrogen peroxide) within the inner mitochondrial membrane. Mitochondrial DNA (mtDNA) is particularly susceptible to oxidative damage, exhibiting an approximately 10-100 fold greater mutation rate than nuclear DNA. Mutated mtDNA may code for abnormal cytochromes of the electron transport chain (ETC) that exacerbates electron 'leakage' and free radical generation within the inner mitochondrial membrane [1]. The oxidative mitochondrial lesions, in turn, promote bioenergetic failure (ATP depletion and deterioration of ATP-dependent processes) and progressive tissue aging [1, 2]. Evidence garnered across the phylogenetic spectrum in support of this theory is reviewed elsewhere [3-5]. Importantly, the model predicts that any injury or disease (genetic, acquired or multifactorial) that augments mitochondrial free radical production might accelerate senescence of the affected tissue or organ. The clinical impression that patients with substance abuse or chronic systemic illness often appear "older than stated age" may be a manifestation of this formulation at the organismal level. Conversely, normal aging tissues harboring an increasingly unfavourable mosaic of healthy and ROS-generating mitochondria may become progressively predisposed to aging-associated conditions such as neurodegeneration, atherosclerosis, and cancer [6]. Changes characteristic of Alzheimer disease (AD) and Parkinson disease (PD) will be invoked to illustrate these principles, although it is acknowledged that many of the features described are ubiquitous to other aging-related neurodegenerative and neuroinflammatory conditions.

2.2.1. Alzheimer Disease

AD is a dementing illness characterized by progressive neuronal degeneration, gliosis, and the accumulation of intracellular inclusions (neurofibrillary tangles) and extracellular deposits of amyloid (senile plaques) in discrete regions of the basal forebrain, hippocampus, and association cortices [7]. Mitochondrial deficits and oxidative stress have been consistently documented in the AD brain and, more enigmatically, in peripheral tissues [8-10].Mitochondrial insufficiency in AD-affected neural tissues is evidenced by (i) deficits in pyruvate dehydrogenase, α-ketoglutarate dehydrogenase and cytochrome c oxidase protein or activity [11], (ii) the presence of excessive mtDNA deletion and missense mutations [12, 13] which correlate with levels of oxidative chemical modifications [14], (iii) attenuated glucose utilization (cerebral metabolism) in positron emission tomographystudies [15, 16] and (iv) altered mitochondrial structure and turnover in the diseased cells [17]. Potential sources of oxidative stress in the AD brain include baseline ROS generation by senescent mitochondria (*vide supra*), β-amyloid-derived H_2O_2 [18], secretion of nitric oxide (NO) and pro-inflammatory cytokines (TNFα, IL-1β) by activated microglia [19] and, as discussed in more detail below, a relative abundance of redox-active tissue iron [6, 20, 21].

2.2.2. Parkinson Disease

Idiopathic Parkinson disease (PD) is an extyrapyramidal (movement) disorder of uncertain etiology that afflicts 1-2% of the population over 65 years of age (Figure 2). PD is characterized pathologically by progressive degeneration of dopaminergic neurons in the substantia nigra pars compacta, formation of α-synuclein-containing fibrillar inclusions (Lewy bodies) in this cell population, and variable depletion of noradrenergic neurons in the locus coeruleus and serotoninergic cells in the median raphé [22]. Mitochondrial insufficiency, predominantly implicating Complex I of the ETC, has been consistently documented in PD-affected neurons, astrocytes and certain peripheral tissues using diverse biochemical, immunohistochemical (IHC) and metabolic neuroimaging techniques [6, 23, 24]. The glial mitochondriopathy may directly or indirectly perpetuate neural injury in the PD nigra by (i) accelerated free radical production within damaged components of the ETC, (ii) suppression of cellular ATP levels and critical ATP-dependent processes such as *de novo* glutathione biosynthesis and uptake of excitotoxic neurotransmitters (glutamate), and (iii) release of cytochrome c and other pro-apoptotic factors [25, 26]. Mitochondrial dysfunction and oxidative stress may also figure prominently in familial PD resulting from mutations in genes coding for LRRK2, parkin, pink1 and α-synuclein proteins [27-35]. Mitochondrial insufficiency and oxidative molecular damage have been implicated in the pathogenesis of other human neurodegenerative disorders - notably amyotrophic lateral sclerosis, progressive supranuclear palsy, frontotemporal degeneration, Huntington disease, Friedreich ataxia and corticobasal degeneration - and occur in cerebrovascular ischemia and hemorrhage (stroke), multiple sclerosis and cerebral malaria [9, 36-39].

Table 1. Proteins implicated in mammalian iron homeostasis. Modified from [53, 89], with permission. For details, see Vol. II, Chapter 19.

Protein	Function
ABCB7	Non-heme Fe export from mitochondria (?)
ABCB10	Mitochondrial transport related to heme synthesis
Ceruloplasmin (Cp)	Ferroxidase activity / Cellular Fe export
DMT1/Nramp2	Membrane transport for Fe^{2+}
Duodenal cytochrome b (Dcytb)	Ferric reductase (provides Fe^{2+} for DMT1 in duodenum)
Ferritin (H and L)	Cellular Fe storage
Ferrochelatase	Fe^{2+} insertion into protoporphyrin IX (heme synthesis)
Ferroportin 1/MTP1/ Ireg1	Cellular Fe export
Frataxin	[Fe-S] cluster synthesis
Heme oxygenases (HO-1 and HO-2)	Recycling of heme Fe / Cell survival
Hemojuvelin (Repulsive Guidance Molecule C)	Unknown/ cardiac and striated muscle Fe metabolism?
Hepcidin	Inhibitor of intestinal Fe absorption and macrophage heme Fe recycling
Hephaestin	Ferroxidase activity / Enterocyte Fe export
HFE	Modulates tissue Fe uptake via interaction with TfR (?)
IRP (1 and 2)	Cellular Fe sensors /Regulators of Fe uptake and storage proteins
Lactoferrin	Fe binding protein / anti-bacterial and anti-viral activities
Melanotransferrin	Unknown / Fe binding protein
Mitochondrial ferritin	Mitochondrial Fe storage (?)
Mitoferrin (1 and 2)	Fe transport to mitochondria
Sideroflexin 1	Mitochondrial transport related to Fe metabolism
Steap3	Endosomal ferrireductase
Transferrin (Tf)	Plasma Fe(III)-carrier
Tf receptor 1 (TfR1)	Membrane receptor for $(Fe)_2$-Tf
Tf receptor 2 (TfR2)	Unknown

2.3. Brain Lipids

The brain is replete with cholesterol and unsaturated fat (e.g. $C_{20:5}$, $C_{22:6}$) and is thus highly vulnerable to lipid peroxidation (Vol. I, Chapter 7). Cholesterol subserves diverse roles in normal mammalian CNS development and function, and in a host of inherited and acquired neurological conditions.

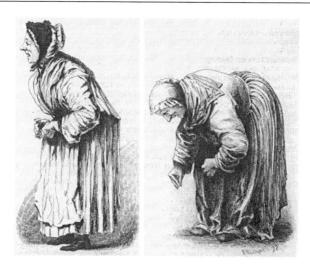

Figure 2. Parkinson disease. Sketches by Paul Richer illustrating the appearance and progression of the disease in an elderly woman in 1874 (*left*) and 1877 (*right*).From [205], with permission.

The human brain contains ~20 mg cholesterol/g tissue, exceeding that of any other organ in the body. Indeed, 25% of the total unesterified body cholesterol resides within the CNS. This holds true regardless of lean body mass because the cholesterol content of the brain is largely autonomous of dietary uptake or hepatic synthesis. Brain cholesterol is mainly synthesized in situ (predominantly within glia) and its metabolism is regulated independently of that in peripheral tissues.

Moreover, cholesterol turnover within the human CNS is slow, exhibiting a half-life of about a year in contrast to that of circulating cholesterol measured in hours [40]. This would permit potentially-deleterious oxidative lipid modifications in brain to persist and accumulate relative to systemic tissues.

Several sites within the cholesterol ring structure and side chain are susceptible to oxidation resulting in the formation of oxidized cholesterol (oxysterols). Enzymatically-generated bioactive oxysterols germane to the CNS include 7-ketocholesterol, 7α- and 7β-hydroxycholesterol, 24-hydroxycholesterol, 25-hydroxycholesterol and 27-hydroxycholesterol. Endogenous tissue cholesterol may also be oxidized non-enzymatically to oxysterols by reactive intermediates generated in the course of lipid peroxidation [41]. Oxysterols may exert important influences within the CNS, which may be either detrimental or beneficial.

As an example of the former, physiologically-relevant concentrations of oxysterols have been shown to induce cytotoxicity/apoptosis in cultured cerebellar granule cells, astrocytes and microglia. In addition, altered patterns of cholesterol hydroxylase expression, and resulting perturbations in neural oxysterol concentrations, may exacerbate neurotoxic amyloid-β deposition in AD tissues.

Alternatively, certain oxysterols may exert salutary effects within the nervous system by suppressing LDL receptor mRNA levels and LDL receptor densities, and opposing the pro-atherogenic effects of oxidized low density lipoprotein. Some regulatory properties of oxysterols may also be mediated through their binding and activation of LXR receptors, followed by interaction of activated LXRs with hormone response elements on target genes [41].

2.4. Oxidizable Neurotransmitters

Neural tissues are enriched for low-molecular-weight compounds, such as dopamine, norepinephrine, and 3-hydroxykynurenine (tryptophan metabolite) and can readily synthesize nitric oxide (a gaseous neurotransmitter/neuromodulator). In turn, *these substances may give rise to a wide array of ROS via enzymatic and autoxidation reactions* [42]. For instance, the breakdown of dopamine by the glial enzyme, monoamine oxidase B yields dihydroxyphenylacetaldehyde, ammonia and the pro-oxidant species, H_2O_2. H_2O_2 may be directly neurotoxic or it may undergo further metabolism to more reactive intermediates such as the hydroxyl radical. The catechol ring of dopamine may also be converted via autoxidation or metal-mediated (pseudo)peroxidase activity to neurotoxic quinones and ortho-semiquinone radicals (Figure 3). Nitric oxide, itself a free radical, can combine with superoxide to generate the neurotoxic species, peroxynitrite ($ONOO^-$). The oxidative bioactivation of dopamine, serotonin and other neurotransmitters has been implicated in the pathogenesis of PD, AD, amyotrophic lateral sclerosis (ALS), Wilson disease, Creutzfeldt-Jakob disease, ischemic stroke, cerebral malaria, HIV encephalopathy, schizophrenia and depression [43-51].

2.5. Transition Metals

Transition metals consist of d-block elements listed between Group IIA and Group IIB of the periodic table. Among them, iron (Fe), copper (Cu), manganese, cadmium and mercury are redox-active (Vol. I, Chapter 5) and are capable of conferring oxidative injury upon deposition within neural tissues. This review will focus primarily on Fe as it is the most abundant transition metal in the CNS and appears to play a role in a wide range of human neurological conditions.

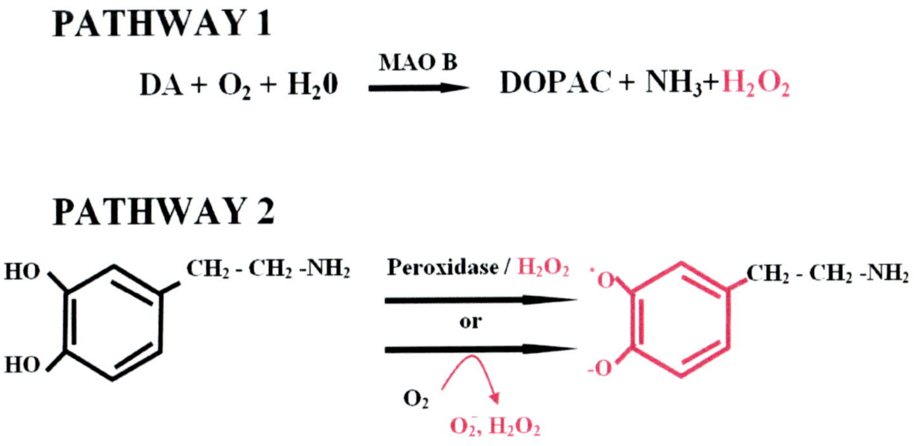

PATHWAY 1

$$DA + O_2 + H_2O \xrightarrow{\text{MAO B}} DOPAC + NH_3 + H_2O_2$$

PATHWAY 2

Figure 3. Oxidative metabolism of dopamine. A. Pathway 1: Monoamine oxidase B (MAO-B)-mediated deamination of dopamine (DA) yields hydrogen peroxide (H_2O_2). B. Pathway 2: In the presence of H_2O_2, the (pseudo)peroxidase activity of ferrous iron (Fe^{2+}) oxidizes DA to dopamine-o-semiquinone radicals. The autoxidation of DA consumes molecular oxygen to yield superoxide, H_2O_2 and dopamine-o-semiquinone radicals. DOPAc, dihydroxyphenylacetaldehyde, NH_3, ammonia. Reactive oxygen species are illustrated in hot pink.

2.5.1. Brain Iron Homeostasis

Brain iron uptake is most efficient during periods of rapid CNS development and continues throughout life [52]. The metal participates in diverse cellular functions including cell proliferation, myelination, electron transport, biogenic amine metabolism, and antioxidant enzyme activity. To enable these vital functions, while concomitantly limiting its propensity to mediate toxic reactions, *iron homeostasis in neural and other tissues is tightly regulated by numerous proteins controlling its absorption, extracellular transport, cellular flux, valence configuration, signalling properties and intracellular* storage [53] (Table 1). The blood-brain barrier (BBB) limits the free passage of transferrin, ceruloplasmin and other proteins from the systemic circulation to the CNS [54]. Blood diferric transferrin binds to transferrin receptors expressed by cerebrovascular endothelial cells at the BBB and the resulting complexes are internalized.

Following dissociation of the complex within endothelial endosomes, apotransferrin is recycled to the circulation and Fe egresses, likely via ferroportin, across the abluminal membrane to the interstitial space. For more details concerning Fe trafficking within and among the various CNS compartments, readers are referred to a review by Moos and colleagues [55]. Little is known regarding mechanisms mediating the release of Fe (and other metals) from the brain parenchyma to the general circulation. In spite of the elaborate regulation of body iron homeostasis (see Vol. II, Chapter 19), the metal progressively accumulates in the aging mammalian CNS. In the senescent human brain, iron storage is prominent in the hippocampus, basal ganglia and certain cerebellar nuclei and less so in the cerebral cortices and other regions [56].

Of note, the brain areas prone to iron sequestration in the course of normal aging are, by and large, those which tend to exhibit pathological metal deposition, oxidative injury and mitochondrial insufficiency in various neurodegenerative disorders of movement and cognition, as described below. Evidence adduced from human neuropathological studies, experimental paradigms of aging-associated neurological disorders, and *in vitro*models of astroglial senescence suggest that *oxidative stress, augmented iron deposition*and *mitochondrial insufficiency in the aging and degenerating CNS may constitute a single neuropathological 'lesion', and that the advent of one component of this triad may obligate the appearance of the others [6].*

2.5.1.1. Disorders of CNS Iron Metabolism

Oxidative stress resulting from perturbations in the levels, distribution or valence of CNS iron has been implicated in a host of genetic and sporadic (acquired) neurological disorders (Table 2).

Iron may promote neural damage in these conditions by mediating (i) the reduction of hydrogen peroxide to highly reactive hydroxyl radicals (Fenton catalysis), (ii) the peroxidatic metabolism of endogenous catechols (e.g. dopamine, 2-hydroxyestradiol) to neurotoxic semiquinone/quinone species and (iii) the bioactivation of pro-toxins (e,g, MPTP) to potent neurotoxins (MPP+) [57, 58]. Attesting to the importance attributed to these reactions, clinical trials have been launched to ascertain the potential therapeutic benefits of metal chelators (e.g deferoxamine, deferiprone, clioquinol) and high-dose antioxidants (e.g. α-tocopherol, CoQ10, idebenone, N-acetylcysteine,) in AD, PD, Friedreich ataxia (FA) and other conditions listed in Table 2.

Table 2. Human neurological conditions featuring aberrant iron homeostasis. FAHN, fatty acid 2-hydroxylase-associated neurodegeneration PKAN, pantothenate kinase2-associated neurodegeneration; PLAN, phospholipase A2G6-associated neurodegeneration. Adapted from [204], with permission.

- CNS senescence
- Cerebral hemorrhage
- Alzheimer disease
- Parkinson disease
- Amyotrophic lateral sclerosis
- Huntington disease
- Progressive supranuclear palsy
- Corticobasal degeneration
- Multiple sclerosis
- Friedreich ataxia
- X-linked sideroblastic anemia with ataxia?
- PKAN (formerly Hallervorden-Spatz)
- PLAN
- FAHN
- Kufor-Rakeb disease
- Aceruloplasminemia
- Neuroferritinopathy
- Superficial siderosis
- Restless legs syndrome
- HIV-1 encephalitis
- Hemochromatosis?

2.5.1.1.1. Sporadic Disorders of Brain Iron Metabolism

Neuropathological, histochemical and neuroimaging studies have consistently revealed excessive deposition of redox-active ironin the basal forebrain and association cortices of patients with sporadicADand in the basal ganglia of subjects with idiopathic PD [20, 21]. Pathological brain iron deposition has also been documented in other sporadic CNS disorders including progressive supranuclear palsy, multiple sclerosis (MS), ischemic stroke, cerebral hemorrhage, cerebral contusion, and HIV-1 encephalitis [59]. In both AD and PD, augmented expression of tissue ferritin, the major intracellular iron storage protein (Vol. II, Chapter 19), parallels the distribution of the surplus iron and largely implicates non-neuronal (glial, endothelial) cellular compartments [6, 20].

Of note, regional concentrations of transferrin binding sites remain unchanged or vary inversely with the elevated iron stores. These observations indicate that the transferrin pathway of iron mobilization, important for normal iron delivery to most peripheral tissues, may contribute little to the pathological deposition of brain iron in these neurodegenerative diseases [60]. Alternate mechanisms for deranged iron compartmentalization in the degenerating CNS have been posited, including the aberrant expression of lactoferrin and melanotransferrin (p97) and their receptors [20, 60, 61], and the heme degrading enzyme, heme oxygenase-1 (HO-1) [59].

2.5.1.1.1.1. The Role of Heme Oxygenase-1

The heme oxygenases (see Vol. II, Chapter 11) are located within the endoplasmic reticulum where they serve, in concert with NADPH cytochrome P450 reductase, to oxidize heme to biliverdin, free ferrous iron and carbon monoxide (CO). Biliverdin is metabolized further to the bile pigment, bilirubin by action of biliverdin reductase [62]. Mammalian cells express at least two isoforms of heme oxygenase, HO-1 (a.k.a. heat shock protein *32*) and HO-2. Whereas HO-2 protein is widely distributed throughout the rodent neuraxis [63], basal HO-1 expression in the normal brain is confined to small groups of scattered neurons and neuroglia [64]. In humans, the *HMOX1* gene is located on chromosome 22q12 and contains four introns and five exons. A 500 bp promoter, a proximal enhancer and two or more distal enhancers occur in the regulatory region of the mammalian *hmox1* gene [65]. Binding sites for the transcription factors AP-1 (Vol. II, Chapter 14), AP-2, nuclear factor kappa B (NF-κB; Vol. II, Chapter 12), HSF and HIF-1 (Vol. II, Chapter 22), as well as metal response elements (MtRE, CdRE) and antioxidant response elements (ARE; Vol. II, Chapter 13) render the *hmox1* gene highly inducible by a wide array of pro-oxidant and inflammatory stimuli including heme, β-amyloid, dopamine, H_2O_2, UV light, transition metals, prostaglandins, pro-inflammatory cytokines and lipopolysaccharide [65, 66]. In the face of oxidative challenge, *induction of HO-1 may protect cells by augmenting the breakdown of pro-oxidant heme and hemoproteins to the radical-scavenging bile pigments, biliverdin and bilirubin* [64, 67-70]. Conversely, in some tissues and under certain experimental conditions, *the heme products, ferrous iron and CO may promote cellular injury by stimulating free radical generation within the mitochondrial and other cellular compartments* [71, 72].

Our laboratory demonstrated that cysteamine, dopamine (DA), β-amyloid and TH1 cytokines (tumor necrosis factor-α, interleukin-1β), up-regulate HO-1 mRNA, protein and/or activity levels in cultured neonatal rat astroglia followed by sequestration of non-transferrin-derived $^{59}Fe/^{55}Fe$ by the mitochondrial compartment [60, 73]. Using various pharmacological approaches, we determined that oxidative stress is a likely common mechanism mediating glial *hmox1* gene induction under these experimental conditions [74, 75]. Co-administration of tin mesoporphyrin (SnMP), a competitive inhibitor of heme oxygenase activity, or dexamethasone, a transcriptional suppressor of the *hmox1* gene, significantly attenuated mitochondrial iron sequestration in cultured astrocytes exposed to the aforementioned stimuli. Similarly, administration of SnMP or dexamethasone abolished the pathological accumulation of mitochondrial ^{55}Fe observed in rat astroglia engineered to over-express the human *hmox1* gene by transient transfection [60, 73, 76]. These findings indicate that up-regulation of HO-1 is a critical event in the cascade leading to excessive mitochondrial iron deposition in oxidatively-challenged astroglia. In astrocytes, up-regulation of HO-1 promotes intracellular OS as evidenced by our observations that a) treatment with SnMP or antioxidants (ascorbate, melatonin or resveratrol) blocked the compensatory induction of the manganese superoxide dismutase (MnSOD) gene in astrocytes challenged with dopamine or transiently transfected with human HO-1 cDNA [72] and b) levels of protein carbonyls (protein oxidation), 8-epiPGF2α (lipid peroxidation), 8-OHdG (nucleic acid oxidation) and a synthetic redox reporter molecule were significantly increased in glial mitochondrial fractions after 3-4 days of HO-1 transfection relative to sham-transfected controls and HO-1-transfected cells receiving SnMP [77, 78]. Treatment with cyclosporin A or trifluoperazine, inhibitors of the mitochondrial permeability transition pore, also curtailed mitochondrial iron trapping in HO-1 transfected glia and cells exposed to DA, TNFα or IL-1β [73, 75].

Conceivably, intracellular oxidative stress accruing from HO-1 activity promotes pore opening [79, 80] and influx of cytosolic iron to the mitochondrial matrix. In turn, the redox-active iron elicits mitochondrial membrane damage and macroautophagy [81]. Numbers of neuroglia immunoreactive for HO-1 in cortical and subcortical regions of the normal human brain increase progressively with advancing age [82]. Moreover, using immunolabeling techniques, we determined that the fractions of GFAP-positive astroglia expressing HO-1 in temporal cortex and hippocampus of subjects with AD and mild cognitive impairment (MCI), PD substantia nigra, and MS spinal white matter are significantly increased relative to non-neurological controls matched for age and post-mortem interval [73, 83, 84]. On the basis of our *in vitro* findings (*vide supra*), we proposed that the augmented glial HO-1 activity may contribute to the transferrin receptor-independent accumulation of CNS iron and mitochondrial insufficiency characteristic of these conditions [6, 85].Using electron spin resonance (ESR) spectrometry, we demonstrated that the glial mitochondrial iron exhibits a pseudo-peroxidase activity that promotes the oxidation of dopamine and other catechols to potentially neurotoxic ortho-semiquinone radicals [58, 86] and facilitates the bioactivation of MPTP to the neurotoxin, MPP+ [57].Furthermore, we observed that neuron-like PC12 cells grown on a substratum of astrocytes pre-loaded with mitochondrial iron by CSH pre-treatment [87] or *hmox1* transfection [77] were far more susceptible to dopamine/H_2O_2-related killing than PC12 cells co-cultured with control, 'iron-poor' astroglia. These observations indicate that metal sequestration by the *glial* compartment may be inimical to nearby *neuronal* constituents and suggest that iron-laden astrocytes may be a pivotal factor predisposing the senescent nervous system to AD, PD and other free radical-mediated neuropathologies. As such, *targeted suppression of glial HO-1 overactivity by pharmacological or other means may ameliorate iron-mediated toxicity and bioenergy deficits in the brains of these patients* [85, 88].

2.5.1.1.2. Genetic Disorders of Brain Iron Metabolism

Recent years have witnessed a growing awareness of heritable disorders of iron homeostasis characterized by pathological deposition of the metal in brain and attendant (often severe) neurological morbidity. In this section, a number of these conditions will be considered in sufficient detail to underscore the biological significance of maintaining rigorous control of brain iron metabolism and the diversity of molecular mechanisms which may compromise iron homeostasis in the human CNS. Interested readers are referred elsewhere [89] for a more comprehensive account of the clinical, molecular and pathological features of these and other genetic disorders impacting brain iron regulation.

2.5.1.1.2.1. Pantothenate Kinase-2 Associated Neurodegeneration

Formerly referred to as the Hallervorden-Spatz syndrome, pantothenate kinase-2 associated neurodegeneration (PKAN) is a form of neurodegeneration with brain iron accumulation (NBIA) resulting from autosomal recessive, loss-of-function mutations in the gene encoding brain-specific mitochondrial pantothenate kinase-2 (*PANK2*) [90-92]. Patients generally present in childhood or young adulthood with combinations of choreoathetosis, dystonia, parkinsonism, spasticity, seizures, mental retardation, dementia, optic atrophy and pigmentary retinopathy [90, 93, 94]. Pathologically, the globus pallidus, substantia nigra and subthalamic nuclei are remarkable for the presence of granular iron deposits within astrocytes, microglial cells and the neuropil [95, 96]. PANK2 catalyzes the phosphorylation of pantothenate (vitamin B_5) in a pathway leading to the synthesis of coenzyme A. Since the resulting phosphopantothenate normally combines with cysteine, in PANK2 deficiency there are elevated concentrations of this amino acid in the basal ganglia of affected persons [97]. Cysteine chelates iron and may be responsible for the regional accumulation of the metal in patients with PKAN. In the presence of excess iron, cysteine may undergo robust autoxidation generating neurotoxic reactive oxygen and sulphur species [98, 99].

2.5.1.1.2.2. Friedreich Ataxia

FA is an autosomal recessive, neurodegenerative disease presenting in the first decades of life with progressive ataxia, dysarthria, sensory loss and cardiomyopathy. In the majority of cases, there is expansion of the GAA trinucleotide repeat in intron 1 of the *FRDA* gene, which codes for the mitochondrial protein, frataxin [100, 101]. Mitochondrial iron overload occurs in the CNS and myocardium of FA patients [100, 102] and in mice with conditional knock-out of the frataxin gene [103]. Frataxin deficiency is associated with inactivation of iron-sulphur (Fe-S)-dependent enzymes such as the aconitases and complexes I-III of the respiratory chain [103]. Frataxin may participate in the assembly or export of Fe-S clusters from mitochondria and influence iron storage within this organelle. Evidence suggests that, as a general rule, iron efflux from mitochondria may require binding of the metal to molecules targeted for delivery to other cellular compartments. For instance, in X-linked sideroblastic anemia with ataxia, mutation of the ATP-binding cassette protein B7 (ABCB7) may predispose to mitochondrial iron trapping by impeding extramitochondrial Fe-S cluster formation [104-107]. By the same token, impaired Fe-S cluster assembly in frataxin-deficient mitochondria [108] may interfere with mitochondrial iron export in FA cells. In patients with FA, oral administration of the antioxidants, co-enzyme Q and idebenone may ameliorate cardiac wall thickness abnormalities, but have thus far shown no significant benefits *vis-a-vis* the disease's neurological manifestations [109]. Of note, in an early-phase clinical trial, *treatment with the membrane permeant iron chelator, deferiprone (3-hydroxy-1,2-dimethylpyridin-4-one) for six months resulted in a significant reduction in cerebellar iron stores (measured by magnetic resonance imaging; MRI) and improved gait ataxia and peripheral neuropathy in several FA subjects* [110].

2.5.1.1.2.3. Neuroferritinopathy

Ferritin is the major intracellular reservoir of metabolically-inert (ferric) iron, with each molecule capable of accommodating up to 4,500 iron atoms in its internal cavity [111, 112]. Fe^{2+} incorporated into the ferritin shell is oxidized by the ferroxidase activity of the molecule's H-subunit to Fe^{3+}, while the L-subunit largely subserves iron-core nucleation. In 2001, Curtis and colleagues [113] reported a novel, dominantly-inherited neurodegenerative condition featuring involuntary movements and surplus iron deposition in the basal ganglia. The genetic defect was mapped to locus 19q13.3 containing the gene for ferritin L-chain and the disease was termed "neuroferritinopathy" [113]. Most affected individuals presented at age 40-55 with rigidity, choreoathetosis, dystonia and spasticity [114, 115]. On neuropathological examination, there is a marked accumulation of ferritin and iron in neurons of the globus pallidus and in oligodendrocytes and microglia of the forebrain and cerebellum. Clinical manifestations appear restricted to the CNS, although intranuclear and intracytoplasmic bodies replete with ferritin and iron have been observed in dermal fibroblasts, renal tubular epithelium, and muscle capillary endothelial cells [116] and some patients may manifest an associated hypoferritinemia [116-118]. Molecular details of the mutations responsible for neuroferritinopathy have been reviewed previously [89]. Several of these mutations extend the amino acid sequence of the ferritin light chain yielding novel polypeptides [113, 116]. The neuroferritinopathy mutations have been shown to alter the C-terminus of L-ferritin, thereby affecting protein folding and stability [119]. "Unshielded" cytosolic iron accruing from the assembly of incompetent holoferritin may promote oxidative tissue damage in patients with neuroferritinopathy. Alternatively, or in addition, mutant L-ferritin may acquire a toxic gain-of-function unrelated to its native biology, as seen in other dominantly-inherited neurodegenerations [113].

2.5.1.1.2.4. Aceruloplasminemia

Ceruloplasmin is a plasma α_2-glycoprotein that contains six copper atoms. Three of these copper atoms form a trinuclear cluster that confers ferroxidase activity capable of oxidizing Fe^{2+} to Fe^{3+} [120, 121]. The ferroxidation of iron by ceruloplasmin may facilitate ferroportin-mediated shedding of iron at the cell surface and loading of (ferric) iron onto transferrin in the extracellular *milieu* [112, 122]. A glycosylphosphatidylinositol (GPI)-anchored form of ceruloplasmin unique to astrocyte membranes has been described which mediates egress of iron from brain tissue and may thereby play a vital role in the maintenance of CNS iron homeostasis [123, 124]. Indeed, adult aceruloplasminemic mice exhibit abnormal iron deposits and free radical injury (lipid peroxidation) in cerebellum, spinal cord and retina [125]. In 1987, Miyajima and co-investigators [126] reported the first case of human aceruloplasminemia, a 52-year-old Japanese woman with diabetes mellitus, extrapyramidal symptoms (involuntary movements), retinal degeneration and undetectable serum ceruloplasmin. A nucleotide sequence analysis of this and subsequent cases revealed loss-of-function mutations (point mutations and splice-variants) in the ceruloplasmin gene on chromosome 3q25, which largely interfere with the proper assembly of the trinuclear copper cluster [127-130]. In homozygous individuals, circulating ceruloplasmin levels and associated ferroxidase activity are negligible and there is severe parenchymal iron overload in the CNS, liver and pancreas.

Treatment of aceruloplasminemia: An understanding of the principal function of ceruloplasmin in iron physiology - its ferroxidase activity - has suggested a novel approach to treatment of aceruloplasminemia. Due to insufficient ferroxidase activity, the iron burden in aceruloplasminemic patients favors the Fe^{2+} state. It is therefore not surprising that early attempts to diminish brain and body iron with the deferoxamine, an Fe^{3+} chelator, were unsuccessful. To circumvent this 'valence' conundrum in an individual with aceruloplasminemia, Yonekawa and colleagues [131] first administered fresh frozen human plasma for 6 weeks to restore circulating ceruloplasmin levels (ferroxidase activity) thereby promoting the conversion of ferrous iron to the ferric state. Subsequently, deferoxamine was administered for an additional 6 weeks to deplete *ferric* iron stores. Although MR images of the brain remained unaltered following this treatment protocol, there was disappearance of abnormal high-voltage sharp waves on electroencephalography and, more importantly, significant improvement of choreoathetosis and ataxia! This case dramatically illustrates how *knowledge of the redox behavior of mutated proteins may translate into rational and potentially effective (neuro)therapeutics.*

2.6. Antioxidant Defenses

Virtually all of the defenses invoked in peripheral tissues to combat oxidative stress are represented within the nervous system. The latter include evolutionarily-conserved antioxidant enzymes (e.g. the superoxide dismutases, catalase, the glutathione peroxidases and various reductases) which operate in concert with a host of non-enzymatic, low-molecular-weight antioxidant compounds (e.g. glutathione, thioredoxin, ascorbate, the tocopherols, uric acid, melatonin, bilirubin) to preserve redox homeostasis (for details see Vol. II, Chapters 1-11). By maintaining transition metals in a relatively low redox state, metal-binding proteins, such as transferrin, ferritin, lactoferrin, ceruloplasmin and the metallothioneins, also contribute substantially to the antioxidant protection of brain and other tissues/body fluids. *Whereas certain antioxidant molecules are relatively abundant in brain parenchyma and CSF (e.g. ascorbate), neural tissues exhibit comparatively low levels of many antioxidant enzymes which may confer susceptibility to oxidative injury.* As such, neural tissues are prime targets of oxidative damage accruing from metabolic disorders such as vitamin B12, vitamin E and thiamine deficiencies, diabetes mellitus, and certain porphyrias (disorders of heme biosynthesis). In some instances, in addition to clinical stabilization resulting from correction or amelioration of the underlying metabolic derangement, there may be further therapeutic benefits from concomitant antioxidant supplementation (e.g α-lipoic acid for diabetic neuropathy [132]). In idiopathic PD, a neurodegenerative disorder, there is an early and profound depletion of intracellular glutathione (GSH) in the affected substantia nigra (midbrain) which may render this region vulnerable to oxidative substrate damage, proteosomal dysfunction, inclusion (Lewy) body formation and degeneration of nigrostriatal dopaminergic circuitry [133]. The up-regulation of the MnSOD gene reported in the PD nigra [134] may, in the absence of commensurate increases in glutathione peroxidase or catalase activity, actually exacerbate the degenerative process by promoting the accumulation of superoxide-derived H_2O_2 (the "SOD paradox"). In such metabolic and degenerative disorders, it is often unclear whether the aberrant antioxidant defences are primary (causative) or reactionary to a more fundamental upstream lesion. In the following subsections, examples are provided illustrating the impact of (i) an antioxidant metabolite deficiency (vitamin E), (ii) mutations in a gene coding for a key antioxidant enzyme (copper-zinc superoxide dismutase; CuZnSOD), and (iii) an antioxidant pharmaceutical (N-acetylcysteine) on human neurological health and wellbeing.

2.6.1. Vitamin E Deficiency

Vitamin E comprises a family of fat-soluble tocopherols (α,β,γ,δ) and tocotrienols (α,β,γ,δ); for details see Vol. II, Chapter 3. α-Tocopherol is the most important biologic chain-breaking antioxidant in humans. Natural sources of vitamin E include grains, seeds, nuts, fruits, mayonnaise, sunflower and olive oils, and green leafy vegetables. After absorption in the small intestine, the vitamin is transported in chylomicrons (large fatty micelles) via the lymphatic circulation to the liver. Hepatocyte α-tocopherol transfer protein (α-TTP) facilitates the secretion of vitamin E within very low density lipoprotein (VLDL) particles to the plasma. Circulating VLDL particles are converted to low density lipoproteins (LDL) which deliver vitamin E to the tissues. Certain tissues, such as brain, uterus and placenta, utilize intracellular α-TTP to properly mobilize and compartmentalize vitamin E [135, 136]. Conditions predisposing to vitamin E deficiency in humans are numerous but may be conveniently classified in two major categories: (i) fat malabsorption and (ii) ataxia with isolated vitamin E deficiency (AVED). Fat malabsorption may occur in persons with enteropathy (e.g. abetalipoproteinemia, celiac disease), hepato-biliary disease (e.g. primary biliary cirrhosis) and pancreatic insufficiency (e.g. chronic pancreatitis). In these conditions, there may be concomitant deficiencies of other lipid-soluble vitamins (A, D and K) [137]. In AVED, a rare autosomal recessive disorder due to mutations in the α-TTP gene, only vitamin E is affected [138, 139]. Vitamin E deficiency is characterized by both neurological and systemic complications, which may take many years to develop and are often mis-diagnosed. Common CNS manifestations of vitamin E deficiency include limb and truncal ataxia (cerebellar dysfunction), epicritic sensory loss (dorsal column disease), and spasticity and hyperreflexia (pyramidal tract involvement). Less commonly, there may be parkinsonism (basal ganglia disorder), cognitive dysfunction, seizures (cortical involvement) and dysautonomia (intermediolateral cell column disease). Involvement of the peripheral nervous system may comprise ptosis, ophthalmoplegia, arreflexia (cranial and peripheral neuropathy) and myopathy. Pigmentary retinopathy and acanthocytosis (burr-shaped erythrocytes) are prominent ophthalmological and hematological signs, respectively, of vitamin E deficiency. Neuroimaging (CT, MRI) may be normal or reveal cerebellar atrophy (Figure 4) and/or abnormal MR (T2) signal intensities in subcortical white matter and dorsal columns [140-143]. At the cellular level, free radical damage accruing from hypovitaminosis E results in axonal degeneration with secondary demyelination in dorsal roots, dorsal columns, Clarke's column and cerebellum; neuronal attrition in ventral horns, brain stem oculomotor and sensory nuclei, and basal ganglia; lipofuscin ("aging pigment") accumulation in neurons, retinal pigment epithelium and skin; and a necrotizing myopathy [144]. *Early recognition of vitamin E deficiency is paramount because the neurological morbidity in both the malabsorption syndromes and AVED can be prevented, slowed, stabilized or even reversed with appropriate and timely replacement therapy* [139, 145].

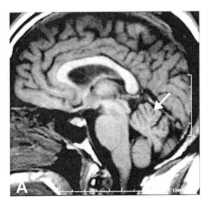
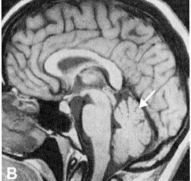

Figure 4. A. Sagittal T1-weighted MRI scan of the brain showing midline cerebellar (vermian) atrophy (arrow) in a 58 year-old man with vitamin E and copper deficiencies due to celiac disease (micronutrient malabsorption syndrome). From [142], with permission. B. Sagittal T1-weighted MRI depicting normal cerebellum (arrow). From http://content.answers.com/main/content/img/oxford/Oxford_Body.

2.6.2. Familial Amyotrophic Lateral Sclerosis

ALS is a fatal neurodegenerative disorder characterized by progressive upper and lower motor neuron loss and weakness of skeletal (voluntary) muscles of the head, neck, trunk and limbs. Pathologically, ALS features degeneration of cortical, brain stem and spinal motor neurons associated with ubiquitinated perikaryal inclusions, mitochondrial and cytoskeletal damage, excitotoxicity and gliosis. As with AD and PD, over 90% of cases are sporadic (non-familial) and <10% are transmitted with high penetrance in an autosomal dominant fashion (familial ALS; FALS). *A major breakthrough in the field occurred in 1993 when it was discovered that (approximately 20% of) FALS may result from mutations in the gene encoding the antioxidant enzyme CuZnSOD or SOD1* [146]. Studies in FALS patients and transgenic mouse models of the disease revealed, quite unexpectedly, that *the activity of SOD1 was not compromised by the mutations! Rather, the defective SOD1 appears to confer a "toxic gain-of-function" akin to that observed in other autosomal dominant neurological disorders.* Although the precise mechanism of this toxicity and its selectivity for motor neurons remains enigmatical, several plausible hypotheses have emerged based on the physico-chemical properties of the altered enzyme and its biological effects in animal models. Of the more than 100 distinct *SOD1* mutations documented, the majority implicate the copper-binding domain of the protein. This may result in "unshielding" of the redox-active copper ion permitting the latter to participate in toxic Fenton reactions ($Cu^1 + H_2O_2 \rightarrow Cu^2 + OH^- + {}^\bullet OH$) [147]. The oxidative insults may promote bioenergetic failure, excitotoxicity, the accumulation of intracellular aggregates, aberrant axonal transport, apoptosis, neuroinflammation and reactive gliosis observed in human and experimental ALS [37, 148, 149]. In addition to Fenton chemistry, *in vitro* biochemical studies suggested that the mutant enzyme may acquire novel peroxidase, superoxide reductase and reverse SOD activity which may contribute to intracellular oxidative stress. Liochev and Fridovich (the latter author is credited with the discovery of SOD in 1969) analyzed the kinetics of these reactions and concluded that the proposed HCO_3^--dependent peroxidase activity ($2H_2O_2 + HCO_3^- \leftrightarrow CO_3^{-\bullet} + O_2^- + 2H_2O + H^+$) may have little biological relevance *in vivo* [150]. Similarly, the reverse SOD reaction ($H_2O_2 + O_2 \rightarrow 2H^+ + 2O_2^-$) was considered to be kinetically unfavorable and unlikely to generate more than trivial amounts of superoxide and superoxide-derived peroxynitrite under *in vivo* conditions. On the other hand, the superoxide reductase reaction mediated by mSOD1 ($RH_2 + O_2^- + H^+ \leftrightarrow RH^\bullet + H_2O_2$) may exacerbate oxidative tissue injury in intact organisms by depletion of cellular reductants (ascorbate, urate) and by monovalent oxidation of reductants to their corresponding free radicals (*ibid.*). Other evidence suggests that the toxic gain-of-function arises primarily from the accumulation of insoluble mutant SOD1 protein in affected motor neurons, implying that mSOD1-related FALS is a protein-misfolding disorder. Some have postulated that absent or attenuated intramolecular disulfide bonding within nascent mSOD1 polypeptides (between Cys-57 and Cys-146) impedes proper insertion of copper ions by "copper chaperone for SOD1 (CCS)" resulting in protein misfolding, monomerization, and the accumulation of immature intermediates [151-153]. The misfolded SOD1polypeptides may induce an endoplasmic reticulum (ER) stress response and dysfunction of the unfolded protein response (UPR), which contribute to the observed cytotoxicity [154]. Intact animal and *in vitro* studies have indicated that oxidized/misfolded SOD1 proteins are selectively toxic to motor neurons and that release of similar intermediates from glial compartments may play a role in the pathogenesis of *sporadic* ALS even in the absence of *SOD1* mutations [155]. Aggregates of misfolded proteins may also hinder the function of the ubiquitin-proteasome system (UPS), as evidenced by early attenuation of protein chaperoning and proteasome-mediated hydrolysis of substrates in lumbar spinal cord of mSOD1 transgenic mice [156]. Finally, mutant SOD1 protein may directly interact with neurofilament-light chain mRNA and the dynein/dynactin complex, thereby compromising the cytoskeleton and axonal transport [157]. The remarkable phenotypic similarity between FALS and sporadic ALS argues strongly for common pathogenetic mechanisms. In this light, *a thorough understanding of the molecular neuropathology devolving from mSOD1 may inform drug development for the far more common sporadic variant of the disease.*

2.6.3. Unverricht-Lundborg Disease

High-dose antioxidants and metal chelators have been administered, with variable success, in patients with a broad spectrum of neurological afflictions, including AD, PD, FA, epilepsy, diabetic neuropathy, ischemic stroke, aneurysmal subarachnoid hemorrhage, and Wilson disease [158]. Notable among these conditions is Unverricht–Lundborg disease (ULD), a form of progressive myoclonic epilepsy (EPM). The progressive myoclonic epilepsies (EPM), characterized by the triad of myoclonus (sudden jerky movements of the head, trunk or limbs), seizures and ataxia, comprise a large group of inherited neurodegenerative diseases that remain poorly understood and largely refractory to treatment. A loss-of-function mutation of the gene encoding cystatin B, an inhibitor of the lysosomal protease, cathepsin B, is responsible for ULD (or EPM1) [159]. ULD features an onset between ages 6–16 years, stimulus-sensitive myoclonus, tonic-clonic seizures and, as the disease progresses, ataxia, dysarthria and mild cognitive dysfunction [160, 161]. In 1996, Hurd et al. reported elevated activity of extracellular superoxide dismutase (EC-SOD) in four patients with ULD relative to control values. Subsequent studies reported a similar trend in EC-SOD, suppressed erythrocyte CuZnSOD levels and low serum total GSH concentrations, without alterations in glutathione peroxidase and catalase activities, in subjects with ULD [162-164].

On the basis of these systemic redox perturbations, several investigators assessed the therapeutic efficacy of high-dose N-acetylcysteine (NAC) in patients with ULD. NAC is a sulfhydryl amino acid derivative (Figure 5) that is approved for use in the U.S. and Canada as a mucolytic agent and as an antidote for acetaminophen poisoning (see Chapter 4 in this Volume). NAC exerts potent antioxidant and anti-apoptotic effects by promoting glutathione synthesis, scavenging hydroxyl radicals and diminishing the production of H_2O_2 [165, 166]. In the first such study, Hurd et al. [164] treated four ULD siblings with 4 to 6 grams of NAC daily in combination with vitamin E, selenium, riboflavin, zinc and magnesium. The patients exhibited a substantial decrease in myoclonus, which was sustained for up to 30 months, and partial normalization of the signature "giant" somatosensory evoked potentials. The investigators concluded that *"NAC may prevent further deterioration in the clinical course of patients with ULD" (ibid.), a condition notorious for its unsatisfactory symptomatic responses to multiple antiepileptic drugs.* Importantly, no adverse effects were noted, save for transient diarrhea in one patient. On the basis of the Hurd report, Selwa administered NAC (6 g/day) and multivitamins to a 40-year-old man with advanced ULD characterized by numerous generalizedtonic-clonic seizures, severeaction myoclonus, ataxia, dysarthria (impaired speech), spasticity and gradual cognitive decline [167]. After one week of therapy, there was dramatic improvement in gait (from largely wheelchair-bound to ambulatory), speech and myoclonus, and cessation of generalized seizure activity. His mother commented that she hadn't "seen him do anything like that since he was a child." In a third report, Ben-Menachem and colleagues treated five EPM patients with NAC (6 g/day) - four with ULD and one with Lafora body disease (or EPM2). Interestingly, NAC greatly improved and stabilized the neurological symptoms in the four ULD subjects (with no overt adverse effects) but not the individual with EPM 2, suggesting that the therapeutic benefits of NAC may be unique to the former condition. Since two of the four ULD subjects received NAC only, the clinical responses documented in the other two individuals concomitantly receiving multiple vitamins, and the cases reported previously by Hurd et al. and Selwa (*vide supra*), were likely due to the NAC rather than to other components of the treatment regimens. In 2002, Edwards et al. reported elevation of serum glutathione levels and improved control of seizures (but not myoclonus or ataxia) following NAC treatment in a patient with ULD [163]. Three other patients with clinically-determined (but not genetically-proven) ULD showed variable responses to NAC. In contradistinction to earlier ULD case series, Edwards and colleagues observed several notable side-effects of NAC, including single instances of neutropenia and sensorineural hearing loss. The latter have not previously been reported as complications of NAC therapy - in fact, *in vitro* experiments suggest that NAC may afford robust *protection* against drug-induced cochlear toxicity [168]. Protracted administration of high-dose NAC elicited no or minimal adverse effects (mainly headache, gastrointestinal disturbances, fatigue) in patients with AD [169] and relapsing-remitting MS (author's unpublished results).

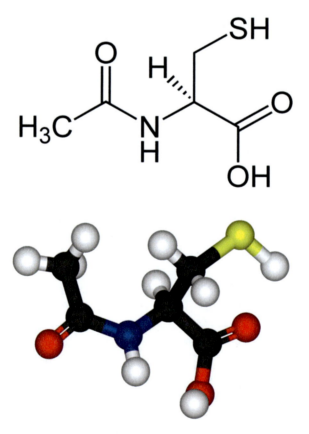

Figure 5. N-acetylcysteine. From commons. wikimedia.org.

The role of oxidative stress in the etiopathogenesis of ULD has recently been corroborated in *cystatin B* knock-out mice, an experimental model of the disease. Groups in Boston, Helsinki and Montreal documented significant reductions in GSH, total SOD activity and glutathione peroxidase activity, and increased HO-1 protein expression (a marker of oxidative stress) and 8-epi PGF2α concentrations (an index of lipid peroxidation), in the cerebellum of cystatin B -/- mice relative to wild-type values [170]. It was also shown that (i) *Cystatin B* knockout or knockdown sensitizes cerebellar granule neurons to oxidative cell death in tissue culture and (ii) the latter effect is mediated by the lysosomal protease, cathepsin B (*ibid.*). Studies are in progress to ascertain whether NAC administration restores cerebellar redox homeostasis and ameliorates behavioral abnormalities in *cystatin B* knock-out mice.

2.7. Excitotoxicity

Excitotoxicity is a mechanism leading to cellular injury and death that is fairly unique to neural tissues. It occurs when post-synaptic glutamate receptors (e.g. NMDA and AMPA receptors) are over-stimulated by the excessive liberation of the endogenous excitatory amino acid, glutamate into the synaptic cleft, or following exposure to exogenous "excitotoxins" such as kainic acid or quinolinic acid. Over-stimulation of the glutamate receptors results in a massive influx of calcium ions, which activate proteases (e.g. calpain), lipases and endonucleases. The latter, in turn, confer damage to mitochondrial and other cellular membranes, the cytoskeleton and nucleic acids leading to cell death by apoptosis or necrosis (Figure 6.A). Excitotoxicity has been implicated in ischemic and traumatic CNS injury (cerebral infarction, spinal cord contusion), neurodegenerative diseases (ALS, AD, PD, Huntington disease), MS, epilepsy, metabolic insults (hypoglycemia), and neurotoxin exposure (domoic acid, BOAA, BMAA) [171-174]. Numerous experiments conducted in intact animals and in cell culture have shown that free radical scavengers and nitric oxide synthase (NOS) inhibitors protect neurons from ischemic and excitotoxic injury. Indeed, *reactive oxygen/nitrogen species appear to play pivotal roles at multiple nodes of the excitotoxicity cascade* (Figure 6.A). The influx of calcium downstream of NMDA receptor stimulation activates nNOS resulting in the production of intracellular NO. The calcium surge leads to the production of superoxide radicals by several mechanisms: (i) calcium-activated proteases convert xanthine dehydrogenase to xanthine oxidase which, in turn, reduces molecular oxygen to superoxide radicals; (ii) calcium-induced phospholipase A2 activity promotes superoxide generation via augmentation of the arachidonate pathway within affected membranes; and (iii) injury to inner mitochondrial membranes exacerbates electron transport infidelity and superoxide formation. Superoxide radicals may dismutate to H_2O_2, a precursor of the highly reactive hydroxyl radical, or combine with NO to yield peroxynitrite (ONOO⁻). Peroxynitrite readily oxidizes proteins, lipids and nucleic acids and may neutralize enzymatic catalysis by interaction with critical sufhydryl moieties and tyrosine nitrosylation [175, 176]. Adding to the complexity, reactive species generated in response to NMDA receptor activation participate in positive and negative servomechanisms that further modulate the excitotoxicity cascade (Figure 6.B). For example, ROS, RNS and arachidonate stimulate TRPM2, a nonspecific, cation-permeable membrane channel, facilitating a second ("delayed") wave of calcium influx and attendant subcellular damage.

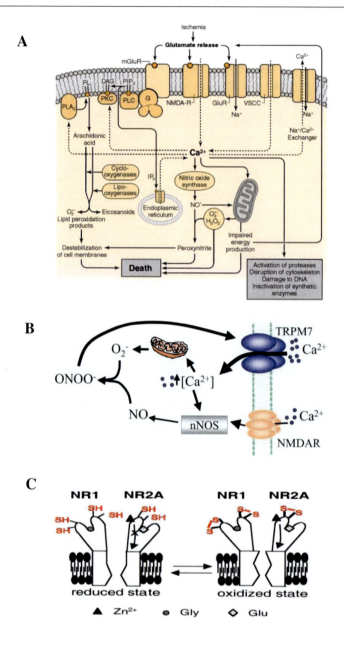

Figure 6. Excitotoxicity and oxidative stress. A. The excitotoxicity cascade. Activation of post-synaptic glutamate (NMDA, AMPA/KA) receptors promotes the intracellular accumulation of calcium (Ca^{++}) and generation of superoxide radical (O$_2^-$), hydrogen peroxide (H$_2$O$_2$), nitric oxide (NO$^{\bullet}$), peroxynitrite (ONOO$^-$) and other reactive species. From [206], with permission. B. NMDA receptor-TRPM7 interactions sustain a positive servomechanism leading to the amplification of intracellular calcium and nitric oxide levels and mitochondrial ROS production. From [171], with permission. C. Redox-sensitive cysteine residues of the NMDA receptor modulate zinc (Zn^{2+})-mediated inhibition of NMDA currents. In the oxidized state (*right*), formation of disulfide bonds between critical cysteine residues induces conformational changes in the NR2A subunit, which facilitate zinc inhibition of channel activity (*arrow*). In the reduced state (*left*), disulfide bonds are converted to free thiol groups, which uncouple inhibition of NMDA-evoked currents from zinc binding (*crossed arrow*). Thus, the vicinal cysteines act as redox sensors, which respectively dampen and augment NMDA channel conductance under oxidizing and reducing conditions. From [207], with permission.

The pro-oxidants similarly engage the monovalent cation channel, TPM7 which promotes sodium loading and associated cytotoxicity [171, 177]. A redox-sensitive site within the NMDA receptor itself contains a cysteine "switch" which regulates the calcium current. The latter is up-modulated when the vicinal cysteines are reduced and suppressed when oxidized (Figure 6.C). Thus, ROS and NO arising from NMDA receptor activation may feed back to the redox-sensitive site to dampen further calcium flux across the NMDA channel [178]. *Some have advocated pharmacological manipulation of the cysteine switch as a potential therapeutic modality to obviate excitotoxicity in cerebral ischemia and other neuropathological states (ibid).*

2.8. Neuroinflammation

The local generation of free radical intermediates is a ubiquitous component of infectious, immunological and inflammatory processes within the nervous system. As in peripheral tissues, reactive species (O_2^-, HOCl, $NO^•$, $ONOO^-$) may serve an adaptive function when released by leukocytes and microglia (the "respiratory burst") to combat invading pathogens, be they bacteria, viruses, fungi, parasites or tumor cells. On the other hand, oxidative stress stemming from these processes and from the action of pro-inflammatory (TH1) cytokines (e.g. TNFα, IL-1β) and arachidonate metabolites may cause "collateral" damage to vulnerable neuronal, glial and microvascular constituents. In some instances, dystrophic inflammatory processes are invoked within the neuraxis in the course of autoimmune attacks, as exemplified by the Guillain-Barré syndrome, acute disseminated encephalomyelitis and MS.

2.8.1. Multiple Sclerosis

MS is a neuroimmunological disease of the human CNS characterised pathologically by dysregulation of cytokine production, inflammation, oligodendroglial degeneration, multifocal demyelination, axonal degeneration and astrogliosis. *Considerable evidence has accumulated implicating pathological iron mobilization and oxidative stress in the pathogenesis of MS and a rodent model of the disease, experimental autoimmune encephalomyelitis (EAE)* [179]. MS patients exhibit pathological brain iron deposition as evidenced on MR imaging by the presence of discrete T1 white matter hypointensities ("black holes"), diffuse T2 hypointensities in deep grey matter, and abnormal R2* sequences. These lesions may have clinical significance insofar as their burden correlates with brain atrophy, cognitive impairment and disability scores [180-183].

Genetic surveys have linked polymorphisms in the genes encoding *NRAMP1* and the *HFE* gene product, proteins involved in cellular iron homeostasis, to MS susceptibility in certain populations, further attesting to the putative role of the transition metal in the pathogenesis of this disease [184, 185]. The iron chelator deferoxamine [186] and the sulfhydryl-containing antioxidant NAC [187] attenuate the induction of EAE in rodents; moreover, in animals with established EAE, behavioral improvement correlated with NAC treatment in a dose- dependent manner [187].

The precise mechanism(s) predisposing to iron accumulation and oxidative stress in MS tissues remains unclear. Experimental studies disclosed that TNFα and IL-1β, pro-inflammatory cytokines elaborated in MS-affected tissues, favor the sequestration of ironby astroglial mitochondria. These effects can be attenuated by co-administration of heme oxygenase inhibitors, mitochondrial permeabilitytransition pore blockers or antioxidants [73]. Since HO-1 is over-expressed in the spinal white matter of MS patients [73], induction of the *HMOX1* gene in MS astrocytes, ostensibly provoked by myelin basic protein [188] or TH1 cytokines [73], may contribute to the pathological iron mobilization and ETC defects reported in the vicinity of MS plaques [73, 179, 189]. In one study [190] (but not in another [191]), suppression of heme oxygenase activity in rodents with EAE ameliorated neural oxidative stress and locomotor deficits. Human MS trials employing antioxidant therapeutics are limited. Odinak et al. [192] administered α-lipoic acid 600 mg/day or an antioxidant cocktail (containing α-lipoic acid 600 mg/day, NAC 1200 mg/day, β-carotene 20 mg/day, α-tocopheryl acetate 80 mg/day, ascorbic acid 200 mg/day, selenium 100 mg/day, and other neuroprotectants) to small groups of patients with relapsing-remitting MS for one month twice yearly. The investigators reported a decline in post-treatment attacks relative to pre-treatment disease activity in the experimental groups but not in control subjects receiving symptomatic management only. The antioxidant-treated groups also exhibited a decline in blood lipid peroxides, increased glutathione levels and enhanced glutathione reductase activity relative to pre-treatment values; and no significant adverse effects attributable to the interventions.

3. Conclusions

Redox Neurology refers to the study of the roles of free radicals, transition metals, oxidative stress and antioxidant defences in diseases of the nervous system. While oxidative stress and free radical damage occur in diseases affecting virtually every organ system, the neuraxis exhibits features rendering it particularly prone to oxidative insults. Prominent among the latter are the high tissue flux of molecular oxygen, abundance of unsaturated fat and redox-active transition metals, presence of oxidizable neurotransmitters and excitotoxic amino acids, and relative dearth of antioxidant enzymes.

Oxidative stress figures centrally in various pathophysiological pathways responsible for an impressive array of adult and pediatric neurological afflictions. The latter may involve excessive generation of reactive chemical species (derived from oxygen, nitrogen, sulphur and chlorine), genetic and acquired dyregulation of CNS iron (and copper) homeostasis, antioxidant deficiencies resulting from inadequate diets or malabsorption states, and toxic gain- or loss-of-function mutations in key antioxidant genes. The successful management of these conditions presupposes a thorough understanding of the underlying molecular pathologies, rational drug design based on salient redox mechanisms and pharmacology, and implementation of effective preventive measures where appropriate.

The academic potential of Redox Neurology is enormous and, as in other biomedical sciences, research opportunities span the full spectrum of basic, translational, clinical and epidemiological studies. Several areas in the redox neurosciences forecasted in 2004 to pre-occupy this nascent field (Table 3) [158] are currently the hub of intense activity word-wide [193-203] and hold great promise for contributing to the public health and welfare.

Table 3. Issues forecasted in 2004 to pre-occupy the field of Redox Neurology (from [158], with permission). Many are currently the focus of intense research activity [193-203]

Neuropathological footprinting: Do different pro-oxidant species engender unique neuropathological profiles within a given region of the neuraxis? Will the same free radical intermediate evoke differential pathological responses in different brain regions?
Oxidative biomarkers: Can biochemical markers in blood or CSF be exploited for the early diagnosis and prognosis of free radical-related neurological disorders? Will oxidatively modified biomolecules provide surrogate markers for monitoring the efficacy of therapeutic interventions?
Redox neuroimaging: Can imaging techniques be adapted for visualization of free radical intermediates/spin traps and oxidative damage in the living brain?
Redox pharmacogenomics: Do specific antioxidant gene polymorphisms modify the natural history of human neurological diseases and individual responses to pharmacotherapy?
Gene and stem cell therapy: Can cell-based delivery of antioxidant genes or their products help restore a favorable redox microenvironment in human neurodegenerative disorders?
"Designer" antioxidants and metal chelators: Will new generations of antioxidants and metal chelators that safely and effectively target the CNS ameliorate oxidative stress-related neurological conditions?
Diet and the environment: Does environmental or dietary exposure to heavy metals or free radical-generating neurotoxins (herbicides/insecticides) constitute a risk factor for human neurodegenerative disorders?

Acknowledgments

Dr. Schipper's laboratory is supported by the Canadian Institutes of Health Research and the Mary Katz Claman Foundation.

References

[1] Linnane AW, Zhang C, Baumer A, Nagley P. Mitochondrial DNA mutation and the ageing process: bioenergy and pharmacological intervention. *Mutat. Res.* 1992;275:195-208.

[2] Samson FE, Nelson SR. The aging brain, metals and oxygen free radicals. *Cell Mol. Biol.* (Noisy-le-grand) 2000;46:699-707.

[3] Finkel T, Holbrook NJ. Oxidants, oxidative stress and the biology of ageing. *Nature,* 2000;408:239-47.

[4] Sohal RS, Mockett RJ, Orr WC. Mechanisms of aging: an appraisal of the oxidative stress hypothesis. *Free Radic. Biol. Med.* 2002;33:575-86.

[5] Hekimi S, Guarente L. Genetics and the specificity of the aging process. *Science,* 2003;299:1351-4.

[6]   Schipper HM. Brain iron deposition and the free radical-mitochondrial theory of ageing. *Ageing Res. Rev.* 2004;3:265-301.

[7]   Selkoe DJ. The molecular pathology of Alzheimer's disease. *Neuron,* 1991;6:487-98.

[8]   Reichmann H, Riederer P. *Mitochondrial disturbances in neurodegeneration.* Philadelphia: *Saunders*; 1994.

[9]   Beal M. *Mitochondrial Dysfunction and Oxidative Damage in Neurodegenerative Diseases*: *Landes*, R.G; 1995.

[10]   Mattson MP. Contributions of mitochondrial alterations, resulting from bad genes and a hostile environment, to the pathogenesis of Alzheimer's disease. *Int. Rev. Neurobiol.* 2002;53:387-409.

[11]   Gibson GE, Sheu KF, Blass JP. Abnormalities of mitochondrial enzymes in Alzheimer disease. *J. Neural. Transm.* 1998;105:855-70.

[12]   Corral-Debrinski M, Horton T, Lott MT, et al. Marked changes in mitochondrial DNA deletion levels in Alzheimer brains. *Genomics,* 1994;23:471-6.

[13]   Tanno Y, Okuizumi K, Tsuji S. mtDNA polymorphisms in Japanese sporadic Alzheimer's disease. *Neurobiol. Aging,* 1998;19:S47-51.

[14]   Bonilla E, Tanji K, Hirano M, Vu TH, DiMauro S, Schon EA. Mitochondrial involvement in Alzheimer's disease. *Biochim. Biophys. Acta,* 1999;1410:171-82.

[15]   Minoshima S, Giordani B, Berent S, Frey KA, Foster NL, Kuhl DE. Metabolic reduction in the posterior cingulate cortex in very early Alzheimer's disease. *Ann. Neurol.* 1997;42:85-94.

[16]   Fukuyama H, Ogawa M, Yamauchi H, et al. Altered cerebral energy metabolism in Alzheimer's disease: a PET study. *J. Nucl. Med.* 1994;35:1-6.

[17]   Hirai K, Aliev G, Nunomura A, et al. Mitochondrial abnormalities in Alzheimer's disease. *J. Neurosci.* 2001;21:3017-23.

[18]   Butterfield DA. Amyloid beta-peptide (1-42)-induced oxidative stress and neurotoxicity: implications for neurodegeneration in Alzheimer's disease brain. *A review. Free Radic. Res.* 2002;36:1307-13.

[19]   McGeer PL, McGeer EG. The inflammatory response system of brain: implications for therapy of Alzheimer and other neurodegenerative diseases. *Brain Res. Brain Res. Rev.* 1995;21:195-218.

[20]   Schipper HM. Glial Iron Sequestration and Neurodegeneration. In: Schipper HM, ed. *Astrocytes in Brain Aging and Neurodegeneration. Austin: R.G. Landes Co.*; 1998:235-51.

[21]   Sayre LM, Smith MA, Perry G. Chemistry and biochemistry of oxidative stress in neurodegenerative disease. *Curr. Med. Chem.* 2001;8:721-38.

[22]   Fahn S. Description of Parkinson's disease as a clinical syndrome. *Ann. N Y Acad. Sci.* 2003;991:1-14.

[23]   Storm T, Rath S, Mohamed SA, et al. Mitotic brain cells are just as prone to mitochondrial deletions as neurons: a large-scale single-cell PCR study of the human caudate nucleus. *Exp. Gerontol.* 2002;37:1389-400.

[24]   Bowen BC, Block RE, Sanchez-Ramos J, et al. Proton MR spectroscopy of the brain in 14 patients with Parkinson disease. *AJNR Am. J. Neuroradiol.* 1995;16:61-8.

[25]   Aschner M. Neuron-astrocyte interactions: implications for cellular energetics and antioxidant levels. *Neurotoxicology,* 2000;21:1101-7.

[26] Ouyang YB, Giffard RG. Bcl-XL maintains mitochondrial function in murine astrocytes deprived of glucose. *J. Cereb. Blood Flow Metab.* 2003;23:275-9.

[27] Clark IE, Dodson MW, Jiang C, et al. Drosophila pink1 is required for mitochondrial function and interacts genetically with parkin. *Nature,* 2006;441:1162-6.

[28] Dagda RK, Cherra SJ, 3rd, Kulich SM, Tandon A, Park D, Chu CT. Loss of PINK1 function promotes mitophagy through effects on oxidative stress and mitochondrial fission. *J. Biol. Chem.* 2009;284:13843-55.

[29] Greene JC, Whitworth AJ, Kuo I, Andrews LA, Feany MB, Pallanck LJ. Mitochondrial pathology and apoptotic muscle degeneration in Drosophila parkin mutants. *Proc. Natl. Acad. Sci. U S A,* 2003;100:4078-83.

[30] Grunewald A, Gegg ME, Taanman JW, et al. Differential effects of PINK1 nonsense and missense mutations on mitochondrial function and morphology. *Exp. Neurol.* 2009;219:266-73.

[31] Martin LJ, Pan Y, Price AC, et al. Parkinson's disease alpha-synuclein transgenic mice develop neuronal mitochondrial degeneration and cell death. *J. Neurosci.* 2006;26:41-50.

[32] Moore DJ, Zhang L, Troncoso J, et al. Association of DJ-1 and parkin mediated by pathogenic DJ-1 mutations and oxidative stress. *Hum. Mol. Genet.* 2005;14:71-84.

[33] Park J, Kim SY, Cha GH, Lee SB, Kim S, Chung J. Drosophila DJ-1 mutants show oxidative stress-sensitive locomotive dysfunction. *Gene,* 2005;361:133-9.

[34] Poon HF, Frasier M, Shreve N, Calabrese V, Wolozin B, Butterfield DA. Mitochondrial associated metabolic proteins are selectively oxidized in A30P alpha-synuclein transgenic mice--a model of familial Parkinson's disease. *Neurobiol. Dis.* 2005;18:492-8.

[35] Zhang Y, Dawson VL, Dawson TM. Oxidative stress and genetics in the pathogenesis of Parkinson's disease. *Neurobiol. Dis.* 2000;7:240-50.

[36] Magrane J, Hervias I, Henning MS, Damiano M, Kawamata H, Manfredi G. Mutant SOD1 in neuronal mitochondria causes toxicity and mitochondrial dynamics abnormalities. *Hum. Mol. Genet.* 2009.

[37] Rothstein JD. Current hypotheses for the underlying biology of amyotrophic lateral sclerosis. *Ann. Neurol.* 2009;65 Suppl 1:S3-9.

[38] Schipper HM. Heme oxygenase-1: Transducer of pathological brain iron sequestration under oxidative stress. In: S. LeVine, Connor JR, Schipper HM, eds. Redox-active Metals in Neurological Disorders. *New York: Ann. NY Acad. Sci.* 1012; 2004:84-93.

[39] Vosler PS, Graham SH, Wechsler LR, Chen J. Mitochondrial targets for stroke: focusing basic science research toward development of clinically translatable therapeutics. *Stroke,* 2009;40:3149-55.

[40] Andersson M, Elmberger PG, Edlund C, Kristensson K, Dallner G. Rates of cholesterol, ubiquinone, dolichol and dolichyl-P biosynthesis in rat brain slices. *FEBS Lett.* 1990;269:15-8.

[41] Vaya J, Schipper HM. Oxysterols, cholesterol homeostasis, and Alzheimer disease. *J. Neurochem.* 2007;102:1727-37.

[42] Siraki AG, O'Brien PJ. Prooxidant activity of free radicals derived from phenol-containing neurotransmitters. *Toxicology,* 2002;177:81-90.

[43] Halliwell B. Role of free radicals in the neurodegenerative diseases: therapeutic implications for antioxidant treatment. *Drugs Aging,* 2001;18:685-716.

[44] Jenner P. Oxidative stress in Parkinson's disease. *Ann. Neurol.* 2003;53 Suppl 3:S26-36; discussion S-8.

[45] Smythies JR. Oxidative reactions and schizophrenia: a review-discussion. *Schizophr. Res.* 1997;24:357-64.

[46] Czub S, Koutsilieri E, Sopper S, et al. Enhancement of central nervous system pathology in early simian immunodeficiency virus infection by dopaminergic drugs. *Acta Neuropathol*, 2001;101:85-91.

[47] Heyes MP, Saito K, Crowley JS, et al. Quinolinic acid and kynurenine pathway metabolism in inflammatory and non-inflammatory neurological disease. *Brain,* 1992;115 (Pt 5):1249-73.

[48] Ste-Marie L, Vachon P, Vachon L, Bemeur C, Guertin MC, Montgomery J. Hydroxyl radical production in the cortex and striatum in a rat model of focal cerebral ischemia. *Can. J. Neurol. Sci.* 2000;27:152-9.

[49] Wichers MC, Maes M. The role of indoleamine 2,3-dioxygenase (IDO) in the pathophysiology of interferon-alpha-induced depression. *J. Psychiatry Neurosci.* 2004;29:11-7.

[50] Mouillet-Richard S, Nishida N, Pradines E, et al. Prions impair bioaminergic functions through serotonin- or catecholamine-derived neurotoxins in neuronal cells. *J. Biol. Chem.* 2008;283:23782-90.

[51] Medana IM, Day NP, Salahifar-Sabet H, et al. Metabolites of the kynurenine pathway of tryptophan metabolism in the cerebrospinal fluid of Malawian children with malaria. *J. Infect. Dis.* 2003;188:844-9.

[52] Morgan EH, Moos T. Mechanism and developmental changes in iron transport across the blood-brain barrier. *Dev. Neurosci.* 2002;24:106-13.

[53] Ponka P. Hereditary causes of disturbed iron homeostasis in the central nervous system. *Ann. N Y Acad. Sci.* 2004;1012:267-81.

[54] Zlokovic BV. The blood-brain barrier in health and chronic neurodegenerative disorders. *Neuron,* 2008;57:178-201.

[55] Moos T, Rosengren Nielsen T, Skjorringe T, Morgan EH. Iron trafficking inside the brain. *J. Neurochem.* 2007;103:1730-40.

[56] Soong NW, Hinton DR, Cortopassi G, Arnheim N. Mosaicism for a specific somatic mitochondrial DNA mutation in adult human brain. *Nat. Genet.* 1992;2:318-23.

[57] DiMonte D, Schipper H, Hetts S, Langston J. Iron-mediated bioactivation of 1-methl-4-phenyl-1,2,3,6-tetrahydropyridine (MPTP) in glial cultures. *Glia,* 1995;15:203-6.

[58] Schipper HM, Kotake Y, Janzen EG. Catechol oxidation by peroxidase-positive astrocytes in primary culture: an electron spin resonance study. *J. Neurosci.* 1991;11:2170-6.

[59] Schipper HM. Heme oxygenase-1: transducer of pathological brain iron sequestration under oxidative stress. *Ann. N Y Acad. Sci.* 2004;1012:84-93.

[60] Schipper HM. Glial HO-1 expression, iron deposition and oxidative stress in neurodegenerative diseases. *Neurotox. Res.* 1999;1:57-70.

[61] Jefferies WA, Food MR, Gabathuler R, et al. Reactive microglia specifically associated with amyloid plaques in Alzheimer's disease brain tissue express melanotransferrin. *Brain Res.* 1996;712:122-6.

[62] Ryter SW, Tyrrell RM. The heme synthesis and degradation pathways: role in oxidant sensitivity. Heme oxygenase has both pro- and antioxidant properties. *Free Radic. Biol. Med.* 2000;28:289-309.

[63] Verma A, Hirsch DJ, Glatt CE, Ronnett GV, Snyder SH. Carbon monoxide: a putative neural messenger. *Science,* 1993;259:381-4.

[64] Baranano DE, Snyder SH. Neural roles for heme oxygenase: contrasts to nitric oxide synthase. *Proc. Natl. Acad. Sci. U S A,* 2001;98:10996-1002.

[65] Dennery PA. Regulation and role of heme oxygenase in oxidative injury. *Curr. Top. Cell Regul.* 2000;36:181-99.

[66] Schipper HM. Heme oxygenase-1: role in brain aging and neurodegeneration. *Exp. Gerontol.* 2000;35:821-30.

[67] Stocker R, Yamamoto Y, McDonagh AF, Glazer AN, Ames BN. Bilirubin is an antioxidant of possible physiological importance. *Science,* 1987;235:1043-6.

[68] Nakagami T, Toyomura K, Kinoshita T, Morisawa S. A beneficial role of bile pigments as an endogenous tissue protector: anti-complement effects of biliverdin and conjugated bilirubin. *Biochim. Biophys. Acta.* 1993;1158:189-93.

[69] Llesuy SF, Tomaro ML. Heme oxygenase and oxidative stress. Evidence of involvement of bilirubin as physiological protector against oxidative damage. *Biochim. Biophys. Acta.* 1994;1223:9-14.

[70] Dore S, Takahashi M, Ferris CD, et al. Bilirubin, formed by activation of heme oxygenase-2, protects neurons against oxidative stress injury. *Proc. Natl. Acad. Sci. U S A,* 1999;96:2445-50.

[71] Zhang J, Piantadosi CA. Mitochondrial oxidative stress after carbon monoxide hypoxia in the rat brain. *J. Clin. Invest.* 1992;90:1193-9.

[72] Frankel D, Mehindate K, Schipper HM. Role of heme oxygenase-1 in the regulation of manganese superoxide dismutase gene expression in oxidatively-challenged astroglia. *J. Cell Physiol.* 2000;185:80-6.

[73] Mehindate K, Sahlas DJ, Frankel D, et al. Proinflammatory cytokines promote glial heme oxygenase-1 expression and mitochondrial iron deposition: implications for multiple sclerosis. *J. Neurochem.* 2001;77:1386-95.

[74] Mydlarski MB, Liang JJ, Schipper HM. Role of the cellular stress response in the biogenesis of cysteamine-induced astrocytic inclusions in primary culture. *J. Neurochem.* 1993;61:1755-65.

[75] Schipper HM, Bernier L, Mehindate K, Frankel D. Mitochondrial iron sequestration in dopamine-challenged astroglia: role of heme oxygenase-1 and the permeability transition pore. *J. Neurochem.* 1999;72:1802-11.

[76] Ham D, Schipper HM. Heme oxygenase-1 induction and mitochondrial iron sequestration in astroglia exposed to amyloid peptides. *Cell Mol. Biol.* (Noisy-le-grand) 2000;46:587-96.

[77] Song W, Su H, Song S, Paudel HK, Schipper HM. Over-expression of heme oxygenase-1 promotes oxidative mitochondrial damage in rat astroglia. *J. Cell Physiol.* 2006;206:655-63.

[78] Vaya J, Song W, Khatib S, Geng G, Schipper HM. Effects of heme oxygenase-1 expression on sterol homeostasis in rat astroglia. *Free Radic. Biol. Med.* 2007;42:864-71.

[79] Petronilli V, Cola C, Massari S, Colonna R, Bernardi P. Physiological effectors modify voltage sensing by the cyclosporin A-sensitive permeability transition pore of mitochondria. *J. Biol. Chem.* 1993;268:21939-45.

[80] Bernardi P. The permeability transition pore. Control points of a cyclosporin A-sensitive mitochondrial channel involved in cell death. *Biochim. Biophys. Acta,* 1996;1275:5-9.

[81] Zukor H, Song W, Liberman A, et al. HO-1-mediated macroautophagy: a mechanism for unregulated iron deposition in aging and degenerating neural tissues. *J. Neurochem.* 2009;109:776-91.

[82] Hirose W, Ikematsu K, Tsuda R. Age-associated increases in heme oxygenase-1 and ferritin immunoreactivity in the autopsied brain. Leg Med (Tokyo) 2003;5 Suppl:S360-6.

[83] Schipper HM. Heme oxygenase expression in human central nervous system disorders. *Free Radic. Biol. Med.* 2004;37:1995-2011.

[84] Schipper HM, Bennett DA, Liberman A, et al. Glial heme oxygenase-1 expression in Alzheimer disease and mild cognitive impairment. *Neurobiol. Aging,* 2006;27:252-61.

[85] Schipper HM, Song W, Zukor H, Hascalovici JR, Zeligman D. Heme oxygenase-1 and neurodegeneration: expanding frontiers of engagement. *J. Neurochem.* 2009;110:469-85.

[86] Schipper HM. Mitochondrial iron deposition in aging astroglia: Mechanisms and disease implications. In: Ebadi M MJ, Chopra RK, ed. Mitochondrial Ubiquinone (Coenzyme Q): *Biochemical, Functional, Medical, and Therapeutic Aspects in Human Health and Disease: Prominent Press*; 2001: 267-80.

[87] Frankel D, Schipper HM. Cysteamine pretreatment of the astroglial substratum (mitochondrial iron sequestration) enhances PC12 cell vulnerability to oxidative injury. *Exp. Neurol.* 1999;160:376-85.

[88] Schipper HM, Gupta A, Szarek W. Suppression of glial HO-1 activitiy as a potential neurotherapeutic intervention in AD. *Curr. Alzheimer. Res.* 2009;6: 424-30.

[89] Schipper HM, Ponka P. Inherited disorders of brain iron homeostasis. In: Yehudah S, Mostofsky DI, eds. *Iron Deficiency and Overload: From Basic Biology to Clinical Medicine.* Totowa, NJ: Human Press Inc.; 2009:251-76.

[90] Hayflick SJ. Neurodegeneration with brain iron accumulation: from genes to pathogenesis. *Semin. Pediatr. Neurol.* 2006;13:182-5.

[91] Johnson MA, Kuo YM, Westaway SK, et al. Mitochondrial localization of human PANK2 and hypotheses of secondary iron accumulation in pantothenate kinase-associated neurodegeneration. *Ann. N Y Acad. Sci.* 2004;1012:282-98.

[92] Zhou B, Westaway SK, Levinson B, Johnson MA, Gitschier J, Hayflick SJ. A novel pantothenate kinase gene (PANK2) is defective in Hallervorden-Spatz syndrome. *Nat. Genet.* 2001;28:345-9.

[93] Hayflick SJ. Unraveling the Hallervorden-Spatz syndrome: pantothenate kinase-associated neurodegeneration is the name. *Curr. Opin. Pediatr.* 2003;15:572-7.

[94] Swaiman KF. Hallervorden-Spatz syndrome. *Pediatr. Neurol.* 2001;25:102-8.

[95] Swaiman KF, Smith SA, Trock GL, Siddiqui AR. Sea-blue histiocytes, lymphocytic cytosomes, movement disorder and 59Fe-uptake in basal ganglia: Hallervorden-Spatz disease or ceroid storage disease with abnormal isotope scan? *Neurology* 1983;33:301-5.

[96] Zupanc ML, Chun RW, Gilbert-Barness EF. Osmiophilic deposits in cytosomes in Hallervorden-Spatz syndrome. *Pediatr. Neurol.* 1990;6:349-52.

[97] Perry TL, Norman MG, Yong VW, et al. Hallervorden-Spatz disease: cysteine accumulation and cysteine dioxygenase deficiency in the globus pallidus. *Ann. Neurol.* 1985;18:482-9.

[98] Yoon SJ, Koh YH, Floyd RA, Park JW. Copper, zinc superoxide dismutase enhances DNA damage and mutagenicity induced by cysteine/iron. Mutat Res 2000;448:97-104.

[99] Berg D, Hochstrasser H. Iron metabolism in Parkinsonian syndromes. *Mov. Disord.* 2006;21:1299-310.

[100] Babady NE, Carelle N, Wells RD, et al. Advancements in the pathophysiology of Friedreich's Ataxia and new prospects for treatments. *Mol. Genet. Metab.* 2007;92:23-35.

[101] Pandolfo M. Friedreich's ataxia: clinical aspects and pathogenesis. *Semin. Neurol.* 1999;19:311-21.

[102] Lamarche JB, Cote M, Lemieux B. The cardiomyopathy of Friedreich's ataxia morphological observations in 3 cases. *Can. J. Neurol. Sci.* 1980;7:389-96.

[103] Puccio H, Simon D, Cossee M, et al. Mouse models for Friedreich ataxia exhibit cardiomyopathy, sensory nerve defect and Fe-S enzyme deficiency followed by intramitochondrial iron deposits. *Nat. Genet.* 2001;27:181-6.

[104] Csere P, Lill R, Kispal G. Identification of a human mitochondrial ABC transporter, the functional orthologue of yeast Atm1p. *FEBS Lett.* 1998;441:266-70.

[105] Kispal G, Csere P, Guiard B, Lill R. The ABC transporter Atm1p is required for mitochondrial iron homeostasis. *FEBS Lett.* 1997;418:346-50.

[106] Napier I, Ponka P, Richardson DR. Iron trafficking in the mitochondrion: novel pathways revealed by disease. *Blood*, 2005;105:1867-74.

[107] Lill R, Muhlenhoff U. Iron-sulfur protein biogenesis in eukaryotes: components and mechanisms. *Annu. Rev. Cell Dev. Biol.* 2006;22:457-86.

[108] Martelli A, Wattenhofer-Donze M, Schmucker S, Bouvet S, Reutenauer L, Puccio H. Frataxin is essential for extramitochondrial Fe-S cluster proteins in mammalian tissues. *Hum. Mol. Genet.* 2007;16:2651-8.

[109] Hart PE, Lodi R, Rajagopalan B, et al. Antioxidant treatment of patients with Friedreich ataxia: four-year follow-up. *Arch. Neurol.* 2005;62:621-6.

[110] Boddaert N, Le Quan Sang KH, Rotig A, et al. Selective iron chelation in Friedreich ataxia: biologic and clinical implications. *Blood,* 2007;110:401-8.

[111] Arosio P, Levi S. Ferritin, iron homeostasis, and oxidative damage. *Free Radic. Biol. Med.* 2002;33:457-63.

[112] Ponka P, Beaumont C, Richardson DR. Function and regulation of transferrin and ferritin. *Semin. Hematol.* 1998;35:35-54.

[113] Curtis AR, Fey C, Morris CM, et al. Mutation in the gene encoding ferritin light polypeptide causes dominant adult-onset basal ganglia disease. *Nat. Genet.* 2001;28:350-4.

[114] Burn J, Chinnery PF. Neuroferritinopathy. *Semin. Pediatr. Neurol.* 2006;13:176-81.

[115] Chinnery PF, Crompton DE, Birchall D, et al. Clinical features and natural history of neuroferritinopathy caused by the FTL1 460InsA mutation. *Brain,* 2007;130:110-9.

[116] Vidal R, Ghetti B, Takao M, et al. Intracellular ferritin accumulation in neural and extraneural tissue characterizes a neurodegenerative disease associated with a mutation in the ferritin light polypeptide gene. *J. Neuropathol. Exp. Neurol.* 2004;63:363-80.

[117] Maciel P, Cruz VT, Constante M, et al. Neuroferritinopathy: missense mutation in FTL causing early-onset bilateral pallidal involvement. *Neurology,* 2005;65:603-5.

[118] Schroder JM. Ferritinopathy: diagnosis by muscle or nerve biopsy, with a note on other nuclear inclusion body diseases. *Acta Neuropathol.* 2005;109:109-14.

[119] Levi S, Cozzi A, Arosio P. Neuroferritinopathy: a neurodegenerative disorder associated with L-ferritin mutation. *Best Pract. Res. Clin. Haematol.* 2005;18:265-76.

[120] Hellman NE, Gitlin JD. Ceruloplasmin metabolism and function. *Annu. Rev. Nutr.* 2002;22:439-58.

[121] Nittis T, Gitlin JD. The copper-iron connection: hereditary aceruloplasminemia. *Semin. Hematol.* 2002;39:282-9.

[122] Schipper HM, Liberman A, Stopa EG. Neural heme oxygenase-1 expression in idiopathic Parkinson's disease. *Exp. Neurol.* 1998;150:60-8.

[123] Patel BN, Dunn RJ, David S. Alternative RNA splicing generates a glycosylphosphatidylinositol-anchored form of ceruloplasmin in mammalian brain. *J. Biol. Chem.* 2000;275:4305-10.

[124] Jeong SY, David S. Glycosylphosphatidylinositol-anchored ceruloplasmin is required for iron efflux from cells in the central nervous system. *J. Biol. Chem.* 2003;278:27144-8.

[125] Patel BN, Dunn RJ, Jeong SY, Zhu Q, Julien JP, David S. Ceruloplasmin regulates iron levels in the CNS and prevents free radical injury. *J. Neurosci.* 2002;22:6578-86.

[126] Miyajima H, Nishimura Y, Mizoguchi K, Sakamoto M, Shimizu T, Honda N. Familial apoceruloplasmin deficiency associated with blepharospasm and retinal degeneration. *Neurology,* 1987;37:761-7.

[127] Daimon M, Kato T, Kawanami T, et al. A nonsense mutation of the ceruloplasmin gene in hereditary ceruloplasmin deficiency with diabetes mellitus. *Biochem. Biophys. Res. Commun.* 1995;217:89-95.

[128] Okamoto N, Wada S, Oga T, et al. Hereditary ceruloplasmin deficiency with hemosiderosis. *Hum. Genet.* 1996;97:755-8.

[129] Yoshida K, Furihata K, Takeda S, et al. A mutation in the ceruloplasmin gene is associated with systemic hemosiderosis in humans. *Nat. Genet.* 1995;9:267-72.

[130] Harris ZL, Takahashi Y, Miyajima H, Serizawa M, MacGillivray RT, Gitlin JD. Aceruloplasminemia: molecular characterization of this disorder of iron metabolism. *Proc. Natl. Acad. Sci. U S A,* 1995;92:2539-43.

[131] Yonekawa M, Okabe T, Asamoto Y, Ohta M. A case of hereditary ceruloplasmin deficiency with iron deposition in the brain associated with chorea, dementia, diabetes mellitus and retinal pigmentation: administration of fresh-frozen human plasma. *Eur. Neurol.* 1999;42:157-62.

[132] van Dam PS. Oxidative stress and diabetic neuropathy: pathophysiological mechanisms and treatment perspectives. *Diabetes Metab. Res. Rev.* 2002;18:176-84.

[133] Martin HL, Teismann P. Glutathione--a review on its role and significance in Parkinson's disease. *FASEB J.* 2009;23:3263-72.

[134] Saggu H, Cooksey J, Dexter D, et al. A selective increase in particulate superoxide dismutase activity in parkinsonian substantia nigra. *J. Neurochem.* 1989;53:692-7.

[135] Kaempf-Rotzoll DE, Traber MG, Arai H. Vitamin E and transfer proteins. *Curr. Opin. Lipidol.* 2003;14:249-54.

[136] Copp RP, Wisniewski T, Hentati F, Larnaout A, Ben Hamida M, Kayden HJ. Localization of alpha-tocopherol transfer protein in the brains of patients with ataxia with vitamin E deficiency and other oxidative stress related neurodegenerative disorders. *Brain Res.* 1999;822:80-7.

[137] Sokol RJ. Vitamin E and neurologic deficits. *Adv. Pediatr.* 1990;37:119-48.

[138] Jackson CE, Amato AA, Barohn RJ. Isolated vitamin E deficiency. *Muscle Nerve,* 1996;19:1161-5.

[139] Mariotti C, Gellera C, Rimoldi M, et al. Ataxia with isolated vitamin E deficiency: neurological phenotype, clinical follow-up and novel mutations in TTPA gene in Italian families. *Neurol. Sci.* 2004;25:130-7.

[140] Aguglia U, Annesi G, Pasquinelli G, et al. Vitamin E deficiency due to chylomicron retention disease in Marinesco-Sjogren syndrome. *Ann. Neurol.* 2000;47:260-4.

[141] Aslam A, Misbah SA, Talbot K, Chapel H. Vitamin E deficiency induced neurological disease in common variable immunodeficiency: two cases and a review of the literature of vitamin E deficiency. *Clin. Immunol.* 2004;112:24-9.

[142] Henri-Bhargava A, Melmed C, Glikstein R, Schipper HM. Neurologic impairment due to vitamin E and copper deficiencies in celiac disease. *Neurology,* 2008;71:860-1.

[143] Vorgerd M, Tegenthoff M, Kuhne D, Malin JP. Spinal MRI in progressive myeloneuropathy associated with vitamin E deficiency. *Neuroradiology,* 1996;38 Suppl 1:S111-3.

[144] Muller DP, Goss-Sampson MA. Neurochemical, neurophysiological, and neuropathological studies in vitamin E deficiency. *Crit. Rev. Neurobiol.* 1990;5:239-63.

[145] Sokol RJ, Butler-Simon N, Conner C, et al. Multicenter trial of d-alpha-tocopheryl polyethylene glycol 1000 succinate for treatment of vitamin E deficiency in children with chronic cholestasis. *Gastroenterology,* 1993;104:1727-35.

[146] Rosen DR, Siddique T, Patterson D, et al. Mutations in Cu/Zn superoxide dismutase gene are associated with familial amyotrophic lateral sclerosis. *Nature,* 1993;362:59-62.

[147] Rakhit R, Chakrabartty A. Structure, folding, and misfolding of Cu,Zn superoxide dismutase in amyotrophic lateral sclerosis. *Biochim. Biophys. Acta,* 2006;1762:1025-37.

[148] Boillee S, Vande Velde C, Cleveland DW. ALS: a disease of motor neurons and their nonneuronal neighbors. *Neuron,* 2006;52:39-59.

[149] Turner BJ, Talbot K. Transgenics, toxicity and therapeutics in rodent models of mutant SOD1-mediated familial ALS. *Prog. Neurobiol.* 2008;85:94-134.

[150] Liochev SI, Fridovich I. Mutant Cu,Zn superoxide dismutases and familial amyotrophic lateral sclerosis: evaluation of oxidative hypotheses. *Free Radic. Biol. Med.* 2003;34:1383-9.

[151] Furukawa Y, O'Halloran TV. Posttranslational modifications in Cu,Zn-superoxide dismutase and mutations associated with amyotrophic lateral sclerosis. *Antioxid. Redox. Signal.* 2006;8:847-67.

[152] Seetharaman SV, Prudencio M, Karch C, Holloway SP, Borchelt DR, Hart PJ. Immature copper-zinc superoxide dismutase and familial amyotrophic lateral sclerosis. *Exp. Biol. Med.* (Maywood) 2009;234:1140-54.

[153] Tiwari A, Hayward LJ. Mutant SOD1 instability: implications for toxicity in amyotrophic lateral sclerosis. *Neurodegener. Dis.* 2005;2:115-27.

[154] Kanekura K, Suzuki H, Aiso S, Matsuoka M. ER stress and unfolded protein response in amyotrophic lateral sclerosis. *Mol. Neurobiol.* 2009;39:81-9.

[155] Kabashi E, Valdmanis PN, Dion P, Rouleau GA. Oxidized/misfolded superoxide dismutase-1: the cause of all amyotrophic lateral sclerosis? *Ann. Neurol.* 2007;62:553-9.

[156] Kabashi E, Durham HD. Failure of protein quality control in amyotrophic lateral sclerosis. *Biochim. Biophys. Acta,* 2006;1762:1038-50.

[157] Andersen PM. Amyotrophic lateral sclerosis associated with mutations in the CuZn superoxide dismutase gene. *Curr. Neurol. Neurosci. Rep.* 2006;6:37-46.

[158] Schipper HM. Redox neurology: visions of an emerging subspecialty. In: S. LeVine, Connor JR, Schipper HM, eds. Redox-active Metals in Neurological Disorders. *New York: Ann. N Y Acad. Sci.* 2004:342-55.

[159] Pennacchio LA, Lehesjoki AE, Stone NE, et al. Mutations in the gene encoding cystatin B in progressive myoclonus epilepsy (EPM1). *Science,* 1996;271:1731-4.

[160] Chew NK, Mir P, Edwards MJ, et al. The natural history of Unverricht-Lundborg disease: a report of eight genetically proven cases. *Mov. Disord.* 2008;23:107-13.

[161] Kalviainen R, Khyuppenen J, Koskenkorva P, Eriksson K, Vanninen R, Mervaala E. Clinical picture of EPM1-Unverricht-Lundborg disease. *Epilepsia,* 2008;49:549-56.

[162] Ben-Menachem E, Kyllerman M, Marklund S. Superoxide dismutase and glutathione peroxidase function in progressive myoclonus epilepsies. *Epilepsy Res.* 2000;40:33-9.

[163] Edwards MJ, Hargreaves IP, Heales SJ, et al. N-acetylcysteine and Unverricht-Lundborg disease: variable response and possible side effects. *Neurology,* 2002;59:1447-9.

[164] Hurd RW, Wilder BJ, Helveston WR, Uthman BM. Treatment of four siblings with progressive myoclonus epilepsy of the Unverricht-Lundborg type with N-acetylcysteine. *Neurology,* 1996;47:1264-8.

[165] Aruoma OI, Halliwell B, Hoey BM, Butler J. The antioxidant action of N-acetylcysteine: its reaction with hydrogen peroxide, hydroxyl radical, superoxide, and hypochlorous acid. *Free Radic. Biol. Med.* 1989;6:593-7.

[166] Ziment I. Acetylcysteine: a drug that is much more than a mucokinetic. *Biomed. Pharmacother,* 1988;42:513-9.

[167] Selwa LM. N-acetylcysteine therapy for Unverricht-Lundborg disease. *Neurology,* 1999;52:426-7.

[168] Feghali JG, Liu W, Van De Water TR. L-n-acetyl-cysteine protection against cisplatin-induced auditory neuronal and hair cell toxicity. *Laryngoscope,* 2001;111:1147-55.

[169] Adair JC, Knoefel JE, Morgan N. Controlled trial of N-acetylcysteine for patients with probable Alzheimer's disease. *Neurology,* 2001;57:1515-7.

[170] Lehtinen MK, Tegelberg S, Schipper H, et al. Cystatin B deficiency sensitizes neurons to oxidative stress in progressive myoclonus epilepsy, EPM1. *J. Neurosci.* 2009;29:5910-5.

[171] Forder JP, Tymianski M. Postsynaptic mechanisms of excitotoxicity: Involvement of postsynaptic density proteins, radicals, and oxidant molecules. *Neuroscience,* 2009;158:293-300.

[172] Kim AH, Kerchner GA, Choi DW. Blocking Excitotoxicity. In: Marcoux FW, Choi D.W., ed. *CNS Neuroprotection.* New York: Springer; 2002:3-36.

[173] Chandrasekaran A, Ponnambalam G, Kaur C. Domoic acid-induced neurotoxicity in the hippocampus of adult rats. *Neurotox. Res*. 2004;6:105-17.

[174] Lindstrom H, Luthman J, Mouton P, Spencer P, Olson L. Plant-derived neurotoxic amino acids (beta-N-oxalylamino-L-alanine and beta-N-methylamino-L-alanine): effects on central monoamine neurons. *J. Neurochem*. 1990;55:941-9.

[175] Kinobe R, Ji Y, Nakatsu K. Peroxynitrite-mediated inactivation of heme oxygenases. *BMC Pharmacol*. 2004;4:26.

[176] Sadidi M, Geddes TJ, Kuhn DM. S-thiolation of tyrosine hydroxylase by reactive nitrogen species in the presence of cysteine or glutathione. *Antioxid. Redox. Signal*. 2005;7:863-9.

[177] Aarts MM, Tymianski M. TRPMs and neuronal cell death. *Pflugers Arch*. 2005;451:243-9.

[178] Choi YB, Lipton SA. Redox modulation of the NMDA receptor. *Cell Mol. Life Sci*. 2000;57:1535-41.

[179] Levine SM, Chakrabarty A. The role of iron in the pathogenesis of experimental allergic encephalomyelitis and multiple sclerosis. *Ann. N Y Acad. Sci*. 2004;1012:252-66.

[180] Bakshi R, Benedict RH, Bermel RA, et al. T2 hypointensity in the deep gray matter of patients with multiple sclerosis: a quantitative magnetic resonance imaging study. *Arch. Neurol*. 2002;59:62-8.

[181] Bakshi R, Dmochowski J, Shaikh ZA, Jacobs L. Gray matter T2 hypointensity is related to plaques and atrophy in the brains of multiple sclerosis patients. *J. Neurol. Sci*. 2001;185:19-26.

[182] Neema M, Arora A, Healy BC, et al. Deep gray matter involvement on brain MRI scans is associated with clinical progression in multiple sclerosis. *J. Neuroimaging*. 2009;19:3-8.

[183] Schenck JF, Zimmerman EA. High-field magnetic resonance imaging of brain iron: birth of a biomarker? *NMR Biomed*. 2004;17:433-45.

[184] Gazouli M, Sechi L, Paccagnini D, et al. NRAMP1 polymorphism and viral factors in Sardinian multiple sclerosis patients. *Can. J. Neurol. Sci*. 2008;35:491-4.

[185] Rubio JP, Bahlo M, Tubridy N, et al. Extended haplotype analysis in the HLA complex reveals an increased frequency of the HFE-C282Y mutation in individuals with multiple sclerosis. *Hum. Genet*. 2004;114:573-80.

[186] Pedchenko TV, LeVine SM. Desferrioxamine suppresses experimental allergic encephalomyelitis induced by MBP in SJL mice. *J. Neuroimmunol*. 1998;84:188-97.

[187] Stanislaus R, Gilg AG, Singh AK, Singh I. N-acetyl-L-cysteine ameliorates the inflammatory disease process in experimental autoimmune encephalomyelitis in Lewis rats. *J. Autoimmune Dis*. 2005;2:4.

[188] Businaro R, Fabrizi C, Caronti B, Calderaro C, Fumagalli L, Lauro GM. Myelin basic protein induces heme oxygenase-1 in human astroglial cells. *Glia,* 2002;37:83-8.

[189] Lu F, Selak M, O'Connor J, et al. Oxidative damage to mitochondrial DNA and activity of mitochondrial enzymes in chronic active lesions of multiple sclerosis. *J. Neurol. Sci*. 2000;177:95-103.

[190] Chakrabarty A, Emerson MR, Levine SM. Heme oxygenase-1 in SJL mice with experimental allergic encephalomyelitis. *Multiple Sclerosis,* 2003;9:372-81.

[191] Liu Y, Zhu B, Luo L, Li P, Paty DW, Cynader MS. Heme oxygenase-1 plays an important protective role in experimental autoimmune encephalomyelitis. *Neuroreport.* 2001;12:1841-5.

[192] Odinak MM, Bisaga GN, Zarubina IV. [New approaches to antioxidant therapy in multiple sclerosis]. Zh Nevrol Psikhiatr Im S S Korsakova 2002;Suppl:72-5.

[193] Fisinin VI, Papazyan TT, Surai PF. Producing selenium-enriched eggs and meat to improve the selenium status of the general population. *Crit. Rev. Biotechnol.* 2009;29:18-28.

[194] Zheng H, Gal S, Weiner LM, et al. Novel multifunctional neuroprotective iron chelator-monoamine oxidase inhibitor drugs for neurodegenerative diseases: in vitro studies on antioxidant activity, prevention of lipid peroxide formation and monoamine oxidase inhibition. *J. Neurochem.* 2005;95:68-78.

[195] Chen B, Caballero S, Seo S, Grant MB, Lewin AS. Delivery of Antioxidant Enzyme Genes Protects Against Ischemia/Reperfusion-Induced Injury to Retinal Microvasculature. *Invest. Ophthalmol. Vis. Sci.* 2009.

[196] Wu J, Hecker JG, Chiamvimonvat N. Antioxidant enzyme gene transfer for ischemic diseases. *Adv. Drug Deliv. Rev.* 2009;61:351-63.

[197] Louboutin JP, Agrawal L, Liu B, Strayer DS. In vivo gene transfer to the CNS using recombinant SV40-derived vectors. *Expert Opin. Biol. Ther.* 2008;8:1319-35.

[198] Ramos-Marquez ME, Siller-Lopez F. Current antioxidant molecular therapies for oxidative stress-related ailments. *Curr. Gene. Ther.* 2008;8:256-63.

[199] Haacke EM, Mittal S, Wu Z, Neelavalli J, Cheng YC. Susceptibility-weighted imaging: technical aspects and clinical applications, part 1. *AJNR Am. J. Neuroradiol.* 2009;30:19-30.

[200] Drechsel DA, Patel M. Role of reactive oxygen species in the neurotoxicity of environmental agents implicated in Parkinson's disease. *Free Radic. Biol. Med.* 2008;44:1873-86.

[201] Madhavan L, Ourednik V, Ourednik J. Neural stem/progenitor cells initiate the formation of cellular networks that provide neuroprotection by growth factor-modulated antioxidant expression. *Stem Cells,* 2008;26:254-65.

[202] Burns DH, Rosendahl S, Bandilla D, Maes OC, Chertkow HM, Schipper HM. Near-infrared spectroscopy of blood plasma for diagnosis of sporadic Alzheimer's disease. *J. Alzheimers Dis.* 2009;17:391-7.

[203] Schipper HM, Kwok CS, Rosendahl SM, et al. Spectroscopy of human plasma for diagnosis of idiopathic Parkinson disease. *Biomarkers in Medicine,* 2008;2:229-38.

[204] Schipper HM. Chapter 123. Metal accumulation during aging. In: Squire LR, ed. *Encyclopedia of Neuroscience.* Oxford: Academic Press; 2009:811-8.

[205] Duvoisin RC. A brief history of parkinsonism. *Neurol. Clin.* 1992;10:301-16.

[206] Dugan LL, Choi DW. Hypoxic-Ischemic Brain Injury and Oxidative Stress. In: Siegal GJ, Agranoff BW, Albers RW, Fisher SK, Uhler MD, eds. *Basic neurochemistry : molecular, cellular and medical aspects.* 6th ed. Philadelphia: Lippincott Williams and Wilkins 1999.

[207] Choi Y, Chen HV, Lipton SA. Three pairs of cysteine residues mediate both redox and Zn^{2+} modulation of the NMDA receptor. *J. Neurosci.* 2001;21:392-400.

In: Principles of Free Radical Biomedicine, Volume III
Editors: K. Pantopoulos and H. M. Schipper

ISBN 978-1-61324-184-4
©2012 Nova SciencePublishers, Inc.

Chapter 11

Redox Ophthalmology

Alex F. Thompson[1] and Leonard A. Levin[1,2,]*

[1]Department of Ophthalmology and Visual Sciences,
University of Wisconsin School of Medicine and Public Health, U.S.A.
[2]Maisonneuve-Rosemont Hospital Research Center and Department of Ophthalmology,
University of Montreal, Canada

Grant Support: CIHR, NIH R01EY012492, R21EY017970, and P30EY016665, Retina Research Foundation, and an unrestricted departmental grant from Research to Prevent Blindness, Inc. LAL is a Canada Research Chair.

1. Age-Related Macular Degeneration

1.1. Clinical Background

Age-related macular degeneration (AMD) is a disease involving the death of photoreceptors and retinal pigmented epithelium (RPE) cells in the macula, the region of retina responsible for fine visual acuity (Figure 1). AMD pathology also includes the formation of drusen, extracellular deposits which accumulate below the RPE [1, 2], and neovascularization, abnormal blood vessels that can leak or bleed, thereby causing severe visual loss. "Dry" AMD is the term used when there is atrophic loss of retina, while "wet" AMD is used when there is neovascularization and consequent leakage or hemorrhage. AMD is the leading cause of legal blindness in the developed world [3], and can significantly affect quality of life, limiting a person's ability to read, drive, or even recognize objects or faces. The molecular etiology of the disease is not fully understood, and as such effective preventative or mitigative treatment options were limited [1, 4] until the introduction of effective drugs for neovascularization [5].

---

*E-mail: leonard.levin@umontreal.ca

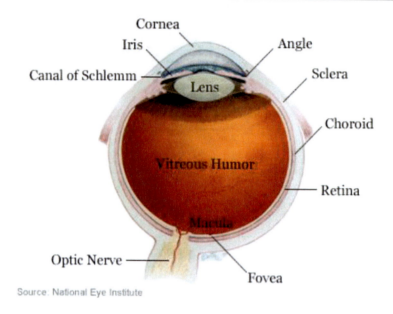

Figure 1. Schematic of the human eye. From the National Eye Institute, USA, with permission.

1.2. Clinical Evidence for Oxidative Stress in AMD Pathogenesis

Multiple clinical and epidemiological studies have linked AMD development and progression to oxidative stress. This should not be surprising, as *the retina is an environment predisposed to the generation of reactive oxygen species (ROS). Oxygen consumption in the retina is greater than other tissues* [6] *and the retina receives high levels of light exposure, which induce the formation of free radicals. The macula in particular is vulnerable to oxidative insult because levels of fatty acids in this area differ from levels in other parts of the human retina* [7]. Macular cells are more likely to experience lipid peroxidation than cells in other retinal areas, and the vulnerability of the macula to oxidative stress increases with age [8, 9] correlating with the strong age association of AMD. In response, levels of the antioxidant α-tocopherol (vitamin E; see Vol. II, Chapter 3) increase in the RPE as a person ages, presumably to combat increasing oxidative damage [10]. Macular pigments such as zeaxanthin and lutein also serve as endogenous antioxidants in the aging retina, with tissue samples from AMD patients showing lower levels of these protective pigments than samples from healthy retinas [11].

Cigarette smoking is the strongest environmental risk factor for AMD [12-14], and is correlated with atrophy and apoptotic death of RPE cells [15]. Smokers have lower levels of macular pigments than non-smokers. The relationship between smoking and pigment concentration is dose-dependent; a greater number of cigarettes smoked per day correlates with a lower level of protective macular pigments [16]. Finally, oxidative stress is a cause of drusen formation, a risk factor for AMD. *Drusen samples from AMD patients are more likely to contain oxidative protein modifications than samples from control eyes, suggesting that oxidative stress may contribute to drusen formation* [2]. Carboxyethylpyrrole adducts indicative of oxidative damage by docosahexaenoic acid have been observed in drusen proteins, including albumin, pyruvate kinase, and glutathione S-transferase [17]. Plasma levels of these adducts are 40% higher in patients with AMD than in age-matched healthy subjects [18].

Light-induced damage has been implicated as a component of AMD pathogenesis. A connection between AMD and excessive light exposure was suggested by findings that the regions of the retina damaged by light exposure in human subjects are the same regions where damage appears in AMD, and that higher levels of ocular melanin correlate with a lower likelihood of AMD development [19]. Spending more time in the sun is significantly correlated with development of AMD [20]. Interestingly, deliberate sun gazing results in macular damage [21, 22], and although it is unlikely that this is a cause of AMD, it can be helpful for understanding disease pathogenesis. Specifically, this connection between light and disease pathology can be exploited to study AMD in animal and cell culture models.

1.3. Experimental Studies of AMD Pathogenesis

Exposure of rats [23, 24], mice [25], or monkeys [22] to constant bright light is commonly used as a model for AMD pathology. The damage induced by light exposure is similar to the damage seen in AMD, and similar mechanisms are thought to underlie both processes [26]. Light induces apoptotic death in photoreceptor cells [27, 28] and a loss of RPE pigment [22]. Light exposure decreases cytochrome c oxidase activity in the retina [24] induces the expression of the antioxidative stress protein heme oxygenase-1 [28] (see also Vol. II, Chapter 11), alters levels of the endogenous redox modulators thioredoxin (Vol. II, Chapter 9) and glutathione (Vol. II, Chapter 1), and results in nuclear translocation of the redox sensitive transcription factor NF-κB [25] (see also Vol. II, Chapter 12). *All of these effects suggest a role for ROS in the signaling of light-induced cell damage.* This connection between photic injury and ROS is further strengthened by the finding that treatment of mice with the thiol antioxidant N-acetylcysteine suppresses changes in levels and activities of redox modulators induced by exposure to bright white light [25].

Animal models are also used to study the role of oxidative stress in cigarette smoking and the development of AMD. Mice exposed to cigarette smoke for 5 hours per day, 5 days per week for 6 months showed ultrastructural changes in the RPE and Bruch's membrane (innermost layer of the choroid; Figure 1) that were not seen in mice exposed only to filtered air. Smoke-exposed mice showed evidence of oxidative DNA damage, and a higher percentage of RPE cells in these mice were identified as apoptotic by terminal dUTP nick end labeling (TUNEL) compared to air-exposed controls [29].

In vitro experiments using immortalized RPE cells (the ARPE-19 cell line) or immortalized photoreceptor cells (the 661W cell line) have examined the mechanistic connection between light exposure and ROS. Early experiments showed light damage in mouse lung cells to be exacerbated by culturing cells in a higher percentage of oxygen, while the damaging effects of light were inhibited by adding catalase or glutathione to the culture medium [30]. The role of mitochondria in light-induced death was explored by manipulating the electron transport chain. Mitochondrial ROS (probably superoxide; O_2^-) generation was demonstrated in ARPE-19 cells exposed to strong blue light: photic injury resulted in production of ROS and cell death in intact cells, but not in Rho^0 cells lacking mitochondrial DNA. Treatment with the synthetic mitochondrially targeted antioxidant MitoQ (see Vol. II,

Chapter 15) is able to prevent light-induced death [3]. In 661W cells, the connection between oxidative stress and photoreceptor apoptosis was explored using a nitric oxide donor. Treatment with this compound resulted in activation of both calpains and caspases, while treatment with an ROS scavenger blocked calpain activation and apoptosis [31]. *Together, these findings implicate significant cell death protease activity downstream of ROS production in injury signaling.*

Neovascularization is responsible for most cases of blindness from AMD. This formation of new blood vessels is partially regulated by changing expression of growth factors [32] which, in turn, are in part regulated by intracellular ROS levels. In ARPE-19 cells, expression of vascular endothelial growth factor (VEGF), connective tissue growth factor (CTGF), and transforming growth factor-β (TGF-β) is upregulated following oxidative stress, induced either by paraquat treatment or a hypoxia/reoxygenation protocol [33, 34]. This suggests that ROS may contribute to neovascularization. Similarly, mice lacking the gene coding for superoxide dismutase 1 (SOD-1; see Vol. II, Chapter 5) are susceptible to neovascularization, which can be prevented by treatment with antioxidants [35].

1.4. Treatment and Prophylaxis

Vitamin E is found naturally in the retina, and appears to play a role in the development of AMD, as areas of the monkey retina where α-tocopherol levels are lowest correlate with areas where the first signs of AMD are likely to develop [36]. Furthermore, monkeys fed vitamin E-deficient diets develop macular degeneration, attributed to lipid peroxidation [37]. Such findings led to experimental studies of natural and synthetic antioxidants in animal models of retinal degeneration. Such drugs been shown to improve both number and functionality of photoreceptors following light damage [28, 38, 39]. RPE cells are also protected by antioxidant treatment. For example, transfection of RPE cells to overexpress catalase protects both RPE cells and neighboring photoreceptors from light-induced death [40].

Given the role for oxidative stress in AMD pathogenesis, antioxidants have been tested as compounds with potential protective or mitigative effects. The largest such study was the Age-Related Eye Disease Study (AREDS), a nationwide clinical trial of 3640 subjects that studied the potential value of antioxidants as a treatment for AMD and associated risk factors. Participants took an oral tablet every day, containing zinc, antioxidants, a combination of zinc and antioxidants, or a placebo. The antioxidants used included vitamin C, vitamin E, and beta-carotene. *For patients who already had intermediate AMD, treatment with antioxidants over seven years reduced their risk of developing advanced AMD by about 17 percent [15] and reduced the risk of vision loss by approximately 10 percent.* These proportions were increased when antioxidant treatment was combined with 80 milligrams per day of zinc.

Improvement in human AMD patients treated with antioxidants is correlated with reduction of plasma glutathione and cysteine oxidation [41]. Since mitochondria have been implicated as a source of ROS in AMD, smaller clinical trials have examined mitotropic compounds (compounds which improve mitochondrial function) as potential treatments. In patients with early AMD, treatment with a mixture of the mitotropic compounds acetyl-L-carnitine, polyunsaturated fatty acids, coenzyme Q_{10}, and vitamin E was more effective than treatment with vitamin E alone. Patients treated with mitotropic compounds improved over time on tests of retinal function, while vision in patients receiving only vitamin E slowly deteriorated. However, these differences between treatments were not significant at any of the follow-up time points in this study [42].

2. Diabetic Retinopathy

2.1. Clinical Background

Diabetic retinopathy is the most common complication of diabetes, affecting approximately 75% of those with diabetes [43, 44]. Diabetic retinopathy is often divided into two types, non-proliferative and proliferative. In patients with non-proliferative diabetic retinopathy, damage to small blood vessels causes microhemorrhages, microaneurysms, and the leakage of fluid, the last resulting in retinal edema. Vision is impaired if edema occurs at the macula. When vascular damage is sufficient to cause retinal ischemia, consequent neovascularization in the retina and into the vitreous (transparent gel-like material that fills the eyeball behind the lens; Figure 1) defines proliferative diabetic retinopathy [45]. The angiogenic cytokine VEGF is seen at greater levels in diabetic patients than controls, and VEGF levels are correlated with the development of proliferative diabetic retinopathy [46]. The neo-vessels can bleed, obscuring vision and leading to subsequent fibrosis that can detach the retina and cause permanent visual loss unless treated.

2.2. Clinical Evidence for Oxidative Stress in the Pathogenesis of Diabetic Retinopathy

Diabetic patients with retinopathy show signs of oxidative stress. Serum levels of malondialdehyde (MDA; indicative of lipid peroxidation), protein carbonyls (oxidation protein products), and 8-hydroxy-2'-deoxyguanosine (8-OHdG; a marker for oxidative DNA) are higher in diabetic patients than control subjects [47]; see also Chapter 9 in this Volume. Diabetic patients with retinopathy have higher levels of these oxidative stress indicators than those without retinal pathology [47].

These differences in serum indicators of oxidative stress are also seen when samples of subretinal fluid are compared, with diabetic patients having higher levels of MDA and protein carbonyls than control subjects. Correspondingly, samples from diabetic patients also contain lower amounts of reduced sulfhydryl proteins and the antioxidant vitamin E [48]. Total antioxidant levels in the vitreous are similarly lower in diabetic patients than control subjects [49]. The lower levels of the antioxidant taurine in patients with diabetic retinopathy may contribute directly to disease pathology [50]. In diabetic retinopathy, retinal endothelial cells and pericytes undergo apoptosis. There is increased terminal dUTP nick end labeling (TUNEL) positivity in endothelial cells and pericytes in diabetic retinas compared to controls [51].

2.3. Experimental Studies of Diabetic Retinopathy Pathogenesis

Diabetic hyperglycemia can be simulated *in vitro* by exposing cultured endothelial cells to high levels of glucose. Glucose exposure results in O_2^- production [52], oxidative DNA damage, and cell death [53]. Treating cultured bovine endothelial cells with glucose dramatically increases ROS production and lipid peroxidation. These effects are diminished by treating the glucose-stressed cells with vitamin E [54]. *Production of ROS connects numerous metabolic changes known to mediate glucose-induced damage in cells [55]. O_2^- is induced by hyperglycemia because high glucose levels result in overproduction of electron donors by the tricarboxylic acid cycle, which disrupts mitochondrial electron transport, leading to increased O_2^- generation by mitochondria [56].*

Peroxynitrite production is also induced with glucose treatment, and is likely involved in cell death signaling. High glucose normally induces apoptosis in cultured retinal endothelial cells, but treatment with the catalyst FeTTPS, which decreases peroxynitrite levels, prevents cell death [57]. MMP2, a matrix metalloproteinase enzyme that degrades extracellular proteins and has known roles in cell signaling, may also be a part of an apoptosis signaling pathway regulated by O_2^-. Stressing cultured retinal endothelial cells with high glucose results in activation of MMP2, and this activation is inhibited the O_2^- scavenger MnTBAP, an SOD mimetic [58]; see also Vol. II, Chapter 6.

In vitro models have also been used to study the role of endogenous antioxidants in diabetic retinopathy. Specifically, SOD appears to have a protective effect against hyperglycemic stress. Overexpressing mitochondrial SOD in cultured bovine retinal endothelial cells limits glucose-induced oxidative stress, evidenced by reduced 8-OHdG and nitrotyrosine levels, and decreases apoptosis [59].

Diabetes can be simulated in rodents by administering streptozotocin. Streptozotocin-treated animals develop neovascularization that closely resembles diabetic retinopathy. Additionally, retinal levels of VEGF and VEGF receptor are increased in these animals compared to controls, mirroring the VEGF elevation seen in human patients with diabetic retinopathy [60, 61]. In mice, streptozotocin treatment results in an increase in O_2^- in the retina, a decrease in mitochondrial glutathione levels, and increased mitochondrial membrane permeability [62]. Treatment with streptozotocin also results in the breakdown of the blood-retina barrier. This is correlated with ROS production, specifically increases in levels of nitric oxide, lipid peroxides, and nitrotyrosine, which is indicative of the presence of peroxynitrite. Pharmacological treatment to inhibit nitric oxide synthase or scavenge peroxynitrite prevents blood-retina barrier breakdown and lipid peroxidation, and limits the increase in VEGF levels normally seen with an increase in ROS [63].

The time course of oxidative stress in diabetes development has been studied in an alternate animal model of diabetes, the BBZ/Wor rat, which develops hyperglycemia spontaneously. In these animals, levels of NADH oxidase, nitric oxide synthase, and peroxynitrite all increase once the rats develop hyperglycemia. *Nitric oxide synthase and peroxynitrite levels are higher in new-onset diabetic rats than rats with chronic diabetes, suggesting that these molecules may play a key role in the initiating pathology of diabetic retinopathy [64].*

2.4. Treatment and Prophylaxis

Preventative measures can delay onset and reduce the severity of diabetic retinopathy. Strict control of blood glucose is important because prolonged elevation of blood glucose is the cause of the vascular dysfunction that defines the first stages of diabetic retinopathy [45]. Control of blood pressure also limits disease progression [65]. Once proliferative retinopathy develops, laser surgery is a common approach used to treat it. However, this technique is not precise enough to avoid destruction of neurons in the retina as well as the targeted vascular tissue. As such, it carries risks of reduced peripheral and night vision, or changed color perception [45].

The development of more specifically targeted pharmaceutical treatments would help reduce the risks of treating diabetic retinopathy. Since VEGF is a critical signaling molecule for neovascularization, it has promise as a target for pharmaceutical intervention. Several methods of inactivating VEGF have been tested in animal models. Chimeric proteins made from immunoglobulin and the extracellular domain of the VEGF receptor have been used to bind and neutralize VEGF in mice with retinopathy induced experimentally by ischemia. This treatment resulted in a dose-dependent reduction in retinal neovascularization [66]. Similarly, intraocular or systemic treatment with a neutralizing antibody against VEGF also blocked proliferative retinopathy in a mouse model [67]. An alternate method to block VEGF signaling is to inhibit phosphorylation by VEGF receptors. This was done using selective kinase inhibitors in mice with experimentally induced retinopathy, and resulted in a reduction in neuovascularization [68]. As a result of these and similar studies, clinical trials of anti-VEGF agents are ongoing, and intravitreal anti-VEGF treatments are currently used in clinical practice [69]. These drugs are not without risk. If anti-angiogenic treatments reach parts of the body besides the eye, they could have damaging effects because vessel growth and repair in the heart and extremities can be impaired in diabetic patients [46].

Because oxidative stress is implicated in the pathogenesis of diabetic retinopathy, antioxidants are being studied as a potentially promising therapy. ROS scavengers have been tested in animal models. Overexpression of mitochondrial SOD, an endogenous scavenger, in mice with streptozotocin-induced diabetes limits DNA and nitrotyrosine levels compared to wild type mice [70]. Treatment with synthetic scavengers, as well, has proven effective in animal studies. The SOD mimetic Tempol, for example, is protective of endothelial cells in diabetic rats [71]. Lowering peroxynitrite levels with the decomposition catalyst FP15 has also proven effective [72, 73]. Lipoic acid is a particularly promising antioxidant treatment as it distributes to the mitochondria, where O_2^- production occurs [74]. Lipoic acid is capable of scavenging hydroxyl radicals, singlet oxygen, and peroxynitrite, and scavenges O_2^- in its reduced form, dihydrolipoic acid [75]. Lipoic acid treatment is protective for retinal vascular tissue in rats with streptozotocin-induced diabetes [74] and reduces vascular damage in diabetic patients in clinical trials [75]. However, not all anti-oxidant trials have been successful. One study found improved retinal blood flow in Type I diabetes patients treated with vitamin E [76], but other studies have repeatedly failed to replicate these results [45].

An alternative to scavenging ROS is using pharmacological agents to reduce their production. Inhibition of NAD(P)H oxidase, for example, reduces generation of O_2^-, prevents an increase in VEGF levels, and obviates blood-retina barrier breakdown in mice with streptozotocin-induced retinopathy [77]. Similarly, inhibition of protein kinase C (PKC) may limit O_2^- generation. LY 333531, a PKC inhibitor, prevents vascular complications in animal models of diabetes [78], and is now being tested in clinical trials [45]. The PKC inhibitor ruboxistaurin has also been shown to reduce retinal complications of diabetes in animal models, and has been shown to diminish vision loss and reduce the need for laser photocoagulation in clinical trials [79].

3. Glaucoma

3.1. Clinical Background

Glaucoma is an optic neuropathy characterized by retinal ganglion cell (RGC) death and degeneration of RGC axons, which form the optic nerve [80] (Figure 1). In many cases optic nerve injury is linked to elevation of intraocular pressure (IOP). Increased IOP can occur if the trabecular meshwork, the tissue responsible for draining aqueous humor from the anterior chamber of the eye, is damaged or blocked. However, not all glaucoma patients present with high IOP, and IOP elevation is not necessarily causative in glaucoma pathogenesis. In fact, depending on the population, 50-90% of glaucoma patients present without elevated IOP, and glaucoma can progress even after IOP is lowered [81-83]. Elevated IOP is capable of causing axonal damage via biomechanical forces, ischemia, and blocking retrograde transport of nutrients and growth factors to RGCs [84, 85]. ROS have been implicated both in damage to the trabecular meshwork [86] and in the signaling of RGC apoptosis [87].

3.2. Clinical Evidence for Oxidative Stress in Glaucoma Pathogenesis

Examination of eyes of human glaucoma patients pre- or post-mortem implicates ROS and oxidative stress in glaucoma pathogenesis. In the trabecular meshwork, oxidative stress is evidenced by increased levels of 8-OH-dG. *Levels of 8-OH-dG are higher in trabecular meshwork tissue samples from primary open-angle glaucoma (POAG) patients than in control subjects, and the level of DNA damage is proportional to the increase in IOP and vision deficiency* [86, 88]. Mitochondrial DNA as well is known to be damaged in the disease, with trabecular meshwork samples from glaucoma patients exhibiting higher numbers of mtDNA mutations than control samples [89]. Similarly, levels of oxidized proteins in trabecular meshwork samples are higher in glaucoma patients than in controls [90].

In addition to the trabecular meshwork, the aqueous humor of glaucoma patients exhibits increased oxidative and decreased antioxidant capacities [91]. In one study, total reactive antioxidant potential in the aqueous humor was 64% lower in POAG patients than in controls, and SOD and glutathione levels were both higher in POAG patients as well [92]. These statistics indicate increased oxidative stress in glaucoma patients.

Finally, oxidative stress is evident in retinal tissue samples. Oxidative stress induces changes in expression of proteins in the retina, including hemoglobin, complement components, and complement regulators, and this is greater in glaucomatous eyes compared than controls [93, 94]. There is upregulation of nitric oxide synthase and presumably an increase in production of nitric oxide in astrocytes at the optic nerve head in patients with glaucoma [95], although the evidence is ambiguous [96]. Post-mortem examination of glaucomatous eyes revealed significant oxidative injury to both blood vessels and glia at the optic nerve head [97].

3.3. Experimental Studies of Glaucoma Pathogenesis

Cultured trabecular meshwork and retinal cells can be used to demonstrate the susceptibility of these tissues to oxidative stress, and also provide a system for screening of therapies to reduce oxidative damage. Human trabecular meshwork cells can be harvested and grown in culture. These cells are more sensitive to oxidative stress than cells from other anterior eye tissues, such as the cornea and iris [98]. Additionally, cultured trabecular meshwork cells of glaucoma patients appear to differ from those of control subjects. Glaucomatous trabecular meshwork cells exhibit higher ROS levels, decreased mitochondrial membrane potential, and increased sensitivity to inhibition of the electron transport chain, which induces production of ROS [99]. Trabecular meshwork cells from glaucoma patients also express less of the antioxidant enzyme peroxiredoxin (Prx; see Vol. II, Chapter 10) than control eyes, and Prx VI decreases the effects of oxidative stress on cultured trabecular meshwork cells [100]. The effect of ROS on trabecular meshwork cells is in part structural; treatment with H_2O_2 limits the ability of these cells to adhere to the extracellular matrix and causes cytoskeletal changes [101].

RGCs harvested from the retina have been used to examine the role of ROS in RGC apoptosis. In some cases RGC-5 cells, a transformed retinal neuronal cell line that shares some features with RGCs [102], have been used for these studies. RGCs are vulnerable to oxidative stress because, like other central nervous system neurons, they exhibit high levels of oxygen consumption and polyunsaturated fatty acids (PUFAs) susceptible to oxidation [87]. Protein oxidation or alteration of gene expression may be involved in ROS-dependent signaling in RGCs. Subjecting RGC-5 cells to hydrostatic pressure to simulate elevated IOP results in altered protein expression, specifically an increase in levels of heme oxygenase-1, an isoform known to be induced by oxidative stress [103]; see also Vol. II, Chapter 11. Subjecting cultured rat RGCs to hypoxia reveals that although caspase activation occurs in apoptotic RGCs, apoptosis has a caspase-independent component [104]. Oxidative modification of lipids may also be a pathway by which ROS signal death in RGCs, a possibility supported by the fact that treatment with the lipid peroxidation inhibitor tirilazadmesylate has a protective effect on primary RGCs stressed with mitochondrial electron transport complex IV inhibition or hypoglycemia [105]. Treatment with a glutathione peroxidase (GPx) mimetic or clorgyline, which can block ROS production by mitochondria, can also be protective for RGCs [106].

In animals, glaucoma can be simulated using a variety of surgical or pharmacological techniques to increase IOP. To simulate the optic neuropathy it is possible to injure the optic nerve directly. Such acute injuries are not typical of human glaucoma, but allow study of some of the earliest events in optic neuropathies. For example, using a rat optic nerve crush model, it has been show that an asynchronous release of O_2^- from mitochondria occurs following damage to RGC axons. Treatment with brain-derived neurotrophic factor, ciliaryneurotrophic factor, forskolin, or insulin did not prevent this O_2^- burst, suggesting that oxidative stress acts as a cell death signal in RGCs, and is not merely a byproduct of neurotrophin deprivation [107]. Redox modulating proteins may then play a role further downstream of O_2^- in cell death signaling. Thioredoxin 1 and thioredoxin 2 are redox-modulating proteins (Vol. II, Chapter 9), and overexpression of these molecules in rat RGCs results in greater numbers of surviving cells after optic nerve transection [108].

Increasing IOP also results in oxidative stress in the eye. This is evidenced indirectly by an increase in levels of heme oxygenase-1 expression within hours of IOP elevation in mice [103]. Increased pressure induces oxidative protein modifications, assessed by protein carbonyl immunoreactivity. Using 2-D gel electorphoresis, approximately 60 proteins in the rat retina underwent oxidative modifications in one study [109]. *Retinal protein samples from rats with experimentally elevated IOP contain significantly more proteins with oxidative modifications than control samples.* Proteins with oxidative modifications after IOP elevation were analyzed by mass spectrometry, and three were identified as glyceraldehyde-3-phosphate dehydrogenase, HSP72, and glutamine synthetase [109]. Oxidative stress induced by elevation of IOP in rats also results in increased expression of hemoglobin, which may alter oxygen transport patterns or act as a free radical scavenger [93]. Finally, overexpression of thioredoxins increases survival in a glaucoma model just as it does after optic nerve transection [110].

3.4. Treatment and Prophylaxis

For glaucoma patients, standard treatment currently focuses on lowering IOP. This treatment isn't sufficient, because glaucoma can progress even without IOP elevation [81-83]. Future treatments will likely need to combine neuroprotection of RGCs with lowering IOP. This, however, can be easier said than done. Neuroprotective treatments have not been as successful in human studies even when they are protective *in vitro* and in animal models [111]. Interestingly, some drugs known to reduce IOP may have some efficacy as neuroprotective treatments. Brimonidine is applied to the eye to lower IOP. However, when given as an intraperitoneal injection to rats with an episceral vein cauterization glaucoma model, brimonidine does not lower IOP but does prevent RGC death [112].

Growth factors are promising compounds to test for neuroprotection, as neurotrophin deprivation is one consequence of axonal injury. Brain-derived neurotrophic factor, for example, is neuroprotective of RGCs, and not only promotes cell survival but also maintains cell structure, improving visual function [113]. Similarly, injecting biodegradable microspheres loaded with glial-derived neurotrophic factor into the vitreous of rats with elevated IOP increased survival of RGC cell bodies and axons [114]. It is also possible to administer growth factors in practical ways, such as eye drops. Nerve growth factor eye drops were protective of RGCs in a rat model of glaucoma and have been shown to improve performance of human glaucoma patients on tests of visual acuity [115], although this study has raised much controversy. Stem cell therapy may, at some point, be an alternative method to supply neurotrophic factors for RGC protection and repair, or even regeneration [116].

Finally, antioxidants have been a logical class of compounds to test as protective agents against ROS-mediated death. The antioxidant N-acetylcysteine limits the oxidative consequences of increasing IOP in a rat glaucoma model [117]. Similarly, subcutaneous implantation of the antioxidant melatonin in rats with elevated IOP prevents the damaging effects of IOP on retinal function as assessed by electroretinography. Melatonin also increases the activity of SOD, decreases nitric oxide synthase activity, and limits lipid peroxidation

[118]. Natural antioxidants in tea, coffee and chocolate are currently being examined for potential benefit in glaucoma patients [119]. The compound resveratrol in particular, which is found in the skin of grapes and in red wine, is protective of primary trabecular meshwork cells exposed to oxidative stress [120].

4. Corneal Diseases

4.1. Clinical Background

As a function of its location at the anterior surface of the eye (Figure 1), the cornea is highly susceptible to oxidative damage from continuous exposure to light and air [121]. The cornea is an avascular structure composed of three cellular layers: an anterior epithelium, the stroma, which contains keratocytes, and a posterior endothelium. The cornea is transparent and uniform to allow light to reach the lens and the retina without inducing distortion. In disease the structure of the cornea is disrupted, impairing this function and resulting in a loss of vision [122]. Examples of corneal disease include keratoconus, characterized by stromal thinning and a conical shaped cornea, Fuch's dystrophy, an inherited degenerative disorder of the corneal endothelium involving increased apoptosis [123], and pterygium, in which connective tissue grows invasively over the cornea [122].

4.2. Clinical Evidence for Oxidative Stress in Pathogenesis of Corneal Diseases

Post-mortem analysis of corneal tissue has connected oxidative stress to several corneal diseases. Accumulation of redox-active iron has been linked to keratoconus [122] and pterygium [124]. Iron deposits could lead to the generation of ROS [122] (see also Vol. I, Chapter 5) and might be responsible for the increased oxidative stress seen in corneal samples of patients with these diseases. In patients without ocular disease, trauma with a metallic object can leave deposits if the foreign body is not immediately removed. Metal deposits that are redox-active induce oxidative stress, increasing the damage done to the cornea [122]. In pterygium, oxidative stress is evidenced by increased 8-OHdG levels seen in samples of abnormal growths but not in samples of unaffected corneal epithelium [125]. MDA levels are significantly higher in corneal samples from patients with keratoconus and Fuch's dystrophy compared to control samples [126]. MDA levels in the aqueous humor of Schnyder corneal dystrophy patients are similarly higher than levels of control samples [127].

If oxidative stress plays a role in corneal disease pathology, the cornea would be expected to possess a system of antioxidant defenses. Tears would be capable of delivering antioxidants to the anterior epithelium, while aqueous humor could supply antioxidants to the posterior endothelium [122]. Indeed, aqueous humor contains cysteine, tyrosine, ascorbic acid, uric acid, and glutathione [128]. It does not, however, have high SOD activity [129]. Similarly, tears contain the non-enzymatic antioxidants cysteine, tyrosine, ascorbic acid, uric acid, and glutathione. The enzymatic antioxidant capacity of tears is more controversial. For example, while initially tears were shown to contain SOD-1 [130], later work found low SOD-1 activity in tear samples [129].

The corneal epithelium, stroma, and endothelium also contain antioxidants. SOD-1, SOD-2, and SOD-3 are found in all three corneal layers [129]. Other antioxidants within the cornea include ferritin, glutathione, GPx, glutathione reductase, ascorbic acid, vitamin E, and catalase [131].

Corneal crystallin proteins may serve as antioxidants in corneal defense [131]. Dysfunction in the expression or the activity of these antioxidants is likely to contribute to the development of corneal disease. In genetic studies, mutations of the gene coding for SOD-1 on chromosome 21 may be linked to inherited cases of keratoconus [132. Corneal samples from Fuch's dystrophy patients show significantly lower expression of antioxidant proteins [133].

4.3. Experimental Studies of Corneal Disease Pathogenesis

In the absence of any external stressor, cultured keratoconus fibroblasts have increased levels of ROS compared to control fibroblasts, indicative of a role for ROS in disease progression. Keratoconus cells are more sensitive to stress (temporary lowering of pH) than control cells.

After stress keratoconus cells have higher caspase activity, decreased mitochondrial membrane potential, and decreased viability [134]. Cultured corneal cells can be subjected to oxidative stress to simulate corneal disease pathologies. A dose-dependent increase in 8-OHdG levels is observed when human corneal endothelial cells from young donors are treated with H_2O_2, and the proliferative capacity of the cells decreases [135].

Similarly, rabbit corneal endothelial cells subjected to ROS generated from xanthine oxidase and hypoxanthine [136] or from UV-B radiation exposure [137] show signs of oxidative damage. Cells die after exposure to xanthine oxidase/hypoxanthine, but can be protected by treatment with the antioxidants purpurogallin, SOD, catalase, or ascorbic acid [136]. Exposure to UV-B radiation induces oxidative stress as evidenced by increased 8-OHdG levels, and treatment with the radical scavenger 4-coumaric acid prevents this damage [137]. Immortalized human corneal epithelial cells undergo injury when exposed to H_2O_2, and are protected by the protein thymosin beta-4, which induces upregulation of the antioxidant enzymes SOD and catalase [138]. *In vivo* experiments have also been used to examine the role of oxidative stress in the development of corneal pathology.

Levels of antioxidant enzymes, including GPx, SOD, and catalase, and levels of non-enzymatic ROS scavengers decrease as the animals age, possibly explaining why some corneal disease are more prominent later in human life [139]. The need for corneal antioxidants has also been studied in genetically modified mice. Knockouts of SOD-1, SOD-3, or both were created, and the corneas assessed. The ablation of SOD-3 resulted in larger mean corneal endothelial cell area, indicative of endothelial cell loss, because these cells have a very limited proliferative capacity [140, 141].

Disruption of both SOD1 and SOD3 resulted in the same increase in mean cell area, and additionally caused the development of irregular cell morphology as the mice aged [141]. Mice of all three knockout types unsurprisingly showed increased levels of O_2^- in the cornea [141].

4.4. Treatment and Prophylaxis

Animal models have additionally been used to explore potential treatment options for corneal disease focused on the modulation of redox state. Treatment with selenium, which contributes to GPx activity (Vol. II, Chapter 8), or vitamin E, improved corneal healing in rabbits with experimentally induced lesions [142]. Similarly, in rats with oxidative stress induced by hypoxia, treatment with para-aminobenzoic acid prevented the rise in peroxide levels normally seen in the cornea under hypoxic conditions. It also lowered MDA levels and stabilized catalase activity [143]. Exposure of rabbit eyes to high-intensity ultrasound energy results in corneal damage mediated by the generation of ROS. Irrigating eyes with solutions containing glutathione or ascorbic acid limited this damage [144]. *Genetic approaches to deliver antioxidants may also be considered as future therapies for corneal diseases. In animal studies, adenoviral delivery of human catalase cDNA resulted in increased survival of rabbit corneal endothelial cells after exposure to H_2O_2* [145].

Although antioxidants have not been investigated extensively in humans as treatment for corneal pathologies, one study has shown that topical vitamin E treatment reduced levels of keratocyte apoptosis after corneal injury [146]. Further exploration of redox modulating therapies for the cornea may be worthwhile.

References

[1]   Ambati J, Ambati BK, Yoo SH, Ianchulev S, Adamis AP. Age-related macular degeneration: etiology, pathogenesis, and therapeutic strategies. *Surv. Ophthalmol.* 2003;48(3):257-93.

[2]   Crabb JW, Miyagi M, Gu X, et al. Drusen proteome analysis: an approach to the etiology of age-related macular degeneration. *Proc. Natl. Acad. Sci. U S A.* 2002;99(23):14682-7.

[3]   King A, Gottlieb E, Brooks DG, Murphy MP, Dunaief JL. Mitochondria-derived reactive oxygen species mediate blue light-induced death of retinal pigment epithelial cells. *Photochem. Photobiol.* 2004;79(5):470-5.

[4]   Roodhooft J. No efficacious treatment for age-related macular degeneration. *Bull. Soc. BelgeOphtalmol.* 2000;276:83-92.

[5]   Brown DM, Regillo CD. Anti-VEGF agents in the treatment of neovascular age-related macular degeneration: applying clinical trial results to the treatment of everyday patients. *Am. J. Ophthalmol.* 2007;144(4):627-37.

[6]   Sickel W. *Retinal metabolism in dark and light.* Berlin: Springer-Verlag; 1972.

[7]   vanKuijk FJ, Buck P. Fatty acid composition of the human macula and peripheral retina. *Invest. Ophthalmol. Vis. Sci.* 1992;33(13):3493-6.

[8]   De La Paz M, Anderson RE. Region and age-dependent variation in susceptibility of the human retina to lipid peroxidation. *Invest. Ophthalmol. Vis. Sci.* 1992;33(13):3497-9.

[9]   Suzuki M, Kamei M, Itabe H, et al. Oxidized phospholipids in the macula increase with age and in eyes with age-related macular degeneration. *Mol. Vis.* 2007;13:772-8.

[10] Organisciak DT, Berman ER, Wang HM, Feeney-Burns L. Vitamin E in human neural retina and retinal pigment epithelium: effect of age. *Curr. Eye Res.* 1987;6(8):1051-5.

[11] Wustemeyer H, Jahn C, Nestler A, Barth T, Wolf S. A new instrument for the quantification of macular pigment density: first results in patients with AMD and healthy subjects. *Graefes Arch. Clin. Exp. Ophthalmol.* 2002;240(8):666-71.

[12] Seddon JM, Willett WC, Speizer FE, Hankinson SE. A prospective study of cigarette smoking and age-related macular degeneration in women. *JAMA* 1996;276(14):1141-6.

[13] Smith W, Assink J, Klein R, et al. Risk factors for age-related macular degeneration: Pooled findings from three continents. *Ophthalmology*, 2001;108(4):697-704.

[14] Tomany SC, Wang JJ, Van Leeuwen R, et al. Risk factors for incident age-related macular degeneration: pooled findings from 3 continents. *Ophthalmology*, 2004;111(7):1280-7.

[15] A randomized, placebo-controlled, clinical trial of high-dose supplementation with vitamins C and E, beta carotene, and zinc for age-related macular degeneration and vision loss: AREDS report no. 8. *Arch. Ophthalmol.* 2001;119(10):1417-36.

[16] Hammond BR, Jr., Wooten BR, Snodderly DM. Cigarette smoking and retinal carotenoids: implications for age-related macular degeneration. *Vision Res.* 1996;36(18):3003-9.

[17] Hollyfield JG, Salomon RG, Crabb JW. Proteomic approaches to understanding age-related macular degeneration. *Adv. Exp. Med. Biol.* 2003;533:83-9.

[18] Gu X, Meer SG, Miyagi M, et al. Carboxyethylpyrrole protein adducts and autoantibodies, biomarkers for age-related macular degeneration. *J. Biol. Chem.* 2003;278(43):42027-35.

[19] Young RW. Solar radiation and age-related macular degeneration. *Surv. Ophthalmol.* 1988;32(4):252-69.

[20] Cruickshanks KJ, Klein R, Klein BE. Sunlight and age-related macular degeneration. The Beaver Dam Eye Study. *Arch. Ophthalmol.* 1993;111(4):514-8.

[21] Ritchey CL, Ewald RA. Sun gazing as the cause of foveomacular retinitis. *Am. J. Ophthalmol.* 1970;70(4):491-7.

[22] Tso MO. Photic maculopathy in rhesus monkey. A light and electron microscopic study. *Invest. Ophthalmol.* 1973;12(1):17-34.

[23] Wiegand RD, Giusto NM, Rapp LM, Anderson RE. Evidence for rod outer segment lipid peroxidation following constant illumination of the rat retina. *Invest. Ophthalmol. Vis. Sci.* 1983;24(10):1433-5.

[24] Chen E. Inhibition of cytochrome oxidase and blue-light damage in rat retina. *GraefesArch. Clin. Exp. Ophthalmol.* 1993;231(7):416-23.

[25] Tanito M, Nishiyama A, Tanaka T, et al. Change of redox status and modulation by thiol replenishment in retinal photooxidative damage. *Invest. Ophthalmol. Vis. Sci.* 2002;43(7):2392-400.

[26] Taylor HR, Munoz B, West S, Bressler NM, Bressler SB, Rosenthal FS. Visible light and risk of age-related macular degeneration. *Trans Am. Ophthalmol. Soc.* 1990;88:163-73; discussion 73-8.

[27] Wu J, Seregard S, Spangberg B, Oskarsson M, Chen E. Blue light induced apoptosis in rat retina. *Eye* (Lond) 1999;13 (Pt 4):577-83.

[28] Organisciak DT, Darrow RM, Barsalou L, et al. Light history and age-related changes in retinal light damage. *Invest. Ophthalmol. Vis. Sci.* 1998;39(7):1107-16.

[29] Fujihara M, Nagai N, Sussan TE, Biswal S, Handa JT. Chronic cigarette smoke causes oxidative damage and apoptosis to retinal pigmented epithelial cells in mice. *PLoS One*, 2008;3(9):e3119.

[30] Parshad R, Sanford KK, Jones GM, Tarone RE. Fluorescent light-induced chromosome damage and its prevention in mouse cells in culture. *Proc. Natl. Acad. Sci. U S A*, 1978;75(4):1830-3.

[31] Sanvicens N, Gomez-Vicente V, Masip I, Messeguer A, Cotter TG. Oxidative stress-induced apoptosis in retinal photoreceptor cells is mediated by calpains and caspases and blocked by the oxygen radical scavenger CR-6. *J. Biol. Chem.* 2004;279(38):39268-78.

[32] Schlingemann RO. Role of growth factors and the wound healing response in age-related macular degeneration. *Graefes Arch. Clin. Exp. Ophthalmol.* 2004;242(1):91-101.

[33] Matsuda S, Gomi F, Oshima Y, Tohyama M, Tano Y. Vascular endothelial growth factor reduced and connective tissue growth factor induced by triamcinolone in ARPE19 cells under oxidative stress. *Invest. Ophthalmol. Vis. Sci.* 2005;46(3):1062-8.

[34] Matsuda S, Gomi F, Katayama T, Koyama Y, Tohyama M, Tano Y. Induction of connective tissue growth factor in retinal pigment epithelium cells by oxidative stress. *Jpn. J. Ophthalmol.* 2006;50(3):229-34.

[35] Dong A, Xie B, Shen J, et al. Oxidative stress promotes ocular neovascularization. *J. Cell Physiol.* 2009;219(3):544-52.

[36] Snodderly DM. Evidence for protection against age-related macular degeneration by carotenoids and antioxidant vitamins. *Am. J. Clin. Nutr.* 1995;62(6 Suppl):1448S-61S.

[37] Hayes KC. Retinal degeneration in monkeys induced by deficiencies of vitamin E or A. *Invest. Ophthalmol.* 1974;13(7):499-510.

[38] Organisciak DT, Wang HM, Li ZY, Tso MO. The protective effect of ascorbate in retinal light damage of rats. *Invest. Ophthalmol. Vis. Sci.* 1985;26(11):1580-8.

[39] Ranchon I, Gorrand JM, Cluzel J, Droy-Lefaix MT, Doly M. Functional protection of photoreceptors from light-induced damage by dimethylthiourea and Ginkgo biloba extract. *Invest. Ophthalmol. Vis. Sci.* 1999;40(6):1191-9.

[40] Rex TS, Tsui I, Hahn P, et al. Adenovirus-mediated delivery of catalase to retinal pigment epithelial cells protects neighboring photoreceptors from photo-oxidative stress. *Hum. Gene. Ther.* 2004;15(10):960-7.

[41] Moriarty-Craige SE, Adkison J, Lynn M, et al. Antioxidant supplements prevent oxidation of cysteine/cystine redox in patients with age-related macular degeneration. *Am. J. Ophthalmol.* 2005;140(6):1020-6.

[42] Feher J, Papale A, Mannino G, Gualdi L, BalaccoGabrieli C. Mitotropic compounds for the treatment of age-related macular degeneration. The metabolic approach and a pilot study. *Ophthalmologica*, 2003;217(5):351-7.

[43] Klein R, Klein BE, Moss SE, Davis MD, DeMets DL. The Wisconsin epidemiologic study of diabetic retinopathy. II. Prevalence and risk of diabetic retinopathy when age at diagnosis is less than 30 years. *Arch. Ophthalmol.* 1984;102(4):520-6.

[44] Sjolie AK, Stephenson J, Aldington S, et al. Retinopathy and vision loss in insulin-dependent diabetes in Europe. The EURODIAB IDDM Complications Study. *Ophthalmology*, 1997;104(2):252-60.

[45] Caldwell RB, Bartoli M, Behzadian MA, et al. Vascular endothelial growth factor and diabetic retinopathy: role of oxidative stress. *Curr. Drug Targets,* 2005;6(4):511-24.

[46] Duh E, Aiello LP. Vascular endothelial growth factor and diabetes: the agonist versus antagonist paradox. *Diabetes,* 1999;48(10):1899-906.

[47] Pan HZ, Zhang H, Chang D, Li H, Sui H. The change of oxidative stress products in diabetes mellitus and diabetic retinopathy. *Br. J. Ophthalmol.* 2008;92(4):548-51.

[48] Grattagliano I, Vendemiale G, Boscia F, Micelli-Ferrari T, Cardia L, Altomare E. Oxidative retinal products and ocular damages in diabetic patients. *Free Radic. Biol. Med.* 1998;25(3):369-72.

[49] Yokoi M, Yamagishi SI, Takeuchi M, et al. Elevations of AGE and vascular endothelial growth factor with decreased total antioxidant status in the vitreous fluid of diabetic patients with retinopathy. *Br. J. Ophthalmol.* 2005;89(6):673-5.

[50] Schaffer SW, Azuma J, Mozaffari M. Role of antioxidant activity of taurine in diabetes. *Can. J. Physiol. Pharmacol.* 2009;87(2):91-9.

[51] Mizutani M, Kern TS, Lorenzi M. Accelerated death of retinal microvascular cells in human and experimental diabetic retinopathy. *J. Clin. Invest.* 1996;97(12):2883-90.

[52] Giugliano D, Ceriello A, Paolisso G. Oxidative stress and diabetic vascular complications. *Diabetes Care,* 1996;19(3):257-67.

[53] Lorenzi M, Montisano DF, Toledo S, Barrieux A. High glucose induces DNA damage in cultured human endothelial cells. *J. Clin. Invest.* 1986;77(1):322-5.

[54] Giardino I, Edelstein D, Brownlee M. BCL-2 expression or antioxidants prevent hyperglycemia-induced formation of intracellular advanced glycationendproducts in bovine endothelial cells. *J. Clin. Invest.* 1996;97(6):1422-8.

[55] Brownlee M. Biochemistry and molecular cell biology of diabetic complications. *Nature,* 2001;414(6865):813-20.

[56] Du XL, Edelstein D, Dimmeler S, Ju Q, Sui C, Brownlee M. Hyperglycemia inhibits endothelial nitric oxide synthase activity by posttranslational modification at the Akt site. *J. Clin. Invest.* 2001;108(9):1341-8.

[57] el-Remessy AB, Bartoli M, Platt DH, Fulton D, Caldwell RB. Oxidative stress inactivates VEGF survival signaling in retinal endothelial cells via PI 3-kinase tyrosine nitration. *J. Cell Sci.* 2005;118(Pt 1):243-52.

[58] Kowluru RA, Kanwar M. Oxidative stress and the development of diabetic retinopathy: contributory role of matrix metalloproteinase-2. *Free Radic. Biol. Med.* 2009;46(12):1677-85.

[59] Kowluru RA, Atasi L, Ho YS. Role of mitochondrial superoxide dismutase in the development of diabetic retinopathy. *Invest. Ophthalmol. Vis. Sci.* 2006;47(4):1594-9.

[60] Gilbert RE, Vranes D, Berka JL, et al. Vascular endothelial growth factor and its receptors in control and diabetic rat eyes. *Lab. Invest.* 1998;78(8):1017-27.

[61] Hammes HP, Lin J, Bretzel RG, Brownlee M, Breier G. Upregulation of the vascular endothelial growth factor/vascular endothelial growth factor receptor system in experimental background diabetic retinopathy of the rat. *Diabetes,* 1998;47(3):401-6.

[62] Kanwar M, Chan PS, Kern TS, Kowluru RA. Oxidative damage in the retinal mitochondria of diabetic mice: possible protection by superoxide dismutase. *Invest. Ophthalmol. Vis. Sci.* 2007;48(8):3805-11.

[63] El-Remessy AB, Behzadian MA, Abou-Mohamed G, Franklin T, Caldwell RW, Caldwell RB. Experimental diabetes causes breakdown of the blood-retina barrier by a

mechanism involving tyrosine nitration and increases in expression of vascular endothelial growth factor and urokinase plasminogen activator receptor. *Am. J. Pathol.* 2003;162(6):1995-2004.

[64] Ellis EA, Guberski DL, Hutson B, Grant MB. Time course of NADH oxidase, inducible nitric oxide synthase and peroxynitrite in diabetic retinopathy in the BBZ/WOR rat. *Nitric. Oxide,* 2002;6(3):295-304.

[65] Tight blood pressure control and risk of macrovascular and microvascular complications in type 2 diabetes: UKPDS 38. UK Prospective Diabetes Study Group. *BMJ,* 1998;317(7160):703-13.

[66] Aiello LP, Pierce EA, Foley ED, et al. Suppression of retinal neovascularization in vivo by inhibition of vascular endothelial growth factor (VEGF) using soluble VEGF-receptor chimeric proteins. *Proc. Natl. Acad. Sci. U S A,* 1995;92(23):10457-61.

[67] Sone H, Kawakami Y, Segawa T, et al. Effects of intraocular or systemic administration of neutralizing antibody against vascular endothelial growth factor on the murine experimental model of retinopathy. *Life Sci.* 1999;65(24):2573-80.

[68] Ozaki H, Seo MS, Ozaki K, et al. Blockade of vascular endothelial cell growth factor receptor signaling is sufficient to completely prevent retinal neovascularization. *Am. J. Pathol.* 2000;156(2):697-707.

[69] Simo R, Hernandez C. Intravitreous anti-VEGF for diabetic retinopathy: hopes and fears for a new therapeutic strategy. *Diabetologia,* 2008;51(9):1574-80.

[70] Kowluru RA, Kowluru V, Xiong Y, Ho YS. Overexpression of mitochondrial superoxide dismutase in mice protects the retina from diabetes-induced oxidative stress. *Free Radic. Biol. Med.* 2006;41(8):1191-6.

[71] Nassar T, Kadery B, Lotan C, Da'as N, Kleinman Y, Haj-Yehia A. Effects of the superoxide dismutase-mimetic compound tempol on endothelial dysfunction in streptozotocin-induced diabetic rats. *Eur. J. Pharmacol.* 2002;436(1-2):111-8.

[72] Sugawara R, Hikichi T, Kitaya N, et al. Peroxynitrite decomposition catalyst, FP15, and poly(ADP-ribose) polymerase inhibitor, PJ34, inhibit leukocyte entrapment in the retinal microcirculation of diabetic rats. *Curr. Eye Res.* 2004;29(1):11-6.

[73] Szabo C, Mabley JG, Moeller SM, et al. Part I: pathogenetic role of peroxynitrite in the development of diabetes and diabetic vascular complications: studies with FP15, a novel potent peroxynitrite decomposition catalyst. *Mol. Med.* 2002;8(10):571-80.

[74] Lin J, Bierhaus A, Bugert P, et al. Effect of R-(+)-alpha-lipoic acid on experimental diabetic retinopathy. *Diabetologia,* 2006;49(5):1089-96.

[75] Packer L, Kraemer K, Rimbach G. Molecular aspects of lipoic acid in the prevention of diabetes complications. *Nutrition,* 2001;17(10):888-95.

[76] Bursell SE, Clermont AC, Aiello LP, et al. High-dose vitamin E supplementation normalizes retinal blood flow and creatinine clearance in patients with type 1 diabetes. *Diabetes Care,* 1999;22(8):1245-51.

[77] Al-Shabrawey M, Bartoli M, El-Remessy AB, et al. Role of NADPH oxidase and Stat3 in statin-mediated protection against diabetic retinopathy. *Invest. Ophthalmol. Vis. Sci.* 2008;49(7):3231-8.

[78] Sheetz MJ, King GL. Molecular understanding of hyperglycemia's adverse effects for diabetic complications. *JAMA,* 2002;288(20):2579-88.

[79] Sun JK, Hamam R, Aiello LP. Clinical trials in protein kinase C-beta inhibition in diabetic retinopathy. In: *Diabetic Retinopathy*: Humana Press; 2009:423-34.

[80] Quigley HA. Open-angle glaucoma. *N. Engl. J. Med.* 1993;328(15):1097-106.

[81] Flammer J. The vascular concept of glaucoma. *Surv. Ophthalmol.* 1994;38 Suppl:S3-6.

[82] Lichter PR, Musch DC, Gillespie BW, et al. Interim clinical outcomes in the Collaborative Initial Glaucoma Treatment Study comparing initial treatment randomized to medications or surgery. *Ophthalmology*, 2001;108(11):1943-53.

[83] Heijl A, Leske MC, Bengtsson B, Hyman L, Hussein M. Reduction of intraocular pressure and glaucoma progression: results from the Early Manifest Glaucoma Trial. *Arch. Ophthalmol.* 2002;120(10):1268-79.

[84] Vrabec JP, Levin LA. The neurobiology of cell death in glaucoma. *Eye* (Lond) 2007;21Suppl 1:S11-4.

[85] Levin LA. Pathophysiology of the progressive optic neuropathy of glaucoma. *Ophthalmol. Clin. North Am.* 2005;18(3):355-64, v.

[86] Izzotti A, Sacca SC, Cartiglia C, De Flora S. Oxidative deoxyribonucleic acid damage in the eyes of glaucoma patients. *Am. J. Med.* 2003;114(8):638-46.

[87] Kumar DM, Agarwal N. Oxidative stress in glaucoma: a burden of evidence. *J. Glaucoma*, 2007;16(3):334-43.

[88] Sacca SC, Pascotto A, Camicione P, Capris P, Izzotti A. Oxidative DNA damage in the human trabecular meshwork: clinical correlation in patients with primary open-angle glaucoma. *Arch. Ophthalmol.* 2005;123(4):458-63.

[89] Izzotti A, Sacca SC, Longobardi M, Cartiglia C. Mitochondrial damage in the trabecular meshwork of patients with glaucoma. *Arch. Ophthalmol.* 2010;128(6):724-30.

[90] Yagci R, Gurel A, Ersoz I, et al. Oxidative stress and protein oxidation in pseudoexfoliation syndrome. *Curr. Eye Res.* 2006;31(12):1029-32.

[91] Zanon-Moreno V, Pinazo-Duran MD. Oxidative stress theory of glaucoma. *J. Glaucoma.* 2008;17:508-9.

[92] Ferreira SM, Lerner SF, Brunzini R, Evelson PA, Llesuy SF. Oxidative stress markers in aqueous humor of glaucoma patients. *Am. J. Ophthalmol.* 2004;137(1):62-9.

[93] Tezel G, Yang X, Luo C, et al. Hemoglobin expression and regulation in glaucoma: insights into retinal ganglion cell oxygenation. *Invest. Ophthalmol. Vis. Sci.* 2010;51(2):907-19.

[94] Tezel G, Yang X, Luo C, et al. Oxidative Stress and the Regulation of Complement Activation in Human Glaucoma. *Invest. Ophthalmol. Vis. Sci.* 2010.

[95] Neufeld AH. Nitric oxide: a potential mediator of retinal ganglion cell damage in glaucoma. *Surv. Ophthalmol.* 1999;43Suppl 1:S129-35.

[96] Pang IH, Johnson EC, Jia L, et al. Evaluation of inducible nitric oxide synthase in glaucomatous optic neuropathy and pressure-induced optic nerve damage. *Invest. Ophthalmol. Vis. Sci.* 2005;46(4):1313-21.

[97] Feilchenfeld Z, Yucel YH, Gupta N. Oxidative injury to blood vessels and glia of the pre-laminar optic nerve head in human glaucoma. *Exp. Eye Res.* 2008;87(5):409-14.

[98] Izzotti A, Sacca SC, Longobardi M, Cartiglia C. Sensitivity of ocular anterior chamber tissues to oxidative damage and its relevance to the pathogenesis of glaucoma. *Invest. Ophthalmol. Vis. Sci.* 2009;50(11):5251-8.

[99] He Y, Leung KW, Zhang YH, et al. Mitochondrial complex I defect induces ROS release and degeneration in trabecular meshwork cells of POAG patients: protection by antioxidants. *Invest. Ophthalmol. Vis. Sci.* 2008;49(4):1447-58.

[100] Fatma N, Kubo E, Toris CB, Stamer WD, Camras CB, Singh DP. PRDX6 attenuates oxidative stress- and TGFbeta-induced abnormalities of human trabecular meshwork cells. *Free Radic. Res.* 2009;43(9):783-95.

[101] Zhou L, Li Y, Yue BY. Oxidative stress affects cytoskeletal structure and cell-matrix interactions in cells from an ocular tissue: the trabecular meshwork. *J. Cell Physiol.* 1999;180(2):182-9.

[102] Krishnamoorthy RR, Crawford MJ, Chaturvedi MM, et al. Photo-oxidative stress down-modulates the activity of nuclear factor-kappaB via involvement of caspase-1, leading to apoptosis of photoreceptor cells. *J. Biol. Chem.* 1999;274(6):3734-43.

[103] Liu Q, Ju WK, Crowston JG, et al. Oxidative stress is an early event in hydrostatic pressure induced retinal ganglion cell damage. *Invest. Ophthalmol. Vis. Sci.* 2007;48(10):4580-9.

[104] Tezel G, Yang X. Caspase-independent component of retinal ganglion cell death, in vitro. *Invest. Ophthalmol. Vis. Sci.* 2004;45(11):4049-59.

[105] Levin LA, Clark JA, Johns LK. Effect of lipid peroxidation inhibition on retinal ganglion cell death. *Invest. Ophthalmol. Vis. Sci.* 1996;37(13):2744-9.

[106] Maher P, Hanneken A. The molecular basis of oxidative stress-induced cell death in an immortalized retinal ganglion cell line. *Invest. Ophthalmol. Vis. Sci.* 2005;46(2):749-57.

[107] Lieven CJ, Hoegger MJ, Schlieve CR, Levin LA. Retinal ganglion cell axotomy induces an increase in intracellular superoxide anion. *Invest. Ophthalmol. Vis. Sci.* 2006;47(4):1477-85.

[108] Munemasa Y, Kim SH, Ahn JH, Kwong JM, Caprioli J, Piri N. Protective effect of thioredoxins 1 and 2 in retinal ganglion cells after optic nerve transection and oxidative stress. *Invest. Ophthalmol. Vis. Sci.* 2008;49(8):3535-43.

[109] Tezel G, Yang X, Cai J. Proteomic identification of oxidatively modified retinal proteins in a chronic pressure-induced rat model of glaucoma. *Invest. Ophthalmol. Vis. Sci.* 2005;46(9):3177-87.

[110] Caprioli J, Munemasa Y, Kwong JM, Piri N. Overexpression of thioredoxins 1 and 2 increases retinal ganglion cell survival after pharmacologically induced oxidative stress, optic nerve transection, and in experimental glaucoma. *Trans. Am. Ophthalmol. Soc.* 2009;107:161-5.

[111] Levin LA, Peeples P. History of neuroprotection and rationale as a therapy for glaucoma. *Am. J. Manag. Care,* 2008;14(1 Suppl):S11-4.

[112] Hernandez M, Urcola JH, Vecino E. Retinal ganglion cell neuroprotection in a rat model of glaucoma following brimonidine, latanoprost or combined treatments. *Exp. Eye Res.* 2008;86(5):798-806.

[113] Weber AJ, Harman CD, Viswanathan S. Effects of optic nerve injury, glaucoma, and neuroprotection on the survival, structure, and function of ganglion cells in the mammalian retina. *J. Physiol.* 2008;586(Pt 18):4393-400.

[114] Jiang C, Moore MJ, Zhang X, Klassen H, Langer R, Young M. Intravitreal injections of GDNF-loaded biodegradable microspheres are neuroprotective in a rat model of glaucoma. *Mol. Vis.* 2007;13:1783-92.

[115] Lambiase A, Aloe L, Centofanti M, et al. Experimental and clinical evidence of neuroprotection by nerve growth factor eye drops: Implications for glaucoma. *Proc. Natl. Acad. Sci. U S A,* 2009.

[116] Bull ND, Johnson TV, Martin KR. Stem cells for neuroprotection in glaucoma. *Prog. Brain Res.* 2008;173:511-9.

[117] Ozdemir G, Tolun FI, Gul M, Imrek S. Retinal oxidative stress induced by intraocular hypertension in rats may be ameliorated by brimonidine treatment and N-acetyl cysteine supplementation. *J. Glaucoma,* 2009;18(9):662-5.

[118] Belforte NA, Moreno MC, de Zavalia N, et al. Melatonin: a novel neuroprotectant for the treatment of glaucoma. *J. Pineal. Res.* 2010;48(4):353-64.

[119] Mozaffarieh M, Grieshaber MC, Orgul S, Flammer J. The potential value of natural antioxidative treatment in glaucoma. *Surv. Ophthalmol.* 2008;53(5):479-505.

[120] Luna C, Li G, Liton PB, et al. Resveratrol prevents the expression of glaucoma markers induced by chronic oxidative stress in trabecular meshwork cells. *Food Chem. Toxicol.* 2009;47(1):198-204.

[121] Wenk J, Brenneisen P, Meewes C, et al. UV-induced oxidative stress and photoaging.*Curr. Probl. Dermatol.* 2001;29:83-94.

[122] Shoham A, Hadziahmetovic M, Dunaief JL, Mydlarski MB, Schipper HM. Oxidative stress in diseases of the human cornea. *Free Radic. Biol. Med.* 2008;45(8):1047-55.

[123] Borderie VM, Baudrimont M, Vallee A, Ereau TL, Gray F, Laroche L. Corneal endothelial cell apoptosis in patients with Fuchs' dystrophy. *Invest. Ophthalmol. Vis. Sci.* 2000;41(9):2501-5.

[124] Hansen A, Norn M. Astigmatism and surface phenomena in pterygium. *ActaOphthalmol.* (Copenh) 1980;58(2):174-81.

[125] Kau HC, Tsai CC, Lee CF, et al. Increased oxidative DNA damage, 8-hydroxydeoxy-guanosine, in human pterygium. *Eye* (Lond) 2006;20(7):826-31.

[126] Buddi R, Lin B, Atilano SR, Zorapapel NC, Kenney MC, Brown DJ. Evidence of oxidative stress in human corneal diseases. *J. Histochem. Cytochem.* 2002;50(3):341-51.

[127] Gatzioufas Z, Charalambous P, Loew U, et al. Evidence of oxidative stress in Schnyder corneal dystrophy. *Br. J. Ophthalmol.* 2010.

[128] Richer SP, Rose RC. Water soluble antioxidants in mammalian aqueous humor: interaction with UV B and hydrogen peroxide. *Vision Res.* 1998;38(19):2881-8.

[129] Behndig A, Svensson B, Marklund SL, Karlsson K. Superoxide dismutase isoenzymes in the human eye. *Invest. Ophthalmol. Vis. Sci.* 1998;39(3):471-5.

[130] Crouch RK, Goletz P, Snyder A, Coles WH. Antioxidant enzymes in human tears. *J. Ocul. Pharmacol.* 1991;7(3):253-8.

[131] Lassen N, Black WJ, Estey T, Vasiliou V. The role of corneal crystallins in the cellular defense mechanisms against oxidative stress. *Semin. Cell Dev. Biol.* 2008;19(2):100-12.

[132] Udar N, Atilano SR, Brown DJ, et al. SOD1: a candidate gene for keratoconus. *Invest. Ophthalmol. Vis. Sci.* 2006;47(8):3345-51.

[133] Gottsch JD, Bowers AL, Margulies EH, et al. Serial analysis of gene expression in the corneal endothelium of Fuchs' dystrophy. *Invest. Ophthalmol. Vis. Sci.* 2003;44(2):594-9.

[134] Chwa M, Atilano SR, Reddy V, Jordan N, Kim DW, Kenney MC. Increased stress-induced generation of reactive oxygen species and apoptosis in human keratoconus fibroblasts. *Invest. Ophthalmol. Vis. Sci.* 2006;47(5):1902-10.

[135] Joyce NC, Zhu CC, Harris DL. Relationship among oxidative stress, DNA damage, and proliferative capacity in human corneal endothelium. *Invest. Ophthalmol. Vis. Sci.* 2009;50(5):2116-22.

[136] Yuen VH, Zeng LH, Wu TW, Rootman DS. Comparative antioxidant protection of cultured rabbit corneal epithelium. *Curr. Eye Res.* 1994;13(11):815-8.

[137] Lodovici M, Raimondi L, Guglielmi F, Gemignani S, Dolara P. Protection against ultraviolet B-induced oxidative DNA damage in rabbit corneal-derived cells (SIRC) by 4-coumaric acid. *Toxicology*, 2003;184(2-3):141-7.

[138] Ho JH, Tseng KC, Ma WH, Chen KH, Lee OK, Su Y. Thymosin beta-4 upregulates anti-oxidative enzymes and protects human cornea epithelial cells against oxidative damage. *Br. J. Ophthalmol.* 2008;92(7):992-7.

[139] Cejkova J, Vejrazka M, Platenik J, Stipek S. Age-related changes in superoxide dismutase, glutathione peroxidase, catalase and xanthine oxidoreductase/xanthine oxidase activities in the rabbit cornea. *Exp. Gerontol.* 2004;39(10):1537-43.

[140] Joyce NC. Proliferative capacity of the corneal endothelium. *Prog. Retin. Eye Res.* 2003;22(3):359-89.

[141] Behndig A. Corneal endothelial integrity in aging mice lacking superoxide dismutase-1 and/or superoxide dismutase-3. *Mol. Vis.* 2008;14:2025-30.

[142] Sieradzki E, Olejarz E, Strauss K, Marzec A, Mieszkowska M, Kaluzny J. [The effect of selenium and vitamin E on the healing process of experimental corneal lesions in the eye of the rabbit]. *Klin. Oczna.* 1998;100(2):85-8.

[143] Akberova SI, MusaevGalbinur PI, Stroeva OG, Magomedov NM, Babaev NF, Galbinur AP. [Comparative evaluation of the antioxidant activity of para-aminobenzoic acid and emoxipin in the cornea and crystalline lens (an experimental study)]. *Vestn. Oftalmol.* 2001;117(4):25-9.

[144] Nemet AY, Assia EI, Meyerstein D, Meyerstein N, Gedanken A, Topaz M. Protective effect of free-radical scavengers on corneal endothelial damage in phacoemulsification. *J. Cataract Refract. Surg.* 2007;33(2):310-5.

[145] Hudde T, Comer RM, Kinsella MT, et al. Modulation of hydrogen peroxide induced injury to corneal endothelium by virus mediated catalase gene transfer. *Br. J. Ophthalmol.* 2002;86(9):1058-62.

[146] Bilgihan K, Adiguzel U, Sezer C, Akyol G, Hasanreisoglu B. Effects of topical vitamin E on keratocyte apoptosis after traditional photorefractive keratectomy. *Ophthalmologica*, 2001;215(3):192-6.

In: Principles of Free Radical Biomedicine, Volume III
Editors: K. Pantopoulos and H. M. Schipper

ISBN 978-1-61324-184-4
©2012 Nova SciencePublishers, Inc.

Chapter 12

Skin Diseases: Role of Reactive Oxygen and Nitrogen

Mohammad Athar,[1,] Arianna L. Kim[2], Levy Kopelovich[3], Craig A. Elmets[1] and David R. Bickers[2]*

[1]Department of Dermatology, University of Alabama at Birmingham,
Birmingham, Alabama, U.S.A.
[2]Department of Dermatology, Columbia University Medical Center,
New York, New York, U.S.A.
[3]Division of Chemoprevention, National Cancer Institute, National Institutes of Health,
Bethesda, Maryland, U.S.A.

1. Skin

The skin is the largest organ, providing an important interface between the environment and the body. It consists of four distinct layers: the epidermis, the basement membrane zone, the dermis, and the subcutaneous layer. Each of these layers contains many specialized cells and structures, which have distinct functions. The epidermis is the outermost layer and continuously differentiates into five layers including: the stratum basale, the stratum spinosum, the stratum granulosum, the stratum lucidum, and the stratum corneum. The epidermis has a thickness of approximately 200 µm, which varies from place to place. The surface consists of dead cells, which are slowly removed and replaced by a continuously growing cell population. The basal layer lies between the epidermis and the dermis. It is estimated that it takes 28 days for a cell to reach from the basal layer to the surface. The human dermis is approximately 1.8 mm thick and is composed of collagen, elastin, etc which are required to make the skin supple. It also contains a network of blood vessels, nerves, sweat glands, oil producing sebaceous glands, and pores. In addition, hair follicles protrude through the dermis and form an interface with the dermal compartment. This interface is

---

*E-mail: mathar@uab.edu

important for regulating hair follicle cycling and hair growth. The area of hypodermis contains muscles, veins, and fat cells. Its thickness varies according to its location on the body. The acid mantle, which lubricates the skin surface, is formed in this layer by the sebum and sweat produced by sweat glands in the dermis. It also maintains skin in a slightly acidic pH; for more details [1].

The major functions of the skin include physical barrier against friction and shearing forces, protection against infection and environmental pollutants, protection against excessive water loss or absorption, temperature regulation, sensation responses, etc. Agents that damage barrier function may lead to the development of various skin disorders and make skin prone to opportunistic infections [2]. In addition, ultraviolet exposure of the skin induces synthesis of vitamin D, which is required for calcium and phosphorous metabolism. Vitamin D is also considered as a chemopreventive agent, particularly against skin cancer [3]. Other important functions performed by skin include antigen presentation, immunological reactions, and wound healing [1]. *Skin also provides an antioxidant barrier. In this regard, sebum functions to provide and replenish vitamin E on the skin surface* [4].

2. Reactive Oxygen and Nitrogen Species

A large number of environmental pollutants, food contaminants, and drugs to which humans are exposed parenterally often manifest their toxicity in skin [5]. These structurally diverse chemicals frequently act through the generation of reactive oxygen species (ROS). ROS include singlet oxygen ($^1O_2$), superoxide anion (O_2^{-}), hydrogen peroxide (H_2O_2), the hydroxyl radical (OH$^-$), etc (for details, see Vol. I, Chapter 2). Among these, $^1O_2$ is generated by the energy transfer to molecular oxygen (O_2) from donor toxicants. Molecular oxygen at ambient temperatures is in the triplet state and is paramagnetic. Superoxideis formed by the univalent reduction of O_2. Its dismutation leads to the formation of H_2O_2, which through catalytic decomposition in the presence of a redox active metal ion, particularly ferrous iron, generates OH (Fenton reaction; see Vol. I, Chapter 5). Cuprous copper can also perform similar catalytic functions.

A physiological source of oxygen radicals in skin is infiltrating activated leukocytes. These cells are capable of generating ROS and other reactive oxidants via NADPH oxidases and myeloperoxidases leading to the formation of O_2^{-} and hypochlorite, respectively [6].

A fundamental purpose for the release of ROS in skin, as in other organs, is to kill invading microorganisms during the inflammatory process. However, an unintended prolonged destruction of normal cells by the locally generated ROS potentially leads to pathologic processes. Antioxidant defense systems have co-evolved with aerobic metabolism to counteract the destructive effects of ROS in normal tissues. Despite these genetically programmed defense mechanisms, ROS-dependent damage of proteins, DNA, and other macromolecules accumulates over the lifetime of aerobic organisms. This damage is thought to contribute to the pathogenesis of skin cancer as well as many other age-related diseases [7, 8]. In this Chapter, we summarize current knowledge related to the roles of ROS in activating signals that are involved in the pathogenesis of inflammatory skin diseases as well as non-melanoma skin cancer.

2.1. The Interaction of $O_2^{\cdot-}$ with NO Generates Peroxynitrite (ONOO⁻)

Nitrate and nitrite, the precursor molecules of nitric oxide (NO) derive from endogenous as well as dietary sources. Vegetables provide most of the dietary nitrate whereas nitrite may come from various canned food items such as meat where it is added as a preservative. Endogenous nitrate and nitrite are produced in mammals via the L-argenine-NO pathway. NO is generated in the body from reactions catalyzed by enzymes known as NO-synthases. These reactions are oxygen-dependent: A five-electron oxidation of the amino acid, L-argenine produces NO and L-citrulline. It is now well established that NO is a critical regulator of vascular homeostasis, neurotransmission, cellular respiration, host defense, and redox signaling (see Vol. I, Chapter 3). In blood, NO reacts with oxyhemoglobin to produce mainly nitrate and methemoglobin. Non-enzymatic NO generation primarily occurs in the human stomach and is highly pH-dependent. However, in other organs a minor nitrite-NO pathway is known to exist and is considered as a back-up system for the generation of NO which is regulated by the physiological oxygen gradient. The expression of NO synthases has been shown in skin as early as 1992 [9]. Since then, investigations have shown the importance of NO in skin physiology. All three isoforms of NO synthase have been identified in skin keratinocytes as well as in fibroblasts [10]. *NO plays an important role in cutaneous inflammation and other immunological responses.* UVA exposure enhances the production of NO in the skin. However, UVB-induced cutaneous erythema formation also requires NO production. The simultaneous production of NO and ROS, particularly superoxide anions, often leads to the formation of the highly reactive peroxynitrite. This induces DNA strain breaks, activation of poly(ADP-ribose) polymerase pathway-dependent necrotic cell death and nitrosation of tyrosine residues in various proteins [11].Cutaneous upregulation of iNOS occurs in the Stevens-Johnson syndrome, an inflammatory skin condition involving toxic epidermal necrolysis [12]. NO regulates the expression of a variety of genes such as Bcl2, VGEF and heme oxygenase in addition to its well known involvement in the activation of cGMP-mediated cell signaling pathway. Besides its deleterious role in tissue injury when combined with ROS, NO augments tissue antimicrobial activity and promotes wound healing of the skin.

3. ROS and Cutaneous Molecular Signaling Pathways

Skin exposure to chemicals, xenobiotics/drugs, or radiation such as ionizing radiation (IR) and/or UV may result in the generation of excessive quantities of ROS that may quickly overwhelm antioxidant defense mechanisms present in the tissue. Other agents known to generate excessive ROS and result in oxidative stress in the skin of experimental animals and humans include gaseous airborne pollutants from automobiles and industries, and contaminants found in food, cosmetics, drugs, etc [13].

In addition, endogenous catabolic pathways in humans and animals lead to the generation of similar oxidative responses. One such example may be heme pathway intermediates that have pro-oxidant effects. However, heme degradation products generated by the enzyme, heme oxygenase can function both as an antioxidant and a pro-oxidant [14] (see also Vol. II,

Chapter 11). *Skin contains an array of cytochrome P-450 enzymes which convert highly hydrophobic and otherwise inert xenobiotics such as polynuclear aromatic hydrocarbons (PAHs) into reactive species via oxidative metabolism. We and others have shown that skin exposure to numerous chemical or physical environmental agents/toxins induce oxidative stress by altering the levels of these* enzymes [6, 15]. One common manifestation of the generation of redox active oxidative metabolites of environmental agents is the enhancement in cutaneous lipid peroxidation which usually occurs with concomitant modulation in levels of antioxidant and drug-metabolizing enzymes [16]. In addition, quinine reductase, an enzyme that transfers electrons from hydroquinones to oxygen, leads to the formation of ROS in normal and neoplastic cutaneous tissue [17].

A number of transcription factors such as activator protein 1 (AP-1) and NF-κB [18] have been implicated in ROS-mediated toxicity. UVA irradiation of skin fibroblasts has been shown to release labile iron, which participates in the activation of NF-κB [19] Another class of enzymes contributing to complex inflammatory responses are the mitogen-activated protein kinases (MAPKs). These kinases are partly regulated by oxidative stress [20]. Solar UV radiation, a major cause of oxidative stress and inflammation in skin, also influences these pathways in a similar manner as ROS. Parenteral administration of antioxidants reverses UVB-induced phototoxicity [21]. We also found that antioxidants or plant extracts containing antioxidant constituents ameliorate perturbations in cell cycle progression and aberrant activity of cell cycle regulatory proteins [22]. Apoptosis regulatory signaling in skin is also impacted by UVB and ROS.

In addition to MAPK, another important trigger of cutaneous inflammatory reactions are the eicosanoids. These clastogenic molecules, including the prostaglandins and the leukotrienes, are generated from arachidonic acid (AA) by the prostaglandin H synthetase catalyzed reaction which produces hydroxyl-endoperoxides. Prostaglandin H synthetase also possesses peroxidase activity which is responsible for co-oxidation of a wide range of substrates, including the PAHs. These chemicals are converted into highly reactive epoxide containing metabolites with a wide mutagenic potential [23].

Besides inflammation, UV induces cutaneous immune suppression and photoaging. In this regard, urocanic acid produced by UV exposure is considered to be a potential mediator of these responses. This is based on the overlapping absorption spectrum of urocanic acid and the action spectrum for UVB-induced immunosuppression. These responses have been associated with a reduction in the numbers of epidermal Langerhans cells. Interestingly, urocanic acid prolongs skin-graft survival time and affects natural killer cell activity [24]. Based on the characteristic production of 5α-cholesterol hydroperoxide, which is a marker of $^1O_2$, it was demonstrated that UVA irradiation-mediated stereochemical-conversion of transurocanic acid generates $^1O_2$ [25].

Other signaling pathways important in the manifestation of immunosuppresive and inflammatory responses in skin are c-jun N-terminal kinase (JNK) signaling. $^1O_2$ is known to initiate JNK signaling, leading to interstitial collagenase production as well as synthesis of pro-inflammatory cytokines such as IL-1 and IL-6 in UVA-irradiated skin cells [26]. However, these responses can also be modulated by endogenously generated chromophores such as nicotinamide adenine dinucleotide (reduced form)/nicotinamide adenine dinucleotide phosphate (reduced form), tryptophan, riboflavin, etc [27].

4. Antioxidant Protection

The temporal regulation of antioxidants in the skin as well as in other organs is required to eliminate ROS or their by-products and to minimize ROS-associated tissue damage. *Glutathione (GSH), alpha-tocopherol or vitamin E, ascorbic acid or vitamin C, glutathione peroxidases (GPxs), glutathione reductase, glutathione S-transferases (GSTs), superoxide dismutases (SODs), catalase, and quinonereductase are the major non-enzymatic and enzymatic antioxidant defenses present in the skin.* Water soluble GSH and ascorbic acid are cytosolic antioxidants, and lipid soluble vitamin E is the protector of the lipid-rich membrane [28, 29]. GSH, present in millimolar concentrations in virtually all normal cells (see Vol. II, Chapter 1), provides a first line of defense against oxidants and is quickly replenished following xenobiotic-dependent decreases in its tissue levels. Diethyl maleate, phorone and L-buthionine-(S,R)-sulfoximine are the model chemical compounds used in experimental animals for tissue GSH depletion [30] and for demonstrating the importance of GSH in oxidant injury. Conversely, N-acetylcysteine or 4-oxothiazoladine carboxylate, which augment tissue GSH levels are also employed to implicate this tripeptide in experimental models [30].

5. ROS and Cutaneous Neoplasms

Skin cancer involves a complex process consisting of multiple stages including, initiation, promotion, and progression, which are mediated by various cellular, biochemical, and genetic factors (see Chapters 6 and 7 in this Volume). ROS and ROS-generated free radicals are known to play a role in all three stages of carcinogenesis [13, 31]. Free radicals in cigarette smoke condensate, for example, manifest tumorigenicity when tested in a skin model of murine carcinogenesis [32]. The structural alterations in DNA that create mutations characterize the initiation stage of carcinogenesis. These genetic alterations in proto-oncogenes and tumor suppressor genes may render epidermal cells resistant to signals for terminal differentiation [33]. At this stage, ROS may also induce extensive DNA damage such as DNA base damage, DNA single-strand and double-strand breaks, crosslinking between DNA and proteins, or DNA and chromosomal aberrations [34], see also Vol. I, Chapter 9. It has been shown that chemical carcinogens capable of generating free radicals often induce the formation of thymine glycol [35], one of the major products of oxidant-based damage in DNA observed following either chemical oxidation or ionizing radiation. ROS induce 8-hydroxyguanosine formation both in genomic and mitochondrial DNA. Elevated levels of 8-hydroxyguanosine in blood and urine of experimental animals and humans are a sensitive biomarker of oxidative DNA damage. Environmental carcinogens, particularly pro-carcinogens, may be activated by ROS before they act as tumor initiators. Peroxyl radicals, which are formed by spontaneous or enzyme-catalyzed oxidation of unsaturated fatty acids, are also known to activate carcinogens such as benzo(a)pyrene, aromatic amines (e.g. naphthylamine, acetylaminofluorene, etc.), amino azo compounds, 4-nitroquinoline-1-oxide, and n-nitro compounds. Azathioprine, a widely used immunosuppressant drug, generates ROS following UVA exposure leading to accumulation of 6-thioguanine in DNA through the generation of guanine sulfonate, a replication-blocking DNA 6-thioguanine photoproduct.

This effect can be bypassed by error-prone Y-family DNA polymerases *in vitro*. Biologically relevant doses of UVA generate ROS in cells in culture with 6-thioguanine-substituted DNA. 6-thioguanine and UVA are synergistically mutagenic. Based on these results, it has been proposed that these treatments carry a risk of future therapy-related cancer and may contribute to the prevalence of skin cancer in azathioprine-treated patients [36]. In addition, other therapeutic modalities can accelerate the initiation of human skin cancer pathogenesis. Examples include PUVA treatment for psoriasis which enhances the risk of nonmelanoma skin cancer [37, 38]. Similarly, chronic immune suppression in organ transplant patients enhances the risk of skin cancers.

The second stage of carcinogenesis, tumor promotion, involves clonal expansion of initiated cells. Free radical involvement in tumor promotion seems likely based on evidence that a number of free radical-generating compounds are known to be tumor promoters. Many of these known tumor promoters have been shown to induce ROS, which, in turn, mimic the biochemical effects of known tumor promoters. In addition, tumor promoters can modulate tissue levels of antioxidants and/or ROS scavengers/detoxifiers and antioxidants [39]. These studies also showed that ROS-dependent modification of DNA and proteins induce specific signaling that modulates responses of initiated cells favoring both proliferation and apoptosis [40].

Examples of these cascades include DNA damage response-dependent signaling characterized by activation of ATM/ATR/ChK1/ChK2/p53 and p53-dependent and independent modulation of intrinsic apoptosis [41]. Recent data show that supraphysiological and physiological levels of p53 exert regulatory effects on the redox status of cells. p53 regulates the expression of both pro-oxidant and antioxidant genes. In addition, p53 also regulates cellular ROS levels by modulating metabolic pathways. Subphysiological levels of p53 are important in suppressing antioxidant genes such as Sestrin1 and 2 and GPx. However, physiological levels of p53 regulate additional metabolic genes such as synthesis of cytochrome c oxidase 2, phosphoglyceratemutase, and TP53-25-induced glycolysis and apoptosis regulator (*TIGAR*). Supraphysiological levels of p53 activate a number of pro-oxidant genes such as quinonereductase, proline oxidase, and MnSOD [42].

Among the early responses in mouse skin exposed to UVB are the induction of both oxidative-stress and enzymes that are considered important in DNA synthesis and proliferation. One such enzyme is ornithine decarboxylase (ODC). ODC drives the production of polyamines, which are potent enhancers of cell proliferation [43]. Antioxidant treatment prior to UVB exposure abrogates both oxidative stress and ODC induction [44]. Various oxidants and free radical-generating chemicals are known to enhance ODC activity in murine skin. ODC induction is regulated by protein kinase C. Both oxidant and non-oxidant tumor promoters and UVB induce protein kinase C although through different underlying mechanisms [45]. ODC induction and augmented polyamine synthesis are associated with important cell survival and cell death regulatory pathways. We showed that ODC is crucial for epidermal carcinogenesis and is involved in the pathogenesis of both basal cell carcinomas (BCCs) and squamous cell carcinomas (SCCs) [46].

In this regard, NF-κB, a ubiquitous transcription factor involved in proliferative signaling and tumor promotion, is activated by oxidants and other stimuli known to generate ROS [47]. The transcriptionally inactive NF-κB exists in the cytoplasm of most cells as homo- or heterodimers of a family of structurally related proteins known as Rel or Rel/NF-κB. Cytoplasmic sequestration of NF-κB is regulated by its binding to an inhibitory protein, IκB.

An upstream IκB kinase signals to induce transcriptional activation of NF-κB by phosphorylating IκB leading to its translocation to the nucleus (see Vol. II, Chapter 12). Interestingly, the promoter region of the ODC gene contains NF-κB response elements suggesting a regulatory role for this transcription factor in ODC induction during tumor promotion [48]. Genetically engineered murine models that overexpress or underexpress various antioxidant enzymes have been developed to investigate the role of oxidative stress in skin carcinogenesis [49-54]. These experiments were not straightforward and generated mixed results. For example, mice overexpressing CuZnSOD or GPx or both did not differ from wild type littermates in terms of two-stage skin chemical carcinogenesis [49, 53], but mice overexpressing MnSOD suppressed the pathogenesis of skin tumors [54]. Furthermore, MnSOD knockout mice did not show increased tumorigenesis [54]. However, depletion of quinonereductase 1 and 2 in skin enhanced cutaneous carcinogenesis [50, 52]. These results indicate that antioxidant responses are required on a temporal basis but a permanent increase or decrease in these molecules may yield unpredictable outcomes.

The third stage of skin carcinogenesis, tumor progression, occurs when benign papillomas or actinic lesions are converted into malignant neoplasms including SCCs and BCCs. In early investigations, we and others have shown that the conversion of papillomas to malignant neoplasm can be accelerated by treating papilloma-bearing mice with free radical-generating compounds [55, 56]. In this regard, our laboratory showed that organic hydroperoxides are effectively metabolized into free radicals by SCC cells [57]. The role of oxidative stress in tumor progression is also supported by studies where modulation of GSH levels in skin altered SCC induction [58]. Furthermore, the free radical scavenger, N-acyl dehydroalanin inhibits carcinogenesis, although it has no effect on 12-O-tetradecanoylphorbol-13-acetate-mediated ornithine decarboxylase (ODC) induction or papilloma formation [59]. Recently, additional ROS-dependent pathways involved in the progression of benign lesions have been identified. These pathways have been shown to enhance the phenomenon known as epithelial- mesencymal transition (EMT). EMT pathways, which are mainly dependent on TGFβ and Rho kinase signaling, alter the phenotype of epithelial cells characterized by high expression of polarity regulating proteins such as E-cadherin to the mesenchymal phenotype characterized by elevated expression of vimentin, alpha smooth muscle actin (α-SMA), and transcription factors twist, slug, snail, etc. This transition confers mobility of transformed epithelial cells allowing them to invade and metastasize to distal sites. Once these cells relocate to distal organs they regain epithelial characteristics through a process known as mesenchymal-epithelial transition (MET). *ROS have been shown to activate signaling cascades regulating EMT [60]. However, it is not known whether redox regulation is evoked in reverse signaling required for MET.*

6. Role of Oxidants in Skin Diseases

6.1. Vitiligo

Vitiligo is a multifactorial disorder characterized by the appearance of white maculae (spots or patches) that may spread over the entire skin. Depigmentation arises from the loss of functioning melanocytes. *It has been shown that impaired antioxidant defenses lead to accumulation of ROS, which affect melanocyte functioning* [61]. Mitochondrial membrane lipid peroxidation may participate in ROS overproduction. A temporal sequence may connect oxidative stress and autoimmunity in this disease. It has recently been shown that methionine sulphoxidereductase is crucial for maintaining redox balance in melanocytes of vitiligo patients [62]. Oral supplementation with pooled antioxidants containing alpha-lipoic acid before and during narrow band UVB significantly improves the latter's clinical effectiveness by reducing vitiligo-associated oxidative stress [63]. It has been proposed that the modification of membrane lipid components in vitiligo cells may be the biochemical basis for the mitochondrial impairment and the subsequent production of intracellular ROS following exposure to mild oxidative stress [63].

6.2. Pathogenesis of Allergic Reactions

During first encounter with antigen, memory T-lymphocytes differentiate into cytokine-producing effector cells. Based on their distinct cytokine expression profiles, Th1 and Th2 cells have been characterized. Th1-lymphocytes secrete IL-2 and IFN-α, whereas Th2-lymphocytes produce IL-4, IL-5, IL-6, IL-10, and IL-13. Th1 and Th2 response configures antigen-presenting cells, which may be modulated by GSH [64]. Positive patch tests in patients with contact allergies to nickel reflect increased tissue iron and an elevated oxidized/reduced GSH ratio, both of which characterize oxidative stress in skin [65]. In an independent study, nickel was found to enhance tissue iron accumulation and generate OH. [66]. These data indicate that ROS may participate in the pathogenesis of allergic skin reactions [67].

Allergic contact dermatitis in response to PAHs requires metabolic activation by cytochrome P450-dependent reactions [68]. Similarly, allergic contact hypersensitivity responses to paraphenylenediamine may be regulated by cytochrome P450-dependent generation of an oxidation product of paraphenylene-diamine known as a Bandrowski base [69]. *It has been reported that ROS upregulate dendritic cell surface markers, including major histocompatibility complex class II molecules, suggesting that interference with redox regulation pathways may interrupt antigen-specific, bidirectional dendritic cell–T-cell communication* [70]. ROS may play an important homeostatic role in the activation of sentinel dendritic cells, linking tissue damage to the initiation of an immune response [29]. 1-fluoro-2,4-dinitrobenzene (DNFB), a skin sensitizer, induces p38 MAPK and extracellular signal-regulated kinase (ERK)1/2 phosphorylation in a dendritic cell line generated from fetal mouse skin which can be blocked by GSH [71].

The production of oxidation products, such as 4-hydroxy-2-nonenal (4-HNE) or malonaldehyde may denature proteins, and influence the release of proinflammatory mediators, such as cytokines, which may be critical to the development of inflammatory skin disease [72]. Activation of NF-κB or AP-1, which are involved in the generation of cytokines by these oxidative metabolites, connects oxidative stress with inflammatory diseases [29]; see also Vol. II, Chapter 21. In this regard, peroxisome proliferator-activated receptors, whose natural ligands are polyunsaturated fatty acids, and their oxidation products may be involved in the pathogenesis of chronic inflammatory skin diseases such as psoriasis and acne, which further strengthens the concept that ROS may drive the development of chronic inflammatory skin disorders [73].

6.3. Varicose Ulcers

Varicose ulcers are another example of potential oxidant stress-driven pathology [74]. These ulcers, characterized by chronic inflammation, carry heme and iron deposits which appear to be associated with infiltrating cells, basement membranes, and fibrin cuffs around blood vessels [75]. Recently, it has been shown that valvular oxidative stress is involved in the development of venous stasis ulcers and venous ulcers [76].

6.4. Drug-Induced Skin Photosensitization

Another category of inflammatory response that involves ROS generation is drug-induced skin photosensitization [29]. Photodynamic therapy (PDT) of cancer often leads to the development of this response. In PDT, porphyrins are used as photosenitizers. Exposure to light following porphyrin administration leads to ROS generation, which can damage or destroy tumor cells [77]. However, a major drawback of this therapy is that many available photosensitizers have long cutaneous half-lives; thus, they can cause protracted and detrimental cutaneous photosensitivity. As determined by electron spin resonance spectroscopy, cutaneous porphyrin photosensitization generates O_2^- and other ROS [77]. In this process, O_2^- generation occurs via activation of cutaneous xanthine oxidase. Support for this concept derives from studies demonstrating that allopurinol, a potent xanthine oxidase inhibitor, blocks porphyrin-mediated photosensitivity responses [78]. Certain other drugs also manifest skin photosensitivity involving generation of ROS [79].

6.5. Acute Inflammation

ROS is a known trigger for the induction and maintenance of inflammatogen-mediated cutaneous inflammation [80]. Leukocyte infiltration is observed in skin exposed to these irritants or other proinflammatory agents. Infiltrating leukocytes produce an oxidative burst which in turn is responsible for the activation of multiple stress-dependent protein kinases. Chemical irritants, allergens and other inflammatory stimuli enhance production of cytokines by infiltrating leukocytes as well as by the afflicted keratinocytes [81]. ROS are known to modulate cysteine-rich redox-sensitive proteins, kinases, phosphatases, and transcription factors [82]. This often results in the phosphorylation-dependent activation of proteins. For example, ROS enhance EGFR phosphorylation and activate ERKs and JNKs [83]. We have shown that UVB activates p38 MAP kinase-dependent signaling which regulates the expression of cyclooxygenase-2 (COX-2) and inflammatory cytokines. p38, ERKs, and JNKs exhibit extensive crosstalk. Interactions between growth factor-activated ERKs and stress-activated JNK and p38 pathways may be detrimental to cell survival in the face of stress [84]. Downstream effectors of the MAPKs include transcription factors such as Elk-1, Ets, CREB, c-Fos and c-Jun. UVA-induced skin inflammation exhibits ROS-dependent activation of NF-κB through the degradation of its regulatory IκBα protein, as observed in other acute inflammatory responses [85]. UVA also releases free iron from body stores which contributes to IκBα-independent NF-κB activation [86]. Parallel to this effect on NF-κB, UVA also activates ERKs, JNKs, and p38 kinases in human skin keratinocytes and fibroblasts [87].

Tumor necrosis factor (TNF) plays an important role in regulating inflammatory responses [88]. It is also considered important in the regulation of cell death and survival pathways. TNF initiates intracellular signaling by binding to its receptor. The formation of TNF receptor complex, which consists of several proteins such as RIP1 kinase, Fas associated death domain (FADD) and pro-caspase-8, initiates an inflammatory process. It also activates two diversely opposite intracellular signaling pathways. One of these is the upregulation of anti-apoptotic genes such as c-FLIP and caspase inhibitor IAPs which are required to antagonize the death pathways. This signaling requires TNF induced activation of transcription factor NF-κB. The other signaling pathway, when activated, leads to elaboration of pro-death signaling mediated through FADD. FADD recruits apoptosis initiating protease, caspase-8, which through autoproteolysis is cleaved and activated and activates executor caspases such as caspase-3. TNF receptor complex also activates NADPH oxidase, which in turn increases ROS production. Persistent ROS production causes prolonged activation of JNK which downregulates the E3 ubiquitin ligase, Itch, which in turn degrades c-FLIP [88]. The degradation of c-FLIP facilitates caspase-8 activation leading to activation of cell death signaling. Recently, the role of TGFB-activated kinase 1 (TAK1) has been shown in regulating TNF-induced cell death through the regulation of ROS mediated via c-jun (see also Vol. II, Chapter 25).

7. Diet and Metabolism

Preventive strategies to reduce the damaging effects of ROS in driving multiple diseases by manipulating the human diet are being extensively investigated worldwide. In this regard, high fat, low calcium and low methionine diet, also known as the McDonald's type diet, is considered to induce ROS in human tissues and may therefore be deleterious under certain circumstances. On the other hand, diets low in fat and high in calcium, folate, and vitamin D are considered to be healthy and possibly a rich source of agents that augment antioxidant mechanisms. In addition, dietary components that have antioxidant properties are considered to be beneficial. For example, tea extracts contain a number of polyphenols, which manifest greater antioxidant activity than do most vegetables and fruits. In *in vitro* assessments, these agents proved to be more potent antioxidants than vitamin C or E or carotenoids. Tea, with a history of consumption dating back several millennia, is considered to be the safest beverage after water. Over the past several decades, our laboratory has been exploring the feasibility of exploiting the potent antioxidant properties of tea and its constituents as skin cancer chemopreventive agents. In this regard, the polyphenolic constituents in tea act as antioxidants and modulate carcinogen metabolism, trap reactive electrophilic metabolites, scavenge free radicals, inhibit cell proliferation, arrest the cell cycle, and induce apoptosis [89]. In early studies, we showed that green tea administration reduces cytochrome P450-dependent mono-oxygenase activity in skin [90]. Interestingly, it was also found to be a potent inducer of phase II detoxification enzymes [91]. The mechanism of this activation was shown to involve its interaction with an antioxidant responsive element (ARE) located at the 5' flanking region of phase II drug-metabolizing genes (see Vol. II, Chapter 13 and Vol. III,

Chapter 16). Our studies also showed that green tea inhibits PAH-induced skin tumor initiating activity by decreasing 7,8-dihydroxy-9,10 epoxy-7,8,9,10 tetrahydrobenzo(a)pyrene formation from benzo(a)pyrene, a known human carcinogen. It also reduces UVB-induced skin photocarcinogenesis in multiple murine models, probably through distinct mechanisms which do not involve phase I and phase II drug metabolism. Both black and green teas and their constituents inhibit molecular events involved in the step-wise progression of skin carcinogenesis and inhibit initiation, promotion, and malignant progression. Oral feeding of green tea to mice enhances regression and retards growth of 7,12-dimethylbenz[a]anthracene- or UVB-initiated and 12-O-tetradecanoylphorbol-13-acetate-promoted skin squamous papillogenesis [6]. We also showed that tea polyphenols (polyphenone E) reduces UVB-induced BCC development in a murine model [92].

The treatment for psoriasis involves administration of photosensitizing drugs known as psoralens followed by exposure to UVA radiation (PUVA). PUVA causes structural changes in DNA as a consequence of generating ROS [93]. PUVA treated patients have been found to be at an increased risk for developing SCCs and melanoma which may be attributable to the mutagenic properties of PUVA treatment [93]. Animal studies have shown that orally administered green tea is effective against PUVA-mediated induction of hyperplasia, hyperkeratosis, erythema, and edema. This treatment also reduces the expression of surrogate biomarkers of skin injury and proliferation such as c-fos, p53, and proliferating cell nuclear antigen [94]. Multiple studies conducted in humans have verified the ability of tea constituents to block carcinogenesis-associated surrogate biomarkers. For example, topical treatment with black tea extracts reduces UVB-induced erythema and edema in human skin [22]. In an independent study, it was shown that green tea abrogates UVB-induced proinflammatory signaling. Binding of epigallocatechin-3-gallate with EGFR was proposed as a mechanism for suppressing extracellular signaling leading to inhibition of cell proliferation and cell cycle arrest [95]. Interestingly, UVB-induced tyrosine phosphorylation of EGFR was also inhibited by black tea. The inhibition of c-fos, c-jun, p53, etc. and the blockade of NF-κB and nitric oxide synthase activity following lipopolysaccharide-induced inflammation by epigallocatechin-3-gallate reflect the importance of these targets in chemoprevention by tea polyphenols [95].

Resveratrol, a constituent present in red wine, is another interesting naturally occurring antioxidant. In murine skin, resveratrol exerts anticarcinogenic effects by multiple mechanisms that ultimately lead to cell cycle arrest followed by apoptosis. In this regard, resveratrol-mediated nuclear translocation of ERKs was associated with an increased p53 phosphorylation (Ser15) [96]. Resveratrol was also shown to induce apoptosis and growth arrest in HCT-116 cells [96]. The anti-inflammatory effects of resveratrol corresponded with non-steroidal anti-inflammatory drugs (NSAIDs) in terms of its ability to enhance the expression of antitumorigenic NAG-1 (NSAID drug-activated gene-1), a member of the transforming growth factor-β superfamily regulated by p53. Studies showing that a dominant-negative mutant of JNK1 or disruption of the Jnk1 or Jnk2 gene markedly inhibits resveratrol-induced p53-dependent transcriptional activation and apoptosis, suggesting that its effects are mediated through JNK activation [96]. Chemopeventive effects of resveratrol in the skin have been investigated in depth by Ahmad et al [97]. We also showed that resveratrol induces senecense in skin carcinoma cells [98]. In addition, we found that resveratrol blocks TGFβ2-dependent tumor progression in UVB-irradiated $p53^{+/-}$ mice [99]. Additional agents with similar antioxidant properties and pharmacological actions include curcumin, silymarin, genistein, apigenin, ascorbic acid, and garlic derivatives. These agents have shown variable efficacy as inhibitors of inflammation as well as of tumorigenesis [100]. They may act on numerous targets and block multiple pathways related to cell cycle regulation, MAPKs, transcription factors such as AP-1 and NF-κB and activate p53-dependent and p53-independent proapoptotic pathways. The multiple targets of action of these agents provide a strong rationale to pursue studies to verify their usefulness in diminishing the risk of human skin cancer.

GSTs are ubiquitously present dimeric enzymes that catalyze the conjugation of GSH to a variety of electrophiles such as arene oxides, unsaturated carbonyls, organic halides, and other substrates (Chapter 16 in this Volume). *A number of dietary natural and synthetic chemical agents including some antioxidants and herbal polyphenols, which are known to have potential cancer chemopreventive properties induce one or many of the GST isozymes both in humans and experimental animals.* Besides being important in metabolic disposition of various xenobiotic chemical compounds including drugs, their levels and activities have been associated with susceptibility to various diseases including cancers. In skin, GSTM1 and GSTT1 genotypes are associated with an increased susceptibility to BCCs and GSTT1 null phenotype was found prevalent in a subgroup of BCC patients who developed multiple clusters of primary tumors [101]. Interestingly, pi class gene product has been linked to JNK inhibition suggesting a role of GSTs in modulating cell signaling [102].

Oxidative stress acts through phospholipase A2-mediated release of membrane-bound AA, which is metabolized to various oxidative products by multiple enzymes including COX and lipoxygenases (LOX). Prostaglandins are produced by COX enzymes whereas hydroxyeicosatetraenoic acids are produced by LOX. These products are important modulators of various physiological responses [103]. In murine models of skin carcinogenesis, their tumor promoting and clastogenic properties have been documented. UVB irradiation induces cutaneous expression of COX. Of the two isoforms of COX that have been cloned and sequenced, COX-1 represents a housekeeping isoform constitutively expressed in most tissues including skin, whereas COX-2 is inducible. Proinflammatory agents and mitogens mediate their effects partly by augmenting the expression of COX-2. The etiologic regulation of COX-2 in skin is evidenced by its upregulation by UVB which is maintained throughout the progression of UVB induced solar keratosis to carcinoma development both in human skin and experimental animals. The effects of its specific and non-specific inhibition of UVB-induced cutaneous neoplasia implicate COX in the pathogenesis of skin cancer [104]. We and others have demonstrated that *COX are important targets for skin cancer chemoprevention* [105]. In this regard, inhibitors of COX such as celecoxib, sulindac, nimesulide, etc have been shown to block both BCCs and SCCs in relevant murine models of skin carcinogenesis [106]. We have also shown that some of these inhibitors diminish BCC development in humans afflicted with basal cell nevus syndrome (BCNS). However, these agents remain much less effective against BCCs than against SCCs [107]. Consistent with these observations, we noted differential expression of COX-2 in the two tumor types. In BCCs COX-2 expression is restricted to tumor stroma whereas in SCCs high COX-2 expression is observed both in tumor and stromal cells [108].

LOX catalyze oxidative metabolism of polyunsaturated fatty acids by the insertion of an oxygen molecule, a reaction which is both regio- and stereo-specific. This leads to generation of 5S-, 8S-, 12S-, 12R, or 15S-hydroperoxyoctadecadienoic acids [103]. The isozymes of LOX that produce these regio- and stereo-specific products are designated as e12S-LOX,

12R-LOX, mouse 8S-LOX and its human orthologue 15S-LOX-2, and eLOX-3. These enzymes are preferentially expressed in both murine and human epidermis [109]. While the isozyme, e12S-LOX is detectable in all cell layers of murine epidermis, other LOX isoforms are mainly detectable in the suprabasal layers. Murine papillomas and SCCs both overexpress the LOX isoforms 8S- and p12S-LOX, which lead to the accumulation of the corresponding metabolites 8S- and 12S-HETE and induce chromosomal damage in primary basal murine keratinocytes. The relatively high levels of these metabolites detectable in tumors lead to DNA *etheno* adduct formation and thereby participate in the generation of endogenous mutagens [110]. To support this thesis, nordihydroguaretic acid, a potent inhibitor of these enzymes, suppresses skin tumor induction in murine models. In addition, the expression level of e12S-LOX can be correlated with skin tumor response in transgenic mouse lines manifesting differential expression of this enzyme. Consistently, low transgene expression is associated with decreased skin tumor response whereas high expressers exhibit greater tumor burden. In contrast, gain-of-function studies with 8S-LOX that generate 8-HETE in normal and tumorigenic keratinocytes result in differentiation and cell cycle arrest and tumor reduction [111].

Conclusions

Skin serves as an important interface between the environment and other body tissues. It provides a protective envelope. However, it remains a major target for environmental toxic agents including ultraviolet radiation and chemicals. Exposure to these agents may alter the structure and function of cutaneous components. The majority of environmental pollutants are either themselves oxidants, tamper down the antioxidant armory, or catalyze the production of ROS through redox reactions. In addition, humans and animals have enzymes which produce ROS as a consequence of the physiological responses that combat invading organisms. In the course of the latter, excessive production of ROS may damage normal tissue. Besides directly injuring tissues through oxidative damage, ROS act by triggering multiple signaling pathways that ultimately lead to proliferation and/or death signals. Many of these responses are involved in the pathogenesis of environment-related cutaneous disorders. Therefore, *understanding of the oxidative stress related pathways involved in the pathogenesis and progression of multiple cutaneous conditions may be important for developing therapeutic and preventive approaches for their management.* In this regard antioxidants have been touted as important protective chemical agents. Their efficacy has mainly been confirmed in cell culture systems and in experimental animal models. These agents are currently used in a variety of cosmetic products. However, it remains to be defined whether these antioxidants protect constituents in cosmetic products from aerial oxidation or also serve to protect skin against environmental toxicants/carcinogen-induced damage.

This review implicates ROS and other oxidant clastogenic and mitogenic moieties in the progression of various cutaneous disorders. The mechanisms by which these reactive species act are also becoming clearer. The molecular signatures unique to oxidative stress mediated regulation, if determined, may be helpful in teasing out the progression of various diseases and may facilitate their effective interception and management.

Acknowledgments

Grant Support from the following awards: P30AR050948, R01 ES015323, R21ES017494, N01-CN-43300.

Abbreviations

AA, arachidonic acid; AP-1, activator protein 1; BCC, basal cell carcinoma; COX, cyclooxygenase; ERK, extracellular signal-regulated kinase; GSH, glutathione; GST, glutathione S-transferase; JNK, c-Jun N-terminal kinase; LOX, lipoxygenase; MAPK, mitogen-activated protein kinase; MMP, matrix metalloprotease; $^1O_2$ singlet oxygen; O^-_2, superoxide anion; O_2, molecular oxygen; ODC, ornithine decarboxylase; OH^-, hydroxyl radical; PUVA, psoralens plus UVA; RNS, reactive nitrogen species; ROS, reactive oxygen species; SCC, squamous cell carcinoma; SOD, superoxide dismutase.

References:

[1]   Bergstresser PR, Costner M. *Anatamy and physiology*. In:Bolognia JL, Jorizzo JL, Rapini RP, eds. Dermatology.2nd ed. Philadelphia, PA: Elsevier, 2008.

[2]   Menon GK, Kligman A, Barrier functions of human skin: A holistic view. Skin Parmacol Physiol 2009;22:178-189.

[3]   Miller J, Gallo RL, Vitamin D and innate immunity. DermatolTher. 2010;23(1):13-22.

[4]   Thiele JJ, Weber SU, Packer L, Sebaceous gland secretion is a major physiologic route of vitamin E delivery to skin. J Invest Dermatol1999; 113(6):1006-10.

[5]   Sander CS, Chang H, Hamm F, Elsner P, Thiele JJ, Role of oxidative stress and the antioxidant network in cutaneous carcinogenesis. Int J Dermatol 2004;43:326–335.

[6]   Bickers DR, Athar M, Oxidative stress in the pathogenesis of skin disease. J Invest Dermatol 2006;126:2565-75.

[7]   Serri F, Bartoli GM, Seccia A, et al. Age-related mitochondrial lipoperoxidation in human skin. J Invest Dermaol 1979; 73:123-125.

[8]   Lopez-Torres M, Shindo Y, Packer L, Effect of age on antioxidants and molecular markers of oxidative damage in murine epidermis and dermis. J Invest Dermatol 1994; 102:476-480.

[9]   Heck DE, Laskin DL, Gardner CR, et al., Epidermal growth factor suppresses nitric oxide and hydrogen peroxide production by keratinocytes. Potential role for nitric oxide in the regulation of wound healing. J Biol Chem 1992;267:21277-80.

[10]   Baudouin JE, Tachon P, Constitutive nitric oxide synthase is present in normal human keratinocytes. J Invest Dermatol 1996; 106:428-31.

[11]   Ahmad R, Rasheed Z, Ahsan H, Biochemical and cellular toxicology of peroxynitrite: implications in cell death and autoimmune phenomenon. IImmunopharma-colImmunotoxicol. 2009; 31(3):388-96.

[12] Lerner LH, Qureshi AA, Reddy BV, Lerner EA, Nitric oxide synthase in toxic epidermal necrolysis and Stevens-Johnson syndrome. J Invest Dermatol 2000, 114; 196-199.

[13] Athar M, Oxidative stress and experimental carcinogenesis. Indian J Exp Biol 2002; 40:656-667.

[14] Ryter SW, Tyrrell RM, The heme synthesis and degradation pathways: role in oxidant sensitivity. Heme oxygenase has both pro-and antioxidant properties. Free Radic Biol Med 2000; 28:289-309.

[15] Baron JM, Wiederholt T, Heise R, Expression and function of cytochrome p450-dependent enzymes in human skin cells. Curr Med Chem 2008; 15:2258-64.

[16] Connor MJ, Wheeler LA, Depletion of cutaneous glutathione by ultraviolet radiation. Photochem Photobiol 1987; 46:239-45.

[17] Long DJ II, Waikel RL, Wang XJ, et al., NAD(P)H:quinineoxidoreductase 1 deficiency and increased susceptibility to 7,12-dimethylbenz[a]-anthracene-induced carcinogenesis in mouse skin. J Natl Cancer Inst 2001; 93;1166-70.

[18] Dhar A, Young MR, Colburn NH, CuZnSOD deficiency leads to persistent and widespread oxidative damage and hepatocarcinogenesis later in life. Mol Cell Biochem 2002; 1234-235:185-93.

[19] Reelfs O, Tyrrell RM, Pourzand C, Ultraviolet A radiation-induced immediate iron release is a key modulation of the activation of NFkB in human skin fibroblasts. J Invest Dermatol 2004;122:1440-1447.

[20] Kim AL, Labasi JM, Zhu Y, et al., Role of p38 MAPK in UVB-induced inflammatory responses in the skin of SKH-1 hairless mice. J Invest Dermatol 2005; 124:1318-25.

[21] Shapira N. Nutritional approach to sun protection: a suggested complement to external strategies. Nutr Rev 2010; 68:75-86.

[22] Bickers DR, Athar M, Novel approaches to chemoprevention of skin cancer. J Dermatol 2000, 27:691-95.

[23] Lee JL, Mukhtar H, Bickers DR, et al., Cyclooxygenases in the skin: pharmacological and toxicological implications. Toxicol Appl Pharmacol 2003; 192:294-306.

[24] Haralampus-Grynaviski N, ransom C, Ye T, et al., Photogeneration and quenching of reactive oxygen species by urocanic acid. J Am Chem Soc 2002; 124:3461-3468.

[25] Hanson K Hanson KM, Simon JD, Epidermal trans-urocanicacidand the UVA-induced photoaging of skin. PrcNatlAcadSci USA 1998; 95:10576-78.

[26] Wiaschek M, Wenk J, Brenneisen P, et al., Singlet oxygen is an early intermediate in cytokine-dependent ultraviolet-A induction of interstitial collagenase in human dermal fibroblasts in vitro. FEBS Lett 1997; 413:239-42.

[27] Kim ST, Li YF, Sancar A, The third chromoophore of DNA photolyase: Trp-277 of Escherichia coli DNA photolyase repairs thymine dimmers by direct electron transfer. Proc Natl Acad Sci USA 1992; 89:900-904.

[28] Amstad P, Peskin A, Shah G, et al. The balance between Cu, Zn-superoxide dismutase and catalase affects the sensitivity of mouse epidermal cells to oxidative stress. Biochemistry 1991; 30:9305-9313.

[29] Briganti S, Picardo M. Antioxidant activity, lipid peroxidation and skin diseases. What's new? J Eur Acad Dermatol Venereol 2003; 17:663-669.

[30] Wu G, Fang YZ, Yang S, et al., Glutathione metabolism and its implications for health. J Nutr 2004; 134:489-92.

[31] Slaga TJ, Multistage skin carcinogenesis: a useful model for the study of the chemoprevention of cancer. Acta Pharmacol Toxicol 1984; 55:107-24.

[32] Curtin GM, Hanausek M, Walaszek Z, et al. Short-term in vitro and in vivo analyses for assessing the tumor promoting potentials of cigarette smoke condensates. Toxicol Sci 2004; 81:14-25.

[33] Descargues P, Sil AK, Karin M, IKKalpha, a critical regulator of epidermal differentiation and a suppressor of skin cancer. EMBO J 2008; 27:2639-47.

[34] Sedelnikova OA, Redon CE, Dickey JS, Role of oxidatively induced DNA lesions in human pathogenesis. Mutat Res 2010; 704:152-159.

[35] Nishigori C, Hattori Y, Toyokuni S, Role of reactive oxygen species in skin carcinogenesis. Antioxid Redox Signal 2004; 6:561-570.

[36] O'Donovan P, Perrett CM, Zhang X, et al., Azathioprine and UVA light generate mutagenic oxidative DNA damage. Science 2005; 309:1871-1874.

[37] Stern RS, Lunder EJ, Risk of squamous cell carcinoma and methoxsalen (psoralen) and UVA radiation (PUVA). A meta-analysis. Arch Dermatol 1998; 134:1582-85.

[38] Parrish JA, Immunosuppression, skin cancer, and ultraviolet A radiation. N Engl J Med 2005; 353:2712-2713.

[39] Rodust PM, Stockfleth E, Ulrich C, et al., UV-induced squamous cell carcinoma - a role for antiapoptotic signaling pathways. Br J Dermatol 2009; 161:107-15.

[40] Liu B, Chen Y, St. Clair DK, ROS and p53: A versatile partnership. Free Radic Biol Med 2008; 44:1529-1535.

[41] Mikkelsen RB, Wardman P, Biological chemistry of reactive oxygen and nitrogen and radiation-induced signal transduction mechanisms. Oncogene 2003; 22:5734-54.

[42] Holley AK, Dhar SK, St Clair DK, Manganese superoxide dismutase versus p53: the mitochondrial center. Ann NY Acad Sci 2010; 1201:72-78.

[43] Pegg AE, Polyamine metabolism and its importance in neoplastic growth and a target for chemotherapy. Cancer Res 1988; 48:759-74.

[44] Black HS, ROS: a step closer to elucidating their role in the etiology of light-induced skin disorders. J Invest Dermatol 2004; 122:13-15.

[45] Janssen YM, Van Houten B, Borm PJ, et al., Cell and tissue responses to oxidative damage. Lab Invest 1993; 69:261-274.

[46] Tang X, Kim AL, Feith DJ, Ornithine decarboxylase is a target for chemoprevention of basal and squamous cell carcinomas in Ptch1+/- mice. J Clin Invest 2004; 113:867-75.

[47] Pasparakis M, Regulation of tissue homeostasis by NF-kappaB signaling: implications for inflammatory diseases. Nat Rev Immunol 2009; 9:778-88.

[48] Kumar AP, Mar PK, Zhao B, Regulation of rat ornithine decarboxylase promoter activity by binding of transcription factor Sp1. J Biol Chem 1995; 270:4341-8.

[49] Lu YP, Lou YR, Yen P, et al., Enhanced skin carcinogenesis in transgenic mice with high expression of glutathione peroxidase or both glutathione peroxidase and superoxide dismutase. Cancer Res 1997; 57:1468-74.

[50] Dalton TP, Chen Y, Schneider SN, et al., Genetically altered mice to evaluate glutathione homeostasis in health and disease. Free Radic Biol Med 2004; 37:1511-1526.

[51] Iskander K, Gaikwad A, Paquet M, et al. Lower induction of p53 and decreased apoptosis in NQO1-null mice lead to increased sensitivity to chemical-induced skin carcinogenesis. Cancer Res 2005; 65:2054-2058.

[52] Iskander K, Paquet M, Brayton C, Jaiswal AK, Deficiency of NRH:quinineoxidoreductase 2 increases susceptibility to 7,12-dimethylbenz(a) anthracene and benzo(a)pyrene-induced skin carcinogenesis. Cancer Res, 2004; 64:5925-5928.

[53] Elchuri S, Oberly TD, Qi W et al., CuZnSOD deficiency leads to persistent and widespread oxidative damage and hepatocarcinogenesis later in life. Oncogene, 2004; 24:367-380.

[54] St Clair D, Zhao Y, Chaiswing L, et al., Modulation of skin tumorigenesis by SOD. Biomed Pharmacother, 2005; 59:209-214.

[55] Athar M, Lloyd JR, Bickers DR, et al., Malignant conversion of UV radiation and chemically induced mouse skin benign tumors by free-radical –generating compounds. Carcinogenesis 1989; 10:1841-45.

[56] Athar M, Agarwal R, Wang ZY, et al., All-trans retinoic acid protects against conversion of chemically induced and ultraviolet B radiation-induced skin papillomas to carcinomas. Carcinogenesis 1991; 2325-9.

[57] Athar M, Mukhtar H, Bickers DR, et al., Evidence for the metabolism of tumor promoter organic hydroperoxides into free radicals by human carcinoma skin keratinocytes: an ESR-spin trapping study. Carcinogenesis 1989c; 10:1499-1503.

[58] Rotstein JB, Slaga TJ, Effect of exogenous glutathione on tumor progression in the murine skin multistage carcinogenesis model. Carcinogenesis 1988; 9:1547-51.

[59] Sander CS, Hamm F, Eisner P, et al., Oxidative stress in malignant melanoma and non-melanoma skin cancer. Br J Dermatol 2003; 148:913-22.

[60] Cannito S, Novo E, di Bonzo LV, et al., Epithelial-mesenchymal transition: from molecular mechanisms, redox regulation to implications in human health and disease. Antioxid Redox Signal, 2010; 12:1383-1430.

[61] Zhou Q, Mrowietz U, Rostami-Yazdi M, Oxidative stress in the pathogenesis of psoriasis. Free Radical Biology Med 2009; 47:891-905.

[62] Zhou Z, Li CY, Li K, et al., Decreased methionine sulphoxidereductase A expression renders melanocytes more sensitive to oxidative stress: a possible cause for melanocyte loss in vitiligo. British Journal of Dermatology 2009; 161:504-509.

[63] Dell'Anna ML, Mastrofrancesco A, Sala R et al., Antioxidants and narrow band-UVB in the treatment of vitiligo: a double-blind placebo controlled trial. Clin Exp Dermatol 2007; 32:631-6.

[64] Kidd P. Th1/Th2 balance: the hypothesis, its limitations, and implications for health and disease. Altern Med Rev 2003; 8:223-246.

[65] Kaur S, Zilmer M, Eisen M, et al., Patients with allergic and irritant contact dermatitis are characterized by striking change of iron and oxidized glutathione status in nonlesional area of the skin. J Invest Dermatol 2001; 116:886-890.

[66] Athar M, Hasan SK, Srivastava RC, et al., Evidence for the involvement of hydroxyl radicals in nickel mediated enhancement of lipid peroxidation: implications for nickel carcinogenesis. Biochem Biophys Res Commun 1987; 147:1276-1281.

[67] Kovacic P, Somanathan R, Dermal toxicity and environmental contamination: electron transfer, reactive oxygen species, oxidative stress, cell signaling, and protection by antioxidants. Rev Environ ContamToxicol 2010; 203:119-38.

[68] Anderson C, Hehr A, Robbins R, et al., Metabolic requirements for induction of contact hypersensitivity to immunotoxicpolyaromatic hydrocarbons. J Immunol 1995; 155:3530-7.

[69] Kawakubo Y, Nakamori M, Schopf E, et al., Acetylator phenotype in patients with a phenylenediamine allergy. Dermatology 1997; 195:43-45.

[70] Del Prete A, Zaccagnino P, Di Pola M, Role of mitochondria and reactive oxygen species in dendritic cell differentiation and functions. Free Radic Biol Med 2008; 44:1443-51.

[71] Matos TJ, Duarte CB, Goncalo M, Role of oxidative stress in ERK and p38 MAPK activation induced by the chemical sensitizer DNFB in a fetal skin dendritic cell line. Immunol Cell Biol 2005; 83:607-614.

[72] Meffert H, Diezel W, Sonnichsen N, Stable lipid peroxidation products in human skin: detection ultraviolet light-induced increase, pathogenic importance. Experientia 1976; 32:1397-98.

[73] Okayama Y, Oxidative stress in allergic and inflammatory skin diseases. Curr Drug Targets Inflamm Allergy 2005; 4:517-19.

[74] Wlaschek M, Scharffetter-Kochanek K, Oxidative stress in chronic venous leg ulcers. Wound Repair Regen 2005; 13:452-61.

[75] Allhorn M, Lundqvist K, Schmidtchen A, et al. Heme-scavenging role of alpha: microglobulin in chronic users. J Invest Dermatol 2003; 121:640-646.

[76] Karatepe O, Unal O, Ugurlucan M, et al., The impact of valvular oxidative stress on the development of venous stasis ulcer valvular oxidative stress and venous ulcers. Angiology 2010; 61:283-8.

[77] Athar M, Mukhtar H, Elmets CA, et al., In situ evidence for the involvement of superoxide anions in cutaneous porphyrin photosensitization. Biochem Biophys Res Commun 1988; 151:1054-1059.

[78] Athar M, Elmets CA, Bickers DR, et al., A novel mechanism for the generation of superoxide anions in hematoporphyrin derivative-mediated cutaneous photo-sensitization. Activation of the xanthine oxidase pathway. J Clin Invest 1989; 83:1137-43.

[79] Onoue S, Tsuda Y, Analytical studies on the prediction of photosensitive/phototoxic potential of pharmaceutical substances. Pharm Res 2006; 23:156-64.

[80] Trenam CW, Blake DR, Morris CJ, Skin inflammation: reactive oxygen species and the role of iron. J Invest Dermatol 1992; 99:675-82.

[81] Pastore S, Mascia F, Mariotti F, et al., ERK1/2 regulates epidermal chemokine expression and skin inflammation. J Immunol 2005; 174:5047-56.

[82] Klaunig JE, Kamendulis LM, Hocevar BA. Oxidative stress and oxidative damage in carcinogenesis. Toxicol Pathol 2010; 38:96-109.

[83] Maziere C, Floret S, Santus R, et al. Impairment of the EGF signaling pathway by the oxidative stress generated with UVA. Free Radic Biol Med 2003; 34:629-636.

[84] Kim AL, Labasi JM, Zhu Y, Role of p38 MAPK in UVB-induced inflammatory responses in the skin of SKH-1 hairless mice. J Invest Dermatol 2005; 124:1318-25.

[85] Junttila MR, Li SP, Westermarck J, Phosphatase-mediated crosstalk between MAPK signaling pathways in the regulation of cell survival. FASEB J 2008; 22:954-65.

[86] Bachelor MA, Bowden GT, UVA-mediated activation of signaling pathways involved in skin tumor promotion and progression. Semin Cancer Biol 2004; 14:131-38.

[87] Bode AM, Dong Z, Mitogen-activated protein kinase activation in UV-induced signal transduction. Sci STKE 2003; 167:1-15.

[88] Croft M. The role of TNF superfamily members in T-cell function and diseases. Nat Rev Immunol 2009; 9:271-85.

[89] Yang CS, Wang X, Lu G, et al., Cancer prevention by tea: animal studies, molecular mechanisms and human relevance. Nat Rev Cancer 2009; 9:429-439.

[90] Khan WA, Wang ZY, Athar M, et al., Inhibition of the skin tumorigenicity of (+/-)-7 beta, 8 alpha-dihydroxy-9 alpha, 10 alpha-epoxy-7,8,9,10-tetrahydrobenzo[a]pyrene by tannic acid, green tea polyphenols and quercetin in Sencar mice. Cancer Lett 1988; 42:7-12.

[91] Na HK, Surh YJ, Modulation of Nrf2-mediated antioxidant and detoxifying enzyme induction bythe green tea polyphenol EGCG. Food ChemToxicol 2008; 46:1271-8.

[92] Hebert JL, Khugyani F, Athar M, et al., Chemoprevention of basal cell carcinomas in the ptc1+/- mouse—green and black tea. Skin Pharmacol Appl Skin Physiol 2001; 14:358-62.

[93] Filipe J, Emerit I, AlaouiYoussefi A, et al., Oxyradical-mediated clastogenic plasma factors in psoriasis: increase in clastogenic activity after PUVA. Photocehm Photobiol 1997; 66:497-501.

[94] Zhao JF, Zhang YJ, Jin XH, et al., Green tea protects against psoralen plus ultraviolet A-induced photochemical damage to skin. J Invest Dermatol 1999; 113:1070-75.

[95] Bowden GT. Prevention of non-melanoma skin cancer by targeting ultraviolet-B-light signaling. Nat Rev Cancer 2004; 4:23-35.

[96] Bode AM, Dong Z, Targeting signal transduction pathways by chemopreventive agents. Mutat Res 2004; 555:33-51.

[97] Ahmad N, Adhami VM, Afaq F, et al. Resveratrol causes WAF-1/p21-mediated G1-phase arrest of cell cycle and induction of apoptosis in human epidermoid carcinoma A431. Cells 2001; 7:1466-73.

[98] Kim AL, Zhu Y, Zhu H. Resveratrol inhibits proliferation of human epidermoid carcinoma A431 cells by modulating MEK1 and AP-1 signalling pathways. Exp Dermatol 2006; 15:538-46.

[99] Kim KH, Back JH, Zhu Y, et al., Resveratrol targets transforming growth factor-beta2 signaling to block UV-induced tumor progression. J Invest Dermatol 2010; [Epub ahead of print].

[100] F' Guyer S, Afaq F, Mukhtar H. Photochemoprevention of skin cancer by botanical agents. Photodermatol Photoimmunol Photomed 2003; 19:56-72.

[101] Ramachandran S, Fryer AA, Smith AG et al., Basal cell carcinomas: association of alleli variants with a high-risk subgroup of patients with the multiple presentation phenotype. Pharmacogenetics 2001: 11:247-54.

[102] Kim SG, Lee SJ, P13K, RSK, and mTOR signal networks for the GST gene regulation. Toxicol Sci 2007; 96:206-13.

[103] Steele VE, Hawk ET, Viner JL, et al., Mechanisms and applications of non-steroidal anti-inflammatory drugs in the chemoprevention of cancer. Mutat Res 2003; 523-524:137-144.

[104] Lee JL, Mukhtar H, Bickers DR, et al., Cyclooxygenases in the skin: pharmacological and toxicological implications. Toxicol Appl Pharmacol 2003; 192:294-306.

[105] An KP, Athar M, Tang X, Cyclooxygenase-2 expression in murine and human nonmelanoma skin cancers: implications for therapeutic approaches. Photochem Photobiol 2002; 76:73-80.

[106] Tang X, Kim AL, Kopelovich L, et al., Cyclooxygenase-2 inhibitor nimesulide blocks ultraviolet B-induced photocarcinogenesis in SKH-1 hairless mice. Photochem Photobiol 2008; 84: 522-7.

[107] Tang JY, Aszterbaum M, Athar M, et al., Basal cell carcinoma chemoprevention with nonsteroidal anti-inflammatory drugs in genetically predisposed PTCH1+/- humans and mice. Cancer Prev Res 2010; 3:25-34

[108] Athar M, An KP, Morel KD, et al., Ultraviolet B (UVB)-induced cox-2 expression in murine skin: an immunohistochemical study. Biochem Biophys Res Commun 2001; 280:1042-7.

[109] Muller K, Siebert M, Heidt M, et al., Modulation of epidermal tumor development caused by targeted overexpression of epidermis-type 12S-lipoxygenase. Cancer Res 2002; 6:229-235.

[110] Nair U, Bartsch H, Nair J, Lipid peroxidation-induced DNA damage in cancer-prone inflammatory diseases: a review of published adduct types and levels in humans. Free Radic Biol Med 2007; 43:1109-20.

[111] Schweiger D, Furstenberger G, Krieg P, Inducible expression of 15-lipoxygenase-2 and 8-lipoxygenase inhibits cell growth via common signaling pathways. J Lipid Res 2007; 48:553-64.

In: Principles of Free Radical Biomedicine, Volume III
Editors: K. Pantopoulos and H. M. Schipper

ISBN 978-1-61324-184-4
©2012 Nova SciencePublishers, Inc.

Chapter 13

Oxidative Stress in Male Reproduction

Rakesh K. Sharma, Aaron Thompson,
*Shiva Kothari and Ashok Agarwal**

Center for Reproductive Medicine, Glickman Urological and Kidney Institute and
Obstetrics and Gynecology and Women's Health Institute,
Cleveland Clinic, Cleveland, Ohio, U.S.A.

1. Introduction

Reactive oxygen species (ROS) have been implicated in the etiopathogenesis of various medical conditions affecting male reproduction such as varicocele, idiopathic infertility, leukocytospermia, and spinal cord injury [1-6]. In addition, a variety of environmental factors including smoking, pollution, and obesity are associated with increased levels of ROS [7]. Spermatozoa undergo one of the most complex maturation processes of any cell prior to achieving competent fertilization abilities. Epididymal priming, post-ejaculatory maturation and sperm-oocyte interactions are all redox-regulated processes.

At physiological concentrations, ROS may enhance and induce the proper activation of key reproductive processes such as capacitation, hyperactivation etc. [5, 8]. Oxidative stress is a consequence of an imbalance between the production of ROS and the body's antioxidant defense mechanisms and has been implicated in the pathogenesis of many other human diseases [1-5, 7, 9, 10] (see also Chapters 1-12 of this Volume). These include atherosclerosis, cancer, diabetes, liver damage, rheumatoid arthritis, cataracts, AIDS, inflammatory bowel disease, central nervous system disorders (Parkinson's disease, motor neuron disease) and conditions associated with premature birth. Recent reports indicate that DNA damage in the spermatozoa of ageing males is associatedwith the appearance of complex polygenic neurological conditionsin the progeny such as epilepsy, schizophrenia, autism and bipolar disease. In light of such considerations, DNA damage in the germline should be regarded as a potential risk factor for the developmentof abnormal human embryos.

---

*Tel: 216-444-9485, Fax: 216-445-6049, E-mail: agarwaa@ccf.org

In this Chapter we address the issue of how DNA damage arises and how such damage should be managed clinically.

The goal of this article is to provide a brief overview of the pathophysiology of ROS generation, highlight its physiological and pathological effects on the male reproductive system, enumerate its importance in the field of assisted reproductive technology, and, finally, propose possible ways of preventing and minimizing oxidative stress with the goal of achieving positive results in infertile couples with male factor infertility.

2. Free Radicals and ROS

Free radicals are a group of highly reactive chemical molecules that have one or more unpaired electrons and that can oxidatively modify biomolecules that they encounter. Generally, free radicals attack the nearest stable molecule, "stealing" its electron. When the "attacked" molecule loses its electron, it often becomes a free radical itself, beginning a chain reaction. Once the process is started, it can cascade and ultimately lead to the disruption of living cells. ROS represent a broad category of molecules comprised of both radical and non-radical derivatives of oxygen, nitrogen and other elements (see Vol. I, Chapters 2 and 3). Some examples of ROS are: superoxide anion ($O_2^{\bullet}$-), hydrogen peroxide (H_2O_2) and hydroxyl radical ($OH^{\bullet}$). Nitric oxide ($NO^{\bullet}$), nitric dioxide ($NO_2^{\bullet}$), and peroxynitrite ($ONOO^-$) are the common reactive nitrogen species (RNS) [3, 4, 9].

3. Physiological versus Pathological ROS

Small amounts of ROS are necessary for spermatozoa to acquire fertilizing capabilities. Low levels of ROS have been shown to be essential for stabilization of the mitochondrial capsule in the mid-piece, acrosome reaction, hyperactivation, motility, oocyte fusion and capacitation [8]. Capacitation has been shown to occur in the female genital tract, a process carried out to prepare the spermatozoa for interaction with the oocyte. During this process, the levels of intracellular calcium, ROS, and tyrosine kinase all increase, leading to an increase in cyclic adenosine monophosphate (cAMP). This increase in cAMP facilitates hyperactivation of spermatozoa, a condition in which they are highly motile. However, only capacitated sperm exhibit hyperactivated motility and undergo a physiological acrosome reaction, thereby acquiring the ability to fertilize. Low concentrations of H_2O_2 have been shown to stimulate sperm capacitation, hyperactivation, acrosome reaction, and oocyte fusion. Other reactive species such as nitric oxide and the superoxide anion have also been shown to promote capacitation and the acrosome reaction [11]. Furthermore, *ROS play an important physiological role, modulating gene and protein activities vital for sperm proliferation, differentiation, and fertilizing function.* In the semen of fertile men, the amount of ROS generation is controlled by seminal antioxidants. *The pathogenic effects of ROS occur when they are produced in excess of the antioxidant capabilities of the male reproductive tract or seminal plasma. Between 30% and 80% of infertile men exhibit elevated ROS levels in their semen [1-6, 9, 12]. Pathological levels can damage DNA and adversely affect fertilizing potential and pregnancy rates (Figure 1).*

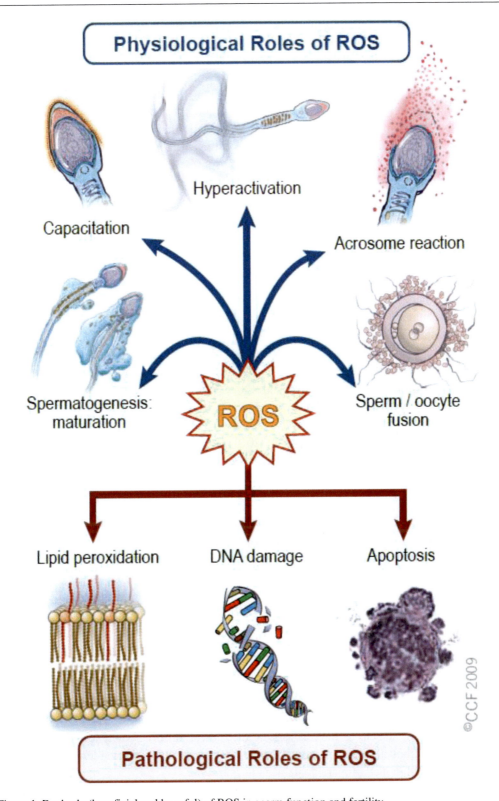

Figure 1. Dual role (beneficial and harmful) of ROS in sperm function and fertility.

4. Endogenous Sources of ROS – Spermatozoa and Leukocytes

ROS production in the male reproductive tract stems from two main sources, leukocytes (mainly granulocytes) and abnormal immature spermatozoa [13-15]. Superoxide is the primary free radical produced, whether by a nicotinamide adenine dinucleotide phosphate reduced NAD(P)H oxidase in the plasma membrane of sperm or leukocytes or by the leakage of electrons from the mitochondrial electron transport chain. The NAD(P)H oxidase of spermatozoa and neutrophils bear several similarities and both result in the extracellular production of ROS.

4.1. Spermatozoa

In spermatozoa, the mitochondria contribute significantly to intracellular ROS production [16]. A nitric oxide synthase (NOS) also exists in the sperm plasma membrane, but its effects are less pronounced. For some time, intracellular superoxide produced during oxidative phosphorylation was the only known source of ROS in spermatozoa.

Production via this mechanism is not unique to spermatozoa, but its effects are more salient because spermatozoa lack the antioxidants and repair mechanisms that are present in somatic cells. The mythic extracellular source of superoxide, long speculated to exist, was only recently identified in immature spermatozoa by polymerase chain reaction (PCR) analysis [17, 18]. This membrane bound enzyme bears similarities to that of leukocytes, except that the responsible enzyme is an NAD(P)H oxidase capable of using either NADH or NADPH as electron donors for the monovalent reduction of molecular oxygen to superoxide; it is estimated to produce ~1000 times less ROS than leukocyte NAD(P)H oxidases [19].

4.2. Leukocytes

Peroxidase-positive leukocytes are major contributors of ROS. In the seminal plasma, 50 to 60 percent of leukocytes are polymorphonuclear (PMN) cells while 40 to 50 percent of leukocytes are macrophages [20], both of which are capable of generating ROS. Leukocytes, which originate from the prostate and seminal vesicles, produce almost three orders of magnitude more ROS than immature spermatozoa and, as such, are the primary producers of ROS in semen.

In fact, leukocytes may even stimulate the production of ROS by sperm [21], thus having both a direct and indirect effect on ROS levels. Activation of ROS-producing leukocytes is the major marker of ROS generation rather than leukocyte concentration *per se*. Leukocytospermia is defined by the World Health Organization (WHO) as $\geq 1x10^6$ white blood cells / mL of semen, or the newly suggested lower cut off of $>0.2 \times 10^6$ white blood cells / mL as the clinicallyrelevant value in the production of ROS. During leukocytospermia, high levels of ROS induce irreparable damage to sperm.

During inflammation and infection, leukocytes produce an oxidative burst that releases various ROS. Included among the latter is the superoxide anion, the hydroxyl radical, and H_2O_2; ROS are also produced via the NADPH oxidase system in the sperm membrane. This

ROS generation serves as a defense mechanism to combat invading pathogens. Leukocytes can produce ROS directly as described above, or indirectly, through the activation of pro-inflammatory cytokines. In fact, levels of interleukin-8, a stimulator of pro-inflammatory cytokines, were correlated with high levels of ROS [22, 23].

Studies have shown that infertile patients generally have higher concentrations of leukocytes, which are also correlated with higher levels of oxidative stress [24]. *In vivo*, leukocytes do not decrease the fertilizing ability of spermatozoa due to protection by the seminal plasma. However, during preparation for assisted reproductive techniques (ART), sperm are washed free of the seminal plasma and are therefore susceptible to leukocyte-induced damage [7].

5. Antioxidants

Antioxidant enzymes in seminal plasma include superoxide dismutase (SOD), catalase and glutathione peroxidase / glutathione reductase. Seminal plasma also contains the nonenzymatic antioxidants, vitamin C and E, urate, ascorbate, pyruvate, glutathione, albumin, transferrin, ceruloplasmin, L-taurine and L- [3, 12, 25]. The total antioxidant capacity (TAC) of fertile men is generally higher than that of infertile men [26].

Even though there have been over 50 studies in the literature analyzing the therapeutic implications of antioxidants in infertility, no consensus is available concerning their efficacy. This may largely be due to variations in study designs and in the types, combinations and doses and of antioxidants used.

Furthermore, studies have shown that both significantly lower and significantly higher activities of SOD or catalase may decrease sperm counts, once again suggesting a dual role of ROS, either physiological or pathological depending on their concentration [7].

6. Oxidative Stress

Oxidative stress is caused by an imbalance between the production of ROS and the antioxidant capacity [1-3, 5, 6, 9, 12, 22, 27]. Virtually every human ejaculate is contaminated with potential sources of ROS. Sperm are particularly susceptible to oxidative damage due to their low cytoplasmic volume, the main source of antioxidants. Mature spermatozoa have transcriptionally inactive DNA and only minimal repair mechanisms for oxidative damage. ROS can result in chromatin cross-linking, DNA strand breaks, DNA base oxidation, chromosome deletions, dicentrics and sister chromatid exchanges. Oxidative stress has been correlated with high frequencies of single and double DNA strand breaks [27-30]. Such damage is not a cause for concern *in vivo* because the collateral peroxidative damage to the sperm plasma membrane ensures that spermatozoa susceptible to oxidative stress are unable to participate in the fertilization process. *Furthermore, seminal plasma contains high levels of antioxidants necessary to protect the sperm from oxidative damage post-ejaculation.* However, during ART such as intracytoplasmic sperm injection (ICSI), these safeguards are bypassed. Therefore, spermatozoa with DNA fragmentation may have adverse consequences if they are used for ART [31-37].

7. Pathology of Oxidative Stress

Male reproductive health is in a state of decline. In a comparison of fertile men from 1940 and 1990, a meta-analysis showed that sperm concentrations dropped 42% in the 50-year span of the study (113×10^6/mL vs. 66×10^6/mL) [38]. Furthermore, there is an increase in the prevalence of testicular cancer, hypospadias, cryptorchidism and poor semen quality referred to as testicular dysgenesis syndrome. In addition, several reproductive disorders may cause infertility by inducing oxidative stress [7].

7.1. Sperm Morphology

The presence of oxidative stress is often correlated with abnormalities in sperm midpiece, most commonly the existence of excess residual cytoplasm, sometimes known as a cytoplasmic droplet. Normally, during late spermatogenesis (spermiogenesis), a spermatozoon rids itself of excess cytoplasm and organelles to become fully mature. Some spermatozoa fail to rid themselves of excessive cytoplasm and retain this even after ejaculation [6]. The abnormal spermatozoa, by way of increased cytoplasmic organelles, contain more mitochondria and a higher concentration of glucose-6-phosphate dehydrogenase (G6PDH), an enzyme responsible for producing NADPH, which is important in the formation of superoxide at the membrane oxidase. Therefore an increase in NADPH leads to augmented ROS production. In this way, excess residual cytoplasm may lead to oxidative stress.

7.2. Sperm Motility

High levels of ROS are correlated with decreased sperm motility [6]. Two mechanisms have been proposed to explain the negative relationship between sperm motility and ROS levels. One hypothesis is that intracellular H_2O_2 can inhibit the activity of glyceraldehyde-3-phosphate dehydrogenase (GPDH), a glycolytic enzyme. GPDH catalyzes the first energy-producing step of glycolysis. As such, GPDH is necessary to generate the energy required for spermatazoa movement, and if damaged, results in immobilization. According to another hypothesis, H_2O_2 promotes lipid peroxidation that destabilizes the plasma membrane rendering the latter abnormally permeable. Molecules of adenosine triphosphate (ATP) and its precursor adenine may then efflux from the cytoplasm to the extracellular space thereby reducing bioenergy substrates available for cell motility.

7.3. Lipid Peroxidation

The plasma membranes of spermatozoa contain abundant polyunsaturated fatty acids (PUFA). The kinks in the fatty acid chains that make up the inner space of the phospholipid bilayer provide the fluidity necessary for flagellar movement and fusion-related events, but also make the sperm unusually susceptible to lipid peroxidation (LPO) [16]. Whenever levels of oxidative stress in the male germ line are high, the peroxidation of unsaturated fatty acids in the sperm plasma membrane leads to lower fertilization rates [39].

Most somatic cells are more prone to oxidative DNA damage than LPO, but the high stability of sperm DNA along with the elevated PUFA content of the plasma membrane makes LPO more detrimental to sperm function. LPO decreases the number of double bonds in fatty acyl side-chain and thereby impacts the fluidity of the plasma membrane (Vol. I, Chapter 7). Sperm with higher levels of PUFA in the plasma membrane are more susceptible to LPO and exhibit lower motility [16]. The relationship between male infertility and LPO is mediated by the negative effects on sperm motility and fusogenicity of the plasma membrane. A high degree of membrane fluidity—normally provided by PUFA—is necessary for proper sperm-oocyte fusion. Lipid peroxidation decreases the fluidity of the membrane and reduces the fusogenic abilities of spermatozoa by removing double bonds from membrane phospholipids, and either removing, truncating, or degrading the fatty acyl side-chain [11, 40]. Thus, *LPO has a two-fold effect on fertility: it decreases motility, thereby reducing the number of sperm that reach the oocyte, and decreases membrane fluidity necessary for sperm-oocyte fusion.* Malondialdehyde (MDA), a by-product of lipid breakdown can be used as a marker to quantify the degree of pre-existing peroxidative damage in biological membranes. LPO of the flagella decreases their flexibility and movement, thus decreasing sperm motility [40]. LPO also results in membrane permeabilization with loss of high-energy substrates (ATP) required for motility as described above [41]. Decreased motility as a result of LPO will prevent an otherwise capable spermatozoon from reaching the oocyte complex for fertilization [7]. This is one mechanism in which excess ROS may cause male infertility.

8. Sperm DNA Damage

Spermatozoa experience both mitochondrial and nuclear DNA damage as a result of oxidative stress. DNA aberrations include cross-links, deletions, structural chromosome rearrangements, fragmentation, single and double strand breaks, and histone and base modifications.

8.1. Mitochondrial DNA Damage

Sperm have very few mitochondria because of a low cytoplasmic volume, yet they have a high demand for ATP. Mitochondrial DNA (mtDNA) is a circular DNA composed of two non-identical strands. It has 16,569 base pairs and is thus much smaller than the nuclear genome. Spermatozoa are particularly prone to incompetence as a result of mtDNA mutations (see Vol. I, Chapter 1 and Vol. II, Chapter 15). In spermatozoa, mitochondrial DNA accumulates mutations at rates 10- to 100-fold greater than nuclear DNA. There are several factors which render mtDNA particularly vulnerable to mutagenesis: (i) The mtDNA is a naked molecule with no protection from basic histone proteins. (ii) The mitochondrial genome lacks a proofreading mechanism. (iii) MtDNA replicates much more rapidly than nuclear DNA. (iv) MtDNA is almost entirely comprised of vulnerable coding regions. (v) MtDNA is located near the inner mitochondrial membrane, the site of the electron transport chain and ROS production [7, 42]. It is at this site that the first ROS-induced oxidative damage occurs. Recently, high levels of seminal ROS, depletion of seminal antioxidant levels, and an increase in mtDNA mutations were all correlated with infertility. The hypothesis is that mtDNA mutations cause inefficient ATP synthesis and greater leakage of electrons from the ETC [43]. Whether enhanced ROS production is a cause or a consequence of mitochondrial dysfunction is unknown. Mitochondrial and nuclear DNA crosstalk is required for ATP production and the maintenance of cellular homeostasis, pre-requisites for successful fertilization. Mutated mtDNA may cause a deficiency in the respiratory chain complexes, resulting in reduced ATP production and an "energy crisis" within the system. In these spermatozoa there is increased electron leakage and ROS are produced at supra-physiological levels. The vicious cycle of net DNA deletion, reduced ATP production, and elevated ROS production is proposed to initiate the apoptotic cascade. Thus supra-physiological ROS levels are correlated to mitochondrial respiratory failure and DNA damage is observed before there is any other indication of apoptosis.

8.2. Nuclear DNA Damage

The exact mechanisms by which chromatin abnormalities/DNA damage arise in human spermatozoa are not completely understood. Three main theories have been proposed: defective sperm chromatin packaging, abortive apoptosis, and oxidative stress [22, 23, 27, 29, 30, 44]. Deficiencies in recombination may also play a role.

8.3. Sperm Chromatin Packaging

Spermatozoa have uniquely compact, stable DNA. Unlike somatic cells, sperm DNA is bound to small cysteine-rich proteins called protamines. The mild oxidation of protamines in the caudal epididymis induces the formation of disulfide bonds and stabilizes nuclear DNA [45-47]. DNA in mammalian sperm is tightly compacted into linear arrays organized as loop domains. In comparison with other species, human sperm chromatin packaging is exceptionally variable both within and between individuals. This variability is largely attributed to its basic protein component. The retention of 15% histones, which are less basic than protamines, leads to the formation of a less-compact chromatin structure [29, 30]. Moreover, in contrast to the bull, cat, boar, and ram, whose spermatozoa contain only one type of protamine (P1), human and mouse spermatozoa contain a second type of protamine called protamine (P2), which is deficient in cysteine residues. Consequently, the disulfide cross-linking responsible for more stable packaging is diminished in human sperm as compared with species containing P1 alone. *Altered P1/P2 ratios and the absence of P2 are associated with male fertility problems* [48, 49]. Immature spermatozoa show high levels of DNA damage and ROS production and are likely to have alterations in protamination and chromatin packaging. DNA fragmentation is characterized by single and double-strand DNA breaks, which are often detected in the ejaculates of subfertile men. Double-stranded breaks can occur naturally in the male germ line in preparation for recombination and during the process of chromatin packaging. However, these strand breaks are physiological and are normally resolved during spermatogenesis. Aberrant recombination-chromatin packaging is more likely to account for unresolved double-strand breaks in the mature human spermatozoa. In abnormal spermatozoa, sensitivity to DNA damage is higher probably as result of failed chromatin condensation, making the DNA more prone to damage [44]. Several studies have shown that oocytes and early embryos can repair sperm DNA damage. Consequently, the biological effect of abnormal sperm chromatin structure depends on the combined effects of sperm chromatin damage and the capacity of the oocyte to repair it. Any errors that may occur during this post-fertilization period of DNA repair have the potential to create mutations that can affect fetal development and, ultimately, the health of the child.

In general, DNA damage has been shown to decrease semen parameters (motility, viability, etc.) and reduce the success of *in vitro* fertilization (IVF). Yet, spermatozoa with DNA damage do retain some capacity for fertilization. Whereas mtDNA damage may be a significant barrier to fertilization *in vivo*, nuclear DNA mutations are more diagnostically relevant for the outcome of assisted reproduction techniques (ART). Damage to nuclear DNA may have a significantly detrimental effect on both ART outcome and increases the risk of transferring a genetic mutation to the offspring.

8.4. Apoptosis

Apoptosis, a form of genetically determined cell-suicide (Vol. II, Chapters 25 and 26), protects an organism by discarding cells with abnormal function, thereby preventing the spread of aberrant cells [50-52]. Spermatogonia, spermatocytes and spermatids have all been shown to undergo apoptosis [27], suggesting that cell-suicide may be an important regulator of spermatogenesis. Testicular germ cell apoptosis occurs in the testis during spermatogenesis as a result of endonuclease activation. This occurs predominantly in the spermatogonia and dividing cells and generates numerous DNA strand breaks in chromatin. The presence of endogenous nucleic acid nicks in ejaculated spermatozoa is characteristic of programmed cell death as seen in apoptosis of somatic cells. Incomplete endogenous nuclease activity creates and ligates nicks during spermiogenesis. A spermatid that has initiated apoptosis may fail to completely activate its endogenous nuclease activity or default in the ligation of DNA nicks.

Evidence suggests that abortive apoptosis occurs in many males who exhibit poor sperm parameters [53]. In certain males, abortive apoptosis may fail in the total clearance of spermatozoa earmarked for elimination by apoptosis. Therefore, the subsequent population of ejaculated spermatozoa presents an array of anomalies that are representative of the characteristics observed in cells undergoing apoptosis.

The incidence of apoptosis in ejaculated sperm is still debatable. Until recently, the inability of a mature spermatozoon to synthesize new proteins was believed to make it impossible for such cells to respond to any of the signals that lead to the programmed death cascade.

However, a number of recent observations have raised the possibility that abortive apoptosis may contribute to DNA damage in human spermatozoa: 1) the detection of Fas on ejaculated spermatozoa [52], 2) the high proportion of spermatozoa with potentially apoptotic mitochondria, and 3) the finding that potential mediators of apoptosis, including endonuclease activity, are present in spermatozoa.

The biochemistry and molecular biology of apoptosis varies somewhat between cells, so although the number of studies addressing the effect of ROS on apoptosis is growing, few have specifically studied sperm. In general, three main pathways exist to initiate apoptosis. The extrinsic pathway is induced by members of the tumor necrosis family (TNF), which upon binding to the 'death receptor' Fas in the plasma membrane, initiate ROS-independent apoptosis.

Table 1. Summary of available tests for the assessment of DNA damage in spermatozoa

	Technique	Assay Principle	Detection method	Measured parameter
	Direct assays			
1.	*In situ* nick translation	Single-strand DNA breaks	Fluorescence microscopy	Percentage cells with incorporated dUTP
2.	TUNEL assay	DNA fragmentation, adds labeled nucleotides to free DNA ends, single- and double-strand DNA breaks	Flow cytometry/fluorescence microscopy	Percentage of cells with labeled DNA
3.	Comet assay	Electrophoresis of a single sperm cell, intact DNA stays in the head, DNA fragments form tails, evaluates DNA integrity, single- and double-strand DNA breaks Alkaline and neutral conditions	Fluorescence microscopy	Percentage of long tails (tail length, % of DNA)
	Indirect assays			
1.	Acridine orange staining	Mild acid treatment, differentiates between single- and double-stranded DNA	Fluorescence microscopy	Percentage of cells with red fluorescence
2.	Sperm chromatin structure assay (SCSA)	Acid DNA denaturation, single or double strand breaks	Flow cytometry	%DFI (ratio of red to red + green fluorescence) population
3.	8-hydroxy-2-deoxyguanosine measurement	Oxidized DNA adducts	HPLC electrochemical detection and flow cytometry	Percentage of DNA adducts formed
4.	DNA breakage Detection-Fluorescence in situ hybridization	DNA breaks, denatures nicked DNA	Fluorescence microscopy and image analyzer	Fluorescence proportional to number of DNA breaks
5.	Sperm chromatin decondensation	Intact spermatozoa with non-fragmented DNA produce characteristic DNA decondensation halo.	Fluorescence microscopy	Percent of sperm with small or absent halos
6.	Chromamycin A3	Indirect visualization of nicked, denatured DNA	Fluorescence microscopy	
7.	Toluidine blue (TB) stain	TB stain is a sensitive structural probe for DNA structure and packaging; it becomes incorporated in the damaged dense chromatin.	Optical microscopy	Light (intact) and dark blue (damaged) stained cells

Only 10% of sperm from healthy donors normally contain the death receptor, but more than 50% of sperm from patients with low sperm concentrations (oligozoospermia) express it [52], indicating that receptor expressivity may regulate apoptosis. Apoptosis occurs when Fas ligand or the agonistic anti-Fas antibody binds to Fas. On the other hand, bcl-2 is an inhibitor of apoptosis, most likely protecting cells by mechanisms that reduce ROS production. Although Fas protein often leads to apoptosis, some of the Fas-labeled cells can escape death by abortive apoptosis. This results in a large population of abnormal spermatozoa in the semen. Failure to clear Fas- positive spermatozoa may be due to a dysfunction at one or more levels: (i) production of spermatozoa may not be adequate to trigger apoptosis in men with hypospermatogenesis and Fas-positive spermatogonia may escape the apoptotic signal. (ii) Fas-positive spermatozoa may accumulate due to failure in activation of Fas-mediated apoptosis.

Significantly higher percentages of Fas-positive spermatozoa are seen in men with oligozoospermia and azoospermia. The intrinsic pathway involves several nuclear transcription factors, the most notable being p53, a mitochondria-dependent pathway for apoptosis that exhibits some redox-regulation and (iii) A less well-known mechanism of apoptosis involves the endoplasmic reticulum and caspase-12 activity. A variety of external factors can stimulate apoptosis by at least one of the aforementioned mechanisms. Such stimuli include ROS, chemotherapeutics, viral infections, radiation, and cytotoxins, all of which are known to have pro-apoptotic effects on spermatozoa.

Intracellular ROS produced by mitochondria are thought to regulate apoptosis. This is supported by the observation that sperm from infertility patients often have significantly higher rates of both apoptosis and ROS than donor sperm. Similar correlation is shown by molecular studies linking ROS levels to caspase activity. Studies using mitochondria-specific antioxidants revealed that low levels of ROS actually inhibit TNF-induced apoptosis by activating nuclear factor-kappa B (NF-κB) [54]. While some studies have found no association between apoptosis and DNA damage, others have demonstrated increased levels of apoptosis in poor quality spermatozoa as measured by the terminal deoxynucleotidyl transferase-mediated deoxyuridine triphosphate-nick end labeling (TUNEL) and comet assays. Apoptosis may also mediate cryoinjury in spermatozoa. Phosphatidylserine (PS), an apoptotic marker, can be used to determine which cells are in the early phases of apoptosis. PS is a type of phospholipid normally present on the inner leaf of the plasma membrane, but becomes externalized early in apoptosis. Sperm destined for cell-suicide can be tagged by annexin V, which binds to the externalized PS [55].

9. Assessment of DNA Integrity

Defects in the chromatin structure of infertile men result in increased DNA instability and sensitivity to denaturing stress. Spermatozoa from infertile men have a higher frequency of chromosomal abnormalities, poor DNA packing quality, increased DNA strand breaks and susceptibility to acid–induced DNA denaturation in situ than spermatozoa from fertile men [23, 27].

Several assays have been developed to evaluate sperm chromatin maturity/DNA integrity (Table 1) [37]. These assays include simple staining techniques such as the acidic aniline blue (AAB) and basic toluidine blue (TB) stains, fluorescent staining techniques such as the sperm chromatin dispersion (SCD) test, chromomycin A_3 (CMA_3), DNA breakage detection – fluorescent *in situ* hybridization assay (DBD–FISH), *in situ* nick translation (NT), and flow cytometric based sperm chromatin structure assay (SCSA). Other assays include combinations of acridine orange staining and TUNEL labeling, and measurement of 8-hydroxy-2-deoxyguanosine by high-performance liquid chromatography. Although studies have shown correlating data sets among SCSA, TUNEL and comet assays, clinical thresholds have been demonstrated only for SCSA and TUNEL. TUNEL assays have correlated with IVF outcome and to a lesser extent with sperm concentration, motility and percentage normal morphology. The SCSA shows strong correlation with exposure to various toxicants, stress conditions and infertility. It is a negative predictor of pregnancy in ART but is poorly correlated with semen parameters [32, 33, 56].

10. Indications for Sperm Chromatin Assessment

Evaluating sperm chromatin is challenging for several reasons: (i) it can be difficult to link the results of chromatin integrity tests to known physiological mechanisms; (ii) the role that sperm chromatin structure assessment plays in clinical practice (especially in ART) is still controversial; and (iii) there is no single standardized method for measuring sperm chromatin integrity.

Sperm chromatin structure is complex and several methods may be necessary to assess it. In addition, a number of confounding factors can complicate the interpretation of the results including heterogeneity in the sperm population and the fact that not all DNA damage is lethal; most DNA contains non-coding regions or introns, and oocytes have the capability to repair sperm DNA damage.

At present, it is clear that sperm chromatin assessment provides good diagnostic and prognostic capabilities for fertility/infertility [32, 33, 35-37, 56].

11. Diagnosis of Male Infertility

Sperm DNA damage has a significant impact on *in vivo* fertilization. Significant differences have been reported in sperm DNA damage levels between fertile and infertile men. Generally spermatozoa from infertile patients are more susceptible to the effects of DNA-damaging agents [14, 57-59].

The probability of fertilization *in vivo* is poor if the proportion of sperm with DNA damage exceeds 30% as detected by the SCSA or 20% as detected by TUNEL. Thus, sperm DNA integrity may be considered an objective marker of sperm function that may serve as a significant prognostic factor for male infertility [32, 33, 56].

Also, reports of a significant increase in DNA damage in sperm from infertile men with normal sperm parameters suggest that analysis of sperm DNA damage may reveal a hidden sperm abnormality in infertile men where fertility is classified as "idiopathic" based on apparently normal standard semen parameters.

12. Disease and Oxidative Stress

Infertility is generally defined as the inability to conceive after one year of unprotected sex. Approximately 15% of couples of reproductive age suffer from some form of infertility, half of which is due to the male factor. *Several conditions and diseases, some reproductive, others not, are associated with elevated levels of ROS and/or decreased antioxidant capabilities. Whether ROS cause or are caused by these conditions is a matter of debate.*

12.1. Idiopathic Infertility

In some cases, despite a battery of tests, the cause of male-factor infertility remains unknown. Idiopathic infertility affects approximately half of all male infertility patients. Despite stemming from an "unknown cause," idiopathic infertility has been recently associated with elevated levels of ROS and decreased antioxidant capacity and may be the result of oxidative stress [14, 60].

12.2. Varicocele

Clinical or subclinical varicocele causes male infertility in about 15% of infertile couples. Patients with varicocele present with dilation and tortuosity of the pampiniform plexus, the vein draining the testicles. Varicocele is a controversial condition. As of yet, there is no agreed upon cause for varicocele. More surprisingly, the consequences and treatments seem to be highly variable. Semen from varicocele patients may exhibit increased levels of ROS, lipid peroxidation, DNA damage, apoptosis, or morphological abnormalities and diminished antioxidant capacity or sperm motility [58, 61]. Many of the abnormal semen characteristics may be interrelated. Increasing degrees of varicocele severity (Grade I, II, or III) are associated with increasing levels of oxidative stress. Also increased levels of nitric oxide have been reported in the spermatic veins of patients with varicocele, which could be responsible for the spermatozoal dysfunction [10, 62]. *Varicocelectomy can reduce oxidative stress and improve sperm motility, concentration, and overall fertility. In addition, because varicocele patients exhibit several characteristics related to oxidative stress, antioxidant treatment may be beneficial in these individuals* [63].

12.3. Leukocytospermia/Genitourinary Tract Infections

The overabundance of white blood cells (WBCs) in the male reproductive tract is often related to genitourinary (GU) infections, including prostate-vesiculo-epididymitis. Leukocytes produced in response to GU pathogens produce high levels of ROS. *Increased levels of ROS in the epididymis may be particularly detrimental because sperm may be stored here for long periods of time while still lacking the antioxidant defenses conferred by the seminal plasma.*

The secondary effects of leukocyte infiltration, rather than the original pathogen, are likely responsible for the negative impact on semen parameters and induction of infertility [7, 14].

12.4 Cancer

Higher rates of apoptosis may be seen in men with testicular cancer than normozoospermic subjects [64]. In addition, if the cancer itself has not negatively affected fertility, often the treatment - radiation, chemotherapy, or alkylating agents - will adversely do. Normally, the effects manifest as DNA damage [65].

Patients with cancer are often referred to sperm banks before chemotherapy, radiation therapy or surgery is initiated. Although pregnancies and births have been reported using cryopreserved sperm from patients with cancer, these semen samples are likely to have decreased fertilization potential.

Evaluating the extent of DNA damage may be helpful in determining how semen should be cryopreserved before starting therapy. It may be prudent to preserve samples showing high sperm concentration and motility and low levels of DNA damage in relatively large aliquots that are more suitable for intrauterine insemination (IUI). In cases where only a single specimen of good sperm quality is available, it should be preserved in multiple small aliquots that are suitable for IVF or ICSI.

12.5. Spinal Cord Injury

Spinal cord damage affecting the lower body often causes infertility. The effects are mediated by increased leukocyte infiltration into the genital tract. Normal neural function n prevents the build-up of sperm in the epididymis through either purposeful or nocturnal emission.

In patients with spinal damage, aberrant neural function prevents the emission of epididymal spermatozoa, resulting in an abnormal accumulation of sperm. An immune response invokes leukocytes to degrade the sperm build-up and induces oxidative stress. Thus, even after patients with spinal cord damage are stimulated to ejaculate, semen parameters and sperm health are often compromised [66].

13. Environmental Factors, Oxidative Stress and Male Infertility

A host of environmental factors have been associated with changes in sperm parameters, particularly estrogens, pesticides, solvents, pthalates, plastics, polychlorinated biphenyls, air pollution, stainless steel welding and tobacco smoke. Most of these agents may not only disrupt hormone levels but also induce oxidative stress, which could damage sperm DNA [7]. *Smoking, alcohol, caffeine consumption and anticancer drugs have been reported to cause aneuploidy in human sperm.*

13.1. Smoking

Tobacco contains numerous substances known to promote ROS and RNS generation, including alkaloids, nitrosamines, nicotine, and hydroxycotinine. These toxic substances induce seminal leukocyte infiltration, thereby increasing ROS levels and decreasing seminal health. In addition, the oxidative properties of smoke deplete seminal antioxidants, further exacerbating the smoke-related decline in sperm health. Reduced sperm count, motility and increased DNA damage have been correlated with cigarette smoking [7, 67]. Fertilization via spermatozoa exhibiting oxidative damage due to smoking may contribute to the incidence of childhood cancers [28].

13.2. Alcohol

The metabolism of alcohol via a variety of processes results in an increase in NADH, a substrate for respiratory chain function. The augmented NADH enhances oxidative phosphorylation and increases the formation of ROS. In addition, acetaldehyde, a metabolic by-product of alcohol, can interact with proteins and lipids to enhance ROS production [7, 68]. Thus *excessive alcohol consumption may induce oxidative stress and reduced fertility.*

13.3. Obesity

High adiposity negatively impacts redox homeostasis of sperm cells. Release of pro-inflammatory cytokines by adipose tissue increases the production of ROS in leukocytes. Furthermore, inguinal or scrotal adipose tissue in morbidly obese men insulates the testicles thereby increasing scrotal temperature which engenders oxidative stress, disrupts spermatogenesis and reduces sperm quality [7].

14. Sperm DNA Damage and Reproductive Outcome

As described above, oxidative stress is major contributor to sperm DNA damage. The influence of sperm DNA damage on reproductive outcomes, both unassisted and assisted, is a subject of intense debate. Studies have shown that fertilization, embryo development and subsequent pregnancy are possible despite high levels of DNA fragmentation in the sperm population. Reports show that couples where husbands display abundant sperm DNA damage have reduced levels of natural fertility; only 10% of couples achieve pregnancy within 1 year when the fraction of denatured DNA exceeds 30% [32, 33, 56]. Furthermore, sperm DNA integrity is poor in those couples whose natural pregnancy results in miscarriage compared to highly fertile couples. A recent meta-analysis showed a strong association between sperm DNA damage and failure to achieve a natural pregnancy [32-34, 56].

A systematic review of the literature suggests that sperm DNA damage is associated with lower natural IUI, and IVF pregnancy rates, but not with ICSI pregnancy rates. The odds ratio

(OR) derived from a recent study indicated that sperm DNA damage is associated with a significantly lower pregnancy rate during IUI (OR, 9.9; 95% confidence interval [CI], 2.37–41.51; $P< 0.001$) [35-37].

The literature also suggests that sperm DNA damage is associated with an increased risk of pregnancy loss in those couples undergoing IVF or ICSI. Numerous studies have examined the influence of sperm DNA integrity on pregnancy rates after standard IVF. In one systematic review and meta-analysis of IVF studies, results indicated that sperm DNA damage is associated, although weakly, with lower IVF pregnancy rates, with a combined OR of 1.57 (95% CI, 1.18–2.07; $P< 0.05$). Another systematic review and meta-analysis of IVF and ICSI studies showed that sperm DNA damage is associated with a significant increase in the rate of pregnancy loss after IVF and ICSI, with a combined OR of 2.48 (95% CI, 1.52–4.04; $P< 0.0001$). However results from another systematic review and meta-analysis of ICSI studies indicated that sperm DNA damage is not associated with ICSI pregnancy rates (combined OR, 1.14; 95% CI, 0.86–1.54, $P = 0.65$) [35-37]. It is possible that the stringent process of sperm and embryo selection at ICSI (in humans) mitigates the potential adverse effect(s) of sperm DNA damage on reproductive outcomes. Sperm DNA damage is an important consideration in ICSI where the natural selection barriers are bypassed. There may be an added risk of iatrogenic transmission of *de novo* genetic abnormalities by the use of sperm with high DNA damage.

Although current data suggest that impaired sperm DNA integrity may have the greatest effect on IUI pregnancy rates and pregnancy loss by IVF and ICSI, further prospective studies are needed before testing should become a routine part of patient management. Furthermore, clear threshold levels of sperm DNA damage beyond which no pregnancy is observed are still lacking. Selection of only high-quality embryos for transfer at IVF may reduce the potential adverse effect of sperm DNA damage on pregnancy rates. On the other hand, the selection process itself (resulting in the loss of embryos) may on occasion lead to reduced pregnancy rates due to fewer embryos available for transfer.

Currently there are no therapies to reduce DNA damage. Therefore there is a strong need to develop therapies for impaired DNA integrity, and subsequent improvements in sperm DNA integrity from such therapies need to be correlated with improved reproductive outcomes.

15. Strategies to Reduce DNA Damage

Baseline levels of DNA integrity in spermatozoa are lower than those of somatic cells. Spermatozoa with good DNA integrity can be obtained by using sperm preparation techniques and antioxidant supplementation alone or in combination [7, 12, 27].

15.1. Separating Spermatozoa with Minimal DNA Damage

This involves the removal of contaminating or activated leukocytes that are more detrimental than dead spermatozoa. It can be accomplished by selectively and efficiently removing contaminating leukocytes using magnetic beads or ferrofluids coated with antibody against the common leukocyte antigen, CD45. This significantly enhances the fertilization capacity of the spermatozoa. *ROS–mediated damage can be reduced by limiting exposure to transition metals in the in vitro culture medium used in ART.* Use of testicular spermatozoa has been shown to be associated with lower amounts of DNA damage. DNA damage is significantly lower in spermatozoa isolated directly from seminal plasma compared to samples prepared from a washed pellet, indicating the importance of implementing strategies that minimize collateral damage. Spermatozoa prepared after swim-up show a negative correlation between DNA fragmentation and fertilization rates following ICSI. Semen samples with morphologically normal spermatozoa and improved DNA integrity can be significantly enhanced after simple preparation techniques such as density gradient centrifugation and glass wool filtration. Different types of sperm preparation techniques should be examined to minimize sperm DNA damage. Decreasing the percentage of spermatozoa with DNA damage following various sperm preparation techniques may be important in increasing fertilization rates above the current rate of 65%-80% after ICSI. For patients with severe oligozoospermia undergoing ICSI, the goal is to maximize sperm recovery rather than sperm function.

15.2. Role of Antioxidants

Ascorbic acid (vitamin C; Vol. II, Chapter 2) is a major contributor to the antioxidant capacity of seminal plasma. Alpha-tocopherol (vitamin E; Vol. II, Chapter 3) can inhibit sperm lipid peroxidation in vitro and protect DNA, making it a potentially useful supplement for sperm preparation media. Administration of low concentrations of vitamins C (350 mg/day) and E (250 mg/day) together in vivo did not prevent DNA sperm damage occurring after ejaculation. However, daily oral supplementation of 1 g vitamins C and E for two months was reported to reduce the number of TUNEL positive spermatozoa from 22.1% to 9.1%, while the amount of spermatozoa with DNA defragmentation remained the same in the placebo group (22.4% to 22.9%). Furthermore a marked improvement of clinical pregnancy (48.2% vs. 6.9%) and implantation (19.6% vs. 2.2%) rates was seen after antioxidant treatment compared with the pre-treatment outcomes of ICSI. In infertile patients with a high level of oxidative DNA damage, the combination of vitamins C and E along with glutathione resulted only in a non-significant increase in sperm concentration. Furthermore combination of vitamins C and E have been reported to show toxic effects. This suggests that there may be a narrow physiological range in which these antioxidants can work synergistically. In another study, supplementing sperm preparation media with a combination of vitamin C and E was associated with decreased ROS production by the sperm. Superoxide supplementation was associated with improved rates of acrosome reaction and preservation of sperm motility. In the clinical ART setting, various antioxidants such as vitamin C, vitamin E, cysteine, taurine and hypotaurine, when added to the culture medium, conferred improvement in the developmental capacity of the embryos by reducing the effects of ROS. Other antioxidants such as urate and N-acetylcysteine (a precursor of glutathione) provided beneficial effects on sperm motility and DNA integrity. Reports have also suggested salutary effects of in vitro supplementation of culture media with ascorbate, urate and alpha-tocopherol on DNA integrity. Sperm freezing and thawing procedures cause a significant and irreversible decrease of motility and metabolic activity of sperm along with disruption of plasma membranes.

Addition of vitamin E (10mmol/L) and rebamipide (300 mmol/L) have been demonstrated to decrease the cryodamage induced during the freeze-thaw procedure and improve post-thaw motility. Furthermore in vitro supplementation of 300 mmol/L of rebamipide in semen samples during incubation ($37^{\circ}C$) and cryopreservation ($-196^{\circ}C$, 3 days) significantly reduced ROS levels.

To the extent that oxidative stress is a critical feature of DNA damage in human spermatozoa, antioxidant administration should be a part of the cure [7, 27]. Recent reports examining DNA damage in spermatozoa following exposure to antioxidant preparations *in vivo* provide some support for this concept. Careful selection and monitoring of patients exhibiting high levels of oxidative stress and DNA damage using robust measurement techniques showed beneficial results with antioxidant regimens. For antioxidants to be effective, it is important to identify whether the source of ROS is extracellular or intracellular. Albumin is effective in neutralizing lipid peroxide-mediated damage to sperm DNA and is also effective in suppressing DNA damage resulting from reduced levels of glutathione. Isoflavones (genistein and equol) conferred significant improvement in sperm DNA damage mediated by H_2O_2. When added at physiological concentrations, genistein appears to be the most potent antioxidant tested, followed by equol, compared with ascorbic acid (10–600 µM) and alpha-tocopherol (1-100 µM). Genistein and equol were more effective in their protective effects when added in combination than when administered individually. These preliminary data suggest that these compounds may play a role in antioxidant protection against sperm DNA damage. However, the beneficial effects of antioxidants have thus far been limited and the topic remains controversial.

Conclusions

The male germ line is highly susceptible to DNA fragmentation. ROS are necessary for various physiological functions but an imbalance in favor of ROS results in oxidative stress. Oxidative stress-induced DNA damage causes promutagenic changes. The latter may not have a negative effect on the quality of the germ line because collateral oxidative injury to the plasma membrane prevents fertilization. There are multiple assays that may be used to evaluate sperm chromatin damage. The importance of assessing sperm for chromatin abnormalities may provide useful information in cases of male idiopathic infertility and in couples pursuing assisted reproduction. It allows the selection of spermatozoa with intact DNA or with the least amount of DNA damage for use in assisted conception. Assessing DNA damage provides better diagnostic and prognostic capabilities than standard sperm parameters for male fertility potential. In addition, the knowledge regarding oxidative stress has given rise to several new treatment modalities currently under investigation for the improvement of male fertility. Moreover, several sperm preparation techniques help by significantly reducing the levels of ambient ROS. Many new antioxidants are now available that can decrease oxidative stress and improve sperm quality. However, the lack of rigorous clinical evidence demonstrating their efficacy remains a concern and approval for their routine use has thus far been denied by the U.S. Food and Drug Administration. Also, threshold ROS levels above which antioxidants might be considered for the management of male infertility should be determined. The doses and treatment durations for these agents should also be ascertained and standardized. With the increased use of ART procedures, efforts should be directed at developing optimum combinations of antioxidants to supplement sperm preparation media. In a clinical context, and also as 'best practice', there is an urgent need to look into other avenues for remediation of sperm DNA damage. Double-blind, randomized, crossover trials are needed to establish the efficacy of antioxidant treatment in reducing DNA damage in the spermatozoa of infertile males. It is vital that such studies be conducted in patients for whom there is good evidence of oxidative stress in their germ line using the most reliable assays available for measuring both oxidative stress and DNA damage.

Acknowledgments

The authors are grateful for research support from the Center for Reproductive Medicine at Cleveland Clinic.

References

[1]   Agarwal A, Saleh RA, Bedaiwy MA. Role of reactive oxygen species in the pathophysiology of human reproduction. *Fertil. Steril.* 2003;79(4):829-43.

[2]   Agarwal A, Sharma RK, Nallella KP, Thomas AJ,Jr, Alvarez JG, Sikka SC. Reactive oxygen species as an independent marker of male factor infertility. *Fertil. Steril.* 2006;86(4):878-85.

[3]   Agarwal A, Cocuzza M, Abdelrazik H, Sharma RK. Oxidative stress measurement in patients with male or female factor infertility. In: Popov I., Lewin G. *Handbook of Chemiluminescent Methods in Oxidative Stress Assessment.* 2008. p. 195 - 218.

[4]   Agarwal A, Varghese AC, Sharma RK. Markers of oxidative stress and sperm chromatin integrity. *Methods Mol. Biol.* 2009;590:377-402.

[5]   Makker K, Agarwal A, Sharma R. Oxidative stress and male infertility. *Indian J. Med. Res.* 2009;129(4):357-67.

[6]   Sharma RK, Agarwal A. Role of reactive oxygen species in male infertility. *Urology,* 1996;48(6):835-50.

[7]   Tremellen K. Oxidative stress and male infertility--a clinical perspective. *Hum. Reprod. Update,* 2008;14(3):243-58.

[8]   Desai N, Sharma R, Makker K, Sabanegh E, Agarwal A. Physiologic and pathologic levels of reactive oxygen species in neat semen of infertile men. *Fertil. Steril.* 2009;92(5):1626-31.

[9]   Agarwal A, Makker K, Sharma R. Clinical relevance of oxidative stress in male factor infertility: an update. *Am. J. Reprod. Immunol.* 2008;59(1):2-11.

[10] Agarwal A, Sharma RK, Desai NR, Prabakaran S, Tavares A, Sabanegh E. Role of oxidative stress in pathogenesis of varicocele and infertility. *Urology,* 2009;73(3):461-9.

[11] Aitken RJ, Clarkson JS, Fishel S. Generation of reactive oxygen species, lipid peroxidation, and human sperm function. *Biol. Reprod.* 1989;41(1):183-97.

[12] Agarwal A, Nallella KP, Allamaneni SS, Said TM. Role of antioxidants in treatment of male infertility: an overview of the literature. *Reprod. Biomed. Online,* 2004;8(6):616-27.

[13] Aitken RJ, Buckingham D, West K, Wu FC, Zikopoulos K, Richardson DW. Differential contribution of leucocytes and spermatozoa to the generation of reactive oxygen species in the ejaculates of oligozoospermic patients and fertile donors. *J. Reprod. Fertil.* 1992;94(2):451-62.

[14] Saleh RA, Agarwal A, Kandirali E, Sharma RK, Thomas AJ, Nada EA et al. Leukocytospermia is associated with increased reactive oxygen species production by human spermatozoa. *Fertil. Steril.* 2002;78(6):1215-24.

[15] Twigg J, Irvine DS, Houston P, Fulton N, Michael L, Aitken RJ. Iatrogenic DNA damage induced in human spermatozoa during sperm preparation: protective significance of seminal plasma. *Mol. Hum. Reprod.* 1998;4(5):439-45.

[16] Koppers AJ, De Iuliis GN, Finnie JM, McLaughlin EA, Aitken RJ. Significance of mitochondrial reactive oxygen species in the generation of oxidative stress in spermatozoa. *J. Clin. Endocrinol. Metab.* 2008;93(8):3199-207.

[17] Banfi B, Molnar G, Maturana A, Steger K, Hegedus B, Demaurex N et al. A Ca(2+)-activated NADPH oxidase in testis, spleen, and lymph nodes. *J. Biol. Chem.* 2001;276(40):37594-601.

[18] Sabeur K, Ball BA. Characterization of NADPH oxidase 5 in equine testis and spermatozoa. *Reproduction,* 2007;134(2):263-70.

[19] Plante M, de Lamirande E, Gagnon C. Reactive oxygen species released by activated neutrophils, but not by deficient spermatozoa, are sufficient to affect normal sperm motility. *Fertil. Steril.* 1994;62(2):387-93.

[20] Wolff H, Anderson DJ. Immunohistologic characterization and quantitation of leukocyte subpopulations in human semen. *Fertil. Steril.* 1988;49(3):497-504.

[21] Ochsendorf FR. Infections in the male genital tract and reactive oxygen species. *Hum. Reprod. Update,* 1999;5(5):399-420.

[22] Agarwal A, Prabakaran SA. Mechanism, measurement, and prevention of oxidative stress in male reproductive physiology. *Indian J. Exp. Biol.* 2005;43(11):963-74.

[23] Agarwal A, Allamaneni SS. Sperm DNA damage assessment: a test whose time has come. *Fertil. Steril.* 2005;84(4):850-3.

[24] Sharma RK, Pasqualotto AE, Nelson DR, Thomas AJ,Jr, Agarwal A. Relationship between seminal white blood cell counts and oxidative stress in men treated at an infertility clinic. *J. Androl.* 2001;22(4):575-83.

[25] Vernet P, Aitken RJ, Drevet JR. Antioxidant strategies in the epididymis. *Mol. Cell Endocrinol.* 2004;216(1-2):31-9.

[26] Mahfouz R, Sharma R, Sharma D, Sabanegh E, Agarwal A. Diagnostic value of the total antioxidant capacity (TAC) in human seminal plasma. *Fertil. Steril.* 2009;91(3):805-11.

[27] Agarwal A, Said TM. Role of sperm chromatin abnormalities and DNA damage in male infertility. *Hum. Reprod. Update,* 2003;9(4):331-45.

[28] Aitken RJ. The Amoroso Lecture. The human spermatozoon--a cell in crisis? *J. Reprod. Fertil.* 1999;115(1):1-7.

[29] Aitken RJ, De Iuliis GN. Origins and consequences of DNA damage in male germ cells. *Reprod. Biomed. Online,* 2007;14(6):727-33.

[30] Aitken RJ, De Iuliis GN. On the possible origins of DNA damage in human spermatozoa. *Mol. Hum. Reprod.* 2010;16(1):3-13.

[31] Bungum M, Humaidan P, Axmon A, Spano M, Bungum L, Erenpreiss J et al. Sperm DNA integrity assessment in prediction of assisted reproduction technology outcome. *Hum. Reprod.* 2007;22(1):174-9.

[32] Evenson DP, Larson KL, Jost LK. Sperm chromatin structure assay: its clinical use for detecting sperm DNA fragmentation in male infertility and comparisons with other techniques. *J. Androl.* 2002;23(1):25-43.

[33] Evenson D, Wixon R. Meta-analysis of sperm DNA fragmentation using the sperm chromatin structure assay. *Reprod. Biomed. Online,* 2006;12(4):466-72.

[34] Carrell DT, Liu L, Peterson CM, Jones KP, Hatasaka HH, Erickson L et al. Sperm DNA fragmentation is increased in couples with unexplained recurrent pregnancy loss. *Arch. Androl.* 2003;49(1):49-55.

[35] Zini A, Meriano J, Kader K, Jarvi K, Laskin CA, Cadesky K. Potential adverse effect of sperm DNA damage on embryo quality after ICSI. *Hum. Reprod.* 2005;20(12):3476-80.

[36] Zini A, Libman J. Sperm DNA damage: clinical significance in the era of assisted reproduction. *CMAJ,*2006;175(5):495-500.

[37] Zini A, Sigman M. Are tests of sperm DNA damage clinically useful? Pros and cons. *J. Androl.* 2009;30(3):219-29.

[38] Carlsen E, Giwercman A, Keiding N, Skakkebaek NE. Evidence for decreasing quality of semen during past 50 years. *BMJ.* 1992;305(6854):609-13.

[39] Lenzi A, Picardo M, Gandini L, Dondero F. Lipids of the sperm plasma membrane: from polyunsaturated fatty acids considered as markers of sperm function to possible scavenger therapy. *Hum. Reprod. Update,* 1996;2(3):246-56.

[40] Jones R, Mann T, Sherins R. Peroxidative breakdown of phospholipids in human spermatozoa, spermicidal properties of fatty acid peroxides, and protective action of seminal plasma. *Fertil. Steril.* 1979;31(5):531-7.

[41] Armstrong JS, Rajasekaran M, Chamulitrat W, Gatti P, Hellstrom WJ, Sikka SC. Characterization of reactive oxygen species induced effects on human spermatozoa movement and energy metabolism. *Free Radic. Biol. Med.* 1999;26(7-8):869-80.

[42] St John JC, Sakkas D, Barratt CL. A role for mitochondrial DNA and sperm survival. *J. Androl.* 2000;21(2):189-99.

[43] Shamsi MB, Kumar R, Bhatt A, Bamezai RN, Kumar R, Gupta NP et al. Mitochondrial DNA Mutations in etiopathogenesis of male infertility. *Indian J. Urol.* 2008;24(2):150-4.

[44] Cocuzza M, Sikka SC, Athayde KS, Agarwal A. Clinical relevance of oxidative stress and sperm chromatin damage in male infertility: an evidence based analysis. *Int. Braz. J. Urol.* 2007;33(5):603-21.

[45] Rousseaux J, Rousseaux-Prevost R. Molecular localization of free thiols in human sperm chromatin. *Biol. Reprod.* 1995;52(5):1066-72.

[46] Saowaros W, Panyim S. The formation of disulfide bonds in human protamines during sperm maturation. *Experientia,* 1979;35(2):191-2.

[47] Ward WS, Coffey DS. DNA packaging and organization in mammalian spermatozoa: comparison with somatic cells. *Biol. Reprod.* 1991;44(4):569-74.

[48] Aoki VW, Liu L, Carrell DT. Identification and evaluation of a novel sperm protamine abnormality in a population of infertile males. *Hum. Reprod.* 2005;20(5):1298-306.

[49] de Mateo S, Gazquez C, Guimera M, Balasch J, Meistrich ML, Ballesca JL et al. Protamine 2 precursors (Pre-P2), protamine 1 to protamine 2 ratio (P1/P2), and assisted reproduction outcome. *Fertil. Steril.* 2009;91(3):715-22.

[50] Rodriguez I, Ody C, Araki K, Garcia I, Vassalli P. An early and massive wave of germinal cell apoptosis is required for the development of functional spermatogenesis. *EMBO J.* 1997;16(9):2262-70.

[51] Sakkas D, Seli E, Bizzaro D, Tarozzi N, Manicardi GC. Abnormal spermatozoa in the ejaculate: abortive apoptosis and faulty nuclear remodelling during spermatogenesis. *Reprod. Biomed. Online,* 2003;7(4):428-32.

[52] Sakkas D, Mariethoz E, St John JC. Abnormal sperm parameters in humans are indicative of an abortive apoptotic mechanism linked to the Fas-mediated pathway. *Exp. Cell Res.* 1999;251(2):350-5.

[53] Wang X, Sharma RK, Sikka SC, Thomas AJ,Jr, Falcone T, Agarwal A. Oxidative stress is associated with increased apoptosis leading to spermatozoa DNA damage in patients with male factor infertility. *Fertil. Steril.* 2003;80(3):531-5.

[54] Hughes G, Murphy MP, Ledgerwood EC. Mitochondrial reactive oxygen species regulate the temporal activation of nuclear factor kappaB to modulate tumour necrosis factor-induced apoptosis: evidence from mitochondria-targeted antioxidants. *Biochem. J.* 2005;389(Pt 1):83-9.

[55] Barroso G, Morshedi M, Oehninger S. Analysis of DNA fragmentation, plasma membrane translocation of phosphatidylserine and oxidative stress in human spermatozoa. *Hum. Reprod.* 2000;15(6):1338-44.

[56] Evenson DP, Jost LK, Marshall D, Zinaman MJ, Clegg E, Purvis K et al. Utility of the sperm chromatin structure assay as a diagnostic and prognostic tool in the human fertility clinic. *Hum. Reprod.* 1999;14(4):1039-49.

[57] Saleh RA, Agarwal A, Nada EA, El-Tonsy MH, Sharma RK, Meyer A et al. Negative effects of increased sperm DNA damage in relation to seminal oxidative stress in men with idiopathic and male factor infertility. *Fertil. Steril.* 2003;79 Suppl 3:1597-605.

[58] Saleh RA, Agarwal A, Nelson DR, Nada EA, El-Tonsy MH, Alvarez JG et al. Increased sperm nuclear DNA damage in normozoospermic infertile men: a prospective study. *Fertil. Steril.* 2002;78(2):313-8.

[59] Saleh RA, Agarwal A, Sharma RK, Said TM, Sikka SC, Thomas AJ,Jr. Evaluation of nuclear DNA damage in spermatozoa from infertile men with varicocele. *Fertil. Steril.* 2003;80(6):1431-6.

[60] Pasqualotto FF, Sharma RK, Kobayashi H, Nelson DR, Thomas AJ,Jr, Agarwal A. Oxidative stress in normospermic men undergoing infertility evaluation. *J. Androl.* 2001;22(2):316-22.

[61] Mostafa T, Anis T, Imam H, El-Nashar AR, Osman IA. Seminal reactive oxygen species-antioxidant relationship in fertile males with and without varicocele. *Andrologia,* 2009;41(2):125-9.

[62] Allamaneni SS, Naughton CK, Sharma RK, Thomas AJ,Jr, Agarwal A. Increased seminal reactive oxygen species levels in patients with varicoceles correlate with varicocele grade but not with testis size. *Fertil. Steril.* 2004;82(6):1684-6.

[63] Marmar JL. The pathophysiology of varicoceles in the light of current molecular and genetic information. *Hum. Reprod. Update,* 2001;7(5):461-72.

[64] Gandini L, Lombardo F, Paoli D, Caponecchia L, Familiari G, Verlengia C et al. Study of apoptotic DNA fragmentation in human spermatozoa. *Hum. Reprod.* 2000;15(4):830-9.

[65] Kobayashi H, Larson K, Sharma RK, Nelson DR, Evenson DP, Toma H et al. DNA damage in patients with untreated cancer as measured by the sperm chromatin structure assay. *Fertil. Steril.* 2001;75(3):469-75.

[66] de Lamirande E, Leduc BE, Iwasaki A, Hassouna M, Gagnon C. Increased reactive oxygen species formation in semen of patients with spinal cord injury. *Fertil. Steril.* 1995;63(3):637-42.

[67] Halliwell B, Cross CE. Oxygen-derived species: their relation to human disease and environmental stress. *Environ. Health Perspect,* 1994;102 Suppl 10:5-12.

[68] Das SK, Vasudevan DM. Alcohol-induced oxidative stress. *Life Sci.* 2007;81(3):177-87.

In: Principles of Free Radical Biomedicine, Volume III
Editors: K. Pantopoulos and H. M. Schipper

ISBN 978-1-61324-184-4
©2012 Nova SciencePublishers, Inc.

Chapter 14

Oxidative Stress
in Female Reproduction

Sajal Gupta, Sarah Brickner, Rathna Shenoy BS,
Chin Kun Baw and Ashok Agarwal[*]

Center for Reproductive Medicine, Glickman Urological and Kidney Institute and
Obstetrics and Gynecology and Women's Health Institute,
Cleveland Clinic, Cleveland, Ohio, U.S.A.

1. Introduction

The Literature suggests that oxidative stress influences the reproductive tract of a woman throughout her entire life span, including the menopausal years. It plays a role in many physiological processes, and, when excessive, can influence various pathophysiological processes in female reproduction by mechanisms such as lipid peroxidation, inhibition of protein synthesis, mitochondrial modification, ATP reduction, and DNA damage. Free radicals affect gametes, embryos, and their environments, including follicular fluid, hydrosalpingeal fluid, and peritoneal fluid. The state of these microenvironments influences pregnancy outcomes by directly affecting oocyte quality, sperm-oocyte interaction, implantation, and early embryo development [6].

2. Redox Homeostasis and Generation of Oxidative Stress

Reactive oxygen species (ROS) and reactive nitrogen species (RNS) induce cellular damage by 'stealing' electrons from nearby molecules, e,g, nucleic acids, lipids, proteins, or

---

[*]Tel: 216-444-9485, Fax: 216-445-6049, E-mail: agarwaa@ccf.org

carbohydrates (Vol. I, Chapters 2-8). Three biologically-important forms of ROS are superoxide ($O_2^{\bullet-}$), hydrogen peroxide (H_2O_2), and hydroxyl radical (HO·). Superoxide is formed via leakage of electrons from the electron transport chain and H_2O_2 is formed from oxidase enzymes or superoxide dismutase (SOD) activity. Hydroxyl radicals are the most reactive of the three and damage DNA through modification of purines and pyrimidines, leading to breaks within the DNA strands (Vol. I, Chapter 9). The imbalance of antioxidants and oxidants also modifies key transcription factors that alter gene expression profiles [7]; see also Vol. II, Chapters 12-14.

ROS have been implicated in signal transduction pathways in processes including, but not limited to, folliculogenesis, oocyte maturation, ovulation, implantation, and pregnancy [39, 42]. However, there is an intricate balance between prooxidants and antioxidants, and disturbance of this balance can result in increased ROS levels and oxidative stress. This may alter various redox pathways and lead to apoptosis in gametes and embryos, potentially engendering oocyte degradation and embryonic fragmentation and wastage [20]. Oxidative stress also plays a role in the menstrual cycle, as it aids in cyclic modulation of the endometrium. In the late secretory phase preceding menstruation, ROS levels increase, implying redox involvement in menstruation. During this phase, lipid peroxide concentrations are elevated and SOD is decreased, which may contribute to endometrium degradation and, consequently, menstruation. Nitric oxide regulates the endometrium's microvasculature, and thus plays a role in menstruation. During menopause, the decline in estrogen levels promotes oxidative stress. Apoptosis can be induced by ROS, decreased antioxidant levels, mitochondrial membrane potential depolarization, proapoptotic protein initiation, and blockage of the electron transport chain (ETC) [6].

Uncontrolled ROS production impacts embryo toxicity and teratogenicity in prenatal development [42-43]. It also may play a large role in endometriosis, polycystic ovarian disease, and spontaneous abortions, as well as conditions arising during pregnancy such as preeclampsia, hydatidiform mole, preterm labor [23], embryopathies, and intrauterine growth retardation. High levels of lipid peroxidation (Vol. I, Chapter 7), which result from excessive ROS generation, can damage lipids and proteins, as well as enzymes and cell membranes. Redox alteration may influence transcription factors and epigenetic mechanisms and lead to a decline in the quality of oocytes and embryos.

Antioxidants, the body's defense mechanism against overproduction of ROS, help prevent and alleviate ROS-induced damage. Both enzymatic and non-enzymatic antioxidants aid in this process. Enzymatic or natural antioxidants include the SODs (Vol. II, Chapter 5), which produce H_2O_2 from $O_2^{\bullet-}$. Catalase (Vol. II, Chapter 7), and glutathione (GSH) related peroxidases (GPx; Vol. II, Chapter 8) break down H_2O_2 [6]. Non-enzymatic antioxidants include GSH (Vol. II, Chapter 1), the main non-enzymatic antioxidant, vitamin C (Vol. II, Chapter 2), vitamin E (Vol. II, Chapter 3), zinc, taurine, hypotaurine, transferrin, and beta-carotene. Large amounts of GSH present in oocytes and embryos provide important cytoprotection. A decrease in GSH can yield elevated H_2O_2 levels and damage to DNA. Vitamin C protects lipoproteins from peroxyl radicals, recycles vitamin E, and decreases sulfydryl stress. Vitamin E directly neutralizes the superoxide anion, hydroxyl radical, and H_2O_2 and is the main chain-breaking antioxidant in membrane lipids. Taurine neutralizes hydroxyl radicals and transferrin binds and limits the toxicity of iron.

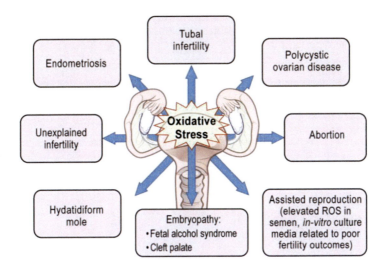

Figure 1. Oxidative stress is associated with a number of different pathologies in women, affecting their fertility and chances of success in assisted reproduction.

This Chapter will review the role of redox status and antioxidants in pregnancy, the impact of oxidative stress in different gynecological conditions, and various physiological roles of ROS in female reproduction. It also describes the role of oxidative stress in embryonic development, its influences in assisted reproductive technology (ART) outcomes, and the therapeutic uses of oral antioxidants as a strategy to modulate the dystrophic effects of ROS in female reproduction (Figure 1).

3. Redox Status and Antioxidants in Pregnancy

3.1. Impact on Pregnancy Outcome

Oxidative stress has been implicated in pregnancy and ROS can regulate many physiological functions in the female reproductive tract. Pregnancy is a state of oxidative stress. During pregnancy, increased production of superoxide occurs. Polymorphonuclear leukocytes are increasingly produced in the first trimester of pregnancy, and in the second and third trimesters, elevated ROS production and oxidative stress are characteristic [4]. ROS can lead to inadequate support needed for continuation of pregnancy by inducing luteal regression and suboptimal luteal hormone levels [6]. Pregnant patients exhibit enhanced lipid peroxidation, ROS, and total antioxidant capacity (TAC) [43]. Superoxide, nitric oxide, vitamin E, and free radicals are elevated in placental mitochondria. Further increases in concentrations of serum malondialdehyde (MDA), a marker of lipid peroxidation, occur during term labor [24]. Nitric oxide has an important role in pregnancy. Preterm pregnant patients have demonstrated higher inducible NOS (iNOS) levels than patients in term labor. NO contributes to uterine inactivity, affects endometrium decidualization, and helps prepare for blastocyst implantation [8]. Low NO levels are necessary for normal ovarian function and implantation, but at high levels, NO hinders sperm motility and implantation, is embryotoxic and leads to lower pregnancy rates [7].

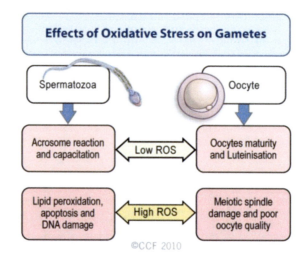

Figure 2. Influences of physiological and pathological levels of reactive oxygen species on sperm function. Low levels of ROS are essential for successful fertilization while high levels may result in poor oocyte quality.

Oxidative stress associated with abnormal placentation and syncitiotrophoblastic damage may be a causative factor in abortion. In normal pregnancies, although oxidative stress markers are elevated in the normal trophoblast, bursts of enhanced free radical production have been implicated in the etiology of early pregnancy loss.

Parental factors also influence pregnancy. Sperm DNA may be damaged when traveling through the seminiferous tubules and epididymis where they are exposed to ROS [10]; see also previous Chapter. The damaged sperm may adversely affect rates of oocyte fertilization. In addition to pregnancy loss, fertilization of oocytes with sperm containing damaged DNA may result in birth defects and embryo developmental arrest (Figure 2).

Recurrent pregnancy loss (RPL) is defined as at least three consecutive pregnancy losses before 20 weeks of gestation [6]. The etiology of RPL is not certain, although oxidative stress is speculated to play a role. RPL is multifactorial and is affected by both genetics and the environment. In a large case controlled study, increased risk of RPL was noted in women with glutathione S-transferase class m1 (GSTM1) null polymorphisms. Pregnant patients experiencing RPL exhibit an association between elevated glutathione levels and poor outcomes, such as abortion [4]. Furthermore, these women express elevated lipid peroxide and lower vitamin E and beta-carotene levels. GSH may represent a protective response against increasing ROS levels. Oxidative stress can also lead to preterm labor by damaging fetal membrane focal collagen.

3.2. Antioxidants and Lipid Peroxidation Status in Diabetes Associated With Pregnancy

Diabetes itself is a state of oxidative stress (see Chapter 9 in this Volume). Low-density lipoprotein (LDL) from pregnant women with diabetes manifests increased susceptibility to oxidative reactions. 6-10% of infants of diabetic mothers express congenital abnormalities, significantly higher rates compared to the general population [43]. Diabetes-complicated pregnancies are also at elevated risk for embryopathies, spontaneous abortions, and perinatal mortality, and both mother and fetus exhibit elevated lipid peroxide (LPO) and protein carbonyl levels [43]. GSH synthesis is suppressed and ROS levels are increased in embryos under hyperglycemic conditions and hyperglycemia-induced oxidative stress contributes to congenital defects in diabetic pregnancies.

4. Changing Dynamics of Oxidative Stress and Antioxidant Status in Preeclampsia

Preeclampsia is an abnormal state of pregnancy characterized by hypertension, fluid retention and albuminuria; it can lead to eclampsia (seizures and coma) if untreated. The cause of preeclampsia is unknown, but increasing evidence suggests a role of oxidative stress in its etiopathogenesis [24]. The pathophysiology of preeclampsia is established in the first trimester of pregnancy. In the first stage of preeclampsia, extravilloustrophoblastwhichplugs in the maternal spiral arteries are dislodged, initiating blood flow into the intervillous space, an oxidative burst and augmented ROS production [6]. Levels of antioxidant defenses are perturbed and production of excess NO^- and O_2^- prevails [43]. The condition also features diminished perfusion of placental tissue, abnormal lipid metabolism, and deranged blood redox homeostasis.

Elevated lipid peroxidation occurs in patients with preeclampsia, as well as elevated protein carbonyl concentrations, plasma MDA levels, and SOD activity [6]. Neutrophil activation may increase ROS production, which in turn leads to further lipid peroxidation [43].

Endothelial cell dysfunction and lipid peroxidation, caused by reduced NO-mediated vascular relaxation and decreased fetoplacental circulation, are characteristic of preeclampsia. Abnormal placentation can lead to placental hypoxia, resulting in oxidative stress. This leads to cytokine and prostaglandin release, triggering endothelial cell dysfunction and possibly preeclampsia [8].

4.1 Dynamics of Redox Changes in Hydatidiform Mole

Hydatidiform mole is a placental defect. It is a grape-like cluster of degenerated placental villi in the uterus, which can involve oxidative stress-induced damage. Patients with complete hydatidiform mole have both lowered antioxidants and decreased total antioxidant capacity (TAC) that can be linked to the pathology of DNA damage [6]. In a study involving 38 patients with complete hydatidiform mole and 31 healthy pregnant women, total plasma antioxidant potential was significantly higher in healthy pregnant women. Mean oxidative stress markers and total plasma peroxide levels were both significantly higher in those with hydatidiform mole [22]. Thus, it was concluded that patients with complete hydatidiform mole experience greater oxidative stress, which may impact the pathogenesis of the disease. In both hydatidiform mole and preeclampsia inflammatory states with increased levels of tumor necrosis factor alpha (TNFα) and Interleukin-6 (IL-6) have been observed. The elaboration of pro-inflammatory cytokines in the face of diminished antioxidant status and elevated oxidative stress markers may contribute to the poor pregnancy outcomes.

5. Oxidative Stress and Other Gynecological Conditions

Endometriosis is a gynecological disorder that affects women typically within their reproductive ages, but may also arise in postmenopausal women. The disease is characterized by uterine and endometrial tissue found outside of the uterus, typically in the peritoneal cavity. However, endometrial tissue has also been found in the pleural cavity, the gluteal muscles, the liver, the bladder, the kidney, and the brain. The endometrial and uterine tissue has the ability to implant within the peritoneal cavity forming intraperitoneal lesions that have been demonstrated to grow and proliferate allowing progression of the disorder. Between 2 and 22% of women will be diagnosed with endometriosis during their reproductive years and 35-50% of them will have associated infertility, one of the secondary problems associated with the disease. Several theories have been proposed to explain the pathogenesis of endometriosis. In 1927,Sampson theorized that endometriosis was the result ofretrograde menstruation, which is the reflux of erythrocytes and endometrial cells and tissue through the oviduct and into the peritoneal cavity where implantation occurs. Along with retrograde menstruation, the refluxed cells must maintain viability and the ability to implant which requires a blood supply. Angiogenic growth factors were found to be up regulated in the peritoneal fluid of women with endometriosis, underscoring the importance of blood supply in the formation and progression of lesions.

The endometrial fragments and erythrocytes refluxed into the peritoneal cavity are regarded as antigenic or foreign objects to the body [18]. Activation of immune cells, such as macrophages, ensues resulting in an inflammatory reaction. The macrophages may phagocytose the foreign objects, but also release ROS such as $O_2^{\bullet-}$, H_2O_2, and hydroxyl radical. In endometriosis, when ROS attack polyunsaturated fatty acids, malondialdehyde (MDA), the stable end product of lipid peroxidation, accumulates in the peritoneal fluid [11]. Other oxidative stress markers such as lipid hydroperoxides (LOOH), and lysophosphatidylcholine collect in the peritoneal fluid eliciting a greater antigenic response [11]. This was shown in a study done in 2009, where peritoneal fluid of women with and without endometriosis was incubated with semen samples [29]. Sperm incubated with peritoneal fluid from women with endometriosis for as little as 1.5 hours had significantly higher sperm DNA damage compared to control specimens [29]. Autoantibodies produced by the body will then form antigen antibody complexes activating more immune cells; these, subsequently release more ROS whichupregulate the activity of transcription factors such as NF-κB [19, 49]. NF-κB has been found to be increased in endometriosis, and can activate genes that express cytokines, growth factors, angiogenic factors, adhesion molecules, and inducible enzymes including nitric oxide synthase and cyclooxygenase [49]; see also Vol. II, Chapter 12.

Levels of iron were found to be increased in the disease process. Iron levels are thought to originate from the erythrocytes found in retrograde menstruation as well as peritoneal lesions [45]. Hemoglobin is heme moiety is degraded by heme oxygenase-1 into iron, bilirubin, and carbon monoxide (Vol. II, Chapter 11). Excess iron, which has the ability to react and cause oxidative stress, is normally bound by ferritin, an iron sequestering protein (Vol. II, Chapter 19). In women with endometriosis, the levels or ferritin and transferrin, were found to be elevated compared to control women [12]. In the face of excessive bleeding, the ferritin system may become overwhelmed, causing iron to be released into the peritoneal fluid [12, 45, 46, 47]. Liberated iron can then cause oxidative stress by reacting with H_2O_2 in the Fenton reaction, generating hydroxyl radical [45, 46, 47]; see also Vol. I, Chapter 5. Iron can also bind to transferrin in the peritoneal fluid, which will then transfer it to the peritoneal lesions that have transferrin receptors. Iron may facilitate proliferation of the lesions and progression of the disease [12, 16, 45, 46, 47].

5.1. Oxidative Stress and Fertility Outcomes with Hydrosalpinx

Hydrosalpinx is the abnormal swelling of the fallopian tube possibly caused by blockage induced by tubal infection. It involves the accumulation of toxic fluid in conditions that lead to an inflammatory reaction. Hydrosalpingeal fluid (HSF) is thought to reduce embryo implantation rates and increase rates of miscarriage [6]. *In vitro* fertilization (IVF) is considered the best option for women with hydrosalpinx. Increased ROS and products of lipid peroxidation exist in the hydrosalpingeal fluid [2], and oxidative stress may mediate the embryotoxic effects. Physiological ROS levels, which do not harm the growing embryo, may be indicative of regular ROS generation by a healthy endosalpinx. Development of blastocysts has been shown to correlate positively with low concentrations of tubal fluid ROS [6]. Thus, low ROS levels may be indicative of normal tubal secretory function. Addtionally, hydrosalpinx can lead to enlarged fallopian tubes that leak fluid, leading to embryotoxic effects. HSF may decrease endometrial integrins, impeding implantation. This implantation rate can be improved with removal of hydrosalpinges.

Inducible nitric oxide (iNOS) activity correlates with resistance to hydrosalpinx and infertility in wild-type mouse strains *in vivo*. The inhibition or deletion of iNOS is associated with augmented post-infection hydrosalpinx formation rates. Studies in mice have shown that iNOS-derived RNS act as a defense mechanism against the development of hydrosalpinx and infertility. Evidence shows that higher *in vivo* production of RNS is correlated with mouse strain-related resistance to hydrosalpinx formation. Nitrogen and oxygen radicals and their combined byproducts, such as peroxynitrite, can induce prostaglandin synthesis, which may regulate inducible nitric oxide synthase (iNOS) activity. NO may also behave as an antioxidant and can participate in the termination of lipid peroxide reactions [6].

5.2. Role of Free Radicals in Unexplained Infertility and Endometriosis-Associated Infertility

Idiopathic infertility is responsible for 3-18% of fertility problems [50]. Infertility may occur due to increased ROS as evidenced by the increased levels of oxidative stress biomarkers in the peritoneal fluid of infertile women [11].

Along with the increased ROS, levels of antioxidants are significantly diminished in these women. The imbalance between the two leads to oxidative stress, which may induce infertility [11]. If ROS are increased in the peritoneal fluid, then it may also affect the fluid in the fallopian tubes, which would lead to fertilization problems as the sperm attempts to penetrate the oocyte [11]. Malondialdehyde levels appear to be elevated in the peritoneal fluid signifying lipid peroxidation. Oxidative stress has also been implicated in endometriosis-associated infertility. If the ROS balance is not maintained, damage to incoming spermatozoa can occur [29]. The ROS can cause damage of the lipid bilayer in the cell membranes of sperm causing loss of fluidity, impeding fertilization. Nuclear DNA damage along with mitochondrial DNA damage can result in detrimental effects such as inability to fertilize properly, implantation failure, and developmental problems [29].

Nitric oxide may play important roles in infertility [38]. In infertile women, activated macrophages have greater NOS activity and NO production. NO may react with $O_2^{\bullet-}$ forming cytotoxicperoxynitrite [38, 51]; see also Vol. I, Chapter 3. Peroxynitrite has a relatively long half-life, and reacts with the amino acid tyrosine to form nitrotyrosine.

Levels of nitrotyrosine were found elevated in the proliferative and secretory phases of the mentstrual cycle of women with adenomyosis [38, 51]. Peroxynitrite may promote DNA damage affecting fertility. Nitric oxide synthase can also be upregulated by the transcription factor NF-κB [49]. High amounts of nitric oxide inhibit sperm movement, and can cause contractile problems [38, 51].

In normal women, endothelial NOS exhibits similar expression patterns as adhesion molecule integrin alpha V beta three [38]. In endometriosis, this relationship appears to be disrupted andas eNOS levels rise, integrin expression diminishes. The adhesion molecule is necessary for implantation to occur, and without it infertility can ensue [38].

Glutathione peroxidase (GPx) activity has been implicated in idiopathic infertility. In one study, selenium and selenium-dependent activity were measured in follicular fluid of women undergoing IVF [18]. Patients with unexplained infertility demonstrated significantly lower concentrations of follicular selenium than those with tubal infertility or couples with male factor infertility. Higher levels of GPx activity were in follicles of oocytes that fertilized, as opposed to those that did not [18].

5.3. Polycystic Ovarian Syndrome

Polycystic ovary syndrome (PCOS) is a syndrome of ovarian dysfunction and infertility. Since it was first reported in 1935, PCOS remains a syndrome but not a disease and no single criterion is sufficient for clinical diagnosis [40]. PCOS also remains a diagnosis of exclusion. Known disorders that mimic the PCOS phenotype should be excluded. The Rotterdam consensus for the diagnosis of PCOS states that two out of the following three criteria must be present: 1) Oligo-ovulation or anovulation, 2) hyperandrogenism and/or hyper-androgenemia, and 3) polycystic ovaries; other etiologies, such as congenital adrenal hyperplasia, androgen-secreting tumors, hypothalamic amenorrhea, hyperprolactinemia, thyroid disease, acromegaly, and Cushing's syndrome, should be excluded. A number of studies have investigated the roles of ROS in PCOS and the results are summarized in tables 1 and 2.

Oxidative Stress in Female Reproduction

Table 1. ROS biomarkers in PCOS patients

Biomarkers	Reference	PCOS patients	Controls	Unit
Malondialdehyde (MDA)	Kuşçu et al., 2009 [27]	0.12*	0.10	n/a
	Sabuncu et al., 2001 [41]	70.9*	62.5	µmol/mol Hb
	Zhang et al., 2008 [52]	12.313*	6.932	µmol/L
	Karadeniz et al., 2008 [25]	5.38	4.475	nmol.mL
Protein carbonyl (PC)	Fenkci et al. [17]	18.01 *	14.19	nmol/L
Nitric oxide (NO)	Nácul et al. [37]	11.5	10.2	µmol/L
	Karadeniz et al., 2008 [25]	9.18	9.21	µmol/L

*p<0.05

Table 2. Antioxidant biomarkers in PCOS patients

Biomarkers	Literature	PCOS patients	Controls	Unit
Total antioxidant capacity (TAC)	Fenkci et al., 2007 [17]	1.15	1.30*	mmol/L
	Verit et al., 2008 [48]	1.8*	1.1	mmol Trolox Eq/L
Superoxide dismutase (SOD)	Kuşçu et al., 2009 [27]	8.0*	7.28	n/a
	Sabuncu et al., 2001 [41]	94.62*	86.53	MU/molHb
	Zhang et al., 2008 [52]	67.32	113.82*	µU/mL
Glutathione peroxidase (GPx)	Sabuncu et al., 2001 [41]	2.88	2.98	MU/molHb
Glutathione (GSH)	Sabuncu et al., 2001 [41]	0.39	0.44*	mol/molHb
	Karadeniz et al., 2008 [25]	10.3*	6.447	Mmol/L

*p<0.05

The results of these studies suggest an association between oxidative stress and PCOS. While the majority of findings are in fair agreement across studies, results may vary as a function of body-mass index, age, degree of insulin resistance, presence of cardiovascular disease, etc. Sabuncu et al. showed that characteristic increases in OS biomarkers and perturbed antioxidant enzyme activities occur in PCOS patients prior to any signs of cardiovascular disease. Fenkci et al. suggested further that decreased antioxidant status and augmented OS may contribute to the increased risk of cardiovascular disease in women with PCOS.

5.4. Oxidative Damage to Ovaries and the Induction of Menopause

Robust SOD activity may be necessary for induction of the AD4-binding protein (AD4BP), a steroidogenesis transcription factor, in ovarian theca and granulosa cells. AD4BP assists in the production of estrogen and progesterone, two essential hormones of the female reproductive system. SOD activity may also influence the function of thecorpus luteum, the tissue that is formed from ruptured follicular cells during each menstrual cycle. The corpus luteum secretes progesterone, the sex hormone responsible for preparing the endometrial lining implantation and pregnancy. SOD activity was demonstrated to be highest during the beginning and middle stages of the luteal phase, commensurate with maximal rates of progesterone secretion. SOD activity and progesterone production decline in parallel during the late luteal phase prior to menstruation. The adverse effects of ROS on epithelial cells surrounding oocytes have been linked to the development of cancer. Most ovarian cancers originate from damage to epithelial cell DNA that normally undergoes repair during the luteal phase [36]. In a study by Murdoch et. al., in humans ands ewes, ovulation-related ovarian epithelial cell damage was assessed by measuring levels of 8-oxoguanine, a marker of oxidative DNA damage [36]. The investigators found that vitamin E administration significantly attenuates 8-oxoguanine concentrations and enhances tumor suppressor responses in these cells [36]. The authors concluded that malignant transformation in ovarian epithelial cells may forestalled by antioxidant exposure.

Perimenopause represents a 4-5 year period of declining estrogen levels, whichends when the menstrual cycle has been arrested for twelve consecutive months (menopause) [35]. Menopause occurs at mean age 51 and is associated with hot flashes, osteoporosis, and cardiovascular disease. Oxidative stress is thought to play a role in the induction of menopause and its major complications [35]. Estrogen, a steroid hormone with documented antioxidant properties, is abundantin premenopausal women, where it protects against cardiovascular disease, in part, by inhibiting the oxidation oflow density lipoproteins [35].Menopause related oxidative stress has also been invoked in the pathogenesis of osteoporosis and the development of hot flashes [28].

Oxidative stress markers are elevated and antioxidant defenses are diminished in post-menoapausal women relative to pre-menopausal controls [43]. For example, post-menopausal women exhibit increased circulating levels of MDA, 4-hydroxynenal, and oxidized lipoproteins concomitant with suppressed GPx activity relative to pre-menopausal values [43]. Antioxidants may be beneficial to postmenopausal women in multiple ways. Consumption of foods rich in vitamins C and E may diminish the risk of cardiovascular mortality in postmenopausal women [31]. A study performed by Meydani in 1999 showed that high dietary levels of vitamins C and E may decrease the risk of cardiovascular events by scavengingfree radicals, and attenuating LDL oxidation, platelet aggregation, and the production of inflammatory cytokines [31]. Health benefits accruing from the supplementation of the post-menopausal diet with soy food and soymilk have been attributed to the high levels of phytoestrogens contained within these foods [31]. Studies have shown that increasing levels of soy compounds suppress levels of oxidized low density lipopoteins, thereby decreasing the incidence of cardiovascular disease [31]. Interestingly, augmented soy intake may also contribute to diminished vertebral bone loss, improved vasodilation, and amelioration of hot flashes in postmenopausal women [28].

6. Oxidative Stress and Embryonic Development

Oxidative stress may severely disrupt the biochemical microenvironments required for normal embryo. In mouse embryos, elevated lipid peroxidation markers correlate with inhibition of embryo growth beyond the two-cell stage and developmental arrest [44]. As mentioned earlier, semen incubated with peritoneal fluid of women with endometriosis exhibits enhanced DNA fragmentation and resultant embryotoxicity [29]. Relative to the nuclear genome, mitochondrial DNA has greater susceptibility to damage by ROS due to lack of histones and other protective mechanisms. Altered mitochondrial DNA can retard embryonic growth, deplete ATP, and engender apoptosis. Furthermore, a rise in ROS may inactivate enzymes critical for life-sustaining biochemical reactions [29]. Antioxidant concentrations are reportedly sub-normal in fragmented embryos, further implicating ROS in the etiopathogenesis of arrested embryonic development [29].

7. Oxidative Stress: Mechanistic Implications for Teratogenesis

Redox-sensitive signal transduction pathways are important for developmental processes, and teratogens may induce teratogenesis through the misregulation of such pathways. Generation of ROS may cause detrimental alterations in the development of the embryo and fetus through cellular lipid, protein, and DNA damage. Cell death or modification, mitotic arrest or delay, and gene-enzyme inhibition may have deleterious effects on growth, differentiation, and morphology, leading to altered organ and tissue development. Postnatal consequences include developmental disease and structurally malformed or functionally incompetent offspring.

Ionizing radiation, hypoxia, alcohol, and cigarette use can lead to teratogenicity. Studies have shown that one of the main mechanisms of fetal damage induced by these factors is embryonic oxidative stress. Tobacco contains ROS and free radical generators, and Graffian follicles of women who actively smoke manifest evidence of impaired redox homeostasis [43]. Cigarette smoking correlates with the intensity of lipid peroxidation in the mature ovarian follicle, and follicular fluid antioxidant status is compromised in smokers [10]. Unfertilized eggs from IVF-embryo transfer in patients who smoke show high diploidy, implying that meiotic immaturity of oocytes is related to smoking and oxidative stress. Similarly, smoking mothers exhibit elevated risk for trisomy [43].

An increase in the occurrence of congenital abnormalities is associated with an age-related decline of oocyte quality. The aging of oocytes correlates with increased levels of oxidative stress, which adversely impacts biochemical pathways subserving pre- and post-implantation embryo development. Disturbances in the latter, in turn, may promote congenital anomalies, behavioral alterations, and learning disabilities.

Diabetes, as mentioned previously, also plays a role in teratogenesis. Congenital anomalies among infants of diabetic mothers occur at a two- to five fold increased rate relative to non-diabetic controls [43]. This teratogenicity mainly targets the central nervous system and the heart. The latter comprise 40% of the perinatal mortality and morbidity associated with pregestational diabetes, but the teratological processes in diabetic pregnancy remain unclear [43]. Arachidonic acid and prostaglandin modifications stimulated by diabetes may contribute to the teratogenesis. Cyclo-oxygenase (COX)-2 activity and COX suppression can hinder morphogenesis, and oxidative stress induced by hyperglycemia may encourage development of congenital malformations.

Placental oxidative stress may also induce teratogenesis. Abnormal placentation may cause enhanced placental oxidative stress, and the inability of the developing embryo to cope with that stress may result in death or congenital anomalies. One way this can occur is through severely impaired trophoblast invasion, which can lead to incomplete plugging of spiral arteries and premature maternal intervillous circulation. The embryo normally develops in a low oxygen environment and this sudden and widespread circulation in the placenta, which takes place around 10-12 weeks of gestation when trophoblast plugs are dislodged, can lead to syncytiotrophoblastic oxidative damage [6]. At this stage of development, the syncytiotrophoblasts lack expression of catalase and MnSODs rendering them vulnerable to oxidative insults. Syncytiotrophoblast degeneration can lead to various congenital anomalies. It increases oxygen tension in the intervillous space at the end of the first trimester. Also, the placenta produces ROS including NO, carbon monoxide, and peroxynitrite. The resulting oxidative stress may predispose to embryonic cytoplasmic fragmentation and apoptosis [7]. Irregular blastocyst apoptosis may result in embryonic death, abortions, or fetal congenital malformations.

By affecting key cellular organelles required for rapid cell division, ROS impedes the development of embryos. Aggregation of cytoskeletal components, condensation of the endoplasmic reticulum, and decreased membrane fluidity which affects embryo cleavage, can occur. Elevated levels of H_2O_2 have been specifically implicated in embryo fragmentation.

8. Oxidative Stress and *in Vitro* Fertilization/ Intracytoplasmic Sperm Injection Outcomes

Oxidative stress generation in IVF culture media may harm post-fertilization development by impacting such cell cleavage rates and blastocyst yield and quality [7]. Sources of ROS in the IVF setting include, but may not be limited to, oocytes, cumulus cell mass, leukocytes, and spermatozoa [13]. ROS may adversely impact sperm-oocyte fusion and fertilization [1]. Concentrations of ROS are higher in embryos cultured *in vitro* compared to those growing *in vivo*.

In assisted reproduction, exogenous sources of ROS include high ambient oxygen concentrations, metal ions, visible light, and dead spermatozoa [13]. The latter contain amine oxidases that catabolize spermine and spermidine, generating H_2O_2 among other products. Spermatozoa are especially susceptible to damage induced by ROS because their plasma membranes contain a large amount of polyunsaturated fatty acids. Also, their cytoplasm is relatively deficient in free radical scavenging enzymes [5]. Embryo development and pregnancy rates may be compromised by time and number of sperm exposed to the oocyte [25].

Visible light induces photodynamic stress, which can cause oxidative damage to unsaturated lipids and sterols within cell membranes. Momentary exposure to light is sufficient to increase significantly H_2O_2 in mouse embryos. Atmospheric oxygen concentrations in the *in vitro* setting are higher than those within the fallopian tubes. ROS generation has been shown to increase under atmospheric oxygen concentration in mouse embryos, and reducing oxygen concentration is associated with enhanced embryo development.

Prolonged sperm-oocyte co-incubation time increases ROS generation. The media composition also plays a major role in the oxidant status of oocytes and preimplantation embryos. O_2 levels are greater in the atmosphere compared to those within culture medium, which leads to increased oxidative insults to the oocytes/embryos in *vitro*. This may lead to two-cell block and embryonic arrest or termination [21].

Relative to patients with unsuccessful pregnancy outcomes, those whose ART procedures yielded viable pregnancies exhibited increased mean levels of GPx activity in follicular fluid and higher total antioxidant capacity (TAC) in day-1 culture media. Elevated day-1 ROS levels in culture media also correlated with late embryonic development, high fragmentation, and morphologically irregular blastocysts [6]. Despite the latter observations, one study suggested that a minimum concentration of follicular fluid ROS is essential for normal pregnancy to ensue.

Gas in culture media balances neutral and ionic bicarbonate concentrations and is important for *in vitro* fertilization In the presence of gametes, oxygen tension in healthy oviducts and uteri is 2%-8%. Overproduction of free radicals may result from elevated oxygen levels (>20%) [26]. Low oxygen concentrations may enhance embryo growth, and improved embryo morphology has been observed in embryos cultured in 5% oxygen (physiological levels) compared to 20% oxygen [26].

Infertile donors exhibit significantly higher levels of spermatozoa with damaged DNA compared with fertile ones [43]. Abnormal chromatin packaging, oxidative stress, and apoptosis are three of many proposed mechanisms to explain the damaged DNA [43]. In cryopreservation, frozen-thawed semen usually affects sperm parameters. Cryopreservation and ROS have been shown to lead to DNA instability in ram sperm.

In ART such as intrauterine insemination (IUI) or IVF, fertilization of "bad sperm" is not possible and avoided because of collateral peroxidative damage to the sperm plasma membrane. However, intracytoplasmic sperm injection (ICSI) circumvents this by direct introduction of the sperm into the oocyte, which evades the natural selection barrier. This can lead to poor results, as the spermatozoa with DNA damage are able to access the egg [30].

9. ROS and *In Vitro* Maturation of Oocytes (IVM)

In vitro maturation (IVM) represents the *in vitro* advancement of an oocyte from the diplotene stage of prophase I to metaphase II. It includes cytoplasmic maturation that encompasses a set of cellular events that have yet to be better defined. IVM is the technique of allowing the ovarian follicles to mature *in vitro*. The same pool of follicles experiences folliculogenesis, oocyte selection, and development in the ovary. As the ovary ages, follicle numbers and quality decrease. IVM can aid in conservation of these scarce follicles as well as production of large quantities of mature oocytes. The major challenge of IVM is relatively low reproductive outcomes. The role of ROS in IVM is controversial. In a study in which cumulus-oocyte complexes (COCs) were matured and SOD, GPx, and catalase activities were measured spectrophotometrically, the enzymes were significantly decreased in denuded oocytes compared with cumulus-intact oocytes. These findings implicate the aforementioned enzymes as key scavengers of ROS during IVM. Cumulus cells also play an important role in protecting oocytes against apoptosis induced by oxidative stress through increasing GSH content in oocytes during IVM.

Oocyte maturation *in vitro* differs from that *in vivo* [3]. A study of bovine oocyte maturation showed that oocytes fertilized *in vivo* yielded a higher number of blastocysts than those fertilized *in vitro*. Another study showed that morulae and blastocysts resulted only from *in vivo*-matured, *in vitro* fertilized oocytes as opposed to *in vitro*-matured, *in vivo* fertilized oocytes [15]. IVM has not yet resulted in favorable outcomes. Successful IVM involves the coordinated maturation of the nucleus and cytoplasm. Reproducing *in vivo* conditions is important in IVM. *In vivo*, gonadotropins, oocyte-cumulus oocyte cell interactions, and various enzyme activities contribute to the intricate process of oocyte maturation. CuZnSOD, MnSOD, and GPx are pivotal players in this process. Procuring, culturing and maturing undeveloped oocytes obviates complications of stimulated cycles and increases the availability of oocytes for ART.

Cellular metabolism and external factors contribute to ROS levels in the culture media. Specifically, ambient oxygen concentration, oocyte handling, visible light, and oocyte metabolism are all known to impact media ROS generation [15]. In the absence of adequate antioxidant defense mechanisms, oocytes are at increased risk for DNA damage or heightened apoptosis rates. Nitric oxide levels in follicular fluid have not been shown to correlate with oocyte maturity or quality. Differences in NO concentrations within follicular fluid among small, medium, and large follicles were not apparent. Poor oocyte quality, however, has been associated with elevated TNFα concentrations in the follicular fluid. TNFαis a cytokine that can induce inflammation as well as programmed cell death. Follicular fluid of oocytes that have been fertilized express significantly higher levels of baseline TAC [2]. Nitrite and nitrate levels were lower in the follicular fluid of follicles containing mature oocytes that had been fertilized compared to those that had not [7].

Data concerning the role of redox balance in meiotic progression are contradictory. During maturation, oocytes face a relatively high risk for aneuploidy. During oocyte development, oxidative stress induces aneuploidy, and it is associated with infertility related to maternal aging [43]. Also, unfertilized oocytes derived from smoking IVF-embryo transfer patients manifest comparatively higher levels of diploidy [43].

Cumulus cells during *in vitro* oocytematuration in cows, as well as in IVM in hamsters produce GSH [18]. Cumulus cells augment the GSH content of oocytes and the latter's defense against OS-related apoptosis. In the human metaphase II oocyte, there is robust expression of CuZnSOD, MnSOD and GPx mRNA. The latter two were also disclosed in the germinal vesicle stage, implying that these enzymes may be markers for oocyte maturation. These findings implicate oxidative stress in oocyte maturation. The oviductal fluid contains GSH, which may play a role in embryo development. Secreted GSH would protect oocytes from the increased ROS levels, which are found during ovulation [18]. During IVM of mouse oocytes, the addition of antioxidants to the culture media significantly decreases the burden of chromosomal abnormalities. Ascorbic acid, urate, isoglavones, taurine, hypotaurine, genistein, and *a*-tocopherol may be particularly useful in this regard.

10. Oral Antioxidants: Therapeutic Considerations

10.1. Endometriosis and Female Infertility

Antioxidant supplementation in the treatment of endometriosis and associated infertility is prevalent in the literature. Antioxidants such as catalase, SOD, GPx, and various types of vitamins, have demonstrated their ability to decrease oxidative stress markers. Injections of SOD and catalase have been shown to prevent the development of endometriotic peritoneal lesions in rabbits. Mier-Cabrera et al., supplemented the diets of women suffering from endometriosis-associated infertility with vitamins C and E [32, 33]. In these women, levels of MDA and lipid hydrperoxides were attenuated by the 4th and 6th months post-treatment, respectively. Women were also examined for conception and delivery of a healthy fetus every three months for a total of nine months after the study had ended. Although women who received antioxidant supplementation had better pregnancy rates, the results did not reach significance [32, 33].

In a second study conducted by the same group, the dietary intake of vitamins A, C, E, zinc, and copper was found to be lower in women with endometriosis than in non-affected controls [32, 33]. Placement of the former on a high antioxidant diet enriched for fruits, vegetables, and seeds resulted ina decline in MDA and lipid hydroperoxide concentrations and enhanced antioxidant levels (25% increase in GPx and 40% elevation in SOD activities) within 3 months of treatment. *These data suggest a possible role for antioxidant therapy in the management of endometriosis.*

10.2. ROS and Idiopathic Infertility

Oxidative stress and ROS have been implicated in the pathogenesis of idiopathic (unexplained) infertility. 8-hydroxy-2'-deoxyguanosine and hexano-lysine, markers of oxidative DNA damage and lipid peroxidation, respectively, were found to be increased in the follicular fluid of women with damaged oocytes and could be attenuated by administration of melatonin and vitamin E [44].

Moreover, melatonin treatment of women who failed to become pregnant in a previous IVF cycle resulted in 11 out of 56 patients becoming pregnant in a subsequent IVF cycle [44]. This contrast with only 6 pregnancies out of 59 control women not receiving melatonin. Melatonin also protected oocytes against the adverse effects of H_2O_2 *in vitro* [44]. Taken together, the results of these studies have prompted some investigators to advocate antioxidant therapy for patients with idiopathic infertility.

10.3. Assisted Reproduction

A randomized, controlled, multi-centre study evaluating the effect of vitamin C supplementation in pregnant women with luteal phase defects demonstrated that pregnancy rates were significantly higher in the treatment group compared to controls [5]. This may provide rationale for the use of vitamin C therapy for ART purposes. Another study demonstrated that patients supplemented with vitamin C had higher vitamin C concentrations in their follicular fluid. The pregnancy rate was elevated in the supplemented group compared to the control group, although the difference (34.2% compared to 23.7%) was not statistically significant [2].

Further evidence is required before antioxidant supplementation should be routinely prescribed in this context. Although mothers with increased plasma vitamins C and E levels had newborns with the greatest birth weights and heights [5], administration of vitamin C may not always be innocuous as the compound may behave as a pro-oxidant and actually promote infertility at high concentrations. .

In animal studies, oral antioxidants have been shown to mediate adverse effects on ovarian and uterine function and reproductive fitness. Oocyte and embryo exposure to ROS produces negative results similar to those of female aging on the quantity and quality of oocytes. Giving mice oral antioxidants has been shown to counteract these negative results [14].

In a double-blind, placebo-controlled pilot study, patients supplemented with vitamin E, iron, zinc, selenium, and L-arginine demonstrated significantly improved ovulation, mean mid-luteal progesterone levels, and pregnancy rates compared to the placebo group [5]. Multivitamin/mineral supplementation during natural pregnancy may also curtail sister chromatic exchange (SCE) rates in the final trimester mediated by steroid hormone-related ROS. *The type, dosage, and duration of antioxidant therapy will require further study before these agents can be safely integrated into routine clinical practice for the management of human infertility.*

10.4. Preeclampsia

Antioxidants have been proposed as a possible solution in the prevention of preeclampsia (see above) but this remains highly controversial. In one clinical trial, antioxidant supplementation of women at high risk for preeclampsia did not diminish the incidence of this condition. In fact, complications including gestational hypertension and low birth weight and the requirement for intravenous antihypertensive medications and magnesium sulfate were more frequent in the antioxidant-treated group [6].

On the other hand, another study determined that vitamin C and E supplementation at 16-22 weeks of pregnancy reduced the incidence of preeclampsia by over 50% relative to untreated controls [5]. Further investigation into the role of antioxidants in the management of preeclampsia is clearly warranted.

11. Strategies to Modulate the Influence of ROS

11.1. Amelioration of Oxidative Stress during *In Vitro* Fertilization/ Intracytoplasmic Sperm Injection

Various strategies have been promulgated to modulate antioxidants and ameliorate oxidative stress during *in vitro* fertilization/intracytoplasmic sperm injection. Spermatozoa used to inseminate oocytes *in vitro* are major contributors of ROS [10].

Although in ICSI only a single spermatozoon is employed, ROS are known to impact the ICSI procedure implicating other potential sources of ROS. Another factor to be considered are the long insemination times. This may increase the possibility of oxidative damage by prolonging the time oocytes are exposed to spermatozoa [10]. Some laboratory investigations have demonstrated beneficial results in IVF by reducing insemination time, while other reports have found no differences. The reduction of pO_2 from 20% to 5% in the mouse model has been linked to improvement of *in vitro* embryo development as well as prevention of the two-cell block [10].

Substandard spermatozoa can release ROS as well as spermine and spermidine, which can promote H_2O_2 production and oxidative damage. Lower sperm concentrations have been reported to enhance fertilization, implantation, embryo quality, and pregnancy rates [10]. Supplementation with catalase or α-tocopherol may protect components of IVF media from lipid peroxidation. Whether such intervention will translate into better pregnancy outcomes remains to be ascertained.

11.2. Optimizing *In Vitro* Culture Media to Overcome Oxidative Stress in Oocyte IVM

Commercial media used during IVF can generate ROS at different rates, depending on their chemical composition. ROS may accumulate at an accelerated pace in culture media lacking antioxidant protection and promote damage to spermatozoa, oocytes, and embryos. Addition of antioxidants to *in vitro* media neutralizes ROS-induced damage and helps preserve spermatozoa and embryo quality [31].

Antioxidants, such as vitamin C, have been shown to enhance the rate of blastocyst development in the mouse embryo model [7] and may combat OS affecting menopause [34]. Furthermore, by simply lowering ambient oxygen tension (e.g. to 5%), blastulation rates of human embryos increased by over 58% [6].

Implantation and clinical pregnancy rates have been demonstrated to be improved when antioxidant-supplemented media are employed in comparison with standard media [2]. However, one must consider that antioxidants may interact with metal ions to *exacerbate* ROS production via Fenton and Haber-Weiss reactions. Media additives may include albumin, which displays potent antioxidant properties.

However, serum preparations may contain abundant amine oxidases, which further contribute to H_2O_2 generation [10]. Adding metal-chelating agents to media could theoretically mitigate oxidant production, although the clinical risks and benefits of this will require stringent empirical testing [5].

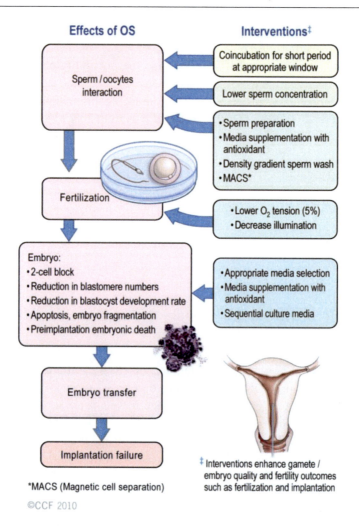

Figure 3. Effects of oxidative stress and interventions to overcome its effects at different ART steps.

Addition of various antioxidants such as beta-mercaptoethanol, taurine, hypotaurine, vitamin E and vitamin C to *in vitro* culture media has been demonstrated to decrease blastocyst degeneration, increase blastocyst development rates and hatching, and reduce embryo apoptosis (Figure 3) [9, 3]. 3 Beta-mercaptoethanol administration may also augment GSH concentrations. Ethylene diaminetetraacetic acid (EDTA) and transferrin may confer protection against developmental arrests.

11.3. Sperm Preparation Techniques for Assisted Reproduction

Inefficient spermatogenesis in men can lead to excessive ROS generation, permeabilization of the plasma membrane and DNA fragmentation. Several approaches may be invoked to circumvent this type of damage (see also previous Chapter). The most common techniques are density gradient centrifugation, swim-up, and one-step wash. Double density gradient centrifugation is useful for isolating mature, leukocyte-free spermatozoa. Seminal plasma is antioxidant-rich and protects spermatozoa from DNA damage and lipid peroxidation [10]. When N-tert-butyl hydroxylamine and SOD/catalase mimetics were added to IVF media, the breakdown of sperm chromatin was blocked [9]. Studies indicate that repeated cycles of centrifugation significantly enhance ROS production in sperm [6]. It is thought that the centrifugation time has a greater impact on ROS generation than the actual force of centrifugation.

Conclusions

Oxidative stress affects multiple physiological processes essential for normal reproductive health in women. ROS impact events across the entire reproductive lifespan from oocyte maturation to fertilization, pregnancy and the menopause. Oxidative stress has been heavily implicated in female infertility and ART outcomes. It appears to also play significant roles in the etiopathogenesis of conditions such as hydatidiform mole, preeclampsia, polycystic ovarian syndrome, and endometriosis, which contribute to poor pregnancy outcomes and fetal morbidity.

Female reproductive tissues produce large amounts of ROS due to steroidogenesis and metabolism [18]. ROS serve as key signal molecules in physiological processes in the female reproductive tract, but they also exacerbate numerous pathological states. Antioxidant supplementation for these reproductive disorders is currently the subject of intense debate and the results to date are controversial. Attempts to simulate physiological redox homeostasis in oocyte IVM, IVF, ICSI, manipulation of culture media, and sperm preparation remain challenging but offer hope for improved ART outcomes.

References

[1] Ali AA, Bilodeau JF, Sirard MA. Antioxidant requirements for bovine oocytes varies during in vitro maturation, fertilization, and development. *Theriogenology*, 2003;59: 939-949.

[2] Allamaneni SS, Agarwal A. Role of free radicals in female reproductive diseases and assisted reproduction. *Reproductive BioMedicine Online,* 2004;9: 338-347.

[3] Agarwal A, Gupta S. The role of free radicals and antioxidants in female infertility and assisted reproduction. *US Genito-Urinary Disease* 2006: 60-5.

[4] Agarwal A, Gupta S. *Role of reactive oxygen species in female reproduction.* Part 1. Oxidative stress: a general overview. AgroFOOD Industry Hi-tech 2005;16: 21-5.

[5] Agarwal A, Gupta S. *Role of reactive oxygen species in female reproduction and the effects of antioxidant supplementation* - Part 2. AgroFOOD Industry Hi-tech 2005;16: 38-41.

[6] Agarwal A, Gupta S, Sekhon L, Shah R. Redox considerations in female reproductive function and assisted reproduction: From molecular mechanisms to health implications. *Antioxidants and Redox Signaling* 2008;10: 1375-1403.

[7] Agarwal A, Gupta A, Sharma R. Oxidative stress and its implications in female infertility a clinician's perspective. *Reproductive BioMedicine Online,* 2005;11: 641-650.

[8] Agarwal A, Gupta A, Sharma RK. Role of oxidative stress in female reproduction. *Reproductive Biology and Endocrinology* 2005;3: 1-21.

[9] Agarwal A, Gupta A, Sikka S. The role of free radicals and antioxidants in reproduction. *Current Opinion in Obstetrics and Gynecology,* 2006;18: 325-332.

[10] Agarwal A, Said TM, Bedaiwy MA, Banerjee J, Alvarez JG. Oxidative stress in an assisted reproductive techniques setting. *Fertility and Sterility,* 2006;86: 503-512.

[11] Arumugam K, Yip YC. Endometriosis and infertility: the role of exogenous lipid peroxides in the peritoneal fluid. *Fertil. Steril.* 1995;63: 198-9.

[12] Arumugam K, Yip YC. De novo formation of adhesions in endometriosis: the role of iron and free radical reactions." *Fertil. Steril.* 1995;64: 62-4.

[13] Attaran M, Pasqualotto E, Falcone T, Goldberg JM, Miller KF, Agarwal A, Sharma RK. The effect of follicular fluid reactive oxygen species on the outcome of in vitro fertilization. *International Journal of Fertility,* 2000;45: 314-320.

[14] Carbone MC, Tatone C, Monache SD, Marci R, Caserta D, Colonna R, Amicarelli F. Antioxidant enzymatic defences in human follicular fluid: characterization and age-dependent changes. *Molecular Human Reproduction,* 2003;9: 639-643.

[15] Combelles CM, Gupta S, Agarwal A. Could oxidative stress influence the in-vitro maturation of oocytes? *Reproductive BioMedicine Online,* 2009;18: 864-880.

[16] Defrere S, Van Langendonckt A, et al. Iron overload enhances epithelial cell proliferation in endometriotic lesions induced in a murine model. *Hum. Reprod.* 2006;21: 2810-2816.

[17] Fenkci V, Fenkci S, Yilmazer M, Serteser M. Decreased total antioxidant status and increased oxidative stress in women with polycystic ovary syndrome may contribute to the risk of cardiovascular disease. *Fertility and Sterility,* 2003;80:123-7.

[18] Fujii J, Iuchi Y, and Okada F. Fundamental roles of reactive oxygen species and protective mechanisms in the female reproductive system. *Reproductive Biology and Endocrinology,* 2005;3: 43.

[19] Gonzalez-Ramos R, Donnez J, et al. Nuclear factor-kappa B is constitutively activated in peritoneal endometriosis. *Mol. Hum. Reprod.* 2007;13: 503-509.

[20] Guérin P, MouatassimSEl, Ménézo Y. Oxidative stress and protection against reactive oxygen species in the pre-implantation embryo and its surroundings. *Human Reproduction Update.* 2001;7: 175-189.

[21] Gupta S, Agarwal A, et al. Role of oxidative stress in endometriosis. *Reprod Biomed Online,* 2006;13: 126-134.

[22] Harma M, Harma M Erel O. Increased oxidative stress in patients with hydatidiform mole. *Swiss Med. Wkly,* 2003; 133:563-6.

[23] Joshi SR, Mehendale SS, Dangat KD, Kilari AS, Yadav HR, Taralekar VS. (2008). High maternal plasma antioxidant concentrations associated with preterm delivery. *Annals of Nutrition and Metabolism,* 2008;53: 276-282.

[24] Jurisicova A, Rogers I, Fasciani A, Casper RF, Varmuza S. Effect of maternal age and conditions of fertilization on programmed cell death during murine preimplantation embryo development. *Molecular Human Reproduction,* 1998;4: 139-145.

[25] Karadeniz M, Erdoğan M, Tamsel S, et al. Oxidative Stress Markers in Young Patients with Polycystic Ovary Syndrome, The Relationship between Insulin Resistances. *Experimental and Clinical Endocrinology and Diabetes*, 2008;116: 231-5.

[26] Krajcir N, Chowdary H, Gupta S, Agarwal A. Female infertility and assisted reproduction: impact of oxidative stress. *Current Women's Health Reviews* 2008;4: 9-15.

[27] Kuşçu NK, Var A. Oxidative stress but not endothelial dysfunction exists in non-obese, young group of patients with polycystic ovary syndrome. *Acta Obstetricia et Gynecologica Scandinavica,* 2009;88: 612-7.

[28] Leal M, Diaz J, et al. Hormone replacement therapy for oxidative stress in postmenopausal women with hot flushes. *Obstet. Gynecol.* 2000;95: 804-9.

[29] Mansour G, Aziz N, et al. The impact of peritoneal fluid from healthy women and from women with endometriosis on sperm DNA and its relationship to the sperm deformity index. *Fertil. Steril.* 2009;92: 61-7.

[30] Martin-Romero FJ, Miguel-Lasobras EM, Dominguez-Arroyo JA, González-Carrera E, Alvarez IS. Contribution of culture media to oxidative stress and its effect on human oocytes. *Reproductive BioMedicine Online,* 2008;17: 652-661.

[31] Meydani, M. Dietary antioxidants of aging and immune endothelial cell interaction. *Mech. AgingDev.* 1999; 11: 123-132.

[32] Mier-Cabrera J, Aburto-Soto T, et al. Women with endometriosis improved their peripheral antioxidant markers after the application of a high antioxidant diet. *Reprod. Biol. Endocrinol.* 2009;7: 54.

[33] Mier-Cabrera J, M. Genera-Garcia, et al. Effect of vitamins C and E supplementation on peripheral oxidative stress markers and pregnancy rate in women with endometriosis. *Int. J. Gynaecol. Obstet.* 2007;100: 252-6.

[34] Miquel J, Ramirez-Bosca A, et al. Menopause: A review on the role of oxygen stress and favorable effects of dietary antioxidants. *Archives of Gerontology and Geriatrics,* 2006; 42: 289–306.

[35] Moreau KL, DePaulis AR, et al. Oxidative stress contributes to chronic leg vasoconstriction in estrogen-deficient postmenopausal women. *J. Appl. Physiol.* 2007;102: 890-5.

[36] Murdoch W J, Martinchick JF. Oxidative damage to DNA of ovarian surface epithelial cells affected by ovulation: carcinogenic implication and chemoprevention. *Exp. Biol. Med.* 2004;229: 546-552.

[37] Nácul AP, Andrade CD, Schwarz P, de Bittencourt PIH, Spritzer PM. Nitric oxide and fibrinogen in polycystic ovary syndrome: Associations with insulin resistance and obesity. *European Journal of Obstetrics and Gynecology,* 2007;133: 191-6.

[38] Osborn B H, Haney AF, et al. Inducible nitric oxide synthase expression by peritoneal macrophages in endometriosis-associated infertility. *Fertil. Steril.* 2002;77: 46-51.

[39] Pasqualotto EB, Agarwal A, Sharma RK, Izzo VM, Pinotti JA, Joshi NJ, Rose BI. Effect of oxidative stress in follicular fluid on the outcome of assisted reproductive procedures. *Fertility and Sterility,* 2004;81(4): 973-6.

[40] The Rotterdam ESHRE/ASRM-sponsored PCOS consensus workshop group. Revised 2003 consensus on diagnostic criteria and long-term health risks related to polycystic ovary syndrome (PCOS). *Human Reproduction,* 2004;19: 41-7.

[41] Sabuncu T, Vural H, Harma M, Harma M. Oxidative stress in polycystic ovary syndrome and its contribution to the risk of cardiovascular disease. *Clinical Biochemistry*, 2001;34: 407-13.

[42] Sharma RK, Agarwal A. Role of reactive oxygen species in gynecologic diseases. *Reproductive Medicine and Biology*, 2004;3: 177-199.

[43] Signorelli SS, Neri S, et al. Behaviour of some indicators of oxidative stress in postmenopausal and fertile women. *Maturitas,* 2006;53: 77-82.

[44] Tamura H, Takasaki A, et al. Oxidative stress impairs oocyte quality and melatonin protects oocytes from free radical damage and improves fertilization rate. *J. Pineal. Res.* 2008;44: 280-7.

[45] Van Langendonckt A, Casanas-Roux F, et al. Iron overload in the peritoneal cavity of women with pelvic endometriosis. *Fertil. Steril.* 2002;78: 712-718.

[46] Van Langendonckt A, Casanas-Roux F, et al. Oxidative stress and peritoneal endometriosis. *Fertil. Steril.* 2002;77(5): 861-870.

[47] Van Langendonckt A, Casanas-Roux F, et al. Characterization of iron deposition in endometriotic lesions induced in the nude mouse model. *Hum. Reprod.* 2004;19: 1265-1271.

[48] Verit FF, Erel O. Oxidative stress in nonobese women with polycystic ovary syndrome: correlations with endocrine and screening parameters. *Gynecologic and Obstetric Investigation*, 2008;65: 233-9.

[49] Viatour P, Merville MP, et al. Phosphorylation of NF-kappaB and IkappaB proteins: implications in cancer and inflammation. *Trends Biochem. Sci.* 2004;30: 43-52.

[50] Wang Y, Sharma RK, et al. Importance of reactive oxygen species in the peritoneal fluid of women with endometriosis or idiopathic infertility. *Fertil. Steril.* 1997;68: 826-830.

[51] Yallampalli C, Dong YL, et al. Role and regulation of nitric oxide in the uterus during pregnancy and parturition. *J. Soc. Gynecol. Investig.* 1998;5: 58-67.

[52] Zhang D, Luo W, Liao H, Wang C, Sun Y. The effects of oxidative stress to PCOS. *Journal of Sichuan University Medical Science Edition* 2008;39: 421.

In: Principles of Free Radical Biomedicine, Volume III
Editors: K. Pantopoulos and H. M. Schipper

ISBN 978-1-61324-184-4
©2012 Nova SciencePublishers, Inc.

Chapter 15

Oxidative Stress in Exercise and Training

*Stelios Kokkoris[1], Theodoros Vassilakopoulos[1] and Sabah N. A. Hussain[2],**

[1]Department of Critical Care and Pulmonary Services, University of Athens Medical School, Evangelismos Hospital, Athens, Greece

[2]Meakins Christine Laboratories, McGill University and Critical Care and Respiratory Divisions, Royal Victoria Hospital, McGill University Health Centre, Montréal, Québec, Canada

1. Introduction

In the last 30 years, the role of reactive oxygen species (ROS) in exercise physiology has received considerable attention. Acute physical exercise induces production of ROS in skeletal muscle via different mechanisms. ROS formation during vigorous physical exertion can result in oxidative stress.

Moreover, the important role of ROS as signaling molecules has been unravelled. ROS modulate contractile function in unfatigued and fatigued skeletal muscle. Furthermore, involvement of ROS in the regulation of gene expression via redox-sensitive transcription pathways represents an important regulatory mechanism, involved in the process of training adaptation.

In this context, the adaptation of endogenous antioxidant systems in response to regular training reflects a potential mechanism responsible for augmented tolerance of skeletal muscle to exercise-induced stress.

---

*E-mail: sabah.hussain@muhc.mcgill.ca

2. Sources of Radicals during Exercise

There are many potential tissue sources of ROS during exercise; however, few studies have investigated the predominant tissues responsible for this production. This is likely due to both the restricted access to most tissues in humans and the complex nature of exercise physiology that involves many organ systems that are linked through the increased metabolic requirements of skeletal muscles. Hence, although many studies have examined whole body markers of free radical activity (such as the release of expired pentane originally reported by Dillard et al. [1]), the majority of reports have assumed that skeletal muscle represents the major source of ROS generation during exercise. It is, however, possible that, in some situations, other tissues such as the heart, lungs, or white blood cells may contribute significantly to total body generation of ROS.

Due to the invasive nature of obtaining tissue samples from exercising humans, many studies have examined whole body footprints of ROS activity. For example, increased lipid [2], DNA [3], and glutathione (GSH) oxidation and net peroxyl radical scavenging capacity (PSC) [4] can be observed in blood, although this has not been documented by all studies [5]. Some authors have suggested that common metabolic changes that occur during most exercise protocols, such as the increased release of catecholamines, may play a role in the increased ROS generation [6], but it is generally accepted that ROS generation occurs predominantly by contracting skeletal and heart muscles. In the following paragraphs, several potential production sites of ROS will be discussed.

2.1. Mitochondria

Mitochondria are generally considered the main site of ROS production in muscle cells [7, 8], and many authors have reiterated early reports that 2–5% of the total oxygen consumed by mitochondria may undergo one electron reduction with the generation of superoxide (O_2^-) [9, 10] (see also Vol. II, Chapter 15). Recent research has identified complexes I and III of the electron transport chain as the main sites of mitochondrial O_2^- production [11, 12]. In complex I, the main site of electron leakage to oxygen appears to be the iron-sulfur clusters, whereas in complex III it is the Q10 semiquinone [12]. Furthermore, complex III releases O_2^- from both sides of the inner mitochondrial membrane [12]. It is unclear if the O_2^- crosses the outer mitochondrial membrane or is dismutated by CuZnSOD located in the mitochondrial intermembrane space. It was initially assumed that the increased ROS generation (50- or 100-fold) that occurs during exercise-related contractile activity is directly related to the elevated oxygen consumption that occurs with increased mitochondrial activity [13, 14]. However, a recent report suggests that mitochondria may not be the dominant source of ROS during exercise [15], and further studies will be required to elucidate fully the role that mitochondria play in contraction-induced production of ROS in skeletal muscle. Brand and colleagues [16] have reassessed the production rate of ROS by mitochondria and concluded that the upper estimate of the total fraction of oxygen utilized that forms O_2^- was approximately 0.15%; this value is considerably lower than the original estimate of 2–5% [16]. This low rate of O_2^- production may implicate uncoupling proteins (specifically UCP3 in skeletal muscle) as regulators of mitochondrial production of ROS [17, 18], acting to protect mitochondria against oxidative damage. In addition, there has been considerable debate concerning the effect of changes in the respiratory state on ROS generation by mitochondria, with growing evidence suggesting that mitochondria produce more ROS during state 4 (basal) respiration compared to state 3 (maximal ADP-stimulated respiration) [18-22]. This is important because during aerobic contractile activity, skeletal muscle mitochondria are predominantly in state 3, and this may limit their generation of ROS during contractions [19-22]. *Overall, these findings suggest that mitochondria are not the primary source of ROS production in skeletal muscle during exercise.* The contribution of mitochondria to ROS production during exercise might be fiber-type specific. Type II skeletal muscle fibers possess unique properties that promote mitochondrial ROS production. Specifically, using an *in situ* approach to measure H_2O_2 release from mitochondria in permeabilized rat muscle fiber bundles, the mitochondrial ROS leak (i.e., H_2O_2 released/O_2 consumed) was two- to threefold greater in type II fibers compared with type I fibers [23]. The underlying mechanism remains unclear, but does not appear to be due to differences in mitochondrial glutathione peroxidase (GPx) activities between type I and II fibers [23].

2.2. Sarcoplasmic Reticulum

Studies have identified NAD(P)H oxidase enzymes associated with the sarcoplasmic reticulum (SR) of both cardiac [24] and skeletal muscle [25]. The O_2^- generated by these enzymes appears to influence calcium release by the SR through oxidation of the ryanodynereceptor [24]. The skeletal muscle enzyme described appears to use preferentially NADH as substrate [25]. Inhibitor studies have indicated that extracellular O_2^- release from stimulated myotubes was reduced by treatment with diphenyleneiodonium (DPI), a nonspecific inhibitor of NAD(P)H oxidases [26], although the NADH oxidase described by Xia et al. [25] is localized to the SR and hence seems unlikely to contribute to the extracellular release.

2.3. Transverse Tubules

The transverse tubules of skeletal muscle contain an NADP(H) oxidase whose activity is increased by depolarization [27, 28]. This enzyme appears to release O_2^- to the cytosol of skeletal muscle cells. Finally, this skeletal muscle-specific NADP(H) oxidase is inhibited by nonspecific inhibitors of this class of enzyme and by prevention of membrane depolarization.

2.4. Plasma Membrane

Several studies revealed that skeletal muscle cells release O_2^- into the extracellular space [26, 29-32]. All cells contain plasma membrane redox systems capable of performing electron transfer across the plasma membrane. An NAD(P)H oxidase complex is constitutively expressed in diaphragm and limb muscles of the rat and is localized to the plasma membrane [33]. The enzyme contains four of the subunits that are found in the enzyme in phagocytic cells ($gp91^{phox}$, $p22^{phox}$, $p47^{phox}$, and $p67^{phox}$), all of which are associated with the cell membrane [34]. Whether this complex predominantly releases O_2^- to the inside or the outside of the plasma membrane has not been definitely ascertained [33]. There are other plasma membrane redox systems that are capable of transferring electrons from intracellular reductants to appropriate extracellular electron acceptors, although no such system has been described in skeletal muscle [35]. Morre [36] has described external NADH oxidase (ECTO-NOX) proteins that exhibit a hydroquinone (NADH) oxidase activity and a protein disulfide-thiol exchange activity. The current view is that these systems accept electrons from the hydroquinones of the plasma membrane and can reduce a number of non-physiological (e.g., ferricyanide and WST-1) and physiological (e.g., protein thiols or oxygen) electron acceptors outside the cell, although oxygen is likely to be a major acceptor *in vivo* [37]. Transfer of electrons from cytosolic NAD(P)H to the plasma membranes has been proposed to occur through either NADH-cytochrome $b5$ oxidoreductase or NAD(P)H quinoneoxidoreductase (NQO1) [37]. Thus, through a series of linked steps, intracellular NAD(P)H can act as substrate for O_2^- generation on the cell surface. The relationship of these processes with skeletal muscle contractions has not been firmly established, but it is likely that these systems are activated during contractile activity or that the substrate level rises to increase electron transfer across the membrane through these systems. The characteristics of the release of O_2^- from skeletal muscle are compatible with the involvement of such pathways.

2.5. Phospholipase A2-Dependent Processes

Phospholipase A2 (PLA2) is an enzyme that cleaves membrane phospholipids to release arachidonic acid, which is a substrate for ROS-generating enzyme systems such as the lipoxygenases [38]. Also, activation of PLA2 can stimulate NAD(P)H oxidases [39], and increased PLA2 activity has been reported to stimulate ROS generation in muscle mitochondria [40] and cytosol [41] and to release ROS into the extracellular space [38]. Both calcium- dependent and independent forms of PLA2 participate in muscle ROS generation. The calcium-independent enzymes (iPLA2) have been shown to regulate cytosolic oxidant activity in skeletal muscle cells [41], while a 14-kDa calcium-dependent isoform (sPLA2) located within mitochondria may stimulate intracellular ROS generation during contractile activity [42]. In non-muscle cells, activity of the third major type of PLA2, cytosolic (cPLA2) that is activated by micromolar concentrations of calcium, has been associated with ROS generation [43]. Reid and colleagues [41] assumed that the calcium-independent PLA2 was a major determinant of ROS activity under resting conditions, whereas during contractions, heat stress, or other processes elevating intracellular calcium, the calcium-dependent PLA2 was activated and stimulated ROS production at supranormal rates.

2.6. Xanthine Oxidase

There has been considerable speculation concerning the role of xanthine oxidase in O_2^- generation by skeletal muscle. Currently, this conjecture is primarily based on the effects of the xanthine oxidase inhibitors allopurinol or oxypurinol [44, 45]. For instance, daily administration of allopurinol to long-distance cyclists during the Tour de France resulted in significant attenuation of plasma activity of creatine kinase and aspartate aminotransferase (indices of tissue damage) and reduction in plasma lipid peroxide levels [44]. Although rat skeletal muscles contain significant levels of xanthine oxidase [46], human skeletal muscle cells *per se* appear to possess low amounts of xanthine dehydrogenase or oxidase [47], although these enzymes will inevitably be present in associated endothelial cells.

In summary, there is clear evidence that O_2^- and H_2O_2 are generated in muscle cells during contractions, and more limited data indicate that hydroxyl radicals may be generated under more specific circumstances. The mitochondria have been considered as the predominant site of ROS generation during activity, yet a number of alternative potential sites of production have been identified. It is still unclear whether all of these sites contribute to the increased ROS levels observed during contractions or whether one site predominates over the others.

It is likely that the multiple sites of generation are active in different situations and that the effects of the ROS generated are relatively localized and important for different functions. For example, localized ROS generation by the sarcoplasmic reticulum or transverse tubule systems may be much more important for the regulation of sarcoplasmic reticulum calcium handling than ROS generated by mitochondria or extracellular oxidases.

3. Markers of Exercise-Induced Oxidative Stress

3.1. Lipidperoxidation

Dillardet al. [48] were the first to report increased expired pentane after 20 minutes of cycle ergometry of moderate intensity. In numerous subsequent studies, exercise-induced lipid peroxidation was assessed by measuring thiobarbituric acid reactive substances-malondialdehyde, lipid hydroperoxides, and F2-isoprostanes in blood, urine, expired air and various tissues, including skeletal muscle [49-53]; see also Vol. I, Chapter 7.

Although the majority of these studies were able to show that exercise induces lipid peroxidation in animal models as well as in humans, the results vary considerably [54]. This is likely due to the variability of exercise protocols and the methods used for assessing oxidative stress in the different studies.

3.2. Protein Oxidation

Initial results from Rezniket al. [55] demonstrated that rats subjected to exhaustive exercise accumulated reactive carbonyl derivates in skeletal muscle, indicating an increased rate of oxidative damage to proteins (see Vol. I, Chapter 6). Similar results were obtained in the hind legs of rats following a three-month period of endurance exercise, which consisted of treadmill running lasting two hours, 3 days a week [56]. Interestingly, immobilization similarly resulted in elevated protein oxidation [57]. The functional significance of exercise-induced protein oxidation in skeletal muscle is still unknown. Nevertheless, there is initial evidence that *protein oxidation may have the potential to exert suppressive effects on exercise performance by affecting contractile elements or by inhibiting enzymes, such as glyceraldehyde phosphate dehydrogenase or mitochondrial ATP synthase* [58].

3.3. DNA modifications

There is growing evidence that exercise is also capable of inducing oxidative modifications of the DNA (see Vol. I, Chapter 9). Most indices of exercise-induced oxidative DNA damage were obtained in peripheral leukocytes [59]. In addition, detection of elevated excretion rates of 8-hydroxy-deoxy-guanosine (8-OhdG) in urine after vigorous or cumulative endurance exercise confirmed the occurrence of oxidative DNA damage secondary to physical exertion [60]. However, analyzing urinary excretion of 8-OHdG does not allow any conclusions regarding the cells in which DNA damage occurs. Nevertheless, and as reflected by increased levels of 8-OHdG in muscle 24 hours after eccentric muscle exercise [61], exercise-related DNA damage does not seem to be restricted to immunocompetent cells. The functional significance of exercise-induced DNA damage is not completely understood and needs to be further elucidated. One may posit on theoretical grounds that accumulating oxidative damage to mitochondrial DNA in muscle cells due to repeated exercise may impact mitochondrial function, and therefore may result in disturbances in cellular energy supply.

4. Oxidative Stress and Physical Activity

4.1. Effects of Aerobic Exercise on ROS Production

In 1982, Davies et al. [62] were the first to show that exercise increases ROS production. Since then, numerous studies have investigated the effects of exercise on oxidative stress. Most of them were carried out using aerobic exercise protocols (running, cycling and swimming) [2, 63-70]. Aerobic exercise increases oxygen consumption (VO_2), which, in turn, may increase ROS production. Therefore, *many studies suggested that such physical activity enhances ROS production both in animals and in humans* [63-71]. However, this effect does not occur with exercise of low intensity (<50% VO_2 max). In this case, the antioxidant capacity is not exhausted and ROS-induced damage does not appear [69]. The greater the exercise intensity, the more robust is the ROS production and associated oxidative stress [67, 69]. This has been confirmed by studies showing correlations between VO_2 and oxidative stress. However, other studies failed to document oxidative stress after intense aerobic exercise [64, 67, 72, 73]. Such contradictory results could be explained by variable antioxidant nutritional status (which is not always controlled in studies), exercise intensity or training level. Notably, these latter studies recruited trained endurance athletes who are likely to be physiologically and biochemically more adept at preventing surges in exercise-related radical production [64, 67, 72, 73]. It should be emphasized that even trained subjects can exhibit oxidative stress [74, 75]. Furthermore, the disparate findings may also be attributed to differing methods used for the measurement of oxidative stress.

4.2. Effects of Anaerobic Exercise on ROS Production

Anaerobic exercise is encountered in various sport activities such as sprints, jumps or resistance training. Research regarding the production of ROS secondary to acute anaerobic exercise is sparse compared to aerobic exercise. However, relevant studies generally show increased oxidative stress after supramaximal anaerobic exercise such as intermittent running, sprints, jumps, resistance exercise (eccentric or concentric) or Wingate tests on a cycle ergometer [76-81].

During anaerobic exercise increased ROS production may be mediated through various pathways in addition to those observed during aerobic exercise [76, 77, 82]. Xanthine oxidase activity, ischemia-reperfusion and the phagocytic respiratory burst have been implicated in ROS production [82].

Moreover, the significant increases in lactic acid, catecholamines and post-exercise inflammation, characteristic of supramaximal anaerobic exercise, can contribute to the production of ROS [51, 82]. It seems plausible that ischemia-reperfusion of the active muscle is heavily involved in oxidative stress during and after anaerobic exercise [82]. Anaerobic exercise significantly enhances the catabolism of purines and induces rapid deoxygenation (associated with ischemia-reperfusion).

Both phenomena are known to increase the activity of xanthine oxidase, which accelerates ROS production [83, 84]. Xanthine oxidase has been demonstrated to generate ROS during ischemia-reperfusion, but direct evidence for its function as a free radical generator in muscle during exercise is lacking. In ischemic tissues, it has been proposed that xanthine dehydrogenase undergoes proteolytic conversion to the oxidase form, which uses O_2 as its electron acceptor [83, 84]. It is known that xanthine oxidase in the presence of the substrates hypoxanthine or xanthine reduces molecular oxygen to $O_2^{\cdot-}$ and H_2O_2. Recently, it has been demonstrated that the enzyme can further reduce H_2O_2 to $OH^{\cdot}$ [84]. The $OH^{\cdot}$ and $O_2^{\cdot-}$ radicals generated by the enzyme may, in turn, react with cellular proteins and membranes causing cellular injury [84].

Another source of ROS production during anaerobic exercise is inflammation and cellular damage, which often take place after intense exercise such as impact sports and eccentric exercises [76, 82, 85-87]. Iron liberation from hemoglobin or ferritin may amplify the inflammatory response and the oxidative stress [85]. Furthermore, a positive correlation between the increase of lactic acid and the rise of oxidative stress markers has been documented [51, 88].

5. Effects of Training on Oxidative Stress

5.1. Aerobic Training and ROS Production

The majority of studies show that endurance training reduces post-exercise oxidative stress and muscular damage [61, 64, 88-92]. These findings are in agreement with the widely-held belief that regular aerobic exercise acts against cell aging and carcinogenesis. This training effect can be sufficiently robust as to obviate oxidative stress in experienced triathletes despite significant triathlon-induced inflammation [93].

However, it has not yet been determined whether this resistance to oxidative stress during exercise after training accrues from a decrease in ROS production or from an increase in the efficiency of antioxidant defence systems.

5.2. Anaerobic Training and ROS Production

Few data concerning the effects of anaerobic training on oxidative stress are available. However, it has been shown that anaerobic-trained subjects develop less oxidative stress and less muscular damage after exercise compared to non-trained individuals [86, 94]. Moreover, these improvements are comparable to those observed in endurance-trained sportsmen [94]. It should be pointed out that these results are controversial, as other studies did not show reduced oxidative stress following an anaerobic training protocol [95, 96]. Methodological differences (population characteristics, training protocols, biological measurements) may explain some of these discrepancies.

5.3. Oxidative Stress and Overtraining

The training program aims to improve individual and team performance. However, it is often difficult to ascertain whether the program applied to individual athletes is well adapted to their physiological needs or engenders deleterious overtraining [97]. This overtraining syndrome is characterised by excessive fatigue, drop in performance and biological modifications [97, 98]. Prolonged periods of intense exercise training and/or intense competition are associated with a variety of hormonal, immunological, hematological and biochemical changes [98, 99]. However, studies on this subject are often contradictory [98]. A period of intense training is associated with decreased antioxidant capacity, increased ROS production and thus commensurate increases in oxidative stress [100]. Although no direct link has been established, the increased oxidative stress has been implicated in the pathogenesis of the overtraining syndrome [101, 102]. Oxidative stress may facilitate development of the overtraining syndrome by incurring cellular metabolic compromise (mitochondrial insufficiency) and muscle damage [101, 103]. In addition, the accumulation of muscular lesions due to overtraining is associated with inflammation (neutrophile activation and cytokine elaboration – see Vol. II, Chapter 21), which may further exacerbate local ROS production and tissue injury [103].

Conclusions

The first evidence that muscular exercise promotes oxidative damage in tissues appeared in 1978 [1]. Since this hallmark report, the field of ROS biology has evolved significantly, and our understanding of the sources and consequences of exercise-induced free radical production has increased markedly. *Current evidence suggests that contracting muscles produce ROS from a variety of cellular locations.* Furthermore, although mitochondria are a potential source of ROS in cells, growing evidence suggests that *these organelles may play less prominent roles in oxidant production by contracting skeletal muscles than was previously thought.* Many early studies investigating exercise and free radical production focused on the damaging effects of oxidants in muscle (e.g., lipid peroxidation). However, a new era in redox biology has risen with an ever-growing number of reports detailing the advantageous biological effects of free radicals. Indeed, it is now clear that ROS are involved in modulation of cell signaling pathways and the control of numerous redox-sensitive transcription factors. Furthermore, *physiological levels of ROS are essential for optimal force production in skeletal muscle. Nonetheless, high levels of ROS promote skeletal muscle contractile dysfunction resulting in muscle fatigue and injury.*

References

[1] Dillard CJ, Litov RE, Savin WM, Dumelin EE, Tappel AL. Effects of exercise, vitamin E, and ozone on pulmonary function and lipid peroxidation. *J. Appl. Physiol.* 1978; 45(6):927-932.

[2] Ashton T, Rowlands CC, Jones E et al. Electron spin resonance spectroscopic detection of oxygen-centred radicals in human serum following exhaustive exercise. *Eur. J. Appl. Physiol. Occup. Physiol.* 1998; 77(6):498-502.

[3] Wierzba TH, Olek RA, Fedeli D, Falcioni G. Lymphocyte DNA damage in rats challenged with a single bout of strenuous exercise. *J. Physiol. Pharmacol.* 2006; 57 Suppl 10:115-131.

[4] Sen CK, Rankinen T, Vaisanen S, Rauramaa R. Oxidative stress after human exercise: effect of N-acetylcysteine supplementation. *J. Appl. Physiol.* 1994; 76(6):2570-2577.

[5] Sahlin K, Ekberg K, Cizinsky S. Changes in plasma hypoxanthine and free radical markers during exercise in man. *Acta Physiol. Scand.* 1991; 142(2):275-281.

[6] Cooper CE, Vollaard NB, Choueiri T, Wilson MT. Exercise, free radicals and oxidative stress. *Biochem. Soc. Trans.* 2002; 30(2):280-285.

[7] Davies KJ, Maguire JJ, Brooks GA, Dallman PR, Packer L. Muscle mitochondrial bioenergetics, oxygen supply, and work capacity during dietary iron deficiency and repletion. *Am. J. Physiol.* 1982; 242(6):E418-E427.

[8] Koren A, Sauber C, Sentjurc M, Schara M. Free radicals in tetanic activity of isolated skeletal muscle. *Comp. Biochem. Physiol. B.* 1983; 74(3):633-635.

[9] Boveris A, Chance B. The mitochondrial generation of hydrogen peroxide. General properties and effect of hyperbaric oxygen. *Biochem. J.* 1973; 134(3):707-716.

[10] Loschen G, Azzi A, Richter C, Flohe L. Superoxide radicals as precursors of mitochondrial hydrogen peroxide. *FEBS Lett.* 1974; 42(1):68-72.

[11] Barja G. Mitochondrial oxygen radical generation and leak: sites of production in states 4 and 3, organ specificity, and relation to aging and longevity. *J. Bioenerg. Biomembr.* 1999; 31(4):347-366.

[12] Muller FL, Liu Y, Van RH. Complex III releases superoxide to both sides of the inner mitochondrial membrane. *J. Biol. Chem.* 2004; 279(47):49064-49073.

[13] Kanter MM. Free radicals, exercise, and antioxidant supplementation. *Int. J. Sport Nutr.* 1994; 4(3):205-220.

[14] Urso ML, Clarkson PM. Oxidative stress, exercise, and antioxidant supplementation. *Toxicology* 2003; 189(1-2):41-54.

[15] Jackson MJ, Pye D, Palomero J. The production of reactive oxygen and nitrogen species by skeletal muscle. *J. Appl. Physiol.* 2007; 102(4):1664-1670.

[16] St-Pierre J, Buckingham JA, Roebuck SJ, Brand MD. Topology of superoxide production from different sites in the mitochondrial electron transport chain. *J. Biol. Chem.* 2002; 277(47):44784-44790.

[17] Brand MD, Affourtit C, Esteves TC et al. Mitochondrial superoxide: production, biological effects, and activation of uncoupling proteins. *Free Radic. Biol. Med.* 2004; 37(6):755-767.

[18] Brand MD, Esteves TC. Physiological functions of the mitochondrial uncoupling proteins UCP2 and UCP3. *Cell Metab.* 2005; 2(2):85-93.

[19] Adhihetty PJ, Ljubicic V, Menzies KJ, Hood DA. Differential susceptibility of subsarcolemmal and intermyofibrillar mitochondria to apoptotic stimuli. *Am. J. Physiol. Cell Physiol.* 2005; 289(4):C994-C1001.

[20] Di MS, Venditti P. Mitochondria in exercise-inducedoxidative stress. *Biol. Signals Recept.* 2001; 10(1-2):125-140.

[21] Herrero A, Barja G. ADP-regulation of mitochondrial free radical production is different with complex I- or complex II-linked substrates: implications for the exercise paradox and brain hypermetabolism. *J. Bioenerg. Biomembr.* 1997; 29(3):241-249.

[22] Kozlov AV, Szalay L, Umar F et al. Skeletal muscles, heart, and lung are the main sources of oxygen radicals in old rats. *Biochim. Biophys. Acta* 2005; 1740(3):382-389.

[23] Anderson EJ, Neufer PD. Type II skeletal myofibers possess unique properties that potentiate mitochondrial H(2)O(2) generation. *Am. J. Physiol. Cell Physiol.* 2006; 290(3):C844-C851.

[24] Cherednichenko G, Zima AV, Feng W, Schaefer S, Blatter LA, Pessah IN. NADH oxidase activity of rat cardiac sarcoplasmic reticulum regulates calcium-induced calcium release. *Circ. Res.* 2004; 94(4):478-486.

[25] Xia R, Webb JA, Gnall LL, Cutler K, Abramson JJ. Skeletal muscle sarcoplasmic reticulum contains a NADH-dependent oxidase that generates superoxide. *Am. J. Physiol. Cell Physiol.* 2003; 285(1):C215-C221.

[26] Pattwell DM, McArdle A, Morgan JE, Patridge TA, Jackson MJ. Release of reactive oxygen and nitrogen species from contracting skeletal muscle cells. *Free Radic. Biol. Med.* 2004; 37(7):1064-1072.

[27] Espinosa A, Leiva A, Pena M et al. Myotube depolarization generates reactive oxygen species through NAD(P)H oxidase; ROS-elicited Ca2+ stimulates ERK, CREB, early genes. *J. Cell Physiol.* 2006; 209(2):379-388.

[28] Hidalgo C, Sanchez G, Barrientos G, racena-Parks P. A transverse tubule NADPH oxidase activity stimulates calcium release from isolated triads via ryanodine receptor type 1 S -glutathionylation. *J. Biol. Chem.* 2006; 281(36):26473-26482.

[29] McArdle A, Pattwell D, Vasilaki A, Griffiths RD, Jackson MJ. Contractile activity-induced oxidative stress: cellular origin and adaptive responses. *Am. J. Physiol. Cell Physiol.* 2001; 280(3):C621-C627.

[30] Reid MB, Haack KE, Franchek KM, Valberg PA, Kobzik L, West MS. Reactive oxygen in skeletal muscle. I. Intracellular oxidant kinetics and fatigue in vitro. *J. Appl. Physiol.* 1992; 73(5):1797-1804.

[31] Reid MB, Shoji T, Moody MR, Entman ML. Reactive oxygen in skeletal muscle. II. Extracellular release of free radicals. *J. Appl. Physiol.* 1992; 73(5):1805-1809.

[32] Zuo L, Christofi FL, Wright VP et al. Intra- and extracellular measurement of reactive oxygen species produced during heat stress in diaphragm muscle. *Am. J. Physiol. Cell Physiol. 2000*; 279(4):C1058-C1066.

[33] Javesghani D, Magder SA, Barreiro E, Quinn MT, Hussain SN. Molecular characterization of a superoxide-generating NAD(P)H oxidase in the ventilatory muscles. *Am. J. Respir. Crit. Care Med.* 2002; 165(3):412-418.

[34] Li JM, Shah AM. Endothelial cell superoxide generation: regulation and relevance for cardiovascular pathophysiology. *Am. J. Physiol. Regul. Integr. Comp. Physiol.* 2004; 287(5):R1014-R1030.

[35] Scarlett DJ, Herst PM, Berridge MV. Multiple proteins with single activities or a single protein with multiple activities: the conundrum of cell surface NADH oxidoreductases. *Biochim. Biophys. Acta* 2005; 1708(1):108-119.

[36] Morre DJ. Quinone oxidoreductases of the plasma membrane. *Methods Enzymol.* 2004; 378:179-199.

[37] de Grey AD. A hypothesis for the minimal overall structure of the mammalian plasma membrane redox system. *Protoplasma* 2003; 221(1-2):3-9.

[38] Zuo L, Christofi FL, Wright VP, Bao S, Clanton TL. Lipoxygenase-dependent superoxide release in skeletal muscle. *J. Appl. Physiol.* 2004; 97(2):661-668.

[39] Zhao X, Bey EA, Wientjes FB, Cathcart MK. Cytosolic phospholipase A2 (cPLA2) regulation of human monocyte NADPH oxidase activity. cPLA2 affects translocation but not phosphorylation of p67(phox) and p47(phox). *J. Biol. Chem.* 2002; 277(28):25385-25392.

[40] Nethery D, Callahan LA, Stofan D, Mattera R, DiMarco A, Supinski G. PLA(2) dependence of diaphragm mitochondrial formation of reactive oxygen species. *J. Appl. Physiol.* 2000; 89(1):72-80.

[41] Gong MC, Arbogast S, Guo Z, Mathenia J, Su W, Reid MB. Calcium-independent phospholipase A2 modulates cytosolic oxidant activity and contractile function in murine skeletal muscle cells. *J. Appl. Physiol.* 2006; 100(2):399-405.

[42] Nethery D, Stofan D, Callahan L, DiMarco A, Supinski G. Formation of reactive oxygen species by the contracting diaphragm is PLA(2) dependent. *J. Appl. Physiol.* 1999; 87(2):792-800.

[43] Muralikrishna AR, Hatcher JF. Phospholipase A2, reactive oxygen species, and lipid peroxidation in cerebral ischemia. *Free Radic. Biol. Med.* 2006; 40(3):376-387.

[44] Gomez-Cabrera MC, Pallardo FV, Sastre J, Vina J, Garcia-del-Moral L. Allopurinol and markers of muscle damage among participants in the Tour de France. *JAMA* 2003; 289(19):2503-2504.

[45] Heunks LM, Machiels HA, de AR, Zhu XP, van der Heijden HF, Dekhuijzen PN. Free radicals in hypoxic rat diaphragm contractility: no role for xanthine oxidase. *Am. J. Physiol. Lung Cell Mol. Physiol.* 2001; 281(6):L1402-L1412.

[46] Judge AR, Dodd SL. Xanthine oxidase and activated neutrophils cause oxidative damage to skeletal muscle after contractile claudication. *Am. J. Physiol. Heart Circ. Physiol.* 2004; 286(1):H252-H256.

[47] Hellsten Y, Apple FS, Sjodin B. Effect of sprint cycle training on activities of antioxidant enzymes in human skeletal muscle. *J. Appl. Physiol.* 1996; 81(4):1484-1487.

[48] Dillard CJ, Litov RE, Tappel AL. Effects of dietary vitamin E, selenium, and polyunsaturated fats on in vivo lipid peroxidation in the rat as measured by pentane production. *Lipids.* 1978; 13(6):396-402.

[49] Alessio HM, Goldfarb AH, Cutler RG. MDA content increases in fast- and slow-twitch skeletal muscle with intensity of exercise in a rat. *Am. J. Physiol.* 1988; 255(6 Pt 1):C874-C877.

[50] Davies KJ, Quintanilha AT, Brooks GA, Packer L. Free radicals and tissue damage produced by exercise. *Biochem. Biophys. Res. Commun.* 1982; 107(4):1198-1205.

[51] Kayatekin BM, Gonenc S, Acikgoz O, Uysal N, Dayi A. Effects of sprint exercise on oxidative stress in skeletal muscle and liver. *Eur. J. Appl. Physiol.* 2002; 87(2):141-144.

[52] Khanna S, Atalay M, Laaksonen DE, Gul M, Roy S, Sen CK. Alpha-lipoic acid supplementation: tissue glutathione homeostasis at rest and after exercise. *J. Appl. Physiol.* 1999; 86(4):1191-1196.

[53] Steensberg A, Morrow J, Toft AD, Bruunsgaard H, Pedersen BK. Prolonged exercise, lymphocyte apoptosis and F2-isoprostanes. *Eur. J. Appl. Physiol.* 2002; 87(1):38-42.

[54] Vollaard NB, Shearman JP, Cooper CE. Exercise-induced oxidative stress:myths, realities and physiological relevance. *Sports Med.* 2005; 35(12):1045-1062.

[55] Reznick AZ, Witt E, Matsumoto M, Packer L. Vitamin E inhibits protein oxidation in skeletal muscle of resting and exercised rats. *Biochem. Biophys. Res. Commun.* 1992; 189(2):801-806.

[56] Witt EH, Reznick AZ, Viguie CA, Starke-Reed P, Packer L. Exercise, oxidative damage and effects of antioxidant manipulation. *J. Nutr.*1992; 122(3 Suppl):766-773.

[57] Tirosh O and Reznick AZ. Chemical bases and biological relevance of protein oxidation. In: Sen CK PLHO, editor. Handbook of Oxidants and Antioxidants in Exercise. Amsterdam.:Elsevier, 2000: 89-114.

[58] Cochrane CG. Mechanisms of cell damage by oxidants. In: Jesaitis AJDEA, editor. The molecular basis of oxidative damage by leukocytes.Boca Raton, Ann Arbor, London, Tokyo.:*CRC-Press*, 1992: 149-162.

[59] Hartmann A.andNiess A.M. DNA damage in exercise. In: C.K.Sen LPOH, editor. Handbook of Oxidants and Antioxidants in Exercise. Amsterdam.:*Elsevier*, 2000: 195-217.

[60] Okamura K, Doi T, Hamada K et al. Effect of repeated exercise on urinary 8-hydroxy-deoxyguanosine excretion in humans. *Free Radic. Res.* 1997; 26(6):507-514.

[61] Radak Z, Kaneko T, Tahara S et al. The effect of exercise training on oxidative damage of lipids, proteins, and DNA in rat skeletal muscle: evidence for beneficial outcomes. *Free Radic. Biol. Med.*1999; 27(1-2):69-74.

[62] Davies KJ, Quintanilha AT, Brooks GA, Packer L. Free radicals and tissue damage produced by exercise. *Biochem. Biophys. Res. Commun.* 1982; 107(4):1198-1205.

[63] Alessio HM. Exercise-induced oxidative stress. *Med. Sci. Sports Exerc.* 1993; 25(2):218-224.

[64] Vasankari TJ, Kujala UM, Vasankari TM, Vuorimaa T, Ahotupa M. Effects of acute prolonged exercise on-serum and LDL oxidation and antioxidant defences. *Free Radic. Biol. Med.* 1997; 22(3):509-513.

[65] Liu ML, Bergholm R, Makimattila S et al. A marathon run increases the susceptibility of LDL to oxidation in vitro and modifies plasma antioxidants. *Am. J. Physiol.* 1999; 276(6 Pt 1):E1083-E1091.

[66] Mastaloudis A, Leonard SW, Traber MG. Oxidative stress in athletes during extreme endurance exercise. *Free Radic. Biol. Med.* 2001; 31(7):911-922.

[67] Palmer FM, Nieman DC, Henson DA et al. Influence of vitamin C supplementation on oxidative and salivary IgA changes following an ultramarathon. *Eur. J. Appl. Physiol.* 2003; 89(1):100-107.

[68] Child RB, Wilkinson DM, Fallowfield JL, Donnelly AE. Elevated serum antioxidant capacity and plasma malondialdehyde concentration in response to a simulated half-marathon run. *Med. Sci. Sports Exerc.* 1998; 30(11):1603-1607.

[69] Lovlin R, Cottle W, Pyke I, Kavanagh M, Belcastro AN. Are indices of free radical damage related to exercise intensity. *Eur. J. Appl. Physiol. Occup. Physiol.* 1987; 56(3):313-316.

[70] Aguilo A, Tauler P, Fuentespina E, Tur JA, Cordova A, Pons A. Antioxidant response to oxidative stress induced by exhaustive exercise. *Physiol. Behav.* 2005; 84(1):1-7.

[71] Vider J, Lehtmaa J, Kullisaar T et al. Acute immune response in respect to exercise-induced oxidative stress. *Pathophysiology* 2001; 7(4):263-270.

[72] Dawson B, Henry GJ, Goodman C et al. Effect of Vitamin C and E supplementation on biochemical and ultrastructural indices of muscle damage after a 21 km run. *Int. J. Sports Med.* 2002; 23(1):10-15.

[73] Chevion S, Moran DS, Heled Y et al. Plasma antioxidant status and cell injury after severe physical exercise. *Proc. Natl. Acad. Sci. U S A* 2003; 100(9):5119-5123.

[74] Pincemail J, Lecomte J, Castiau J et al. Evaluation of autoantibodies against oxidized LDL and antioxidant status in top soccer and basketball players after 4 months of competition. *Free Radic. Biol. Med.* 2000; 28(4):559-565.

[75] Palazzetti S, Richard MJ, Favier A, Margaritis I. Overloaded training increases exercise-induced oxidative stress and damage. *Can. J. Appl. Physiol.* 2003; 28(4):588-604.

[76] McBride JM, Kraemer WJ, Triplett-McBride T, Sebastianelli W. Effect of resistance exercise on free radical production. *Med. Sci. Sports Exerc.* 1998; 30(1):67-72.

[77] Groussard C, Rannou-Bekono F, Machefer G et al. Changes in blood lipid peroxidation markers and antioxidants after a single sprint anaerobic exercise. *Eur. J. Appl. Physiol.* 2003; 89(1):14-20.

[78] Frank J, Pompella A, BiesalskiHK.Histochemical visualization of oxidant stress. *Free Radic. Biol. Med.* 2000; 29(11):1096-1105.

[79] Chen SS, Chang LS, Wei YH. Oxidative damage to proteins and decrease of antioxidant capacity in patients with varicocele. *Free Radic. Biol. Med.* 2001; 30(11):1328-1334.

[80] Goldfarb AH, Bloomer RJ, McKenzie MJ. Combined antioxidant treatment effects on blood oxidative stress after eccentric exercise. *Med. Sci. Sports Exerc.* 2005; 37(2):234-239.

[81] Ramel A, Wagner KH, Elmadfa I. Plasma antioxidants and lipid oxidation after submaximal resistance exercise in men. *Eur. J. Nutr.* 2004; 43(1):2-6.

[82] Sahlin K, Cizinsky S, Warholm M, Hoberg J. Repetitive static muscle contractions in humans--a trigger of metabolic and oxidative stress? *Eur. J. Appl. Physiol. Occup. Physiol.* 1992; 64(3):228-236.

[83] Goldfarb AH. Nutritional antioxidants as therapeutic and preventive modalities in exercise-induced muscle damage. *Can. J. Appl. Physiol.* 1999; 24(3):249-266.

[84] Heunks LM, Vina J, van Herwaarden CL, Folgering HT, Gimeno A, Dekhuijzen PN. Xanthine oxidase is involved in exercise-induced oxidative stress in chronic obstructive pulmonary disease. *Am. J. Physiol.* 1999; 277(6 Pt 2):R1697-R1704.

[85] Childs A, Jacobs C, Kaminski T, Halliwell B, Leeuwenburgh C. Supplementation with vitamin C and N-acetyl-cysteine increases oxidative stress in humans after an acute muscle injury induced by eccentric exercise. *FreeRadic. Biol.Med.* 2001; 31(6):745-753.

[86] Ortenblad N, Madsen K, Djurhuus MS. Antioxidant status and lipid peroxidation after short-term maximal exercise in trained and untrained humans. *Am. J. Physiol.* 1997; 272(4 Pt 2):R1258-R1263.

[87] Saxton JM, Donnelly AE, Roper HP. Indices of free-radical-mediated damage following maximum voluntary eccentric and concentric muscular work. *Eur. J. Appl. Physiol. Occup. Physiol.* 1994; 68(3):189-193.

[88] Clarkson PM. Antioxidants and physical performance. *Crit. Rev. Food Sci. Nutr.* 1995; 35(1-2):131-141.

[89] Leeuwenburgh C, Hansen PA, Holloszy JO, Heinecke JW. Hydroxyl radical generation during exercise increases mitochondrial protein oxidation and levels of urinary dityrosine. *Free Radic. Biol. Med.* 1999; 27(1-2):186-192.

[90] Tessier F, Margaritis I, Richard MJ, Moynot C, Marconnet P. Selenium and training effects on the glutathione system and aerobic performance. *Med Sci. Sports Exerc.* 1995; 27(3):390-396.

[91] Miyazaki H, Oh-ishi S, Ookawara T et al. Strenuous endurance training in humans reduces oxidative stress following exhausting exercise. *Eur. J. Appl. Physiol.* 2001; 84(1-2):1-6.

[92] Elosua R, Molina L, Fito M et al. Response of oxidative stress biomarkers to a 16-week aerobic physical activity program, and to acute physical activity, in healthy young men and women. *Atherosclerosis* 2003; 167(2):327-334.

[93] Margaritis I, Tessier F, Richard MJ, Marconnet P. No evidence of oxidative stress after a triathlon race in highly trained competitors. Int J Sports Med 1997; 18(3):186-190.

[94] Selamoglu S, Turgay F, Kayatekin BM, Gonenc S, Yslegen C. Aerobic and anaerobic training effects on the antioxidant enzymes of the blood. *Acta Physiol. Hung.* 2000; 87(3):267-273.

[95] Rall LC, Roubenoff R, Meydani SN, Han SN, Meydani M. Urinary 8-hydroxy-2'-deoxyguanosine (8-OHdG) as a marker of oxidative stress in rheumatoid arthritis and aging: effect of progressive resistance training. *J. Nutr. Biochem.* 2000; 11(11-12):581-584.

[96] Vincent KR, Vincent HK, Braith RW, Lennon SL, Lowenthal DT. Resistance exercise training attenuates exercise-induced lipid peroxidation in the elderly. *Eur. J. Appl. Physiol.* 2002; 87(4-5):416-423.

[97] Fry RW, Morton AR, Keast D. Overtraining in athletes. An update. *Sports Med.* 1991; 12(1):32-65.

[98] Rowbottom DG, Keast D, Goodman C, Morton AR. The haematological, biochemical and immunological profile of athletes suffering from the overtraining syndrome. *Eur. J. Appl. Physiol. Occup. Physiol.* 1995; 70(6):502-509.

[99] Urhausen A, Kindermann W. Diagnosis of overtraining: what tools do we have? *Sports Med.* 2002; 32(2):95-102.

[100] Balakrishnan SD, Anuradha CV. Exercise, depletion of antioxidants and antioxidant manipulation. *Cell Biochem. Funct.* 1998; 16(4):269-275.

[101] McKenzie DC. Markers of excessive exercise. Can J ApplPhysiol 1999; 24(1):66-73.

[102] Petibois C, Cazorla G, Poortmans JR, Deleris G. Biochemical aspects of overtraining in endurance sports: a review. *Sports Med.* 2002; 32(13):867-878.

[103] Tiidus PM. Radical species in inflammation and overtraining. *Can. J. Physiol. Pharmacol.* 1998; 76(5):533-538.

In: Principles of Free Radical Biomedicine, Volume III
Editors: K. Pantopoulos and H. M. Schipper

ISBN 978-1-61324-184-4
©2012 Nova SciencePublishers, Inc.

Chapter 16

Reactive Metabolites and Oxygen Species in Toxicology

Jennifer J. Schlezinger[1] and Koren K. Mann[2,]*

[1]Department of Environmental Health, Boston University School of Public Health,
Boston, MA, U.S.A.
[2]Segal Cancer Centre at the Lady Davis Institute for Medical Research and Department of
Oncology, McGill University, Montréal, QC, Canada

1. Introduction

Toxicology is defined as the study of adverse effects of chemicals or xenobiotics [1]. By the strictest definition, xenobiotics are substances foreign to the organism, but in fact, endogenous substances also can have toxic effects at increased doses. *The basic tenet in toxicology is attributed to Paracelsus: "All things are poison and nothing without poison. Solely the dose determines that a thing is not a poison."* Therefore, the study of toxicology aims to define the dose at which deleterious effects are observed and to determine the mechanism of action of toxicants, usually through examination of a particular physiologic response.

The study of toxicology dates back to earliest times as knowledge of animal and plant-derived poisons was used in hunting and warfare. Modern toxicology has evolved rapidly during the last hundred years due to the exponential increase in industrial production of chemicals including drugs, pesticides, plastics and munitions. Toxicology is an applied science that is truly multi-disciplinary and utilizes many basic sciences to address hypotheses. This Chapter is designed to provide an understanding of the contribution of reactive species to toxicological mechanisms.

---

*E-mail: koren.mann@mcgill.ca

2. Biotransformation

During a lifetime, organisms are exposed to innumerable compounds that may not resemble anything previously encountered. In order to protect from this onslaught, organisms have evolved specific mechanisms to remove these xenobiotic substances. Often, elimination of these compounds involves conversion from a lipophilic compound to a more hydrophilic derivative that can be excreted. In addition, this "detoxification" process may lead to the production of free radicals and reactive intermediates. This process is known as biotransformation and is enzymatically catalyzed. Without this process, xenobiotics could accumulate within organisms, resulting in death. Many years ago, it was recognized that *non-water soluble xenobiotics were conjugated to functional groups to facilitate excretion*. In 1947, R.T. Williams proposed a two-step biotransformation process in which non-polar compounds acquired a functional group in the first step and then were conjugated to larger functional groups that significantly increased the hydrophilicity of the compound in the second step. The enzymes required for biotransformation are generally divided into two groups: phase I and phase II enzymes. Phase I involves reactions that add or reveal functional groups through a process of hydrolysis, reduction and oxidation. These reactions, in general, do not result in a significant increase in hydrophilicity. In contrast, phase II reactions commonly add large bulky functional groups resulting in a large increase in hydrophilicity, which facilitates excretion.

3. Cytochrome P450 Enzymes

Phase 1 metabolism is catalyzed by a family of enzymes, called the cytochrome P450s or CYPs, which has 57 members in humans [2]. CYP enzymes are associated with the endoplasmic reticulum and are highly expressed in the liver and small intestine. Expression may be either constitutively maintained (eg. CYP2E1 [3]) or induced (e.g. CYP1A1 [4]; and CYP3A4 [5]). In general, constitutively expressed CYPs metabolize endogenous substrates, while the expression of CYPs that metabolize exogenous substrates is inducible. Transcriptional activation of CYP1A1, the enzyme largely responsible for biotransformation of polycyclic aromatic hydrocarbons (PAHs, e.g. benzo[a]pyrene (B[a]P)) and halogenated aromatic hydrocarbons (HAHs, e.g. tetrachlorodibenzo-*p*-dioxin (TCDD)), is dependent upon the signaling cascade induced by the aryl hydrocarbon receptor (AhR) (Figure 1) (reviewed in [6, 7]). In the absence of a ligand, the AhR is found in the cytoplasm in a complex with heat shock protein 90 (hsp90), p23, and aryl hydrocarbon receptor–interacting protein (AIP) [8]. Upon ligand binding, hsp90 dissociates and the complex translocates to the nucleus [7]. The ligandedAhR forms a heterodimeric complex with the aryl hydrocarbon nuclear translocator/hypoxia-inducible factor 1β (ARNT/HIF-1β) protein [9]. This AhR/ARNT complex binds to specific response elements (AhR response elements; AhREs) in the promoters of genes in the "AhR gene battery" such as *Cyp1a1* and *Cyp1b1*. The extent of AhR-induced gene expression is governed, in part, by AhR export from the nucleus followed by proteasomal degradation [10]. In addition, AhR activation induces transcription of the AhR repressor (AhRR), a protein with a potent repressor domain capable of binding ARNT in the absence of agonist [11, 12]. The AhRR forms a feedback mechanism to inhibit

AhRtransactivation and gene induction [12]. Although primarily considered in the context of xenobiotics, the AhR pathway plays important roles in addition to the activation of the detoxification enzymes. These roles include regulation of cell cycle, induction of apoptosis, and generation of immune responses [7, 12, 13]. The AhR is required for the biotransformation of B[a]P to its highly reactive, carcinogenic intermediates, but likely also plays a role in non-xenobiotic-mediated tumorigenesis [14]. In addition to the AhR, CYP enzymes are transcriptionally activated by several nuclear receptors. The pregnane X receptor (PXR in mouse or the steroid and xenobiotic receptor (SXR in humans) and the constitutive androstane receptor (CAR) are ligand-activated transcription factors linked to induction of proteins involved in multiple aspects of xenobiotic metabolism and transport [15], including members of the CYP2B and CYP3A families [5, 16]. PXR is a nuclear protein, and CAR is cytoplasmic protein. Each, when activated, heterodimerizes with retinoid X receptor α, binds to response elements (DR-3, DR-4 and ER-6) in CYP gene promoter regions, and activates transcription [17, 18,19]. In addition, PXR interacts with other nuclear receptors to modulate the transcriptional activation of CYP enzymes. For example, PXR activation leads to inhibition of farnesoid X receptor (FXR)-dependent activation of CYP7A1 [20]. PXR target genes overlap significantly with constitutive androstane receptor (CAR) targets. While some genes are enhanced by either PXR or CAR activation, others are differentially regulated [21, 22].

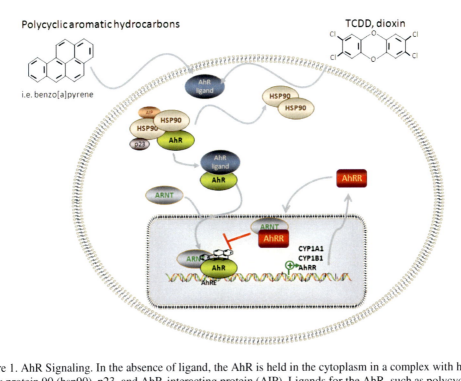

Figure 1. AhR Signaling. In the absence of ligand, the AhR is held in the cytoplasm in a complex with heat shock protein 90 (hsp90), p23, and AhR-interacting protein (AIP). Ligands for the AhR, such as polycyclic aromatic hydrocarbons or TCDD, diffuse across the membrane and once in the cytoplasm, bind the AhR. Upon ligand binding, the AhR is released from the cytoplasmic complex and translocates to the nucleus. In the nucleus, the AhR binds to AhR response elements (AhRE) as a heterodimer with the AhR nuclear translocator (ARNT). The AhR/ARNT complex acts as a transcription factor to induce expression of many genes called the "AhR gene battery" that includes the AhR repressor (AhRR). The AhRR binds ARNT and inhibits AhR-mediated transcription.

Approximately 75% of drugs are metabolized by CYP enzymes and 95% of those require only 5 different CYPs [23]. Thus, the activity of CYP enzymes can dramatically affect the activity of drugs. The individual sensitivity to drugs has been attributed to polymorphisms in the CYP genes that make an enzyme more or less active. Increased activity will increase drug clearance, while decreased drug activity can increase the half-life of the drug. This can impact metabolism of xenobiotics, but also those endogenous compounds that require CYP-dependent modification, such as steroids. For example, St. John's Wort is an over-the-counter "herbal" supplement taken by many people for relief of depression, although clinical trials have not supported this claim [24]. St. John's Wort is a potent inducer of CYP3A4 [25], the most abundant of the CYP enzymes, which is responsible for biotransformation of more than 50% of prescription medications [26]. This induction of CYP3A4 leads to many drug-drug interactions and taking St. John's Wort can significantly alter the efficacy of other drugs including HIV protease inhibitors, anti-neoplastic drugs, and hormonal contraceptives [27].

At the core of all CYPs is a heme group containing an iron atom that accepts electrons and donates them to an oxygen molecule, making it highly reactive. The oxygen radical can then react with a wide variety of endogenous and xenobiotic compounds [28]. The general form of the CYP reaction is as follows [29]; however, it should be noted that CYPs catalyze a number of simple reactions (e.g. C-hydroxylation, heteroatom oxygenation, dealkylation, epoxide formation, and 1,2-migration), as well as complex reactions. In the resting state, the heme iron of the CYP prosthetic group is in a low spin state (Fe^{3+})(Figure 2). Once a substrate binds, the iron is converted to a high spin state and to a redox potential that favors reduction. The iron is reduced by electrons donated from the flavoprotein NADPH-cytochrome P450 reductase.

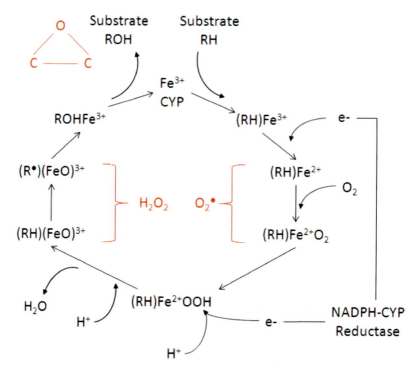

Figure 2. Generalized catalytic cycle for cytochrome P450s. Reactive intermediates and reactive oxygen species are indicated in red [29, 31].

Oxygen binds. Addition of a proton and a second electron converts the complex to a peroxide. The oxygen-oxygen double bond is cleaved by the introduction of a second proton. A substrate radical is formed, hydroxylated and released. One atom of molecular oxygen is reduced to water, while the other oxidizes the substrate.

During the biotransformation process, both reactive intermediates and reactive oxygen species (ROS) can be formed. For instance, among a number of possible substrate modifications catalyzed by CYPs, the introduction of oxygen onto the substrate can create an epoxide. The epoxide is formed by three atoms, resulting in a highly strained ring that is more reactive than other ethers [30]. In addition, *because coupling of electron transfer from NADPH and substrate oxidation tends to be highly inefficient, superoxide anion (O_2^-) and H_2O_2 are common by-products of the CYP catalytic cycle* [31]. This process is amplified during the oxidation of slowly metabolized substrates of CYP1As, such as planar polychlorinated biphenyls [32-34]. In contrast, CY2E1 produces significant ROS, even in the absence of substrate [35]. *Oxidative stress induced by substrates for CYP1A1 and CYP2E1 are hypothesized to contribute to the toxicity induced by these compounds in vivo* [36, 37].

4. Phase II Enzymes

A phase II reaction usually follows a phase I reaction and results in a water-soluble compound that can be excreted via the urine or bile. Phase II enzymes reactions can include acetylation, methylation, glutathione conjugation, glucuronidation, or amino acid conjugation. Expression of many phase II enzymes is induced by Nrf2 activation as discussed in Vol. II, Chapter 13. Nrf2 is sequestered in the cytoplasm by Keap1 protein that recruits CUL3 as an ubiquitin E3 ligase. This results in proteasomal degradation of Nrf2 and constitutively low Nrf2 activation. In the presence of ROS, Nrf2 protein levels are stabilized by the release of Keap1, whereby Nrf2 translocates to the nucleus and binds as heterodimeric complexes with the small Maf proteins to antioxidant response elements (AREs) in the promoters of many phase II enzymes such as γ-glutamylcysteine synthase (GCLC) and NAD(P)H:quinoneoxidoreductase 1 (NQO1). GCLC is the rate-limiting enzyme in glutathione synthesis (Vol. II, Chapter 1). NQO1 reduces quinones to hydroquinones thereby, preventing the one-electron reduction of quinones to produce reactive species [38]. In addition to Nrf2 regulation, the AhR gene battery discussed above contains several phase II enzymes such as NQO1, UDP-glucuronosyltransferase 1a6 (Ugt1a6), and glutathione S-transferase omega I. The Nrf2 and AhR gene batteries are linked by multiple mechanisms, including induction of Nrf2 expression by the AhR, indirect activation of Nrf2 by ROS produced by CYP1A1, and coordinate activation of genes whose promoters contain both AhREs and AREs [39].

It is the uncoupling of phase I and phase II that results in the accumulation of reactive intermediates. This can occur when a xenobiotic is a mono-inducer of the biotransformation system. For example, many drugs induce expression of CYP3A4, a phase I cytochrome P450, without induction of phase II enzymes. This results in the generation of large amounts of intermediate metabolites with reactive functional groups [40]. In the absence of increased phase II enzyme-mediated conjugation, these reactive intermediates can cause damage to nucleic acids, proteins, or lipids. This is in contrast to multi-inducers that result in phase I and

II enzyme induction and a more efficient detoxification process [41]. Polymorphisms in both phase I (e.g. CYP1A1) and phase II (e.g. glutathione S-transferase) enzymes are linked with cancer risk [42-44].

5. Phase III?

Although controversial, some investigators have added a phase III to the xenobiotic excretion process. This phase consists of the export of the conjugated xenobiotics from the cell via specific antiporters or ATP-dependent pumps whose activity results in decreased intracellular xenobiotic concentrations. Examples of such transporters include P-glycoprotein (P-gp; ABCB1), multi-drug resistance protein 1 (MRP1; ABCC1), and MRP2 (ABCC2). Interestingly, phase III transport, expression and activity is often linked to that of phase I enzymes.

For example, P-gp and CYP3A4 are located in close proximity within cells of the small intestine, such that P-gp is located on the apical membrane of the brush border and CYP3A4 is located in the endoplasmic reticulum just below the brush border [45]. Furthermore, P-gp and CYP3A4 have extensive overlap in substrates resulting in common inhibitors [46] and potentiation of CYP3A4-mediated drug clearance by P-gp*in vitro* [47].

Each toxic compound goes through a specific biotransformation process during which reactive species can be generated. The previous discussion is only a general schematic of the detoxification process. Some compounds require only one phase in biotransformation while others require all three or could be biotransformed using several different mechanisms. For some toxic compounds, free radical production is the main contributory factor to toxicity, but the role for free radicals produced by other compounds remains undefined. *Halliwell and Gutteridge have defined 6 ways that reactive species can be involved in the toxic actions of compounds* [48].

1. The toxicant itself is a reactive compound.
2. The toxicant is biotransformed to a reactive species.
3. The toxicant is capable of redox cycling and therefore generates $O_2^{\cdot-}$.
4. The toxicant alters the antioxidant state of the cell, thereby rendering it susceptible to secondary reactive species.
5. The toxicant affects a normal cellular process that results in generation of reactive species.
6. The toxicant or its biotransformation products can result in an immune response that generates reactive species.

In addition, a combination of these properties may occur. This is particularly prevalent in the case of complex mixture exposure where an organism may be exposed to multiple toxic compounds at once, each of which can produce reactive species by a different mechanism. The rest of this Chapter will discuss several specific examples of biotransformation and the production of reactive species within the process. This is by no means an exhaustive list, but is meant to illustrate the different mechanisms by which reactive species are produced in an effort to eliminate toxic compounds.

6. Specific Examples of Biotransformation

6.1. Polycyclic Aromatic Hydrocarbons (PAHs)

PAHs are prevalent organic contaminants of oil and tar, and are by-products of burning carbon-based compounds such as fossil fuels. These compounds consist of fused aromatic rings and are highly lipophilic. This characteristic allows them to easily diffuse across membranes.

Exposure to PAHs results in activation of the CYP1A/B family of enzymes. The best described PAH biotransformation process is that of B[a]P, a PAH found in charcoal-broiled food, cigarette smoke, and fossil fuel exhaust. The biotransformation of B[a]P is complex and defined elsewhere [49, 50], but here, we will highlight the reactions leading to formation of the ultimate carcinogen (Figure 3).

First, B[a]P is metabolized by CYP1A1, 1A2, or 1B1 to form B[a]P-epoxides, and a subsequent reaction catalyzed by epoxide hydrolases results in formation of the B[a]P-dihydrodiols. Formation of the most toxic intermediates requires further biotransformation. A specific dihydrodiol, B[a]P-7,8-dihydrodiol can be further metabolized by CYP enzymes to form B[a]P-7,8-dihydrodiol-9,10-epoxide (BPDE). BPDE is the ultimate carcinogen that covalently binds to DNA causing DNA damage or can non-covalently intercalate into DNA [50].

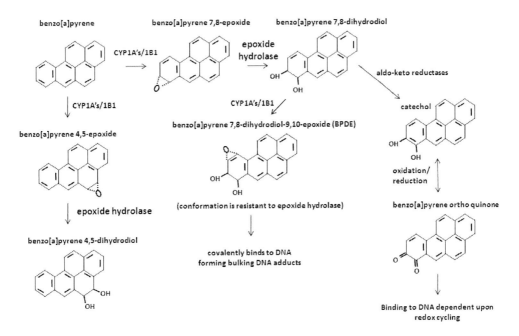

Figure 3. Biotransformation of benzo[a]pyrene (B[a]P). B[a]P is a substrate for CYP1A1/1A2 and CYP1B1. The cytochrome-mediated reaction results in the formation of an epoxide that is further transformed to a dihydrodiol by epoxide hydrolase. Importantly, the B[a]P 7,8-dihydrodiol is also a substrate for CYP1A's and CYP1B1, whose action results in formation of the 7,8-dihydriol-9,10-epoxide (BPDE). BPDE is resistant to further action by epoxide hydrolase, but forms bulky DNA adducts. The 7,8-dihydrodiol is also a substrate of aldo-ketoreductases resulting in the formation of catechol. In a redox-cycling reaction between catechol and B[a]P orthoquinone, further reactive species are formed.

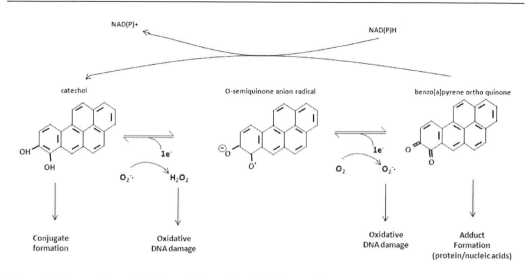

Figure 4. Redox cycling of B[a]P metabolites. Catechol is formed from aldoketoreductase action on B[a]P 7,8-dihydrodiol. Catechol is unstable and undergoes a one-electron oxidation to form a semi-quinone radical. This reaction produces H_2O_2. The semi-quinone is further oxidized to B[a]P ortho-quinone and $O_2^{-\cdot}$. B[a]P orthoquinone can form adducts with proteins and nucleic acids or in an NAD(P)H-dependent reaction, form catechol to compleate the redox cycle.

In addition, aldo-ketoreductases can convert the B[a]P-7,8-dihydrodiol to reactive quinones [51] (Figure 4). This process involves the NADP+-dependent oxidation of the dihydrodiol to form a ketol, which spontaneously rearranges to form a catechol. Catechol is not stable and undergoes a one-electron oxidation to form a semi-quinone and H_2O_2. A subsequent electron oxidation event results in production of the ortho-quinone and $O_2^{-\cdot}$. Importantly, the ortho-quinone species can undergo reduction reactions forming both the semi-quinone and further, catechol, establishing a redox cycle that is capable of producing significant ROS. The ortho-quinone compounds are highly reactive and form DNA adducts.

Exposure to B[a]P is often through inhalation and many studies have shown that exposure to mixtures containing B[a]P is linked to lung cancer [52-55]. When BPDE binding to DNA occurs in specific tumor suppressors or oncogenes, mutations occur and in the absence of sufficient repair mechanisms, result in increased transformation and the development of tumors. BPDE-DNA adducts can alter topoisomerase cleavage activity [56, 57], which has implications for the use of toposiomerase poisons as chemotherapeutics for B[a]P-induced tumors.

6.2. Carbon Tetrachloride

Carbon tetrachloride (CCl_4) is a clear, colorless liquid. Human exposure to CCl_4 is mainly via inhalation, and it is quickly absorbed via the gastrointestinal and respiratory tracts. Production of CCl_4 began in the early 1900s and continued until the Montréal Protocol of 1990 and its subsequent amendments established the phase-out of production and use of carbon tetrachloride and of chlorofluorocarbons (CFCs) by major manufacturing countries by 1996. CCl_4 was included in this ban due to its ozone-depletion properties. Most of the CCl_4 was used in the production of CFCs for use as refrigerants. CCl_4 was also employed in fire extinguishers and as flame retardants, because it is non-flammable, and as a solvent. Today, CCl_4 is used experimentally as a representative of the haloalkane family of compounds that also includes chloroform. CCl_4 is an effective laboratory model for hepatoxicity, which illustrates the main paradigm of toxicology in that the dose makes the poison. Low dose exposure results in transient liver toxicity followed by regeneration, while high dose or longer duration of exposure results in permanent, severe outcomes including fatty liver degeneration, cirrhosis and cancer [58]. Many mechanisms of action have been described for CCl_4-induced hepatotoxicity and the ultimate outcome is likely a combination of all these mechanisms.

Biotransformation of CCl_4 is initiated by cytochrome P450 enzyme-mediated transfer of an electron to the C-Cl bond that results in formation of the trichloromethyl radical, $CCl_3 \cdot$. This reaction is mediated by CYP2E1 and at higher doses CYP2B1/2 [58]. Interestingly, CCl_4 exposure has been linked to formation of CCl_3-CYP enzymes complexes and, thus, the suicide-inactivation of CYP2E1 [59, 60]. The $CCl_3 \cdot$ radical is highly reactive and rapidly forms complexes with proteins, nucleic acids and lipids resulting in haloalkylation. In the presence of oxygen, the $CCl_3 \cdot$ radical is converted to the trichloromethylperoxy radical, $CCl_3OO \cdot$. $CCl_3OO \cdot$ is even more reactive than the $CCl_3 \cdot$ and causes lipid peroxidation resulting in dissolution of membranes and generation of further reactive compounds. In addition, CCl_4-induced hepatic injury results in inflammatory cytokine release from Kupffer cells, the resident macrophages in the liver. These cytokines include TNFα, IL-1, IL-6, IL-10, and TGF-β and their upregulation is associated with a decreased antioxidant capacity via decreased glutathione levels and an increase in NF-κB activity [61]. The release of these cytokines may contribute to the fibrosis associated with CCl_4 exposure.

Regardless of the contribution of each of these mechanisms to CCl_4-induced hepatotoxicity, oxidative stress is clearly a mediator of injury. Compounds that protect against hepatotoxicity also inhibit CCl_4-induced CYP2E1 activity and oxidative stress [62, 63]. Ginsan, a polysaccharide extracted from Panax ginseng, downregulates CYP2E1, upregulates antioxidant enzymes, and blunts the inflammatory response, all resulting in protection of the liver in CCl_4-exposed mice [64]. Pretreatment with vitamin A [65] or E [66, 67] can reduce the oxidative stress and hepatotoxicity associated with CCl_4 exposure in a variety of species. These results indicate that CCl_4-induced oxidative stress results in liver damage that can be reversed by treatment with a variety of antioxidant compounds and phytochemicals.

6.3. Arsenic

Importantly, not all reactive species produced by toxicants are the result of CYP-mediated reactions. Some contaminants, such as arsenic, induce ROS production from cellular sources. Exposure to arsenic is primarily through contaminated drinking water, where the arsenic is derived from geological sources and/or potentially enriched by human manipulations. Chronic arsenic exposure is linked to an increased risk of cancer, peripheral vascular disease, neuropathies, atherosclerosis, and diabetes. A recent report has shown that chronic arsenic exposure increases the susceptibility of mice to death caused by influenza [68]. Arsenic exists as arsenate (As^{5+}) and arsenite (As^{3+}). Inorganic arsenic enters cells via two families of transporters: the aquaglyceroporins and the GLUT permeases [69]. Once inside the cell, two pathways have been proposed for arsenic biotransformation: 1) reduction and oxidative methylation and 2) glutathionylation and subsequent methylation (Figure 5)

[70]. Arsenate is rapidly reduced to arsenite either non-enzymatically by glutathione or enzymatically by glutathione-S-transferase (GST) [71]. Arsenic (III) methyltransferase (As3mt) utilizes S-adenosylmethionine as a methyl donor and catalyzes both the methylation reaction and the reduction of methylated arsenates to methylated arsenites [71]. Interestingly, polymorphisms in both As3mt and GST are linked to the efficiency of the arsenic methylation reaction [72, 73]. The triglutathionylated-As^{3+} species is a target for the ABCC1 exporter, which removes arsenic from the cell [74].

A major component in arsenic-induced toxicity is the generation of ROS that results in oxidative stress and subsequent stress signaling. Arsenic exposure promotes activation of the NADPH oxidase complex and generation of $O_2^{-}\cdot$ through increased p47 phosphorylation [75], translocation of p47, Rac1, and p67 to the membrane-bound complex [75], and activation of cdc42 [76]. A role for mitochondrially-generated ROS is implicated by the absence of arsenic genotoxicity in cells lacking mitochondria [77] and the loss of cytochrome C oxidase function and oxygen consumption following arsenic exposure [78]. Co-treatment with N-acetylcysteine, a compound that results in increased glutathione synthesis, inhibits many of the toxic effects of arsenic, while inhibition of glutathione synthesis enhances arsenic's effects. The results of arsenic-induced oxidative stress include oxidative DNA damage, lipid peroxidation, protein carbonylation, and reduction of glutathione levels. Arsenic is a potent inducer of the Nrf2 signaling cascade, likely through the action of ROS. As discussed above, ROS result in stabilization of the Nrf2 protein and transcription of Nrf2-target genes including heme oxygenase-1 (Vol. II, Chapter 11). Also, arsenic exposure results in activation of stress-induced kinases, particularly the MAP kinases p38 and c-jun N-terminal kinase (JNK). Interestingly, these two kinases appear to work in opposite directions such that inhibition of JNK inhibits arsenic-induced apoptosis [79], while inhibition of p38 promotes arsenic-induced apoptosis [80].

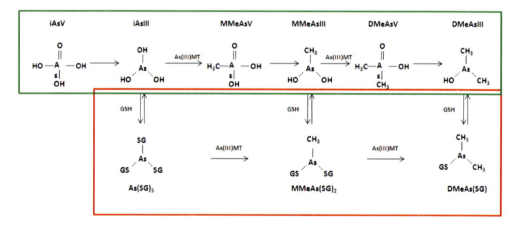

Figure 5. Arsenic biotransformation. There are two proposed pathways for arsenic biotransformation. Reduction and oxidative methylation (green square) occurs when arsenate (AsV) is converted to arsenite (AsIII) As(III) is methylated by arsenic(III)methyltransferase and oxidized to monomethylarsenate (MMeAsV). The methylated arsenate undergoes a similar reaction to form dimethylated arsenicals. At each step in this pathway, the arsenite (III) species can undergo glutathionylation and methylation (red square), such that As(III)MT replaces a glutathione group on triglutathionylatedarsenite (As(SG)$_3$) to form diglutathionylated, monomethylarsenite (MMeAs(SG)$_2$). Further methylation, forms the glutathionylated, dimethylatedarsenite (DMeAs(SG)).

6.4. Complex Mixtures

Exposure to chemical mixtures is prevalent, examples of which include diesel exhaust particles, mineral oil, and coal tar. Cigarette smoke is an example of a complex mixture to which a significant proportion of the population is exposed. Tobacco smoking is thought to be the cause of 30% of cancer-related deaths in the industrial world [81]. Smoking also is linked to an increase in mortality from chronic obstructive pulmonary disease and cardiovascular diseases [82]. Not only is the primary smoker at risk, but exposure to environmental tobacco smoke ("second-hand smoke") is linked to an increased risk of cancer [83, 84], pulmonary [85], and cardiovascular disease [86]; see also Chapter 1 in this Volume. Cigarette smoke contains over 3500 identified compounds including at least 55 known carcinogens [87]. These include metals (e.g. arsenic, nickel, cadmium and chromium), polycyclic aromatic hydrocarbons (e.g. B[a]P), aldehydes, and nitrosamines (e.g. 4-(methylnitrosamino)-1-(3-pyridyl)-1-butanone(NNK)) [87]. Importantly, cigarette smoke contains several of the compounds already discussed that generate reactive species (e.g. B[a]P and arsenic), but also contains/generates additional reactive species.

Cigarette smoke contains both particulate and gas phase contaminants. The particulate, or tar, phase is that which gets trapped when the smoke passes through a filter (generally larger than 0.1 μM in size) [88]. Over 3000 different compounds have been identified in the particulate phase of cigarette smoke [88]. The free radicals in the particulate phase are long-lived and can be detected using electron spin resonance spectroscopy [88]. These free radicals have been defined as mostly quinones that can either oxidize hydrocarbons also found in cigarette smoke or can bind to DNA directly [89]. Furthermore, this particulate phase contains free radicals derived from interactions of quinones/hydroquinones with the smokestream, independent of hydrocarbons [88]. Thus, reactive species are generated not only from constituents of the particulate phase already discussed (e.g. arsenic), but also those formed during combustion of the tobacco. Condensates of this tar phase cause free radical injury in cell culture, while simultaneously inhibiting expression of antioxidant enzymes [90]. The particulate phase can inhibit the mitochondrial electron transport chain and cause increased hydroxyl radical formation [91]. The gas phase is defined as that which passes through a filter. The free radicals in the gas phase are short-lived and at lower concentrations. Gas phase radicals include superoxide anion and nitric oxide [89]. These radicals cannot be detected by electron spin resonance, but require spin-trapping [88]. Although exposure to cigarette smoke involves both phases simultaneously, it is important to note that each phase may be contributing different toxicities, potentially based on their free radical properties.

Risk assessment for these exposures is difficult, because in many cases, the complete list of constituent chemicals in unknown. Another complication for risk assessment is the sequential or multiple exposures to single agents and mixtures. A distinction is made between simple mixtures (a few defined chemicals) and complex mixtures (usually more than 10 chemicals). Nevertheless, several questions arise when considering the toxicity of mixtures. Which components of a mixture result in a toxic outcome? Does the whole equal more than the sum of its component parts? In the past, the toxicity of a mixture was believed to be the sum of the toxicity associated with each individual chemical. Clearly, this could be problematic if there was a toxic interaction, where one compound affects the toxicity of another compound. While understanding the particular mechanism of action of a single chemical is essential, this mechanism of action may be altered in the presence of other toxic compounds.

Conclusions

Understanding the mechanism by which a compound adversely affects the organism is key to finding successful interventions, as well as to defining exposure limits. For each toxicant, the involvement of reactive species is different. Some compounds are themselves reactive species, while others change the oxidant/antioxidant balance within the cell, creating an environment in which additional reactive species could be more harmful.

References

[1]   Klaassen C. *Casarett and Doull's Toxicology: The Basic Science of Poisons.* New York: McGraw-Hill; 2001.

[2]   Park JY, Shigenaga MK, Ames BN. Induction of cytochrome P4501A1 by 2,3,7,8-tetrachlorodibenzo-p-dioxin or indolo(3,2-b)carbazole is associated with oxidative DNA damage. *Proc. Natl. Acad. Sci. U S A.* 1996;93:2322-2327.

[3]   Gonzalez FJ, Lee YH. Constitutive expression of hepatic cytochrome P450 genes. *Faseb J.* 1996;10:1112-1117.

[4]   Whitlock JP, Jr. Induction of cytochrome P4501A1. *Annu. Rev. Pharmacol. Toxicol.* 1999;39:103-125.

[5]   Lehmann JM, McKee DD, Watson MA, Willson TM, Moore JT, Kliewer SA. The human orphan nuclear receptor PXR is activated by compounds that regulate CYP3A4 gene expression and cause drug interactions. *J. Clin. Invest.* 1998;102:1016-1023.

[6]   Bock KW, Kohle C. The mammalian aryl hydrocarbon (Ah) receptor: from mediator of dioxin toxicity toward physiological functions in skin and liver. *Biol. Chem.* 2009;390:1225-1235.

[7]   Stevens EA, Mezrich JD, Bradfield CA. The aryl hydrocarbon receptor: a perspective on potential roles in the immune system. *Immunology.* 2009;127:299-311.

[8]   Bell DR, Poland A. Binding of aryl hydrocarbon receptor (AhR) to AhR-interacting protein. The role of hsp90. *J. Biol. Chem.* 2000;275:36407-36414.

[9]   Reyes H, Reisz-Porszasz S, Hankinson O. Identification of the Ah receptor nuclear translocator protein (Arnt) as a component of the DNA binding form of the Ah receptor. *Science.* 1992;256:1193-1195.

[10] Davarinos NA, Pollenz RS. Aryl hydrocarbon receptor imported into the nucleus following ligand binding is rapidly degraded via the cytosplasmic proteasome following nuclear export. *J. Biol. Chem.* 1999;274:28708-28715.

[11] Evans BR, Karchner SI, Allan LL, Pollenz RS, Tanguay RL, Jenny MJ, Sherr DH, Hahn ME. Repression of aryl hydrocarbon receptor (AHR) signaling by AHR repressor: role of DNA binding and competition for AHR nuclear translocator. *Mol. Pharmacol.* 2008;73:387-398.

[12] Hahn ME, Allan LL, Sherr DH. Regulation of constitutive and inducible AHR signaling: complex interactions involving the AHR repressor. *Biochem. Pharmacol.* 2009;77:485-497.

[13] Ray S, Swanson HI. Activation of the aryl hydrocarbon receptor by TCDD inhibits senescence: a tumor promoting event? *Biochem. Pharmacol.* 2009;77:681-688.

[14] Schlezinger JJ, Liu D, Farago M, Seldin DC, Belguise K, Sonenshein GE, Sherr DH. A role for the aryl hydrocarbon receptor in mammary gland tumorigenesis. *Biol. Chem.* 2006;387:1175-1187.

[15] Kliewer SA, Goodwin B, Willson TM. The nuclear pregnane X receptor: a key regulator of xenobiotic metabolism. *Endocr. Rev.* 2002;23:687-702.

[16] Faucette SR, Zhang TC, Moore R, Sueyoshi T, Omiecinski CJ, LeCluyse EL, Negishi M, Wang H. Relative activation of human pregnane X receptor versus constitutive androstane receptor defines distinct classes of CYP2B6 and CYP3A4 inducers. *J. Pharmacol. Exp. Ther.* 2007;320:72-80.

[17] Goodwin B, Hodgson E, Liddle C. The orphan human pregnane X receptor mediates the transcriptional activation of CYP3A4 by rifampicin through a distal enhancer module. *Mol. Pharmacol.* 1999;56:1329-1339.

[18] Handschin C, Meyer UA. Induction of drug metabolism: the role of nuclear receptors. *Pharmacol. Rev.* 2003;55:649-673.

[19] di Masi A, Marinis ED, Ascenzi P, Marino M. Nuclear receptors CAR and PXR: Molecular, functional, and biomedical aspects. *Mol. Aspects Med.* 2009;30:297-343.

[20] Staudinger JL, Goodwin B, Jones SA, Hawkins-Brown D, MacKenzie KI, LaTour A, Liu Y, Klaassen CD, Brown KK, Reinhard J, Willson TM, Koller BH, Kliewer SA. The nuclear receptor PXR is a lithocholic acid sensor that protects against liver toxicity. *Proc. Natl. Acad. Sci. U S A.* 2001;98:3369-3374.

[21] Maglich JM, Stoltz CM, Goodwin B, Hawkins-Brown D, Moore JT, Kliewer SA. Nuclear pregnane x receptor and constitutive androstane receptor regulate overlapping but distinct sets of genes involved in xenobiotic detoxification. *Mol. Pharmacol.* 2002;62:638-646.

[22] Savas U, Griffin KJ, Johnson EF. Molecular mechanisms of cytochrome P-450 induction by xenobiotics: An expanded role for nuclear hormone receptors. *Mol. Pharmacol.* 1999;56:851-857.

[23] Guengerich FP. Cytochrome p450 and chemical toxicology. *Chem. Res. Toxicol.* 2008;21:70-83.

[24] Effect of Hypericumperforatum (St John's wort) in major depressive disorder: a randomized controlled trial. *Jama.* 2002;287:1807-1814.

[25] Roby CA, Anderson GD, Kantor E, Dryer DA, Burstein AH. St John's Wort: effect on CYP3A4 activity. *Clin. Pharmacol. Ther.* 2000;67:451-457.

[26] Keshava C, McCanlies EC, Weston A. CYP3A4 polymorphisms--potential risk factors for breast and prostate cancer: a HuGE review. *Am. J. Epidemiol.* 2004;160:825-841.

[27] Mannel M. Drug interactions with St John's wort : mechanisms and clinical implications. *Drug. Saf.* 2004;27:773-797.

[28] Goodsell DS. The molecular perspective: cytochrome p450. *Oncologist.* 2001;6:205-206.

[29] Isin EM, Guengerich FP. Complex reactions catalyzed by cytochrome P450 enzymes. *Biochim. Biophys. Acta.* 2007;1770:314-329.

[30] Guengerich FP. Cytochrome P450 oxidations in the generation of reactive electrophiles: epoxidation and related reactions. *Arch. Biochem. Biophys.* 2003;409:59-71.

[31] Zangar RC, Davydov DR, Verma S. Mechanisms that regulate production of reactive oxygen species by cytochrome P450. *Toxicol. Appl. Pharmacol.* 2004;199:316-331.

[32] Schlezinger JJ, White RD, Stegeman JJ. Oxidative inactivation of cytochrome P-450 1A (CYP1A) stimulated by 3,3',4,4'-tetrachlorobiphenyl: production of reactive oxygen by vertebrate CYP1As. *Mol. Pharmacol.* 1999;56:588-597.

[33] Schlezinger JJ, Struntz WD, Goldstone JV, Stegeman JJ. Uncoupling of cytochrome P450 1A and stimulation of reactive oxygen species production by co-planar polychlorinated biphenyl congeners. *Aquat .Toxicol.* 2006;77:422-432.

[34] Schlezinger JJ, Keller J, Verbrugge LA, Stegeman JJ. 3,3',4,4'-Tetrachlorobiphenyl oxidation in fish, bird and reptile species: relationship to cytochrome P450 1A inactivation and reactive oxygen production. *Biochem. Physiol. C Toxicol. Pharmacol.* 2000;125:273-286.

[35] Ekstrom G, Ingelman-Sundberg M. Rat liver microsomal NADPH-supported oxidase activity and lipid peroxidation dependent on ethanol-inducible cytochrome P-450 (P-450IIE1). *Biochem. Pharmacol.* 1989;38:1313-1319.

[36] Goldstone HM, Stegeman JJ. Molecular mechanisms of 2,3,7,8-tetrachlorodibenzo-p-dioxin cardiovascular embryotoxicity. *Drug Metab. Rev.* 2006;38:261-289.

[37] Cederbaum AI, Lu Y, Wu D. Role of oxidative stress in alcohol-induced liver injury. *Arch. Toxicol.* 2009;83:519-548.

[38] Vasiliou V, Ross D, Nebert DW. Update of the NAD(P)H:quinoneoxidoreductase (NQO) gene family. *Hum. Genomics.* 2006;2:329-335.

[39] Kohle C, Bock KW. Coordinate regulation of Phase I and II xenobiotic metabolisms by the Ah receptor and Nrf2. *Biochem. Pharmacol.* 2007;73:1853-1862.

[40] Prestera T, Zhang Y, Spencer SR, Wilczak CA, Talalay P. The electrophile counterattack response: protection against neoplasia and toxicity. *Adv. Enzyme Regul.* 1993;33:281-296.

[41] Talalay P, Fahey JW, Holtzclaw WD, Prestera T, Zhang Y. Chemoprotection against cancer by phase 2 enzyme induction. *Toxicol. Lett.* 1995;82-83:173-179.

[42] Taspinar M, Aydos SE, Comez O, Elhan AH, Karabulut HG, Sunguroglu A. CYP1A1, GST gene polymorphisms and risk of chronic myeloid leukemia. *Swiss. Med. Wkly.* 2008;138:12-17.

[43] Nock NL, Tang D, Rundle A, Neslund-Dudas C, Savera AT, Bock CH, Monaghan KG, Koprowski A, Mitrache N, Yang JJ, Rybicki BA. Associations between smoking, polymorphisms in polycyclic aromatic hydrocarbon (PAH) metabolism and conjugation genes and PAH-DNA adducts in prostate tumors differ by race. *Cancer Epidemiol. Biomarkers Prev.* 2007;16:1236-1245.

[44] Yang M, Choi Y, Hwangbo B, Lee JS. Combined effects of genetic polymorphisms in six selected genes on lung cancer susceptibility. *Lung Cancer.* 2007;57:135-142.

[45] Watkins PB. The barrier function of CYP3A4 and P-glycoprotein in the small bowel. *Adv. Drug Deliv. Rev.* 1997;27:161-170.

[46] Wacher VJ, Wu CY, Benet LZ. Overlapping substrate specificities and tissue distribution of cytochrome P450 3A and P-glycoprotein: implications for drug delivery and activity in cancer chemotherapy. *Mol. Carcinog.* 1995;13:129-134.

[47] Chan LM, Cooper AE, Dudley AL, Ford D, Hirst BH. P-glycoprotein potentiates CYP3A4-mediated drug disappearance during Caco-2 intestinal secretory detoxification. *J. Drug Target.* 2004;12:405-413.

[48] Halliwell B, Gutteridge JMC. *Free Radicals in Biology and Medicine.* Oxford: Oxford University Press; 2007.

[49] Agency for Toxic Substances and Disease Registry. Toxicological profile for Polycyclic Aromatic Hydrocarbons (PAHs). In: US Department of Health and Human Services PHS, ed.; 1995.

[50] Gelboin HV. Benzo[alpha]pyrene metabolism, activation and carcinogenesis: role and regulation of mixed-function oxidases and related enzymes. *Physiol. Rev.* 1980;60:1107-1166.

[51] Penning TM, Burczynski ME, Hung CF, McCoull KD, Palackal NT, Tsuruda LS. Dihydrodiol dehydrogenases and polycyclic aromatic hydrocarbon activation: generation of reactive and redox active o-quinones. *Chem. Res. Toxicol.* 1999;12:1-18.

[52] Gao YT, Blot WJ, Zheng W, Fraumeni JF, Hsu CW. Lung cancer and smoking in Shanghai. *Int. J. Epidemiol.* 1988;17:277-280.

[53] Zhong L, Goldberg MS, Parent ME, Hanley JA. Risk of developing lung cancer in relation to exposure to fumes from Chinese-style cooking. *Scand. J. Work Environ. Health.* 1999;25:309-316.

[54] Mooney LA, Madsen AM, Tang D, Orjuela MA, Tsai WY, Garduno ER, Perera FP. Antioxidant vitamin supplementation reduces benzo(a)pyrene-DNA adducts and potential cancer risk in female smokers. *Cancer Epidemiol. Biomarkers Prev.* 2005;14:237-242.

[55] Vyskocil A, Viau C, Camus M. Risk assessment of lung cancer related to environmental PAH pollution sources. *Hum. Exp. Toxicol.* 2004;23:115-127.

[56] Khan QA, Kohlhagen G, Marshall R, Austin CA, Kalena GP, Kroth H, Sayer JM, Jerina DM, Pommier Y. Position-specific trapping of topoisomerase II by benzo[a]pyrenediol epoxide adducts: implications for interactions with intercalating anticancer agents. *Proc. Natl. Acad. Sci. U S A,.* 2003;100:12498-12503.

[57] Pommier Y, Kohlhagen G, Laco GS, Kroth H, Sayer JM, Jerina DM. Different effects on human topoisomerase I by minor groove and intercalated deoxyguanosine adducts derived from two polycyclic aromatic hydrocarbon diol epoxides at or near a normal cleavage site. *J. Biol. Chem.* 2002;277:13666-13672.

[58] Weber LW, Boll M, Stampfl A. Hepatotoxicity and mechanism of action of haloalkanes: carbon tetrachloride as a toxicological model. *Crit. Rev. Toxicol.* 2003;33:105-136.

[59] Dai Y, Cederbaum AI. Inactivation and degradation of human cytochrome P4502E1 by CCl4 in a transfected HepG2 cell line. *J. Pharmacol. Exp. Ther.* 1995;275:1614-1622.

[60] Tierney DJ, Haas AL, Koop DR. Degradation of cytochrome P450 2E1: selective loss after labilization of the enzyme. *Arch. Biochem. Biophys.* 1992;293:9-16.

[61] Luckey SW, Petersen DR. Activation of Kupffer cells during the course of carbon tetrachloride-induced liver injury and fibrosis in rats. *Exp. Mol. Pathol.* 2001;71:226-240.

[62] Bhadauria M, Nirala SK, Shrivastava S, Sharma A, Johri S, Chandan BK, Singh B, Saxena AK, Shukla S. Emodin reverses CCl induced hepatic cytochrome P450 (CYP)

enzymatic and ultrastructural changes: The in vivo evidence. *Hepatol. Res.* 2009;39:290-300.

[63] Bhadauria M, Nirala SK, Shukla S. Propolis protects CYP 2E1 enzymatic activity and oxidative stress induced by carbon tetrachloride. *Mol. Cell Biochem.* 2007;302:215-224.

[64] Shim JY, Kim MH, Kim HD, Ahn JY, Yun YS, Song JY. Protective action of the immunomodulatorginsan against carbon tetrachloride-induced liver injury via control of oxidative stress and the inflammatory response. *Toxicol. Appl. Pharmacol*;242:318-325.

[65] Wang L, Potter JJ, Rennie-Tankersley L, Novitskiy G, Sipes J, Mezey E. Effects of retinoic acid on the development of liver fibrosis produced by carbon tetrachloride in mice. *Biochim. Biophys. Acta.* 2007;1772:66-71.

[66] Yonezawa LA, Kitamura SS, Mirandola RM, Antonelli AC, Ortolani EL. Preventive treatment with vitamin E alleviates the poisoning effects of carbon tetrachloride in cattle. *J. Vet. Med. A Physiol. Pathol. Clin. Med.* 2005;52:292-297.

[67] MacDonald-Wicks LK, Garg ML. Vitamin E supplementation in the mitigation of carbon tetrachloride induced oxidative stress in rats. *J. Nutr. Biochem.* 2003;14:211-218.

[68] Kozul CD, Ely KH, Enelow RI, Hamilton JW. Low-dose arsenic compromises the immune response to influenza A infection in vivo. *Environ. Health Perspect.* 2009;117:1441-1447.

[69] Rosen BP, Liu Z. Transport pathways for arsenic and selenium: a minireview. *Environ. Int.* 2009;35:512-515.

[70] Kumagai Y, Sumi D. Arsenic: signal transduction, transcription factor, and biotransformation involved in cellular response and toxicity. *Annu. Rev. Pharmacol. Toxicol..* 2007;47:243-262.

[71] Schuhmacher-Wolz U, Dieter HH, Klein D, Schneider K. Oral exposure to inorganic arsenic: evaluation of its carcinogenic and non-carcinogenic effects. *Crit. Rev. Toxicol.* 2009;39:271-298.

[72] Agusa T, Iwata H, Fujihara J, Kunito T, Takeshita H, Minh TB, Trang PT, Viet PH, Tanabe S. Genetic polymorphisms in glutathione S-transferase (GST) superfamily and arsenic metabolism in residents of the Red River Delta, Vietnam. *Toxicol. Appl. Pharmacol*;242:352-362.

[73] Chung CJ, Hsueh YM, Bai CH, Huang YK, Huang YL, Yang MH, Chen CJ. Polymorphisms in arsenic metabolism genes, urinary arsenic methylation profile and cancer. *Cancer Causes Control.* 2009;20:1653-1661.

[74] Leslie EM, Haimeur A, Waalkes MP. Arsenic transport by the human multidrug resistance protein 1 (MRP1/ABCC1). Evidence that a tri-glutathione conjugate is required. *J. Biol. Chem.* 2004;279:32700-32708.

[75] Lemarie A, Bourdonnay E, Morzadec C, Fardel O, Vernhet L. Inorganic arsenic activates reduced NADPH oxidase in human primary macrophages through a Rho kinase/p38 kinase pathway. *J. Immunol.* 2008;180:6010-6017.

[76] Qian Y, Liu KJ, Chen Y, Flynn DC, Castranova V, Shi X. Cdc42 regulates arsenic-induced NADPH oxidase activation and cell migration through actin filament reorganization. *J. Biol. Chem.* 2005;280:3875-3884.

[77] Liu SX, Davidson MM, Tang X, Walker WF, Athar M, Ivanov V, Hei TK. Mitochondrial damage mediates genotoxicity of arsenic in mammalian cells. *Cancer. Res.* 2005;65:3236-3242.

Reactive Metabolites and Oxygen Species in Toxicology

[78] Partridge MA, Huang SX, Hernandez-Rosa E, Davidson MM, Hei TK. Arsenic induced mitochondrial DNA damage and altered mitochondrial oxidative function: implications for genotoxic mechanisms in mammalian cells. *Cancer Res.* 2007;67:5239-5247.

[79] Davison K, Mann KK, Waxman S, Miller WH. JNK activation is a mediator of arsenic trioxide-induced apoptosis in acute promyelocytic leukemia cells. *Blood.* 2004;103:3496-3502.

[80] Verma A, Mohindru M, Deb DK, Sassano A, Kambhampati S, Ravandi F, Minucci S, Kalvakolanu DV, Platanias LC. Activation of Rac1 and the p38 mitogen-activated protein kinase pathway in response to arsenic trioxide. *J. Biol. Chem.* 2002;277:44988-44995.

[81] Vineis P, Alavanja M, Buffler P, Fontham E, Franceschi S, Gao YT, Gupta PC, Hackshaw A, Matos E, Samet J, Sitas F, Smith J, Stayner L, Straif K, Thun MJ, Wichmann HE, Wu AH, Zaridze D, Peto R, Doll R. Tobacco and cancer: recent epidemiological evidence. *J. Natl. Cancer Inst.* 2004;96:99-106.

[82] Ezzati M, Lopez AD. Estimates of global mortality attributable to smoking in 2000. *Lancet.* 2003;362:847-852.

[83] Dockery DW, Trichopoulos D. Risk of lung cancer from environmental exposures to tobacco smoke. *Cancer Causes Control.* 1997;8:333-345.

[84] Johnson KC, Hu J, Mao Y. Passive and active smoking and breast cancer risk in Canada, 1994-97. *Cancer Causes Control.* 2000;11:211-221.

[85] Bates MN, Fawcett J, Dickson S, Berezowski R, Garrett N. Exposure of hospitality workers to environmental tobacco smoke. *Tob. Control.* 2002;11:125-129.

[86] Bonita R, Duncan J, Truelsen T, Jackson RT, Beaglehole R. Passive smoking as well as active smoking increases the risk of acute stroke. *Tob. Control.* 1999;8:156-160.

[87] Hecht SS. Tobacco smoke carcinogens and lung cancer. *J. Natl. Cancer Inst.* 1999;91:1194-1210.

[88] Church DF, Pryor WA. Free-Radical Chemistry of Cigarette Smoke and Its Toxicological Implications. *Environ. Health Perspect.* 1985;64:111-126.

[89] Pryor WA, Hales BJ, Premovic PI, Church DF. The radicals in cigarette tar: their nature and suggested physiological implications. *Science.* 1983;220:425-427.

[90] Russo M, Cocco S, Secondo A, Adornetto A, Bassi A, Nunziata A, Polichetti G, De Felice B, Damiano S, Seru R, Mondola P, Di Renzo G. Cigarette Smoke Condensate Causes a Decrease of the Gene Expression of Cu-Zn Superoxide Dismutase, Mn Superoxide Dismutase, Glutathione Peroxidase, Catalase, and Free Radical-Induced Cell Injury in SH-SY5Y Human Neuroblastoma Cells. *Neurotox. Res.* 2009.

[91] Pryor WA, Arbour NC, Upham B, Church DF. The inhibitory effect of extracts of cigarette tar on electron transport of mitochondria and submitochondrial particles. *Free Radic. Biol. Med.* 1992;12:365-372.

Index

#

21st century, 201

A

acanthocytosis, 243
acarbose, 204, 221
access, 66, 174, 182, 341, 352
accounting, 97
acetaldehyde, 77, 79, 89, 99, 319
acetaminophen, 59, 63, 91, 104, 245
acetic acid, 79
acetone, 90
acetylation, 371
acid, 9, 11, 15, 17, 18, 19, 20, 36, 75, 81, 84, 85, 87,
    110, 115, 117, 124, 125, 130, 133, 136, 137, 139,
    140, 141, 142, 157, 165, 169, 178, 191, 199, 203,
    204, 205, 208, 212, 213, 218, 222, 223, 224, 225,
    226, 237, 242, 247, 250, 254, 260, 261, 269, 273,
    274, 275, 279, 283, 286, 288, 289, 292, 297, 298,
    299, 301, 303, 310, 314, 315, 321, 325, 340, 342,
    346, 354, 355, 362, 379, 382
acidic, 68, 286, 315
acidosis, 91
acne, 292
acquired immunity, 14
acromegaly, 336
acrosome, 306, 321
active site, 146, 153
active transport, 174
activity level, 238
acute infection, 66
acute lung injury, 27
acute lymphoblastic leukemia, 168
acute promyelocytic leukemia, 383

acute renal failure, 54
acute respiratory distress syndrome, 26, 27
adaptation, 75, 158, 168, 209, 216, 351
adaptations, 193, 218
additives, 345
adduction, 147
adenine, 69, 71, 72, 74, 77, 78, 79, 80, 93, 148, 163,
    170, 189, 288, 308, 310
adenocarcinoma, 25, 156
adenomyosis, 336
adenosine, 74, 77, 81, 93, 120, 306, 310
adenosine triphosphate, 74, 77, 93, 120, 310
ADH, 77, 78, 79
adhesion, 11, 93, 94, 108, 132, 145, 147, 148, 160,
    163, 213, 334, 336
adhesions, 172, 348
adipocyte, 69
adiponectin, 69, 75, 81, 91, 99, 100, 217
adipose, 75, 83, 91, 102, 201, 215, 216, 319
adipose tissue, 75, 83, 91, 102, 215, 217, 319
adiposity, 215, 319
adjunctive therapy, 89
ADP, 129, 222, 223, 279, 287, 353, 360
adult respiratory distress syndrome, 26
adulthood, 35, 239
adults, 23, 95, 104, 111, 113, 165, 201, 220
advancement, 341
adventitia, 170, 180, 187
adverse effects, 38, 123, 130, 155, 245, 250, 279,
    338, 343, 344, 367
aerobic exercise, 356, 357
aflatoxin, 88
age, 39, 56, 70, 98, 174, 179, 204, 217, 231, 232,
    239, 240, 264, 265, 274, 275, 276, 277, 286, 298,
    337, 338, 339, 348
age-related diseases, 286
aggressiveness, 126, 137, 144, 159

aging process, 225, 231, 251
agonist, 142, 173, 278, 368
agranulocytosis, 38
AIDS, 305
air pollutants, 3, 18
airflow obstruction, 9
airway epithelial cells, 21, 24, 25
airway hyperresponsiveness, 9, 18
airway inflammation, 16, 17, 18, 19, 20
airways, 1, 7, 9, 11, 18, 20, 23, 26
alanine, 261
albumin, 58, 59, 108, 110, 116, 141, 214, 264, 309, 345
albuminuria, 107, 333
alcohol abuse, 83, 90, 99
alcohol consumption, 76, 77, 79, 80, 81, 82, 83, 88, 90, 98, 100, 319
alcoholic cirrhosis, 80, 83, 90, 99, 101
alcoholic liver disease, 95, 98, 99, 100, 101, 104
alcoholics, 88, 90, 100
alcoholism, 83
aldehydes, 88, 89, 377
aldosterone, 170
alkaloids, 154, 155, 319
alkylation, 92
allele, 34, 43, 79
allergens, 8, 10, 11, 293
allergic asthma, 18, 19
allergic inflammation, 9, 18
allergic rhinitis, 8, 9, 17, 18
allergy, 27, 302
alpha-tocopherol, 121, 137, 194, 219, 227, 259, 289, 321, 322
ALS, 235, 244, 247, 259
alters, 14, 76, 89, 97, 98, 227, 265, 372
alveoli, 3, 7, 15
ambient air, 3, 9
amenorrhea, 336
American Heart Association, 199, 219, 227
amine, 236, 340, 345
amines, 289
amino, 13, 49, 50, 112, 146, 173, 189, 204, 240, 241, 245, 247, 250, 261, 287, 289, 336, 371
amino acid, 13, 146, 189, 204, 240, 241, 245, 247, 250, 261, 287, 336, 371
amino acids, 146, 189, 250, 261
amino groups, 112
ammonia, 235
ammonium, 58
amyotrophic lateral sclerosis, 232, 235, 253, 259, 260
analgesic, 91
anatomic site, 150

anchorage, 151, 160
androgen, 336
anemia, 30, 34, 35, 37, 40, 41, 46, 90
aneuploidy, 318, 342
angina, 197
angiogenesis, 90, 103, 140, 143, 157, 173, 179, 211
angiotensin converting enzyme, 173
angiotensin II, 180, 183, 184, 185, 186, 187, 188, 189, 190, 191, 193, 195, 196, 208, 214, 222
angiotensin receptor antagonist, 219
angiotensin receptor blockers, 173
aniline, 315
anorexia, 92
anorexia nervosa, 92
antagonism, 196
antibody, 23, 85, 109, 113, 114, 269, 279, 314, 320, 334
anti-cancer, 123, 125, 127, 129, 130, 131, 142
anticancer activity, 156, 167
anticancer drug, 155, 156, 318
antiepileptic drugs, 245
antigen, 18, 32, 42, 75, 76, 88, 89, 98, 115, 286, 292, 295, 321, 334
antigen-presenting cell, 292
antihypertensive agents, 182
antihypertensive drugs, 173
anti-inflammatory agents, 15
anti-inflammatory drugs, 304
antioxidant defense, 1, 3, 8, 12, 24, 51, 75, 101, 130, 178, 202, 216, 217, 219, 273, 287, 289, 291, 305, 317, 333, 338, 342
anti-oxidant therapies, 143
antioxidative activity, 219
antipyretic, 91
antitumor, 142
antiviral therapy, 72
anxiety, 55
aorta, 171, 222
APL, 156, 168
apoptosis, 3, 10, 11, 12, 16, 20, 21, 23, 52, 53, 60, 62, 67, 68, 69, 73, 75, 86, 89, 91, 93, 94, 99, 105, 111, 116, 117, 121, 125, 127, 128, 129, 130, 131, 132, 136, 137, 138, 139, 140, 142, 146, 151, 152, 153, 155, 160, 165, 166, 167, 168, 175, 208, 209, 210, 220, 222, 229, 234, 244, 247, 266, 267, 268, 270, 271, 273, 275, 276, 277, 281, 282, 283, 290, 294, 295, 301, 303, 312, 313, 314, 315, 317, 318, 326, 330, 339, 340, 341, 342, 346, 362, 369, 376, 383
apoptotic pathways, 151
aqueous humor, 270, 273, 280, 282
ARDS, 15, 26
aromatic hydrocarbons, 90, 288, 368

aromatic rings, 373
arrest, 47, 142, 146, 294, 295, 297, 303, 332, 339, 341
arrests, 346
arsenic, 153, 166, 168, 375, 376, 377, 382, 383
arterial hypertension, 83, 183
arteries, 118, 170, 172, 176, 178, 180, 184, 191, 192, 195, 196, 333, 340
arterioles, 107
artery, 110, 111, 114, 133, 180, 181
arthritis, 31, 55
aryl hydrocarbon receptor, 368, 378, 379
asbestos, 14, 26
asbestosis, 15
ascites, 59, 140
ascorbic acid, 198, 203, 250, 273, 274, 275, 289, 296, 322
Asia, 79, 135
aspartate, 39, 207, 355
aspiration, 15, 55
assessment, 314, 316, 324, 325, 377, 381
asthenia, 39
asthma, 8, 9, 10, 11, 13, 15, 16, 17, 18, 19, 20, 27, 229
asthmatic airways, 9, 19
astrocytes, 128, 232, 234, 238, 239, 240, 250, 253, 254, 270
astrogliosis, 249
asymptomatic, 51, 54, 56
ataxia, 36, 46, 55, 232, 236, 237, 240, 242, 243, 245, 257, 259
atherogenesis, 179, 180, 181, 190, 197, 222
atherosclerosis, 139, 150, 169, 170, 171, 173, 174, 175, 176, 178, 179, 180, 181, 182, 183, 185, 189, 192, 194, 196, 197, 232, 305, 375
atherosclerotic plaque, 162, 197
atherosclerotic vascular disease, 198
athletes, 356, 358, 363, 364, 365
atmosphere, 341
atoms, 37, 240, 241, 371
ATP, 36, 46, 74, 77, 85, 87, 92, 93, 94, 123, 129, 153, 156, 207, 211, 231, 232, 240, 310, 311, 329, 339, 356, 372
atrophy, 239, 243, 249, 261, 264
attachment, 114
atypical pneumonia, 15
autism, 305
autoantibodies, 276, 363
autoimmune diseases, 67
autoimmune hepatitis, 54
autoimmunity, 292
automobiles, 287
autopsy, 35

autosomal dominant, 34, 38, 45, 244
autosomal recessive, 32, 36, 46, 50, 239, 240, 243
awareness, 239
axonal degeneration, 243, 249
axons, 270, 271, 272
Azathioprine, 289, 300

B

background radiation, 26
bacteremia, 30
bacteria, 3, 6, 16, 190, 249
bacterial infection, 11, 22
bacterial pathogens, 11
ban, 374
banks, 318
barriers, 320
basal cell carcinoma, 290, 298, 303
basal cell nevus syndrome, 296
basal forebrain, 232, 237
basal ganglia, 52, 236, 237, 240, 243, 256, 257
basal layer, 285
basal metabolic rate, 215
base, 129, 289, 292, 309, 311
base pair, 311
basement membrane, 108, 112, 147, 176, 285, 293
batteries, 371
BBB, 236
behavioral change, 54
behaviors, 143, 156
Belgium, 95
beneficial effect, 65, 150, 158, 181, 182, 183, 218, 321, 322
benefits, 150, 215, 219, 225, 240, 338, 345
benign, 56, 148, 163, 291, 301
benign prostatic hyperplasia, 148
benign tumors, 301
benzo(a)pyrene, 289, 295, 301, 381
beta-carotene, 164, 165, 224, 227, 266, 330, 332
bias, 150
bicarbonate, 12, 341
bile, 50, 51, 238, 255, 371
bilirubin, 174, 238, 242, 255, 335
biliverdin, 180, 238, 255
biliverdin reductase, 238
bioavailability, 38, 174, 176, 181, 219
biochemistry, 252, 313
bioenergy, 239, 251, 310
biological activities, 16
biological activity, 155, 199
biological systems, 65, 76
biomarkers, 26, 47, 158, 159, 212, 227, 251, 276, 295, 335, 337, 364

biomass, 10
biomolecules, 251, 306
biopsy, 35, 39, 47, 54, 56, 57, 66
biosynthesis, 36, 37, 49, 126, 137, 173, 232, 242, 253
Birmingham, Alabama, 285
birth weight, 344
births, 50, 318
black hole, 249
black tea, 295, 303
bladder cancer, 139
bleeding, 335
blepharospasm, 258
blindness, x, 201, 266
blood, 1, 2, 4, 6, 11, 29, 30, 35, 36, 37, 56, 67, 71, 93, 94, 103, 132, 133, 134, 147, 154, 169, 170, 171, 172, 174, 177, 178, 179, 181, 182, 184, 185, 186, 192, 193, 195, 196, 198, 199, 201, 206, 212, 213, 222, 225, 236, 250, 251, 254, 262, 263, 266, 267, 268, 269, 271, 278, 279, 280, 285, 287, 289, 293, 308, 333, 334, 352, 355, 363, 364
blood flow, 67, 93, 94, 133, 213, 225, 269, 279, 333
blood plasma, 4, 6, 154, 262
blood pressure, 169, 171, 172, 174, 177, 178, 179, 181, 182, 184, 185, 186, 192, 193, 195, 196, 198, 199, 222, 269, 279
blood supply, 134, 334
blood transfusion, 29, 30, 36, 37
blood transfusions, 29, 36
blood vessels, 132, 133, 134, 147, 170, 184, 185, 263, 266, 267, 271, 280, 285, 293
blood-brain barrier, 35, 236, 254
body fluid, 242
body mass index, 39
body weight, 205
bonding, 244
bonds, 7, 248, 311, 312, 325
bone, 33, 180, 338
bone marrow, 180
bowel, 380
brain, 35, 50, 52, 128, 132, 170, 185, 230, 232, 233, 234, 236, 237, 238, 239, 241, 242, 243, 244, 249, 251, 252, 253, 254, 255, 256, 258, 261, 271, 334, 360
brain stem, 185, 243, 244
breakdown, 211, 235, 238, 268, 269, 278, 311, 325, 347
breast cancer, 132, 138, 140, 141, 148, 149, 155, 156, 158, 163, 164, 168, 383
breast carcinoma, 140
breathing, 5
breathlessness, 9
bronchial asthma, 7, 10, 11

bronchial epithelial cells, 24
bronchial epithelium, 20, 23, 25
bronchial hyperresponsiveness, 12
bronchiectasis, 23
bronchioles, 3
bronchitis, 27
bronchoscopy, 7
bronchus, 7
Brownlee and co-workers, 202
by-products, 195, 215, 289, 371, 373

C

Ca^{2+}, 142, 173, 176, 182, 360
cadmium, 235, 377
caffeine, 318
calcium, 69, 73, 75, 89, 93, 94, 97, 173, 176, 188, 189, 192, 213, 247, 248, 249, 286, 294, 306, 353, 354, 355, 360
calcium channel blocker, 173
caloric intake, 216
caloric restriction, 225
cancer, 14, 26, 30, 41, 87, 88, 90, 103, 104, 123, 126, 127, 132, 135, 136, 137, 138, 139, 143, 144, 149, 150, 151, 154, 155, 156, 157, 158, 162, 164, 165, 167, 168, 229, 232, 286, 289, 293, 296, 300, 304, 305, 318, 327, 338, 350, 372, 375, 377, 380, 381, 382, 383
cancer cells, 135, 139, 143, 144, 149, 151, 155, 156, 157, 158, 167, 168
capillary, 107, 108, 109, 110, 111, 113, 114, 115, 116, 119, 241
capsule, 107, 306
carbohydrate, 102, 207, 209, 225
carbohydrates, 330
carbon, 1, 24, 180, 238, 255, 335, 340, 373, 374, 381, 382
carbon dioxide, 1
carbon monoxide, 24, 180, 238, 255, 335, 340
carbon tetrachloride, 374, 381, 382
carboxyl, 49
carboxylic acid, 100, 127
carcinogen, 14, 66, 89, 131, 294, 297, 373
carcinogenesis, 14, 88, 95, 98, 99, 103, 124, 135, 140, 150, 289, 290, 291, 295, 296, 298, 299, 300, 301, 302, 357, 381
carcinogenicity, 16
carcinoma, 139, 140, 141, 142, 147, 151, 155, 164, 295, 296, 301, 303, 304
cardiomyopathy, 31, 33, 36, 37, 46, 213, 240, 257
cardiovascular disease, 18, 171, 174, 178, 181, 182, 185, 197, 198, 199, 224, 337, 338, 348, 350, 377
cardiovascular function, 164

cardiovascular physiology, 193
cardiovascular risk, 179, 180, 197
cardiovascular system, 182
carotene, 149, 150, 159, 199, 250, 276
carotenoids, 223, 276, 277, 294
caspases, 126, 127, 136, 153, 266, 277, 294
catabolism, 180, 357
catalase, 13, 75, 79, 82, 85, 111. 112, 114, 115, 125, 126, 130, 147, 149, 151, 153, 173, 174, 178, 179, 213, 214, 218, 242, 245, 265, 266, 274, 275, 309, 330, 340, 342, 343, 345, 347
catalysis, 236, 247
catalyst, 268, 269, 279
catalytic activity, 126, 153, 215
cataract, 38, 39, 47
catecholamines, 352, 357
catheter, 133
cation, 247, 249
cattle, 382
Caucasian population, 12
Caucasians, 32, 40
causal relationship, 69, 204, 206
cauterization, 272
C-C, 375
CD95, 52, 62
cDNA, 238, 275
cell biology, 122, 132, 220, 278
cell culture, 11, 38, 73, 117, 132, 247, 265, 297, 377
cell cycle, 127, 128, 138, 288, 294, 295, 297, 303, 369
cell death, 10, 11, 12, 15, 21, 22, 62, 73, 92, 100, 104, 123, 126, 127, 128, 129, 131, 132, 135, 136, 143, 147, 151, 152, 153, 155, 156, 157, 158, 161, 182, 214, 229, 247, 253, 256, 261, 265, 268, 271, 280, 281, 287, 290, 294, 298, 313, 342, 348
cell differentiation, 173
cell division, 124, 127, 129, 132, 137, 340
cell fate, 143
cell killing, 151
cell line, 24, 39, 47, 62, 128, 141, 144, 148, 149, 151, 155, 156, 159, 166, 168, 265, 271, 281, 292, 381
cell lines, 39, 47, 141, 144, 149, 151, 155, 156, 159, 166, 168
cell membranes, 65, 124, 330, 336, 340
cell signaling, 17, 116, 119, 121, 146, 160, 167, 172, 268, 287, 296, 302, 359
cell surface, 42, 45, 241, 354, 361
cellular homeostasis, 312
central nervous system, 29, 45, 53, 60, 184, 231, 254, 256, 258, 271, 305, 339
central obesity, 83
cerebellum, 241, 243, 247

cerebral contusion, 237
cerebral hemorrhage, 237
cerebrospinal fluid, 254
ceruloplasmin, 35, 40, 45, 51, 56, 57, 236, 241, 242, 258, 309
challenges, 10, 27
channel blocker, 182
chaperones, 73
chelates, 240
chemical, 11, 16, 79, 80, 132, 135, 136, 157, 161, 232, 244, 250, 288, 289, 291, 296, 297, 301, 302, 306, 345, 377, 379
chemical properties, 244
chemical reactions, 79
chemicals, 10, 77, 126, 130, 286, 287, 288, 290, 297, 367, 377
chemokines, 11, 101
chemoprevention, 143, 150, 161, 295, 296, 299, 300, 304, 349
chemopreventive, 143, 286, 294, 296, 303
chemopreventive agents, 294, 303
chemotaxis, 69, 85, 93, 94
chemotherapeutic agent, 153, 158
chemotherapy, 143, 154, 167, 300, 318, 380
childhood, 239, 319
children, 7, 15, 19, 22, 24, 27, 54, 111, 254, 259
chlorine, 11, 250
chloroform, 375
cholangiocarcinoma, 54, 63
cholestasis, 55, 259
cholesterol, 83, 114, 116, 181, 184, 186, 204, 212, 233, 234, 253, 288
chorea, 258
choreoathetosis, 239, 240, 242
choroid, 265
chromium, 377
chromosomal abnormalities, 315, 342
chromosome, 32, 33, 34, 35, 44, 46, 50, 238, 241, 274, 277, 309, 311
chronic active hepatitis, 54, 103
chronic granulomatous disease, 172, 178
chronic liver diseases, viii, 29, 38, 39, 66, 67, 71, 88
chronic lymphocytic leukemia, 153, 156, 166, 167
chronic obstructive pulmonary disease, 8, 20, 21, 27, 364, 377
cigarette smoke, 3, 9, 11, 12, 15, 16, 20, 21, 26, 265, 277, 289, 300, 373, 377
cigarette smoking, 14, 20, 25, 265, 276, 319
circulation, 30, 51, 55, 58, 147, 148, 236, 242, 333, 340
cirrhosis, 31, 54, 58, 61, 66, 67, 70, 88, 90, 95, 102, 103, 104, 375
cities, 20

citrulline, 287
classes, 77, 379
claudication, 361
cleavage, 213, 340, 374, 381
clinical application, 151, 262
clinical diagnosis, 336
clinical examination, 39
clinical presentation, 54
clinical symptoms, 31, 33
clinical syndrome, 252
clinical trials, 86, 153, 155, 158, 215, 219, 236, 266, 269, 270, 370
clone, 137
cloning, 46
clusters, 46, 240, 296, 352
CNS, 29, 31, 35, 45, 231, 233, 234, 235, 236, 237, 239, 240, 241, 243, 247, 249, 250, 251, 258, 260, 262, 296
CO_2, 4
coal, 377
coal tar, 377
cocaine, 25
coding, 14, 70, 232, 242, 266, 274, 311, 316
codon, 103
codon 249, 103
coenzyme, 78, 240, 266
coffee, 273
cognition, 236
cognitive dysfunction, 243, 245
cognitive impairment, 239, 249, 256
collaboration, 17, 95
collagen, 58, 68, 69, 85, 89, 102, 108, 114, 121, 176, 213, 285, 332
collateral, 249, 309, 321, 322, 341
collateral damage, 321
colon, 131, 147, 150, 151, 165
colon cancer, 131, 151, 165
color, 269
colorectal adenocarcinoma, 126, 137
colorectal cancer, 159
coma, 333
combination therapy, 156
combined effect, 313
combustion, 377
communication, 141, 292
community, 16, 17, 164
competition, 358, 363, 378
competitors, 364
complement, 107, 108, 109, 114, 116, 255, 270, 299
complex interactions, 379
complexity, 143, 230, 247
complications, 3, 6, 7, 30, 59, 60, 66, 67, 70, 83, 112, 117, 122, 198, 202, 205, 207, 209, 210, 211, 212,

213, 214, 215, 219, 220, 221, 224, 243, 246, 269, 278, 279, 338, 342, 344
composition, 6, 67, 68, 136, 187, 207, 275, 341, 345
compounds, 38, 89, 110, 150, 155, 156, 158, 167, 202, 204, 219, 235, 242, 266, 272, 277, 289, 290, 291, 296, 301, 322, 338, 368, 370, 372, 373, 374, 375, 377, 378
conception, 322, 343
condensation, 128, 313, 340
conditioning, 216
conductance, 12, 23, 25, 248
conference, 165
configuration, 236
congenital adrenal hyperplasia, 336
congenital malformations, 340
Congress, 220
conjugated bilirubin, 255
conjugation, 151, 296, 371, 380
connective tissue, 49, 67, 70, 266, 273, 277
consensus, 309, 336, 349
conservation, 341
constituents, 13, 239, 249, 288, 294, 295, 297, 377
consumption, 11, 13, 15, 20, 52, 78, 81, 90, 99, 103, 164, 198, 199, 219, 227, 231, 264, 294, 318
contact dermatitis, 292, 301
contraceptives, 370
control group, 344
control measures, 95
controlled studies, 150
controlled trials, 150
controversial, 30, 82, 87, 89, 273, 316, 317, 322, 341, 344, 347, 358, 372
contusion, 247
convergence, 86
conversion rate, 207
cooking, 381
coordination, 26, 37, 154
COPD, 10, 11, 12, 13, 14, 15, 16, 21, 22, 27
copper, 45, 49, 50, 51, 52, 53, 55, 56, 57, 58, 59, 60, 61, 62, 63, 125, 162, 235, 241, 242, 243, 244, 250, 258, 259, 286, 343
cornea, 55, 271, 273, 274, 275, 282, 283
coronary arteries, 180, 187
coronary artery disease, 165, 182, 199, 212
coronary heart disease, 198, 199, 223, 227
corpus luteum, 338
correlation, 18, 61, 97, 124, 127, 131, 139, 144, 148, 205, 280, 315, 316, 321
correlations, 350, 356
cortex, 112, 239, 252, 254
corticobasal degeneration, 233
corticosteroid therapy, 19
cosmetic, 297

cosmetics, 287
coughing, 9
counterbalance, 68
CPI, 157
creatine, 21, 213, 355
creatinine, 279
Creutzfeldt-Jakob disease, 235
cryopreservation, 322, 341
cryptorchidism, 310
crystal structure, 161
crystalline, 283
CSF, 11, 242, 251
culture, 109, 116, 117, 139, 203, 247, 254, 255, 265, 271, 277, 290, 321, 340, 341, 342, 345, 346, 347, 349
culture media, 203, 321, 340, 341, 342, 345, 346, 347, 349
culture medium, 117, 265, 321, 341
curcumin, 15, 295
cure, 322
CVD, 225
cycles, 5, 342, 347
cycling, 50, 51, 195, 213, 286, 356, 372, 373, 374
cyclins, 132, 181
cyclooxygenase, 72, 110, 170, 293, 298, 334
cyclophosphamide, 154
cyclosporine, 178
cysteine, 50, 53, 82, 146, 147, 153, 155, 162, 167, 240, 248, 249, 257, 260, 261, 262, 266, 273, 277, 282, 293, 312, 321, 364
cysteine-rich protein, 53, 312
cystic fibrosis, 7, 8, 17, 22, 23, 24, 25, 27
cystine, 277
cytoarchitecture, 213
cytochrome, 51, 73, 77, 78, 79, 84, 88, 92, 99, 101, 109, 119, 124, 126, 152, 166, 170, 205, 232, 233, 238, 265, 276, 288, 290, 292, 294, 299, 354, 368, 370, 371, 373, 375, 376, 378, 379, 380, 381
cytochrome p450, 299, 379
cytochromes, 231
cytokines, 10, 11, 17, 30, 52, 67, 68, 72, 73, 76, 77, 80, 83, 85, 87, 88, 91, 94, 101, 117, 129, 130, 147, 159, 171, 173, 180, 193, 210, 215, 232, 238, 249, 250, 255, 288, 292, 293, 309, 319, 334, 338, 375
cytometry, 208, 314
cytoplasm, 77, 147, 290, 310, 340, 342, 368, 369, 371
cytoplasmic tail, 32
cytosine, 14, 25, 126, 137
cytoskeleton, 187, 245, 247
cytotoxicity, 65, 124, 125, 131, 141, 142, 156, 167, 168, 192, 218, 234, 244, 249

D

damages, 92, 278
data set, 316
database, 96
deaths, 143, 377
decomposition, 155, 192, 269, 279, 286
defects, 30, 33, 35, 37, 41, 43, 125, 172, 202, 207, 208, 209, 212, 250, 332, 333, 343
defence, 21, 100, 358
defense mechanisms, 159, 178, 282, 286, 287, 305, 342
deficiencies, 242, 243, 250, 259, 277
deficiency, 9, 12, 13, 22, 29, 30, 35, 41, 43, 45, 46, 87, 103, 125, 131, 148, 164, 172, 181, 190, 205, 240, 242, 243, 257, 258, 259, 260, 270, 299, 301, 312, 359
degradation, 32, 34, 45, 46, 61, 67, 69, 99, 109, 152, 162, 171, 176, 210, 255, 293, 294, 299, 330, 368, 371, 381
Delta, 382
dementia, 239, 258
demyelination, 243, 249
denaturation, 314, 315
dendritic cell, 11, 13, 292, 302
deoxyribonucleic acid, 280
dephosphorylation, 50, 146, 161, 215, 216
depolarization, 330, 353, 360
deposition, 31, 39, 55, 67, 72, 73, 86, 90, 109, 114, 115, 169, 176, 234, 235, 236, 237, 238, 239, 240, 249, 252, 254, 255, 256, 258, 350
deposits, 35, 37, 46, 54, 72, 113, 114, 232, 240, 241, 257, 263, 273, 293
depression, 59, 235, 254, 370
deprivation, 31, 271, 272
depth, 158, 295
derivatives, 27, 51, 130, 140, 147, 163, 296, 306
dermis, 285, 298
destruction, 11, 202, 219, 269, 286
detectable, 5, 162, 297
detection, 6, 17, 55, 101, 121, 204, 226, 302, 313, 314, 315, 356, 359
detoxification, 53, 155, 219, 294, 368, 369, 372, 379, 381
developed countries, 66
developing countries, 30, 66, 201
developmental change, 254
developmental process, 339
deviation, 124, 131, 140
diabetes, 31, 33, 39, 72, 88, 117, 150, 165, 170, 179, 181, 194, 201, 202, 204, 205, 206, 207, 208, 209, 211, 212, 214, 215, 218, 219, 220, 221, 222, 223,

224, 225, 226, 227, 229, 241, 242, 258, 267, 268, 269, 270, 277, 278, 279, 305, 332, 340, 375
diabetes mellitus, 31, 33, 72, 88, 91, 150, 170, 179, 201, 202, 220, 221, 223, 224, 226, 227, 229, 241, 242, 258, 278
diabetic nephropathy, 117, 118, 119, 120, 122, 224
diabetic neuropathy, 242, 245, 258
diabetic patients, 201, 204, 205, 206, 212, 213, 215, 218, 226, 267, 269, 278
diabetic retinopathy, 224, 225, 267, 268, 269, 277, 278, 279
diacylglycerol, 207, 223, 224
diagnostic criteria, 55, 349
dialysis, 59
diaphragm, 21, 108, 353, 361
diarrhea, 245
dichotomy, 158
diet, 15, 81, 112, 114, 120, 132, 141, 171, 181, 182, 186, 190, 194, 199, 202, 205, 207, 215, 219, 222, 224, 294, 338, 343, 349
dietary fat, 140
dietary intake, 226, 343
dietary iron absorption, 29, 30, 35, 37
diffusion, 17, 38
dilation, 175, 317
dimethylsulfoxide, 114
dioxin, 378
diplotene, 341
direct action, 110, 209
disability, 30, 66, 249
discomfort, 4, 5, 6, 7, 8
disease activity, 99, 250
disease gene, 61
disease model, 202
disease progression, 30, 39, 54, 63, 116, 269, 274
diseases, 1, 8, 10, 21, 23, 33, 38, 39, 65, 66, 67, 87, 88, 107, 112, 115, 119, 120, 123, 150, 189, 202, 207, 229, 250, 258, 262, 273, 275, 282, 294, 296, 297, 303, 305, 317, 347, 350
disequilibrium, 32, 93, 94
disorder, 8, 9, 36, 38, 50, 52, 55, 60, 86, 219, 232, 242, 243, 244, 256, 258, 273, 291, 334
dispersion, 315
disposition, 296
dissociation, 147, 215, 236
distribution, 61, 75, 136, 164, 236, 237, 380
diversity, 34, 79, 239
DNA, 3, 7, 14, 25, 26, 47, 51, 53, 57, 71, 73, 75, 76, 79, 81, 88, 89, 92, 97, 98, 99, 103, 127, 128, 129, 135, 137, 138, 146, 147, 148, 155, 156, 158, 161, 162, 167, 173, 176, 181, 182, 204, 208, 210, 212, 221, 223, 231, 251, 257, 265, 267, 268, 269, 270, 278, 280, 282, 283, 286, 287, 289, 290, 295, 297,

299, 300, 304, 305, 306, 309, 311, 312, 313, 314, 315, 316, 317, 318, 319, 320, 321, 322, 324, 325, 326, 327, 329, 330, 332, 333, 334, 336, 338, 339, 341, 342, 343, 346, 349, 352, 356, 359, 362, 373, 374, 376, 377, 378, 380
DNA breakage, 314, 315
DNA damage, 14, 25, 26, 47, 71, 73, 88, 89, 97, 103, 129, 138, 147, 155, 167, 181, 182, 204, 257, 265, 268, 270, 278, 280, 282, 283, 289, 290, 300, 304, 305, 311, 312, 313, 314, 315, 316, 317, 318, 319, 320, 321, 322, 324, 325, 326, 327, 329, 333, 334, 336, 338, 339, 341, 342, 343, 347, 356, 359, 362, 373, 376, 378
DNA lesions, 300
DNA polymerase, 75, 290
DNA repair, 89, 128, 313
DNA sequencing, 57
DNA strand breaks, 309, 313, 315
docetaxel, 139, 155
docosahexaenoic acid, 125, 139, 140, 142, 264
dogs, 132
donors, 82, 101, 207, 268, 274, 308, 314, 324, 341
dopamine, 53, 62, 235, 236, 238, 239, 255
dopaminergic, 232, 242, 254
dosage, 344
dosing, 219
double bonds, 124, 126, 311
down-regulation, 86, 160, 166
drinking water, 58, 114, 375
Drosophila, 253
drug delivery, 380
drug design, 250
drug interaction, 370, 378
drug metabolism, 295, 379
drug resistance, 158, 372
drug therapy, 22
drugs, 30, 41, 66, 86, 90, 92, 117, 123, 128, 129, 130, 135, 142, 154, 156, 168, 182, 254, 262, 263, 266, 269, 272, 286, 287, 293, 295, 296, 367, 370, 371
drusen, 263, 264
duodenum, 73, 233
dusts, 10
dyes, 203
dysarthria, 55, 240, 245
dyslipidemia, 83, 181
dysphagia, 55
dystonia, 55, 239, 240

E

EAE, 249, 250
E-cadherin, 291

Index

ECM, 52, 67, 68, 73, 86, 91, 175

edema, 94, 267, 295

editors, 221, 223

egg, 341

eicosapentaenoic acid, 125, 126, 139, 140, 142

ejaculation, 309, 310, 321

elaboration, 294, 334, 358

elastin, 67, 176, 285

electroencephalography, 241

electron, 50, 53, 62, 73, 74, 77, 85, 123, 124, 126, 145, 154, 170, 171, 172, 178, 207, 217, 231, 236, 239, 247, 254, 265, 268, 271, 276, 287, 293, 299, 302, 306, 308, 311, 330, 352, 353, 357, 360, 371, 374, 375, 377, 383

electrons, 123, 154, 171, 172, 288, 306, 308, 312, 329, 354, 370

electrophoresis, 208

electroretinography, 272

elucidation, 127

embryos, 306, 313, 320, 321, 329, 330, 333, 339, 340, 341, 345

emission, 318

emphysema, 12, 21

encephalitis, 237

encephalomyelitis, 249, 261

encephalopathy, 235

encoding, 12, 33, 34, 91, 147, 172, 239, 244, 245, 249, 257, 260

endocrine, 39, 350

endocrine glands, 39

endometriosis, 330, 334, 335, 336, 339, 343, 347, 348, 349, 350

endonuclease, 313

endoplasmic reticulum (ER), 32, 65, 74, 117, 244

endothelial cells, 25, 68, 69, 93, 94, 108, 115, 117, 122, 131, 132, 141, 147, 159, 162, 173, 176, 181, 185, 188, 189, 203, 206, 207, 208, 210, 220, 222, 236, 241, 267, 268, 269, 274, 275, 278, 355

endothelial dysfunction, 169, 171, 176, 177, 178, 179, 180, 182, 183, 185, 186, 187, 190, 194, 196, 212, 220, 223, 225, 279, 349

endothelium, 132, 141, 147, 170, 176, 183, 184, 185, 186, 199, 207, 209, 213, 273, 274, 282, 283

endotoxemia, 80, 99

endurance, 218, 355, 356, 357, 358, 363, 364, 365

energy, 50, 99, 157, 168, 205, 213, 217, 224, 225, 252, 275, 286, 310, 311, 312, 325, 356

energy expenditure, 217, 225

energy supply, 356

energy transfer, 286

enlargement, 111

entrapment, 279

environment, 98, 251, 252, 264, 285, 297, 332, 340, 378

environmental contamination, 302

environmental factors, 219, 305, 318

environmental stress, 327

environmental tobacco, 377, 383

enzymatic activity, 16, 128, 382

enzyme, 2, 9, 11, 12, 13, 46, 77, 82, 85, 87, 90, 100, 102, 108, 128, 129, 131, 145, 146, 148, 163, 171, 172, 174, 177, 180, 189, 196, 205, 207, 208, 209, 219, 235, 236, 237, 240, 242, 244, 257, 262, 268, 271, 287, 289, 290, 297, 303, 308, 310, 337, 339, 342, 353, 354, 357, 368, 370, 371, 375, 380, 381

enzyme induction, 303, 372, 380

enzyme inhibitors, 219

enzymes, 2, 9, 11, 13, 16, 17, 21, 50, 65, 67, 69, 75, 76, 77, 82, 85, 100, 114, 115, 120, 121, 123, 125, 129, 136, 147, 148, 149, 150, 151, 155, 158, 163, 164, 169, 170, 177, 179, 180, 181, 183, 205, 211, 213, 215, 217, 218, 222, 240, 242, 250, 252, 261, 274, 282, 283, 287, 288, 290, 291, 294, 296, 297, 299, 309, 330, 339, 340, 342, 353, 354, 355, 356, 362, 364, 368, 370, 371, 372, 373, 375, 377, 379, 381

eosinophils, 2, 5, 8, 9, 18

EPA, 125, 126, 131, 132, 134, 142

epidemiology, 95

epidermis, 285, 297, 298, 304

epididymis, 312, 317, 318, 324, 332

epididymitis, 317

epilepsy, 245, 247, 260, 305

epithelia, 16, 22

epithelial cells, 2, 5, 8, 11, 13, 14, 17, 20, 21, 25, 61, 108, 109, 112, 113, 114, 116, 117, 119, 121, 122, 274, 275, 277, 283, 291, 338, 349

epithelial lining fluid, 19, 22

epithelium, 2, 9, 11, 12, 20, 26, 163, 241, 243, 263, 273, 274, 276, 277, 283

equilibrium, 39

equipment, 4, 6

erythrocytes, 4, 205, 213, 243, 334

erythroid cells, 35, 46

erythropoietin, 30

ESR, 239, 301

essential fatty acids, 135, 139, 140, 141

ester, 109

estrogen, 190, 330, 338, 349

ETA, 177, 194

ethanol, 79, 80, 98, 99, 100, 103, 380

ethanol metabolism, 100

ethers, 371

ethnicity, 195

etiology, 66, 67, 88, 95, 225, 232, 263, 275, 300, 332

etiopathogenesis, 16, 247, 305, 325, 333, 339, 347

Europe, 79, 277

evidence, 3, 13, 15, 19, 43, 50, 51, 53, 54, 55, 59, 75, 87, 88, 90, 91, 94, 99, 102, 116, 117, 133, 138, 143, 144, 148, 149, 150, 156, 170, 171, 177, 178, 179, 180, 182, 184, 191, 192, 202, 207, 210, 211, 212, 214, 217, 218, 219, 225, 244, 249, 265, 270, 280, 281, 290, 302, 322, 325, 326, 333, 339, 344, 353, 355, 356, 357, 358, 362, 364, 382, 383

evil, 162

evoked potential, 245

evolution, 83

exchange of oxygen, 1

excision, 148

excitotoxicity, 244, 247, 248, 249, 260

excitotoxins, 247

exclusion, 40, 336

excretion, 13, 50, 51, 56, 58, 116, 121, 167, 214, 356, 362, 368, 372

execution, 128, 153

exercise, 21, 37, 46, 182, 193, 202, 215, 216, 218, 225, 226, 351, 352, 355, 356, 357, 358, 359, 360, 362, 363, 364, 365

exercise performance, 356

exertion, 351, 356

exons, 238

experimental autoimmune encephalomyelitis, 249, 261, 262

experimental condition, 238

exporter, 376

exposure, 1, 8, 10, 14, 15, 16, 17, 18, 19, 20, 26, 52, 53, 78, 80, 87, 99, 100, 126, 128, 130, 162, 203, 219, 231, 247, 251, 264, 265, 268, 273, 274, 275, 286, 287, 288, 289, 290, 292, 295, 316, 321, 322, 338, 340, 344, 372, 374, 375, 376, 377, 378, 381, 382

expressivity, 314

extracellular antioxidants, 1

extracellular matrix, 52, 67, 109, 117, 147, 169, 171, 175, 271

extracts, 288, 294, 295, 383

extravasation, 147

F

fallopian tubes, 335, 336, 341

families, 44, 57, 127, 259, 369, 375

family history, 178

family members, 152

fasting, 92, 201, 202, 218, 220, 225, 226

fasting glucose, 220

fat, 13, 81, 83, 85, 86, 99, 100, 101, 186, 190, 202, 205, 213, 224, 225, 233, 242, 250, 286, 294

fat intake, 205

fatty acids, 85, 86, 87, 90, 91, 110, 124, 125, 126, 127, 130, 131, 132, 135, 136, 138, 139, 140, 141, 142, 201, 203, 206, 207, 209, 210, 216, 222, 225, 264, 289, 311

fears, 279

femur, 133

ferric state, 241

ferritin, 38, 39, 47, 72, 97, 233, 237, 240, 242, 256, 257, 258, 274, 335, 357

fertility, 307, 311, 312, 316, 317, 318, 319, 322, 326, 331, 335, 336

fertilization, 305, 309, 311, 312, 313, 316, 318, 319, 321, 322, 332, 335, 336, 340, 341, 344, 345, 347, 348, 350

fetal development, 313

fetus, 333, 339, 343

fiber, 37, 353

fiber bundles, 353

fibers, 353

fibrin, 293

fibrinogen, 349

fibroblast growth factor, 70

fibroblasts, 10, 11, 128, 129, 135, 138, 145, 159, 160, 172, 207, 241, 274, 282, 287, 288, 294, 299

fibrogenesis, 16, 42, 61, 67, 68, 69, 72, 85, 96, 97, 101

fibrosarcoma, 140, 148, 163

fibrosis, 12, 15, 23, 24, 26, 31, 39, 47, 54, 66, 67, 69, 70, 72, 83, 84, 85, 87, 95, 96, 101, 175, 179, 186, 267, 375, 381, 382

fibrous cap, 179, 181

filament, 382

filters, 3

filtration, 108, 109, 110, 321

fish, 100, 131, 140, 142, 380

fish oil, 100, 131, 140, 142

fission, 253

fitness, 344

flame, 375

flame retardants, 375

flavopiridol, 139

flexibility, 311

fluid, 38, 59, 174, 267, 278, 329, 333, 334, 335, 336, 339, 341, 342, 348, 349, 350

fluorescence, 203, 214, 314

focal segmental glomerulosclerosis, 111

folate, 294

follicle, 286, 339, 341

follicles, 336, 339, 341, 342

follicular fluid, 329, 336, 339, 341, 342, 343, 344, 348, 349

food, 57, 58, 59, 205, 221, 286, 287, 338, 373

force, 225, 347, 359

Ford, 260, 381

forebrain, 241

formation, 14, 49, 67, 69, 71, 72, 73, 77, 79, 82, 83, 85, 87, 90, 92, 93, 103, 111, 113, 114, 115, 117, 121, 122, 124, 125, 129, 130, 131, 133, 142, 145, 146, 151, 152, 154, 171, 172, 177, 179, 180, 183, 186, 202, 203, 204, 207, 208, 209, 212, 213, 221, 232, 234, 240, 242, 247, 248, 262, 263, 264, 266, 278, 286, 287, 288, 289, 291, 294, 295, 297, 310, 312, 319, 325, 327, 334, 335, 348, 351, 361, 370, 373, 375

fragments, 314, 334

frameshift mutation, 33

France, 226, 354, 361

free radicals, 16, 51, 52, 65, 80, 82, 92, 98, 101, 120, 123, 125, 126, 127, 128, 129, 130, 131, 132, 135, 138, 140, 157, 174, 178, 182, 190, 202, 205, 218, 222, 226, 229, 244, 250, 251, 253, 264, 289, 291, 294, 301, 306, 329, 331, 341, 347, 348, 359, 361, 362, 368, 372, 377

freezing, 321

friction, 286

fructose, 223

fruits, 149, 182, 219, 242, 294, 343

funding, 201

fungi, 249

fusion, 306, 310, 311, 340

G

gadolinium, 155, 156, 167

gait, 36, 240, 245

gallbladder, 168

gametes, 329, 330, 341

gamma globulin, 115

gamma-tocopherol, 219

ganglion, 270, 280, 281

gastrointestinal bleeding, 66

gel, 208, 267, 272

gene expression, 14, 16, 21, 44, 62, 67, 76, 97, 127, 158, 161, 168, 183, 189, 222, 255, 271, 282, 330, 351, 368, 378

gene mutations, 29, 102, 104

gene promoter, 14, 369

gene regulation, 98, 229, 303

gene therapy, 60, 185

gene transfer, 63, 262, 283

genes, 14, 30, 43, 52, 53, 62, 70, 75, 77, 87, 88, 97, 102, 128, 132, 144, 145, 146, 147, 151, 153, 157, 158, 160, 162, 172, 174, 185, 210, 211, 217, 226, 232, 234, 249, 250, 251, 252, 256, 287, 289, 290, 294, 334, 360, 368, 369, 370, 371, 376, 378, 379, 380, 382

genetic alteration, 289

genetic background, 202

genetic defect, 60, 240

genetic disorders, 239

genetic factors, 289

genetic information, 326

genetic mutations, 14

genetic predisposition, 14

genetic testing, 56, 61

genetics, 42, 103, 253, 332

genome, 57, 60, 70, 71, 75, 96, 127, 173, 231, 311

genotoxic stresses, 89

genotype, 23, 32, 33, 40, 61, 227

genotyping, 40

germ cells, 324

germ line, 311, 312, 322

Germany, 201

gestation, 332, 340

ginseng, 375

gland, 298, 379

glaucoma, 270, 271, 272, 280, 281, 282

glia, 234, 239, 271, 280

glial cells, 52, 128, 138

glioblastoma, 128

glioma, 126, 137, 139, 162

globus, 240, 241, 257

glomerulonephritis, 109, 114, 115, 119, 120, 121, 122, 229

glomerulus, 107, 108, 119

glucocorticoid receptor, 146

glucose, 84, 85, 117, 122, 157, 182, 195, 201, 202, 203, 206, 208, 209, 211, 212, 215, 218, 220, 221, 222, 226, 227, 232, 253, 268, 269, 278, 310

glucose disposal, 202

glucose tolerance, 201, 221, 222, 227

glucose tolerance test, 222, 227

GLUT, 375

glutamate, 232, 247, 248

glutamine, 272

glutathione, 6, 11, 13, 15, 17, 19, 21, 22, 23, 25, 27, 71, 72, 74, 77, 82, 92, 100, 112, 125, 126, 130, 137, 146, 148, 149, 151, 153, 154, 164, 166, 167, 173, 174, 179, 182, 189, 205, 208, 209, 210, 217, 218, 221, 226, 232, 242, 245, 247, 250, 260, 261, 264, 265, 266, 268, 270, 271, 273, 274, 275, 283, 289, 298, 299, 300, 301, 309, 321, 322, 330, 332, 352, 353, 362, 364, 371, 372, 375, 376, 382

glutathione peroxidase (GPx), 82, 112, 114, 115, 125, 148, 149, 151, 174, 179, 209, 213, 216, 218, 271, 274, 275, 289, 290, 291, 330, 336, 337, 338, 341, 342, 343, 353

glycerol, 207
glycol, 163, 259, 289
glycolysis, 156, 168, 211, 290, 310
glycosylation, 211, 223
grants, 119, 183
granules, 36
gray matter, 261
Greece, 32, 351
growth, 3, 11, 14, 16, 26, 35, 37, 67, 69, 70, 91, 96, 102, 116, 117, 123, 124, 125, 126, 127, 128, 130, 131, 132, 135, 136, 137, 140, 141, 144, 145, 146, 147, 148, 151, 155, 156, 157, 158, 160, 161, 164, 165, 166, 169, 173, 175, 176, 183, 190, 191, 196, 215, 229, 262, 266, 269, 270, 272, 277, 278, 279, 286, 293, 295, 298, 300, 304, 334, 339, 341
growth arrest, 295
growth factor, 11, 14, 26, 67, 69, 70, 91, 96, 102, 116, 117, 125, 135, 137, 144, 145, 147, 155, 157, 160, 164, 173, 176, 190, 191, 215, 262, 266, 270, 272, 277, 278, 279, 293, 298, 334
growth rate, 124, 126, 135, 136
guanine, 204, 289

H

hair, 260, 285
hair follicle, 285
hairless, 299, 302, 304
half-life, 51, 151, 234, 336, 370
halogenation, 111
halos, 314
haptoglobin, 219, 227
harmful effects, 3
hazards, 14
HBV, 38, 66, 72, 75, 76, 88, 89
HBV infection, 72
HCC, 66, 75, 87, 88, 89, 90, 103, 104
HE, 23, 79, 162, 383
head and neck cancer, 167
headache, 246
healing, 275, 283
health, 18, 27, 30, 34, 41, 66, 201, 218, 224, 225, 226, 242, 254, 300, 301, 310, 313, 318, 319, 347, 349
health care, 30
health effects, 18
health problems, 201
health risks, 349
heart attack, 201
heart disease, 185, 202, 229
heart failure, 37, 39, 150
heat shock protein, 53, 60, 62, 211, 238, 368, 369
heavy drinking, 104

heavy metals, 251
hematuria, 107, 114
heme, 35, 36, 37, 45, 46, 75, 87, 94, 170, 180, 209, 233, 237, 238, 242, 250, 255, 256, 258, 261, 265, 271, 272, 287, 293, 299, 334, 370, 376
heme degradation, 287
heme oxygenase, 35, 45, 75, 170, 180, 209, 237, 238, 250, 255, 256, 258, 261, 265, 271, 272, 334, 376
hemochromatosis, 29, 31, 32, 33, 34, 35, 38, 39, 40, 41, 42, 43, 44, 45, 47, 73, 89, 104
hemoglobin, 270, 272, 357
hemolytic anemia, 35, 37, 54
hemorrhage, 233, 237, 263
hepatic encephalopathy, 59, 91
hepatic fibrosis, 38, 70, 85, 96
hepatic injury, 91, 105, 375
hepatic necrosis, 99
hepatic stellate cells, 52, 67, 72, 96, 102
hepatitis, 38, 39, 47, 54, 62, 66, 70, 71, 72, 73, 74, 75, 76, 83, 85, 88, 89, 95, 96, 97, 98, 99, 103, 104
hepatocarcinogenesis, 88, 89, 90, 91, 136, 299, 301
hepatocellular carcinoma, 31, 42, 54, 66, 95, 100, 102, 103, 104
hepatocytes, 50, 51, 52, 53, 57, 58, 59, 60, 67, 68, 73, 75, 77, 79, 82, 84, 85, 88, 89, 98, 99, 100, 103, 104
hepatoma, 91, 124, 136, 139, 149, 157, 167, 168
hepatomegaly, 39, 54
hepatorenal syndrome, 66
hepatotoxicity, 92, 104, 375
heredity, 195
heterogeneity, 44, 103, 316
heterozygote, 57
high fat, 171, 209, 215, 294
high risk patients, 198
hippocampus, 232, 236, 239, 261
histidine, 204
histological examination, 53
histone, 47, 73, 97, 217, 311
histone deacetylase, 47, 73, 97
histones, 312, 339
history, 66, 95, 103, 104, 178, 251, 257, 260, 262, 276, 294
HIV, 235, 237, 370
HIV-1, 237
HLA, 42, 261
HO-1, 35, 87, 180, 233, 237, 238, 239, 247, 250, 254, 256
HO-2, 209, 233, 238
homeostasis, 3, 16, 19, 29, 31, 32, 33, 34, 38, 41, 44, 50, 53, 61, 62, 72, 85, 93, 94, 139, 153, 168, 193, 211, 230, 233, 236, 237, 239, 241, 242, 247, 249,

250, 253, 254, 255, 256, 257, 287, 300, 319, 333, 339, 347, 362

homopolymers, 39

hormone, 30, 32, 33, 69, 99, 173, 225, 234, 318, 331, 338, 379

hormone levels, 318, 331

hormones, 83, 215, 338

hospitality, 383

host, 1, 8, 16, 21, 30, 60, 71, 72, 75, 124, 126, 172, 207, 212, 233, 236, 242, 287, 318

hub, 250

human brain, 132, 231, 234, 236, 239, 254

human health, 301

human immunodeficiency virus, 98

human leukemia cells, 125, 168

human neutrophils, 24

human subjects, 217, 265

hunting, 367

hybrid, 148

hydatidiform mole, 330, 333, 347, 348

hydrocarbons, 302, 377

hydrogen, 3, 16, 17, 19, 20, 23, 26, 27, 47, 81, 82, 110, 120, 123, 159, 163, 166, 170, 185, 186, 189, 191, 192, 195, 218, 231, 235, 236, 248, 260, 282, 283, 286, 298, 306, 330, 359

hydrogen peroxide, 3, 16, 17, 19, 20, 23, 26, 27, 47, 81, 110, 120, 123, 159, 163, 166, 170, 185, 186, 189, 191, 192, 195, 218, 231, 235, 236, 248, 260, 282, 283, 286, 298, 306, 330, 359

hydrolysis, 245, 368

hydroperoxides, 204, 206, 221, 223, 291, 301, 334, 355

hydrophilicity, 38, 368

hydroquinone, 3, 354

hydroxyl, 9, 25, 77, 79, 81, 108, 111, 114, 115, 120, 123, 135, 235, 236, 245, 247, 260, 269, 286, 288, 298, 301, 306, 308, 330, 334, 335, 355, 377

hyperandrogenism, 336

hypercalciuria, 55

hypercholesterolemia, 179

hyperglycaemia, 207

hyperglycemia, 86, 117, 206, 207, 209, 210, 211, 212, 220, 224, 268, 278, 279, 333, 340

hyperinsulinemia, 84, 86, 91

hyperlipidemia, 39, 83

hyperplasia, 91, 138, 295

hyperprolactinemia, 336

hypersensitivity, 108, 292, 302

hypersplenism, 90

hypertension, 39, 169, 171, 172, 174, 175, 176, 177, 178, 179, 181, 182, 183, 184, 185, 186, 188, 189, 190, 191, 192, 193, 194, 195, 196, 198, 199, 219, 222, 223, 282, 333, 344

hypertonic saline, 7

hypertriglyceridemia, 83

hypertrophy, 46, 175, 176, 177, 183, 184, 186, 188, 191, 193, 213

hyperuricemia, 39

hypodermis, 286

hypoglycemia, 91, 247, 271

hypogonadism, 31, 32

hypoparathyroidism, 55

hypospadias, 310

hypothesis, 83, 137, 150, 202, 205, 207, 215, 218, 219, 251, 301, 310, 312, 361

hypoxemia, 90

hypoxia, 77, 159, 161, 164, 168, 193, 197, 210, 255, 266, 271, 275, 333, 339, 368

hypoxia-inducible factor, 164, 197, 368

I

iatrogenic, 231, 320

ICAM, 11, 162, 210

identification, 40, 142, 183, 281

idiopathic, 15, 26, 42, 116, 120, 121, 237, 242, 258, 262, 305, 316, 317, 322, 326, 336, 343, 350

IFN, 292

IL-13, 68, 292

IL-8, 11, 73, 75, 84, 85

illumination, 276

image, 314

images, 241

imbalances, 12

immobilization, 310, 355

immune response, 2, 8, 10, 14, 18, 19, 26, 72, 75, 91, 132, 292, 318, 363, 369, 372, 382

immune system, 15, 77, 84, 378

immunity, 11, 26, 164

immunocompetent cells, 356

immunodeficiency, 254, 259

immunofluorescence, 113

immunoglobulin, 8, 88, 109, 112, 269

immunoglobulin superfamily, 112

immunohistochemistry, 83, 115

immunoreactivity, 256, 272

immunosuppression, 60, 288

impotence, 39

improvements, 150, 320, 358

in situ hybridization, 314, 315

in vitro, 24, 89, 117, 120, 131, 132, 136, 139, 140, 141, 142, 148, 161, 162, 167, 168, 181, 192, 197, 218, 236, 239, 244, 246, 262, 268, 272, 281, 290, 294, 299, 300, 313, 321, 340, 341, 342, 344, 345, 346, 347, 348, 360, 363 in vivo, 41, 82, 89, 91, 100, 116, 118, 131, 132, 137, 138, 139, 141, 160, 162, 166, 168, 171, 190, 193, 244, 279, 300, 309, 313, 316, 321, 322, 335, 340, 342, 354, 362, 382

incidence, 10, 55, 58, 66, 88, 90, 103, 149, 150, 158, 159, 165, 313, 319, 338, 344

incubation time, 341

India, 123, 135

indirect effect, 308

individuals, 6, 7, 9, 12, 17, 29, 39, 51, 53, 54, 56, 57, 59, 66, 81, 83, 91, 179, 198, 202, 219, 227, 240, 241, 246, 261, 312, 317, 358

inducer, 87, 93, 94, 294, 370, 371, 376

inducible enzyme, 334

induction, 17, 30, 47, 52, 53, 75, 79, 88, 90, 93, 94, 98, 114, 115, 116, 117, 127, 139, 148, 151, 152, 155, 162, 164, 166, 189, 208, 209, 210, 220, 238, 249, 250, 255, 290, 291, 293, 295, 297, 299, 301, 302, 303, 318, 338, 369, 370, 371, 379

industrialized countries, 66

industries, 287

ineffectiveness, 219

infants, 23, 25, 332, 339

infarction, 247

infection, 13, 16, 23, 25, 26, 38, 41, 66, 70, 71, 72, 73, 88, 286, 308, 335, 382

infertility, 55, 229, 305, 306, 309, 310, 311, 312, 315, 316, 317, 318, 322, 323, 324, 325, 326, 334, 335, 336, 342, 343, 344, 347, 348, 349, 350

inflammation, 4, 7, 8, 9, 11, 12, 14, 15, 16, 17, 18, 19, 21, 26, 27, 30, 34, 35, 43, 54, 71, 72, 73, 75, 80, 81, 83, 87, 99, 101, 105, 110, 114, 148, 163, 169, 175, 176, 178, 180, 183, 184, 189, 192, 193, 199, 202, 224, 227, 249, 287, 288, 293, 295, 296, 302, 308, 342, 350, 357, 358, 365

inflammatory bowel disease, 229, 305

inflammatory cells, 52, 148, 176, 218

inflammatory disease, 13, 99, 196, 261, 292, 300, 304

inflammatory mediators, 159

inflammatory responses, 9, 10, 11, 12, 110, 288, 293, 294, 299, 302

influenza, 8, 17, 375, 382

infrared spectroscopy, 262

ingestion, 57, 88, 90, 91

ingredients, 205

inguinal, 319

inhaled air, 1, 3, 6

inheritance, 34

inherited disorder, 49

inhibition, 39, 52, 69, 75, 82, 89, 91, 98, 116, 124, 127, 130, 137, 145, 147, 151, 158, 160, 168, 175, 180, 181, 182, 192, 207, 209, 215, 216, 219, 224,

248, 262, 269, 271, 279, 281, 295, 296, 329, 335, 339, 369, 376

inhibitor, 52, 81, 99, 111, 126, 131, 147, 155, 156, 160, 167, 177, 178, 193, 203, 210, 211, 222, 223, 238, 245, 262, 269, 271, 279, 293, 294, 297, 304, 314, 353

initiation, 58, 59, 67, 68, 88, 132, 142, 143, 144, 147, 150, 158, 289, 292, 295, 330

injections, 281

injure, 108, 271

injuries, 120, 271

injury, 3, 9, 15, 21, 25, 35, 38, 45, 49, 51, 52, 53, 55, 56, 58, 59, 60, 63, 67, 69, 76, 80, 81, 82, 85, 87, 89, 90, 91, 93, 94, 96, 97, 98, 99, 100, 102, 105, 107, 108, 109, 110, 111, 113, 114, 115, 116, 117, 119, 120, 121, 129, 137, 138, 169, 172, 175, 176, 181, 182, 183, 202, 209, 229, 231, 232, 235, 236, 238, 241, 242, 244, 247, 255, 256, 258, 265, 270, 271, 272, 274, 275, 280, 281, 283, 287, 289, 295, 322, 357, 358, 359, 363, 364, 375, 377, 380, 381, 382

innate immunity, 26, 298

inner ear, 172

inositol, 142, 176

insertion, 7, 233, 244, 296

insulin, 38, 39, 66, 69, 70, 75, 81, 83, 84, 85, 86, 88, 91, 97, 100, 101, 102, 104, 160, 175, 185, 201, 202, 203, 204, 208, 209, 210, 212, 213, 215, 216, 217, 218, 221, 222, 223, 225, 226, 271, 277, 337, 349

insulin dependent diabetes, 202

insulin resistance, 38, 66, 75, 83, 84, 86, 88, 91, 101, 102, 185, 202, 209, 210, 212, 213, 215, 216, 218, 221, 223, 225, 226, 337, 349

insulin sensitivity, 75, 86, 87, 100, 215, 217, 218, 226

insulin signaling, 85, 102, 215, 216

integration, 60

integrin, 122, 147, 162, 336

integrins, 335

integrity, 10, 11, 69, 81, 90, 127, 182, 283, 314, 315, 316, 319, 320, 321, 323, 325

interface, 114, 285, 297

interference, 151, 292

interferon, 72, 97, 254

interleukin-8, 25, 309

internalization, 71, 145, 160

interstitial lung disease, 15

intervention, 218, 229, 251, 256, 269, 345

intestine, 37, 43

intima, 118, 179, 180

intoxication, 67

intramuscular injection, 58

intraocular, 269, 270, 279, 280, 282

intraocular pressure, 270, 280

intrauterine growth retardation, 330

introns, 238, 316

invading organisms, 297

iodine, 111, 115

ion channels, 174, 175

ion transport, 50

ionizing radiation, 128, 138, 155, 287, 289

ions, 6, 12, 77, 123, 244, 247

iris, 271

iron, 29, 30, 31, 32, 33, 34, 35, 36, 37, 38, 39, 40, 41, 42, 43, 44, 45, 46, 47, 71, 72, 73, 77, 84, 86, 87, 88, 89, 90, 91, 94, 96, 97, 101, 102, 103, 104, 108, 114, 119, 141, 180, 230, 232, 233, 235, 236, 237, 238, 239, 240, 241, 249, 250, 252, 253, 254, 255, 256, 257, 258, 261, 262, 273, 286, 288, 292, 293, 299, 301, 302, 330, 334, 344, 348, 350, 352, 359, 370

iron regulatory pathways, 29

iron transport, 46, 254

iron-related disorders, 29, 41

irradiation, 128

ischemia, 15, 67, 93, 94, 105, 233, 249, 254, 269, 270, 357, 361

islands, 14

isoniazid, 92

isotope, 256

isozyme, 297

isozymes, 296

issues, 101, 102, 148

Italy, 29, 32, 65, 135

J

Jordan, 17, 282

K

K^+, 176

keratinocytes, 145, 160, 287, 293, 297, 298, 301

kidney, 35, 50, 55, 58, 75, 107, 110, 111, 113, 114, 115, 116, 117, 119, 120, 122, 134, 170, 185, 189, 201, 213, 214, 222, 334

kidney failure, 111, 113, 201

kidneys, 111

kill, 16, 127, 135, 157, 167, 286

kinase activity, 86, 146, 153, 160, 183, 191, 215, 224

kinetics, 244, 360

kinks, 310

Krebs cycle, 77

kynurenine pathway, 254

L

labeling, 265, 267, 315, 316

lactic acid, 37, 46, 357

lactoferrin, 237, 242

laminar, 280

Langerhans cells, 288

L-arginine, 13, 171, 208, 344

larynx, 3

lateral sclerosis, 237, 260

Latin America, 20

LDL, 179, 180, 184, 196, 205, 206, 212, 213, 223, 234, 243, 332, 338, 362, 363

lead, 10, 12, 29, 33, 35, 38, 40, 54, 55, 60, 67, 71, 72, 73, 75, 83, 85, 93, 108, 110, 114, 119, 123, 129, 130, 151, 157, 171, 179, 180, 183, 215, 273, 286, 287, 291, 295, 297, 301, 306, 310, 313, 320, 330, 331, 332, 333, 335, 336, 339, 340, 341, 346, 368

leakage, 123, 170, 231, 263, 267, 308, 312, 330, 352

lean body mass, 234

learning, 339

learning disabilities, 339

legal blindness, 263

legs, 237, 355

lending, 126

lens, 39, 47, 55, 267, 273, 283

leptin, 69, 216

lesions, 88, 103, 107, 111, 118, 122, 179, 180, 213, 231, 249, 261, 275, 283, 291, 334, 343, 348, 350, 358

leukemia, 153, 155, 166, 380

leukotrienes, 131, 133, 134, 288

liberation, 247, 357

lifetime, 286, 368

ligand, 145, 151, 176, 314, 368, 369, 378

light, 39, 53, 157, 219, 241, 245, 257, 258, 264, 265, 266, 273, 275, 276, 277, 293, 300, 302, 303, 305, 326, 340, 342

linoleic acid, 83, 125, 139, 141, 178

lipases, 247

lipid metabolism, 85, 333

lipid oxidation, 4, 13, 85, 87, 363

lipid peroxidation, 15, 24, 51, 52, 71, 72, 73, 79, 81, 82, 83, 85, 86, 87, 91, 94, 100, 103, 104, 114, 118, 121, 122, 124, 125, 126, 127, 130, 131, 132, 135, 136, 137, 138, 140, 141, 154, 164, 169, 174, 176, 178, 182, 233, 234, 238, 241, 247, 264, 266, 267, 268, 271, 272, 275, 276, 281, 288, 292, 299, 301, 302, 310, 317, 321, 323, 329, 330, 331, 333, 334, 335, 336, 339, 343, 345, 347, 355, 359, 361, 362, 363, 364, 375, 376, 380 lipid peroxides, 124, 126, 127, 129, 130, 131, 137, 250, 268, 348

lipids, 4, 51, 65, 76, 77, 110, 133, 174, 180, 199, 210, 212, 247, 271, 319, 329, 330, 340, 362, 371, 375

lipolysis, 85, 202

lipoprotein synthesis, 202

lipoproteins, 184, 243, 330, 338

liquid chromatography, 316

lithium, 132, 133, 134, 141

liver, 17, 29, 31, 35, 38, 39, 42, 43, 47, 49, 50, 51, 52, 53, 54, 55, 56, 57, 58, 59, 60, 61, 62, 63, 65, 66, 67, 69, 70, 71, 72, 73, 75, 76, 77, 80, 81, 82, 83, 84, 85, 86, 87, 88, 89, 90, 91, 93, 94, 95, 96, 97, 98, 99, 100, 101, 102, 103, 104, 105, 124, 125, 126, 128, 136, 137, 138, 147, 149, 161, 168, 202, 215, 241, 242, 305, 334, 362, 368, 375, 378, 379, 380, 381, 382

liver cancer, 90

liver cells, 51, 53, 57, 60

liver cirrhosis, 54, 66, 88, 100

liver damage, 38, 85, 94, 104, 305, 375

liver disease, 29, 31, 38, 39, 55, 56, 59, 65, 66, 67, 71, 72, 80, 83, 84, 85, 87, 88, 95, 98, 99, 101, 102, 104

liver enzymes, 102

liver failure, 52, 54, 55, 59, 60, 63, 67, 91, 104

liver function tests, 57, 85

liver transplant, 54, 59, 60, 66, 93, 101

liver transplantation, 54, 59, 60, 66, 93, 101

localization, 98, 128, 188, 256, 325

loci, 43

locomotor, 250

locus, 32, 33, 44, 232, 240

longevity, 216, 359

longitudinal study, 104

lovastatin, 116

low-density lipoprotein, 171, 179, 186, 196

low-grade inflammation, 181

luciferase, 163

lumen, 3, 6, 9, 11

lung cancer, 14, 16, 25, 26, 150, 155, 159, 160, 167, 374, 380, 381, 383

lung disease, 12, 15, 22, 25, 26

lung function, 12, 19, 22, 23

Luo, 262, 280, 350

lupus, 115

lutein, 264

lymph, 147, 324

lymph node, 324

lymphocytes, 2, 5, 10, 11, 13, 98, 155, 218, 292

lymphoid, 173

lymphoid tissue, 173

lymphoma, 88, 130, 155, 156, 158, 168

lysine, 89, 110, 343

lysosome, 53

M

macromolecules, 99, 108, 209, 286

macrophages, 2, 5, 9, 11, 13, 30, 31, 34, 35, 37, 68, 73, 75, 88, 109, 116, 119, 132, 142, 159, 179, 180, 196, 218, 229, 308, 334, 336, 349, 375, 382

macular degeneration, 229, 263, 266, 275, 276, 277

magnesium, 226, 245, 344

magnetic resonance, 39, 240, 261

magnetic resonance imaging, 39, 240, 261

magnitude, 9, 308

major depressive disorder, 379

major histocompatibility complex, 32, 43, 292

majority, 3, 5, 8, 13, 32, 36, 41, 77, 126, 143, 240, 244, 297, 337, 352, 355, 357

malabsorption, 13, 30, 243, 250

malaria, 233, 235, 254

malignancy, 144, 148

malignant cells, 148, 149

malignant growth, 144, 147

malignant melanoma, 151, 156, 301

malignant tumors, 137

malnutrition, 13

mammalian brain, 258

mammalian cells, 98, 116, 125, 207, 382, 383

mammalian tissues, 257

mammals, 287

man, 98, 173, 225, 243, 245, 359

management, 16, 39, 40, 41, 59, 86, 93, 101, 102, 104, 127, 155, 220, 250, 297, 320, 322, 343, 344

manganese, 125, 137, 138, 166, 235, 238, 255

manipulation, 151, 159, 249, 347, 362, 365

mantle, 286

manufacturing, 374

mapping, 44

marijuana, 25

marrow, 180

Maryland, 23, 285

mass, 231, 272, 337, 340

mass spectrometry, 272

mastectomy, 164

matrix, 11, 67, 68, 69, 75, 107, 111, 114, 147, 148, 162, 175, 176, 183, 189, 192, 194, 196, 197, 239, 268, 278, 281, 298

matrix metalloproteinase, 11, 147, 162, 175, 176, 183, 189, 192, 194, 196, 197, 268, 278

matter, 3, 9, 52, 249, 261, 317

maturation process, 305

MBP, 261

MCP, 67, 69, 70, 176, 180, 213

MCP-1, 67, 69, 176, 180, 213

measurement, 56, 57, 192, 220, 314, 316, 322, 323, 324, 356, 361

measurements, 23, 358

meat, 262, 287

media, 170, 180, 321, 323, 341, 342, 345, 347

median, 204, 232

mediation, 114, 121, 183, 192

medical, 40, 59, 60, 230, 262, 305

medical history, 40

medication, 219

medicine, 7, 159, 189, 198, 221, 229

melanin, 265

melanoma, 126, 132, 142, 147, 148, 149, 150, 151, 155, 160, 162, 163, 164, 165, 286, 295, 301, 303

melatonin, 238, 242, 272, 343, 350

mellitus, 91, 150, 170, 201, 202, 221, 227, 258, 278

membrane permeability, 51, 92, 268

membranes, 17, 38, 51, 71, 73, 76, 85, 114, 124, 125, 135, 241, 247, 311, 354, 357, 373, 375

membranous glomerulonephritis, 115, 121

membranous nephropathy, 109, 113, 116, 117, 120, 121

memory, 292

menopause, 330, 338, 345, 347

menstruation, 330, 334, 338

mental retardation, 239

mercury, 235

mesangial cells, 107, 109, 110, 115, 117, 118, 122

mesangial proliferative glomerulonephritis, 121

mesothelioma, 149

messengers, 140, 144, 145, 215

meta-analysis, 25, 150, 165, 198, 224, 225, 300, 310, 319, 320

Metabolic, 104, 252, 302

metabolic changes, 268, 352

metabolic disorder, 66, 242

metabolic disorders, 66, 242

metabolic pathways, 212, 290

metabolic syndrome, 39, 83, 86, 97, 101, 117, 207, 209, 211, 217, 220, 222, 225, 227

metabolism, 16, 30, 34, 37, 41, 43, 46, 49, 50, 60, 65, 75, 76, 77, 79, 81, 84, 90, 99, 100, 103, 124, 133, 134, 135, 136, 137, 139, 157, 167, 168, 182, 194, 201, 211, 213, 215, 217, 224, 225, 226, 232, 233, 234, 235, 236, 239, 252, 254, 257, 258, 275, 286, 288, 294, 296, 300, 301, 319, 325, 342, 347, 368, 370, 379, 380, 381, 382

metabolites, 1, 20, 89, 92, 120, 132, 139, 217, 249, 288, 292, 294, 297, 371, 374

metabolized, 77, 108, 109, 133, 231, 238, 291, 296, 370, 371, 373

metabolizing, 136, 205, 288, 294

metabolome, 142

metal ion, 50, 53, 162, 286, 340, 345

metal ions, 162, 340, 345

metalloproteinase, 68, 70

metals, 53, 87, 235, 236, 250, 251, 377

metaphase, 341, 342

metastasis, 14, 141, 143, 147, 148, 151, 162, 163, 164, 165, 166

metformin, 86, 204, 220

methylation, 25, 87, 126, 137, 371, 375, 376, 382

methylprednisolone, 111

MHC, 32, 42, 43

mice, 17, 21, 22, 26, 32, 33, 35, 36, 43, 44, 45, 46, 47, 80, 81, 86, 87, 88, 89, 97, 99, 102, 103, 112, 125, 128, 136, 140, 141, 147, 148, 151, 156, 163, 164, 169, 171, 172, 174, 177, 178, 179, 180, 181, 184, 185, 186, 188, 193, 196, 197, 204, 213, 215, 216, 218, 240, 241, 245, 247, 253, 261, 265, 266, 268, 269, 272, 274, 277, 278, 279, 283, 291, 295, 299, 300, 301, 302, 303, 304, 335, 344, 375, 382

microcirculation, 90, 93, 94, 279

microenvironments, 219, 329, 339

micronutrients, 27, 165

microorganisms, 172, 286

microscopy, 53, 110, 113, 314

microsomes, 124, 136

microspheres, 272, 281

midbrain, 242

migration, 69, 148, 163, 173, 175, 176, 179, 370, 382

mild asthma, 19

mild hypertensive, 199

milligrams, 266

mineralocorticoid, 177

minimal change disease, 111, 115, 116

miscarriage, 319, 335

Misregulation of systemic iron homeostasis, 29, 31

mitochondria, 10, 16, 29, 36, 53, 63, 65, 73, 75, 77, 85, 89, 98, 123, 124, 130, 135, 154, 178, 182, 183, 186, 192, 199, 206, 207, 216, 231, 232, 233, 240, 250, 253, 256, 265, 266, 268, 269, 271, 278, 302, 308, 310, 311, 313, 315, 326, 331, 352, 354, 355, 358, 360, 376, 383

mitochondrial damage, 231, 255

mitochondrial DNA, 81, 99, 148, 164, 252, 254, 261, 265, 289, 311, 325, 336, 339, 356, 383

mitogen, 69, 91, 118, 146, 170, 174, 186, 191, 288, 298, 383

mitogens, 296

mitosis, 69, 131

MMP, 68, 69, 70, 147, 148, 175, 176, 189, 298

MMP-2, 189

MMP-9, 147, 148

MMPs, 11, 67, 68, 69, 175, 179
models, 11, 33, 36, 38, 39, 43, 46, 52, 53, 60, 85, 87, 88, 91, 107, 109, 111, 112, 115, 117, 119, 120, 130, 145, 148, 149, 156, 158, 169, 177, 178, 182, 192, 195, 207, 236, 244, 257, 259, 265, 266, 268, 269, 270, 272, 275, 289, 291, 295, 296, 297, 355
modifications, 114, 146, 204, 232, 234, 259, 264, 272, 311, 340, 356, 358, 371
mole, 333
molecular biology, vii, 313
molecular mass, 38, 146
molecular oxygen, 3, 51, 108, 207, 231, 235, 247, 250, 286, 298, 308, 357, 371
molecular pathology, 45, 252
molecular weight, 6, 7, 8, 161
molecules, 11, 37, 38, 50, 51, 58, 60, 65, 77, 79, 82, 108, 109, 122, 132, 147, 151, 169, 170, 171, 174, 176, 204, 229, 240, 242, 260, 268, 272, 287, 288, 291, 292, 306, 329, 334, 347, 351
monolayer, 11
morbidity, 66, 239, 243, 339, 347
morphogenesis, 340
morphological abnormalities, 317
morphology, 253, 274, 316, 339, 341
mortality, 66, 80, 103, 104, 149, 150, 164, 165, 198, 333, 338, 339, 377, 383
mosaic, 232
motif, 50, 146
motor neuron disease, 305
motor neurons, 244, 259
motor skills, 55
movement disorders, 59
MRI, 240, 243, 259, 261
mRNA, 37, 39, 47, 73, 100, 126, 128, 137, 172, 173, 180, 189, 234, 238, 245, 342
mRNAs, 145
mtDNA, 148, 231, 232, 252, 270, 311, 313
mucosa, 3, 6, 9, 79
multiple factors, 158
multiple myeloma, 156
multiple nodes, 247
multiple sclerosis, 233, 237, 255, 261, 262
multiplication, 131
muscles, 12, 21, 244, 286, 334, 352, 353, 355, 358, 360, 361
mutagenesis, 44, 88, 162, 311
mutant, 32, 36, 37, 45, 62, 136, 241, 244, 259, 295
mutation, 14, 34, 39, 42, 43, 44, 45, 46, 50, 60, 163, 231, 240, 245, 251, 254, 257, 258, 261, 313
mutation rate, 231
mutations, 12, 26, 29, 30, 32, 33, 34, 35, 36, 38, 39, 40, 42, 47, 50, 56, 57, 61, 73, 87, 88, 90, 97, 101,

102, 104, 164, 231, 232, 239, 241, 242, 243, 244, 250, 253, 259, 260, 270, 274, 289, 311, 313, 374
myelin, 250
myelin basic protein, 250
myelodysplastic syndromes, 37
myocardial infarction, 198
myocardium, 240
myoclonus, 245, 260
myofibroblasts, 115
myoglobin, 55
myopathy, 12, 37, 46, 243
myosin, 213

N

NaCl, 7
NAD, 18, 77, 78, 79, 96, 120, 130, 162, 165, 166, 183, 184, 185, 186, 187, 188, 189, 193, 194, 195, 197, 199, 205, 206, 222, 269, 299, 308, 353, 354, 360, 361, 371, 374, 380
NADH, 77, 115, 171, 183, 185, 187, 207, 211, 268, 279, 308, 319, 353, 354, 360, 361
National Health and Nutrition Examination Survey, 201
National Institutes of Health, 165, 285
natural killer cell, 218, 288
natural pregnancy, 319, 344
natural selection, 320, 341
nausea, 91
necrosis, 54, 60, 67, 99, 100, 125, 129, 132, 151, 153, 159, 179, 238, 247, 294, 314, 326
negative effects, 181, 311
negative relation, 205, 310
neoangiogenesis, 88, 90
neonates, 231
neoplasm, 291
neovascularization, 263, 266, 267, 268, 269, 277, 279
nephritic syndrome, 107
nephritis, 109, 113, 114, 115, 119, 120, 121
nephrolithiasis, 55, 63
nephropathy, 113, 114, 115, 116, 117, 121, 202, 211
nephrosis, 111, 114, 120
nephrotic syndrome, 107, 111, 113, 117, 120
nerve, 46, 211, 213, 214, 257, 258, 270, 271, 281
nerve biopsy, 258
nerve growth factor, 281
nervous system, 229, 231, 234, 239, 242, 249, 250
neural function, 318
neurobiology, 280
neuroblastoma, 133, 149, 155
neurodegeneration, 53, 125, 232, 237, 239, 252, 255, 256

neurodegenerative diseases, 237, 245, 247, 252, 253, 254, 262

neurodegenerative disorders, 231, 232, 236, 251, 254, 259

neurofibrillary tangles, 232

neuroglioma, 135

neuroimaging, 232, 237, 251

neuroinflammation, 244

neurological disease, 56, 251, 254, 259

neuronal apoptosis, 193

neuronal cells, 254

neurons, 53, 127, 231, 232, 238, 240, 243, 244, 247, 252, 255, 260, 261, 269, 271

neuropathologies, 239

neuropathy, 202, 270, 271, 280

neuroprotection, 262, 272, 281, 282

neuroscience, 230

neurotoxicity, 62, 252, 261, 262

neurotransmission, 287

neurotransmitter, 49, 53, 235

neurotransmitters, 232, 235, 250, 253

neurotrophic factors, 272

neutral, 314, 341

neutropenia, 38, 246

neutrophils, 2, 5, 9, 11, 13, 15, 16, 24, 88, 93, 94, 109, 111, 159, 162, 207, 308, 324, 361

New England, 159, 195, 196, 198, 199

New Zealand, 91

NH2, 152

nickel, 292, 301, 377

nicotinamide, 69, 71, 72, 74, 77, 78, 79, 80, 93, 148, 163, 170, 218, 226, 288, 308

nicotine, 319

nigrostriatal, 242

nitric oxide, 18, 19, 20, 23, 67, 68, 72, 74, 92, 93, 97, 126, 148, 169, 170, 171, 180, 184, 185, 186, 190, 192, 193, 195, 199, 203, 205, 206, 208, 217, 220, 232, 235, 247, 248, 255, 266, 268, 270, 272, 278, 279, 280, 287, 295, 298, 306, 308, 317, 331, 334, 335, 336, 349, 350, 377

nitric oxide synthase, 23, 72, 93, 97, 170, 171, 180, 186, 195, 203, 206, 208, 217, 220, 247, 255, 268, 270, 272, 278, 279, 280, 295, 298, 308, 334, 335, 349

nitrite, 24, 148, 287

nitrogen, 1, 2, 16, 21, 65, 71, 72, 93, 162, 169, 202, 219, 229, 247, 250, 261, 298, 300, 306, 329, 360

nitrogen dioxide, 219

nitrosamines, 88, 90, 319, 377

NMR, 261

NO synthases, 287

nodules, 90, 124

non-enzymatic antioxidants, 273, 330

non-insulin dependent diabetes, 201, 221

non-polar, 368

nonsense mutation, 33, 258

nonsmokers, 10, 14, 20, 264

non-steroidal anti-inflammatory drugs, 295, 304

norepinephrine, 235

normal aging, 232, 236

Nrf2, 15, 146, 147, 162, 209, 210, 211, 303, 371, 376, 380

NSAIDs, 295

nuclear genome, 311, 339

nuclear membrane, 130

nuclear receptors, 369, 379

nucleation, 240

nuclei, 54, 128, 236, 240, 243

nucleic acid, 25, 238, 247, 313, 329, 371, 374, 375

nucleotide sequence, 241

nucleotides, 314

nucleus, 53, 76, 125, 128, 147, 153, 172, 252, 291, 342, 368, 369, 371, 378

null, 43, 112, 180, 181, 296, 301, 332

nutrient, 30, 93

nutrients, 61, 94, 202, 270

nutrition, 66, 95, 185, 195

nutritional status, 356

O

obesity, 39, 66, 91, 102, 104, 216, 220, 225, 305, 349

obstruction, 10, 14, 24, 25

obstructive lung disease, 15

occlusion, 93, 132, 133, 134, 142

oculomotor, 243

OH, 51, 81, 108, 123, 169, 174, 183, 191, 244, 270, 286, 292, 298, 306, 357

oil, 100, 132, 141, 142, 285, 373, 377

oleic acid, 141

oligodendrocytes, 241

oligodendroglia, 128, 138

oligomerization, 153

oligozoospermia, 314, 315, 321

olive oil, 242

omega-3, 141

oncogenes, 14, 144, 145, 157, 374

oncogenesis, 103

oocyte, 305, 306, 311, 313, 329, 330, 332, 336, 339, 340, 341, 342, 347, 350

opportunities, 27, 250

optic nerve, 270, 271, 272, 280, 281

organ, 38, 49, 54, 57, 93, 150, 231, 234, 250, 285, 290, 339, 352, 359

organelles, 124, 219, 310, 340, 358

organism, 37, 313, 367, 372, 378

organs, 3, 11, 14, 35, 49, 59, 156, 169, 213, 286, 287, 289, 291

ornithine, 290, 291, 298, 300

osmotic stress, 210

osteogenic sarcoma, 139

osteoporosis, 55, 338

ovarian cancer, 155, 338

ovaries, 336

overlap, 56, 369, 372

overproduction, 12, 39, 148, 223, 268, 292, 330

overtraining, 358, 365

oviduct, 334

ovulation, 330, 336, 338, 342, 344, 349

oxidant-enhancing strategies, 143

oxidation, 3, 5, 12, 14, 19, 50, 51, 75, 77, 79, 81, 84, 85, 87, 103, 112, 116, 117, 118, 121, 123, 145, 146, 152, 153, 160, 161, 162, 176, 184, 190, 204, 205, 207, 212, 213, 215, 218, 221, 225, 234, 238, 239, 244, 254, 266, 267, 271, 277, 287, 288, 289, 292, 297, 309, 312, 338, 352, 353, 355, 362, 363, 368, 371, 374, 380

oxidation products, 19, 292

oxidative damage, 24, 25, 51, 53, 148, 149, 152, 153, 155, 158, 163, 173, 174, 182, 183, 187, 189, 212, 223, 231, 242, 251, 255, 257, 264, 271, 273, 274, 277, 280, 283, 297, 298, 299, 300, 301, 302, 309, 312, 319, 340, 345, 353, 355, 356, 358, 361, 362

oxidative destruction, 171

oxidative reaction, 72, 332

oxidative stress, 4, 11, 12, 13, 17, 18, 19, 21, 22, 24, 26, 38, 47, 52, 57, 61, 62, 65, 66, 71, 72, 73, 74, 75, 76, 77, 79, 80, 81, 83, 84, 85, 86, 87, 88, 89, 91, 92, 93, 94, 96, 97, 98, 99, 100, 103, 112, 116, 117, 121, 125, 128, 129, 130, 137, 138, 144, 146, 147, 148, 149, 150, 151, 152, 153, 154, 155, 157, 158, 160, 162, 167, 168, 169, 171, 174, 175, 176, 177, 178, 179, 180, 181, 182, 183, 184, 185, 189, 190, 191, 192, 194, 195, 197, 199, 202, 204, 205, 206, 207, 209, 210, 212, 215, 216, 218, 220, 221, 222, 223, 225, 227, 229, 232, 236, 238, 239, 242, 244, 247, 248, 249, 250, 251, 252, 253, 254, 255, 259, 260, 262, 264, 265, 266, 267, 268, 269, 270, 271, 272, 273, 274, 275, 277, 278, 279, 281, 282, 283, 287, 288, 290, 291, 292, 293, 297, 298, 299, 301, 302, 306, 309, 310, 311, 312, 317, 318, 319, 322, 323, 324, 325, 326, 327, 329, 330, 331, 332, 333, 334, 335, 336, 337, 338, 339, 340, 341, 342, 343, 344, 346, 348, 349, 350, 351, 355, 356, 357, 358, 359, 360, 362, 363, 364, 375, 376, 380, 382

oxygen, 1, 15, 17, 21, 24, 25, 27, 51, 65, 77, 84, 93, 94, 108, 119, 120, 121, 122, 130, 135, 136, 137, 139, 160, 162, 165, 172, 182, 183, 185, 186, 192, 197, 202, 207, 211, 217, 222, 223, 226, 235, 250, 251, 265, 269, 271, 272, 277, 286, 287, 288, 296, 298, 299, 305, 306, 323, 324, 329, 335, 340, 341, 342, 345, 349, 352, 354, 356, 359, 360, 361, 370, 371, 375, 376

oxygen consumption, 271, 352, 356, 376

oxyhemoglobin, 287

ozone, 3, 9, 20, 359, 374

P

P13K, 303

p21WAF1/CIP1, 128

p53, 88, 103, 116, 127, 128, 129, 130, 135, 138, 146, 155, 162, 167, 191, 290, 295, 300, 301, 315

Pacific, 135

paclitaxel, 139, 141, 155, 158, 168

pain, 91

pancreas, 31, 35, 241

pancreatic cancer, 141, 151, 155, 165, 166

pancreatic insufficiency, 13, 243

pancreatitis, 55, 243

paracentesis, 59

parallel, 115, 338

parasites, 249

parenchyma, 15, 31, 93, 94, 236, 242

parenchymal cell, 31, 35, 37

parkinsonism, 239, 243, 262

participants, 361

pathogenesis, 9, 20, 25, 27, 30, 31, 41, 46, 49, 51, 66, 70, 71, 76, 80, 81, 83, 84, 87, 88, 89, 91, 94, 96, 111, 113, 115, 117, 119, 121, 122, 177, 178, 192, 197, 207, 219, 225, 231, 232, 235, 244, 249, 252, 253, 256, 257, 261, 265, 266, 269, 270, 275, 280, 286, 290, 291, 292, 296, 297, 298, 300, 301, 305, 323, 333, 334, 338, 343, 358

pathogens, 2, 3, 8, 30, 65, 229, 249, 309, 317

pathology, 16, 80, 213, 253, 254, 263, 265, 267, 268, 273, 274, 293, 333

pathophysiological, 15, 81, 191, 202, 224, 250, 258, 329

pathophysiological roles, 15

pathophysiology, 1, 42, 67, 94, 105, 172, 183, 187, 209, 211, 212, 254, 257, 306, 323, 326, 333, 361

pathways, 29, 36, 45, 62, 67, 76, 81, 86, 87, 88, 97, 102, 108, 117, 118, 123, 127, 137, 144, 145, 146, 150, 152, 155, 166, 168, 180, 189, 191, 192, 195, 209, 211, 222, 223, 250, 255, 257, 287, 288, 290, 291, 292, 293, 294, 296, 297, 299, 303, 314, 330, 339, 351, 354, 357, 359, 375, 376, 382

PCR, 252, 308

penetrance, 32, 244

peptide, 32, 44, 51, 252

peptides, 6, 255

perfusion, 105, 114, 217, 333
perinatal, 333, 339
peripheral nervous system, 229, 243
peripheral neuropathy, 240, 243
peripheral vascular disease, 375
peritoneal cavity, 334, 350
permeability, 22, 73, 80, 81, 99, 108, 110, 111, 152, 209, 238, 255, 256
permeable membrane, 247
permission, 110, 113, 233, 234, 237, 243, 248, 251, 264
permit, 234
peroxidation, 24, 51, 76, 84, 85, 87, 90, 101, 110, 114, 124, 125, 127, 130, 131, 135, 136, 138, 140, 148, 204, 212, 220, 304, 311, 331, 333
peroxide, 17, 19, 94, 138, 160, 179, 192, 262, 275, 322, 330, 332, 333, 335, 355, 371
peroxynitrite, 16, 92, 93, 94, 169, 192, 194, 235, 244, 247, 248, 268, 269, 279, 287, 298, 306, 335, 340
persistent asthma, 19
PET, 252
pH, 274, 286, 287
phagocyte, 116, 141, 185
pharmaceutical, 242, 269, 302
pharmacogenomics, 251
pharmacology, 250
pharmacotherapy, 251
phenol, 253
phenotype, 19, 31, 32, 33, 39, 43, 44, 45, 61, 67, 68, 69, 126, 137, 148, 149, 151, 158, 166, 177, 188, 259, 291, 296, 302, 303, 336
phenotypes, 34, 39, 122
pheochromocytoma, 138
Philadelphia, 62, 63, 119, 223, 252, 262, 298
phlebotomy, 31, 34, 86, 89
phosphate, 36, 69, 71, 72, 74, 93, 148, 163, 170, 182, 189, 199, 207, 272, 288, 308, 310, 356
phosphatidylcholine, 100
phosphatidylserine, 326
phospholipids, 16, 77, 83, 101, 124, 275, 311, 325, 354
phosphorous, 286
phosphorylation, 50, 76, 85, 91, 93, 94, 98, 117, 130, 132, 138, 139, 142, 145, 146, 152, 160, 170, 175, 176, 187, 188, 191, 207, 210, 211, 215, 217, 240, 269, 292, 293, 295, 308, 319, 361, 376
photorefractive keratectomy, 283
photosensitivity, 293
physical activity, 199, 225, 356, 364
physical environment, 288
physical exercise, 12, 215, 217, 226, 351, 363
physiological, 34, 187, 190, 192, 256, 306, 335, 360

physiological factors, 231
physiological mechanisms, 316
physiology, 183, 187, 225, 241, 287, 298, 324, 351, 352
PI3K, 145, 155, 160, 173
pigmentation, 31, 39, 258
pigs, 161, 181
pilot study, 121, 277, 344
placebo, 27, 102, 150, 198, 226, 266, 276, 301, 321, 344
placenta, 50, 243, 340
plaque, 179, 180, 181
plasma levels, 24, 51, 205
plasma membrane, 11, 32, 50, 75, 113, 124, 145, 188, 208, 209, 213, 308, 309, 310, 311, 314, 315, 321, 322, 325, 326, 340, 341, 346, 353, 361
plasmapheresis, 59
plasminogen, 148, 211, 222, 223, 279
plastics, 318, 367
platelet activating factor, 109
platelet aggregation, 93, 94, 338
platelets, 94, 111
platform, 157
platinum, 154, 168
Platinum, 154
playing, 58
pleural cavity, 334
plexus, 317
PM, 18, 160, 163, 164, 222, 224, 260, 300, 349, 360, 361, 364, 365
pneumonia, 8, 15, 17, 24
point mutation, 32, 39, 241
poison, 367, 375
Poland, 378
polarity, 291
polarization, 19
pollen, 2, 18
pollutants, 9, 10, 11, 14, 286, 287, 297
pollution, 11, 305, 318, 381
polyamine, 290
polyamines, 290
polychlorinated biphenyl, 318, 371, 380
polycyclic aromatic hydrocarbon, 368, 369, 377, 380, 381
polycystic ovarian syndrome, 347
polymerase, 71, 129, 173, 210, 211, 222, 223, 279, 287, 308
polymerase chain reaction, 308
polymorphism, 12, 22, 23, 25, 261
polymorphisms, 178, 195, 219, 249, 251, 252, 332, 370, 376, 379, 380, 382
polypeptide, 257, 258
polypeptides, 4, 77, 241, 244

406 Index

polyphenols, 294, 295, 296, 303

polysaccharide, 375

polyunsaturated fat, 124, 139, 141, 142, 198, 266, 271, 292, 296, 310, 325, 334, 340, 362

polyunsaturated fatty acids, 124, 139, 141, 142, 198, 266, 271, 292, 296, 310, 325, 334, 340

population, 12, 17, 20, 22, 38, 44, 61, 66, 79, 86, 98, 104, 150, 182, 195, 196, 198, 201, 219, 220, 232, 262, 270, 285, 313, 314, 315, 316, 319, 325, 332, 358, 377

porphyria, 38

porphyrins, 293

portal hypertension, 59, 90

positive correlation, 144, 357

positron, 232

positron emission tomography, 232

preeclampsia, 178, 179, 196, 330, 333, 344, 347

pregnancy, 181, 198, 306, 316, 319, 320, 321, 325, 329, 330, 331, 332, 333, 334, 338, 340, 341, 343, 344, 345, 347, 349, 350

premature death, 201

preparation, 309, 312, 320, 321, 322, 324, 347

preservation, 321

preservative, 287

preterm delivery, 348

prevention, 82, 95, 131, 143, 149, 150, 158, 159, 164, 165, 179, 182, 183, 196, 198, 215, 220, 221, 226, 262, 277, 279, 303, 324, 344, 345, 353

preventive approach, 297

primary biliary cirrhosis, 243

primary function, 12

primary tumor, 147, 148, 296

priming, 18, 305

principles, 229, 230, 232

pro-atherogenic, 205, 234

probability, 316

proband, 56, 57

probe, 314

producers, 171, 308

professionals, 199, 227

progenitor cells, 30, 199, 210, 262

progesterone, 338, 344

prognosis, 88, 164, 168, 251

programming, 177, 192

progressive supranuclear palsy, 232, 237

pro-inflammatory, 11, 12, 97, 176, 210, 211, 213, 232, 238, 249, 250, 288, 309, 319, 334

proliferation, 10, 30, 68, 69, 87, 91, 96, 102, 114, 115, 117, 122, 124, 127, 128, 131, 132, 137, 139, 140, 143, 144, 145, 149, 157, 158, 160, 165, 173, 176, 179, 189, 210, 211, 213, 236, 290, 294, 295, 297, 303, 306, 335, 348

proline, 290

promoter, 14, 73, 98, 103, 126, 238, 291, 300, 301

propane, 141

prophase, 341

prophylaxis, 218, 226

prostaglandins, 93, 94, 110, 131, 133, 134, 135, 139, 238, 288

prostate cancer, 148, 151, 159, 163, 165, 166, 379

prostate carcinoma, 159

protease inhibitors, 370

protection, 47, 58, 60, 82, 112, 136, 198, 199, 205, 213, 217, 242, 246, 260, 272, 277, 278, 279, 280, 283, 286, 299, 302, 309, 311, 322, 345, 346, 348, 375, 380

protective mechanisms, 339, 348

protective role, 53, 180, 219, 262

protein folding, 241

protein kinase C, 86, 117, 118, 142, 173, 188, 207, 222, 223, 224, 269, 279, 290

protein kinases, 139, 191, 210, 288, 293

protein misfolding, 244

protein oxidation, 12, 162, 179, 221, 238, 280, 355, 362, 364

protein synthesis, 53, 329

proteins, 4, 6, 14, 21, 24, 32, 36, 46, 50, 53, 59, 60, 61, 68, 71, 72, 73, 75, 76, 77, 79, 83, 88, 89, 92, 101, 109, 116, 117, 121, 122, 123, 129, 132, 142, 145, 146, 152, 153, 155, 158, 161, 169, 173, 179, 185, 210, 212, 213, 221, 232, 233, 236, 242, 244, 247, 249, 253, 257, 259, 260, 264, 267, 268, 269, 270, 271, 272, 274, 279, 281, 286, 287, 288, 289, 290, 291, 292, 293, 294, 311, 313, 319, 329, 330, 350, 352, 354, 355, 357, 360, 361, 362, 363, 369, 371, 374, 375

proteinuria, 110, 111, 113, 114, 115, 116, 117, 118, 119, 120, 121

proteoglycans, 67, 108, 109

proteolytic enzyme, 11

proteome, 275

protons, 174

proto-oncogene, 89, 183, 289

proximal tubules, 22

Pseudomonas aeruginosa, 3, 13, 16, 24, 25

psoriasis, 290, 292, 295, 301, 303

psychosis, 55

PTEN, 146, 161

pterygium, 273, 282

ptosis, 243

puberty, 202

public health, 250

pulmonary diseases, 1, 3, 6, 7, 8, 10, 15

pulmonary hypertension, 182, 193

pumps, 372

purines, 171, 330, 357

Q

quadriceps, 21
quality control, 260
quality of life, 30, 263
quantification, 39, 276
quercetin, 303
quinolinic acid, 247
quinone, 3, 137, 162, 236, 374
quinones, 235, 371, 374, 377, 381

R

race, 364, 380
radiation, 123, 130, 135, 147, 155, 162, 167, 210, 274, 276, 287, 295, 297, 299, 300, 301, 315, 318, 339
radiation therapy, 318
radical formation, 51, 60, 77, 377
radical mechanism, 98, 140
radical reactions, 348
radicals, 9, 16, 51, 52, 65, 77, 79, 80, 82, 105, 111, 114, 115, 120, 121, 123, 125, 128, 129, 135, 138, 139, 154, 182, 190, 194, 202, 222, 235, 236, 239, 245, 247, 260, 269, 286, 289, 301, 306, 329, 330, 335, 338, 355, 357, 359, 360, 361, 362, 377, 383
radio, 111, 115
radiotherapy, 143, 147
radon, 14
rapidly progressive glomerulonephritis, 107
rat kidneys, 115
reactions, 16, 36, 79, 83, 87, 112, 123, 127, 171, 235, 236, 244, 254, 286, 287, 288, 292, 297, 335, 339, 345, 368, 370, 371, 373, 374, 375, 379, 380
reactive nitrogen species (RNS), 1, 169, 202, 306, 329
reactive oxygen, 1, 16, 24, 37, 47, 51, 68, 71, 72, 74, 77, 78, 80, 84, 93, 97, 107, 119, 122, 123, 125, 135, 136, 139, 142, 143, 159, 160, 161, 162, 163, 166, 167, 168, 169, 170, 180, 183, 186, 189, 190, 192, 195, 196, 199, 202, 220, 222, 225, 229, 240, 247, 262, 264, 275, 282, 286, 298, 299, 300, 302, 323, 324, 325, 326, 327, 332, 347, 348, 350, 351, 360, 361, 370, 371, 380
reactive oxygen species (ROS), 1, 51, 107, 143, 169, 202, 222, 264, 286, 351, 371
reactivity, 37, 175
reading, 76

receptors, 14, 26, 69, 75, 80, 81, 100, 144, 145, 147, 152, 155, 157, 173, 180, 207, 209, 234, 236, 237, 247, 248, 269, 278, 292, 335, 369, 379
recognition, 15, 42, 60, 243
recombinant DNA, 7
recombination, 312
recommendations, 205
recovery, 8, 59, 69, 321
recurrence, 148, 164
recycling, 174, 208, 233
red blood cells, 37
red wine, 273, 295
redistribution, 61, 86
reduced lung function, 22
reflexes, 63
regeneration, 21, 52, 105, 138, 272, 375
Registry, 381
regression, 178, 182, 295, 331
relatives, 40, 57
relaxation, 176, 209, 211, 212, 223, 333
relevance, 135, 139, 146, 148, 208, 244, 280, 303, 323, 325, 361, 362
relief, 370
remediation, 323
remission, 116
remodelling, 326
renin, 112, 170, 177, 179, 185, 186, 208, 214, 222
repair, 10, 11, 14, 21, 25, 60, 128, 158, 210, 269, 272, 308, 309, 313, 316, 338, 374
replication, 73, 89, 140, 289
repression, 146
repressor, 368, 369, 378, 379
reproduction, 305, 313, 322, 323, 325, 326, 329, 331, 340, 347, 348, 349
reproductive age, 317, 334
reptile, 380
reptile species, 380
requirements, 30, 43, 302, 347, 352
RES, 71
resection, 93
residues, 89, 94, 110, 146, 147, 155, 162, 204, 206, 248, 262, 287, 312
resistance, 69, 83, 86, 91, 102, 124, 126, 127, 138, 153, 166, 168, 172, 174, 178, 184, 190, 191, 192, 195, 196, 201, 202, 215, 216, 223, 225, 335, 357, 358, 363, 364, 382
resolution, 8, 61, 69, 70
respiration, 49, 51, 157, 168, 215, 287, 353
respiratory distress syndrome, 15
respiratory failure, 12, 26, 312
respiratory syncytial virus, 8
respiratory tract, 1, 2, 3, 4, 5, 6, 7, 8, 9, 10, 11, 12, 14, 15, 16, 17, 18, 20, 374

response, 10, 13, 20, 22, 24, 25, 30, 32, 34, 36, 38, 42, 43, 47, 51, 53, 62, 67, 68, 72, 73, 75, 76, 86, 93, 97, 103, 108, 109, 111, 117, 122, 128, 132, 137, 146, 147, 149, 151, 153, 155, 158, 159, 162, 172, 177, 179, 188, 190, 192, 193, 203, 206, 209, 211, 215, 217, 218, 225, 227, 234, 238, 244, 247, 252, 255, 260, 264, 277, 290, 292, 293, 297, 317, 332, 334, 351, 357, 363, 367, 368, 369, 371, 375, 380, 382, 383

responsiveness, 22, 219

restoration, 81

resveratrol, 238, 273, 295

retardation, 35

reticulum, 32, 65, 72, 74, 76, 84, 98, 102, 117, 122, 130, 142, 167, 172, 231, 238, 244, 315, 340, 353, 355, 360, 368, 372

retina, 241, 263, 264, 265, 266, 267, 268, 269, 270, 271, 272, 273, 275, 276, 278, 279, 281

retinal ischemia, 267

retinitis, 276

retinoblastoma, 126, 137, 181

retinol, 165

retinopathy, 202, 211, 240, 243, 267, 268, 269, 277, 278, 279

rhabdomyolysis, 55, 63

rheumatoid arthritis, 305, 364

rhinitis, 8, 17, 18

rhinovirus infection, 18

rhythm, 39

riboflavin, 245, 288

ribose, 129, 222, 223, 279, 287

rings, 55, 56, 57

risk, 6, 9, 10, 12, 14, 15, 18, 21, 22, 25, 55, 60, 66, 67, 73, 75, 83, 84, 86, 88, 89, 90, 95, 144, 150, 159, 164, 165, 185, 195, 198, 199, 201, 212, 219, 221, 224, 227, 231, 251, 264, 266, 269, 276, 277, 279, 290, 295, 296, 303, 305, 313, 320, 332, 333, 337, 338, 339, 342, 344, 348, 350, 372, 375, 377, 379, 380, 381, 383

risk assessment, 377

risk factors, 10, 14, 18, 66, 83, 84, 86, 88, 90, 95, 185, 266, 379

risks, 269, 345

RNA, 70, 71, 193, 258

RNA splicing, 258

RNAs, 151

rodents, 173, 249, 250, 268

ROOH, 204, 212

roots, 243

Rouleau, 260

ruthenium, 167

S

safety, 27, 58, 60, 156, 165

saliva, 6

salts, 132

sarcoidosis, 15, 26

saturated fat, 99

saturation, 31, 32, 33, 34, 40, 43, 86, 90

scar tissue, 69

scatter, 137

scavengers, 111, 125, 150, 182, 219, 247, 269, 274, 283, 290, 342

schizophrenia, 235, 254, 305

school, 54

school performance, 54

science, 165, 253, 367

sclerosis, 118, 237

scrotal, 319

sebum, 286

secrete, 292

secretion, 10, 12, 47, 69, 97, 133, 147, 202, 212, 218, 226, 232, 243, 298, 338

seizure, 246

selectivity, 244

selenium, 112, 114, 120, 150, 159, 164, 245, 250, 262, 275, 283, 336, 344, 362, 382

semen, 306, 308, 310, 313, 315, 316, 317, 318, 322, 323, 324, 325, 327, 334, 339, 341

seminal vesicle, 308

seminiferous tubules, 332

senescence, 138, 161, 181, 229, 231, 236, 237, 379

sensation, 286

sensing, 32, 33, 44, 62, 87, 168, 211, 256

sensitivity, 45, 56, 126, 129, 137, 153, 155, 156, 158, 166, 168, 217, 255, 271, 299, 301, 313, 315, 370

sensitization, 188

sensorineural hearing loss, 246

sensors, 146, 233, 248

sepsis, 15

serine, 30, 41, 86, 162, 210

serotonin, 93, 94, 105, 235, 254

serum, 4, 24, 34, 35, 38, 39, 40, 43, 51, 56, 57, 71, 72, 73, 75, 80, 85, 90, 97, 101, 114, 116, 142, 165, 179, 241, 245, 246, 267, 331, 345, 359, 362, 363

serum albumin, 116

serum ferritin, 34, 38, 39, 72, 90

serum transferrin, 43

severe asthma, 19

sex, 43, 70, 193, 317, 338

shear, 173

sheep, 113

shock, 53, 210

showing, 116, 134, 147, 151, 178, 205, 243, 264, 295, 318, 356
siblings, 56, 104, 245, 260
sickle cell, 37
side chain, 234
side effects, 8, 60, 156, 260
sideroblastic anemia, 36, 46, 237, 240
signal transduction, 102, 117, 132, 135, 155, 161, 173, 185, 223, 300, 303, 330, 339, 382
signaling pathway, 30, 69, 73, 81, 144, 146, 152, 157, 158, 166, 174, 175, 191, 197, 209, 210, 215, 268, 288, 294, 297, 300, 302, 303, 304
signalling, 67, 68, 102, 161, 222, 236, 303
signals, 116, 130, 140, 145, 153, 223, 286, 289, 291, 297, 313
signs, 54, 56, 91, 243, 266, 267, 274, 337
silver, 110
Sinai, 220
single test, 56
sinuses, 3
siRNA, 177
sister chromatid exchange, 309
skeletal muscle, 4, 12, 55, 81, 161, 190, 202, 215, 217, 225, 226, 231, 351, 352, 353, 354, 355, 359, 360, 361, 362
skin, 31, 39, 140, 150, 164, 243, 273, 285, 286, 287, 288, 289, 290, 291, 292, 293, 294, 295, 296, 297, 298, 299, 300, 301, 302, 303, 304, 378
skin cancer, 150, 286, 290, 294, 296, 299, 300, 301, 303, 304
skin diseases, 286, 292, 299, 302
slit lamp, 55, 57
slit lamp examination, 55
small intestine, 161, 242, 368, 372
smoke exposure, 18
smoking, 9, 10, 11, 14, 15, 18, 20, 21, 26, 27, 98, 179, 264, 276, 305, 319, 339, 342, 377, 380, 381, 383
smoking cessation, 11, 20
smooth muscle, 9, 11, 68, 127, 169, 171, 172, 176, 178, 179, 181, 183, 187, 188, 189, 191, 192, 193, 195, 197, 203, 207, 210, 211, 213, 220, 224, 291
smooth muscle cells, 10, 11, 127, 169, 171, 172, 178, 179, 183, 187, 188, 189, 191, 192, 195, 197, 207, 211, 213, 220
SNS, 170
soccer, 363
sodium, 114, 186, 199, 249
solar keratosis, 296
solid tumors, 155, 156, 157, 167
solution, 110, 111, 132, 344
solvents, 90, 318
somatic cell, 129, 308, 311, 312, 313, 320, 325

somatic mutations, 148
soymilk, 338
spasticity, 55, 239, 240, 243, 245
spectroscopy, 252, 293, 377
speculation, 354
speech, 245
sperm, 305, 306, 307, 308, 309, 310, 311, 312, 313, 314, 315, 316, 317, 318, 319, 320, 321, 322, 323, 324, 325, 326, 327, 329, 331, 332, 334, 336, 340, 341, 344, 345, 347, 349
sperm function, 307, 311, 316, 321, 323, 325, 332
spermatid, 313
spermatogenesis, 310, 312, 313, 319, 326, 346
spin, 129, 239, 251, 254, 293, 301, 359, 370, 377
spinal cord, 241, 245, 247, 305, 318, 327
spinal cord injury, 305, 327
spleen, 35, 73, 324
sponge, 148
spontaneous abortion, 330, 333
Sprague-Dawley rats, 141
Spring, 224
sputum, 4, 6, 7, 13, 17, 22, 24, 27
squamous cell, 290, 298, 300
squamous cell carcinoma, 290, 298, 300
stability, 45, 139, 162, 197, 210, 241, 311
stabilization, 60, 213, 242, 306, 376
stable asthma, 18, 19
stable complexes, 37
standardization, 96
stasis, 293, 302
state, 25, 39, 50, 51, 52, 77, 79, 128, 130, 144, 146, 147, 148, 159, 160, 162, 165, 174, 189, 201, 241, 242, 248, 275, 286, 310, 329, 331, 332, 333, 353, 370, 372
states, 39, 40, 81, 117, 183, 202, 209, 211, 221, 249, 250, 333, 336, 347, 359
statin, 279
statistics, 103, 270
status asthmaticus, 19
steel, 318
sterile, 4, 7
steroids, 370
sterols, 340
Stevens-Johnson syndrome, 287, 299
stimulant, 116
stimulus, 60, 69, 146, 245
stoichiometry, 37
stomach, 77, 149, 287
storage, 30, 42, 49, 53, 57, 59, 233, 236, 237, 240, 256
striatum, 254
stroke, 177, 184, 193, 194, 233, 235, 237, 245, 253, 383

stroma, 144, 273, 274, 296
stromal cells, 296
structural changes, 53, 295
structural gene, 70
structural protein, 71, 74, 75, 88, 109
structure, 11, 42, 49, 61, 85, 107, 162, 169, 196, 232, 234, 272, 273, 281, 297, 312, 314, 315, 316, 325, 326, 327, 361
style, 381
subarachnoid hemorrhage, 245
substance abuse, 231
substitution, 32, 33, 34
substitutions, 32, 34
substrate, 9, 86, 90, 91, 104, 125, 129, 171, 174, 180, 182, 208, 231, 242, 319, 353, 354, 370, 371, 373, 380
substrates, 85, 90, 146, 204, 215, 217, 245, 288, 296, 310, 311, 357, 360, 368, 371, 372
suicide, 313, 315, 375
sulfate, 99, 108, 344
sulfur, 12, 36, 37, 46, 94, 229, 257, 352
sulphur, 46, 240, 250
Sun, 163, 166, 168, 276, 279, 350
superoxide anion, 3, 8, 9, 21, 26, 92, 108, 123, 183, 185, 189, 192, 193, 203, 281, 286, 287, 298, 302, 306, 308, 330, 371, 377
superoxide dismutase (SOD) mimetics, 169
supplementation, 15, 30, 59, 63, 103, 150, 164, 165, 174, 196, 198, 212, 219, 221, 223, 224, 226, 227, 242, 276, 279, 282, 292, 320, 321, 338, 343, 344, 347, 349, 359, 360, 362, 363, 382
suppression, 51, 86, 126, 132, 140, 149, 151, 166, 232, 239, 250, 288, 290, 340
supraventricular tachycardia, 56
surgical removal, 148, 151, 164
surplus, 217, 237, 240
surveillance, 95
survival, 14, 63, 100, 123, 126, 142, 143, 145, 151, 155, 156, 157, 158, 168, 233, 272, 275, 278, 281, 288, 290, 293, 294, 303, 325
susceptibility, 14, 23, 52, 109, 124, 184, 204, 223, 242, 249, 271, 275, 296, 299, 301, 315, 332, 339, 360, 363, 375, 380
sweat, 285
swelling, 110, 335
Switzerland, 95
sympathetic nervous system, 170
symptomatic treatment, 59
symptoms, 8, 18, 35, 39, 40, 54, 56, 91, 241, 246
syndrome, 15, 38, 47, 55, 86, 104, 111, 225, 231, 237, 239, 243, 249, 256, 257, 259, 280, 310, 336, 348, 349, 350, 358, 365
synergistic effect, 88, 156

synthesis, 13, 23, 45, 46, 53, 60, 68, 69, 86, 90, 94, 109, 127, 132, 141, 174, 176, 202, 233, 234, 240, 245, 255, 286, 288, 290, 299, 312, 333, 335, 371, 376
systolic blood pressure, 193

T

T cell, 10, 19, 42, 108, 111, 142
tamoxifen, 141
tar, 3, 373, 377, 383
target, 34, 49, 81, 132, 139, 142, 150, 152, 157, 161, 183, 199, 210, 215, 229, 234, 251, 269, 297, 300, 369, 376
techniques, 1, 3, 4, 5, 6, 39, 203, 232, 239, 251, 271, 309, 313, 315, 320, 321, 322, 325, 346, 348
technologies, 158
technology, 148, 157, 306, 325, 331
teens, 32
telomere, 129, 138, 181
telomere shortening, 129, 138, 181
temperature, 286, 319
tension, 340, 341, 345
termination codon, 33
testicular cancer, 310, 318
testing, 56, 320, 345
testis, 313, 324, 326
tetrachlorodibenzo-p-dioxin, 368, 378, 380
TGF, 37, 67, 68, 69, 70, 72, 73, 84, 85, 91, 93, 94, 115, 117, 118, 173, 266, 291, 295, 375
thalassemia, 46
therapeutic agents, 198
therapeutic approaches, 119, 143, 304
therapeutic benefits, 236, 242, 246
therapeutic effects, 112, 174
therapeutic interventions, 251
therapeutic use, 331
therapeutics, 242, 250, 253, 259
therapy, 15, 22, 30, 36, 37, 47, 58, 59, 60, 63, 66, 72, 87, 89, 97, 102, 121, 130, 139, 141, 155, 166, 182, 198, 220, 243, 245, 251, 252, 260, 262, 269, 272, 281, 290, 293, 318, 325, 343, 344, 349
thermoregulation, 30
thiazolidinediones, 86
thinning, 273
thiobarbituric acid-reactive substances (TBARS), 169
threonine, 210
threshold level, 320
thrombin, 173
thromboxanes, 133, 134
thymine, 289, 299
thyroid, 172, 189, 336

tics, 18

TIMP, 69, 70

TIMP-1, 69, 70

tin, 238

tissue, 11, 12, 25, 33, 35, 37, 44, 49, 52, 58, 65, 69, 80, 84, 116, 117, 119, 124, 126, 128, 132, 136, 148, 154, 156, 172, 177, 202, 207, 210, 211, 212, 214, 217, 229, 231, 232, 233, 234, 237, 241, 244, 247, 250, 254, 255, 258, 264, 269, 270, 273, 281, 287, 288, 289, 290, 292, 297, 300, 319, 333, 334, 338, 339, 352, 355, 358, 362, 380

tissue homeostasis, 300

TLR, 74, 75

TNF, 11, 67, 68, 70, 72, 73, 74, 75, 80, 81, 83, 84, 85, 86, 87, 91, 93, 94, 101, 126, 130, 131, 146, 173, 186, 216, 239, 294, 303, 314, 315, 342

tobacco, 20, 25, 66, 90, 318, 377, 383

tobacco smoke, 20, 90, 318, 383

tocopherols, 174, 223, 242

tonic, 245

tonic-clonic seizures, 245

toxic aldehydes, 180

toxic effect, 321, 367, 376

toxic substances, 319

toxicity, 51, 52, 53, 59, 61, 62, 63, 81, 82, 91, 92, 103, 124, 126, 156, 157, 168, 239, 244, 246, 253, 259, 260, 286, 288, 302, 330, 371, 372, 375, 376, 377, 378, 379, 380, 382

toxicology, 62, 298, 367, 375, 379

toxin, 24, 111

TP53, 290

trachea, 3

trafficking, 34, 43, 236, 254, 257

training, 218, 226, 351, 356, 357, 358, 362, 363, 364

transaminases, 81, 85

transcription, 10, 14, 37, 47, 53, 62, 73, 75, 80, 86, 87, 91, 97, 98, 127, 144, 146, 153, 155, 157, 158, 159, 161, 165, 168, 170, 174, 175, 191, 209, 210, 211, 223, 238, 265, 288, 290, 291, 293, 294, 296, 300, 315, 330, 334, 336, 338, 351, 359, 368, 369, 376, 382

transcription factors, 10, 14, 75, 91, 98, 144, 146, 153, 157, 158, 161, 168, 170, 174, 175, 191, 211, 223, 238, 288, 291, 293, 296, 315, 330, 334, 359, 369

transducer, 73, 254

transduction, 123, 144, 145, 191

transection, 272, 281

transfection, 60, 128, 238, 239, 266

transferrin, 31, 32, 33, 34, 35, 40, 42, 43, 44, 86, 90, 236, 237, 238, 239, 241, 242, 257, 309, 330, 335, 346

transformation, 89, 94, 115, 127, 145, 149, 151, 157, 158, 160, 165, 187, 338, 374

transforming growth factor, 37, 67, 68, 70, 72, 84, 93, 96, 115, 118, 173, 211, 266, 295, 303

transfusion, 60

transfusional siderosis, 29, 36, 37, 38, 39

transgene, 72, 297

transition metal, 156, 229, 235, 238, 242, 249, 250, 321

transition metal ions, 156

translation, 39, 70, 132, 142, 314, 315

translocation, 76, 86, 98, 128, 138, 142, 147, 172, 187, 207, 265, 291, 295, 326, 361, 376

transmission, 32, 33, 34, 320

transplant, 63, 290

transplantation, 59, 60, 67

transport, 22, 24, 50, 73, 74, 85, 87, 123, 124, 126, 145, 154, 157, 170, 171, 178, 207, 225, 231, 233, 236, 244, 247, 265, 268, 270, 271, 272, 308, 311, 330, 352, 360, 369, 372, 377, 382, 383

trauma, 15, 93, 148, 163, 273

treatment, 7, 9, 27, 29, 30, 34, 36, 38, 54, 55, 57, 58, 59, 60, 62, 63, 80, 81, 87, 88, 95, 101, 112, 114, 115, 116, 121, 124, 129, 135, 139, 143, 145, 146, 147, 155, 158, 167, 183, 184, 194, 195, 201, 202, 204, 213, 218, 219, 224, 238, 239, 240, 241, 245, 246, 249, 250, 253, 257, 258, 259, 263, 265, 266, 268, 269, 271, 272, 274, 275, 277, 280, 282, 290, 295, 301, 314, 317, 318, 321, 322, 324, 343, 353, 363, 375, 376, 382

tremor, 55

trial, 26, 27, 150, 155, 157, 164, 165, 167, 196, 198, 199, 224, 226, 227, 240, 259, 260, 266, 275, 276, 301, 344, 379

tricarboxylic acid, 207, 268

tricarboxylic acid cycle, 207, 268

Trientine, 57, 58

triggers, 1, 37, 76, 77, 85, 92, 98, 145

triglycerides, 75, 86

triphenylphosphine, 221

trisomy, 339

tryptophan, 204, 235, 254, 288

tuberculosis, 10, 26

tumor, 14, 26, 67, 68, 72, 74, 80, 84, 88, 90, 93, 99, 100, 103, 123, 124, 125, 126, 127, 129, 130, 131, 132, 133, 134, 135, 136, 137, 139, 140, 141, 142, 143, 144, 145, 146, 147, 148, 149, 151, 155, 156, 158, 159, 161, 162, 163, 164, 167, 168, 173, 189, 249, 289, 290, 291, 293, 295, 296, 297, 300, 301, 303, 304, 314, 333, 338, 374, 379

tumor cells, 123, 124, 125, 126, 127, 129, 130, 131, 132, 134, 135, 136, 139, 140, 141, 142, 144, 147, 148, 149, 159, 163, 167, 168, 249, 293

tumor development, 127, 140, 141, 304
tumor growth, 132, 148, 149, 151, 155, 163, 164
tumor invasion, 144
tumor metastasis, 147, 148, 162, 163, 164
tumor necrosis factor, 67, 68, 72, 74, 80, 84, 93, 99,
    100, 137, 140, 142, 146, 173, 189, 333
tumor progression, 148, 159, 291, 295, 301, 303
tumorigenesis, 26, 141, 145, 146, 164, 291, 296, 301,
    369, 379
tumors, 87, 93, 125, 126, 129, 131, 135, 136, 138,
    142, 144, 148, 149, 151, 156, 158, 159, 164, 166,
    291, 297, 336, 374, 380
tumour growth, 159, 163
tungsten, 114
turnover, 232, 234
twist, 291
type 1 diabetes, 220, 223, 226, 279
type 2 diabetes, 66, 83, 91, 102, 199, 201, 202, 205,
    212, 217, 218, 219, 223, 224, 225, 227, 279
tyrosine, 76, 94, 98, 116, 145, 146, 152, 153, 160,
    161, 170, 174, 175, 176, 190, 191, 192, 204, 215,
    216, 247, 261, 273, 278, 279, 287, 295, 306, 336
tyrosine hydroxylase, 261

U

ubiquitin-proteasome system, 245
UK, 136, 221, 279
ulcer, 302
ultrasound, 275
ultrastructure, 110, 119
UN, 139, 140, 142
underlying mechanisms, 290
UNESCO, 220
uniform, 150, 273
United, 91, 104, 185, 191, 196, 198, 201
United Kingdom, 91
United States, 91, 104, 185, 191, 196, 198, 201
unstable angina, 197
upper airways, 18
upper and lower airways and lungs, 1
upper respiratory tract, 3, 6, 8
uric acid, 94, 174, 242, 273
urine, 38, 56, 57, 289, 355, 356, 371
urokinase, 148, 279
US Department of Health and Human Services, 381
USA, 42, 43, 44, 45, 119, 123, 138, 140, 264, 285,
    299, 367
uterus, 243, 333, 334, 350
UV, 238, 274, 282, 287, 288, 300, 301, 303
UV light, 238
UV radiation, 288, 301
UVA irradiation, 288

UVB irradiation, 296

V

valence, 236, 241
valine, 204
valuation, 259
vapor, 5
variables, 39
variations, 100, 309
vascular cell adhesion molecule, 176
vascular endothelial growth factor (VEGF), 179,
    211, 266, 279
vascular system, 174
vascular wall, 171, 177, 179
vasculature, 170, 172, 176, 192, 207, 208, 211, 212,
    213
vasoconstriction, 90, 93, 94, 349
vasodilation, 338
vasodilator, 176
vasomotor, 185, 194
vasospasm, 133
VCAM, 176, 210
vector, 151
vegetables, 149, 182, 219, 224, 242, 294, 343
vein, 222, 272, 317
very low density lipoprotein, 243
vesicle, 342
vessels, 132, 133, 134, 142, 147, 176, 181, 183, 267
Vietnam, 382
viral gene, 71
viral infection, 9, 315
virology, 71
virus infection, 97, 103, 254
virus replication, 96
viruses, 3, 8, 9, 11, 18, 38, 66, 67, 70, 88, 96, 249
visceral adiposity, 201
vision, 266, 267, 269, 270, 273, 276, 277
visions, 260
visual acuity, 263, 272
visualization, 251, 314, 363
vitamin A, 150, 164, 375
vitamin B1, 242
vitamin B12, 242
vitamin C, 182, 199, 210, 213, 215, 227, 266, 289,
    294, 309, 321, 330, 343, 344, 345, 346, 363, 364
vitamin D, 286, 294
vitamin E, 13, 51, 59, 62, 82, 115, 125, 126, 127,
    130, 149, 150, 156, 159, 165, 198, 199, 203, 208,
    210, 213, 214, 215, 218, 219, 221, 224, 226, 227,
    242, 243, 245, 259, 264, 266, 267, 268, 269, 274,
    275, 277, 279, 283, 286, 289, 298, 321, 330, 331,
    332, 338, 343, 344, 346, 359, 362, 382

vitamin supplementation, 198, 381
vitamins, 25, 167, 179, 181, 184, 194, 196, 198, 209, 212, 224, 243, 246, 276, 277, 321, 338, 343, 344, 349
vitiligo, 292, 301
VLDL, 243
vulnerability, 52, 129, 149, 256, 264

W

walking, 21
water, 4, 5, 82, 107, 155, 174, 286, 294, 368, 371
water vapor, 4
weakness, 36, 244
weapons, 17
weight gain, 215
weight loss, 215
welding, 318
welfare, 250
Western countries, 66
wheezing, 9
white blood cell count, 324
white blood cells, 308, 317, 352
white matter, 239, 243, 249, 250
WHO, 95
wild type, 128, 148, 180, 269, 291

Wisconsin, 263, 277
withdrawal, 83
wool, 321
workers, 202, 383
World Health Organization, 17, 66, 308
World Health Organization (WHO), 66, 308
worldwide, 30, 66, 88, 91, 143, 294
wound healing, 16, 67, 277, 286, 287, 298

X

xenografts, 155

Y

Yale University, 49
yeast, 36, 61, 257
yield, 171, 211, 235, 247, 291, 330, 340
young women, 79

Z

zinc, 53, 58, 62, 63, 77, 125, 137, 161, 242, 245, 248, 257, 259, 266, 276, 330, 343, 344